Denver Health Medical Center
HANDBOOK OF SURGICAL CRITICAL CARE
The Practice and the Evidence

Denver Health Medical Center
HANDBOOK OF SURGICAL CRITICAL CARE
The Practice and the Evidence

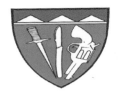

Fredric M. Pieracci, MD, FACS
Ernest E. Moore, MD, FACS

Denver Health Medical Center, USA
University of Colorado Health Sciences Center, USA

World Scientific

NEW JERSEY · LONDON · SINGAPORE · BEIJING · SHANGHAI · HONG KONG · TAIPEI · CHENNAI

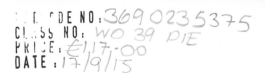
Published by

World Scientific Publishing Co. Pte. Ltd.

5 Toh Tuck Link, Singapore 596224

USA office: 27 Warren Street, Suite 401-402, Hackensack, NJ 07601

UK office: 57 Shelton Street, Covent Garden, London WC2H 9HE

Library of Congress Cataloging-in-Publication Data
Denver Health Medical Center handbook of surgical critical care : the practice and the evidence /
[edited by] Fredric M. Pieracci, Ernest E. Moore.
    p. ; cm.
  Handbook of surgical critical care
  Includes bibliographical references and index.
  ISBN 978-9814602181 (hardcover : alk. paper)
  I. Pieracci, Fredric M., editor. II. Moore, Ernest Eugene, editor. III. Denver Health, issuing body.
IV. Title: Handbook of surgical critical care.
  [DNLM: 1. Surgical Procedures, Operative--Handbooks. 2. Critical Care--Handbooks.
3. General Surgery--Handbooks. WO 39]
  RD51.5
  617.028--dc 3
                    2014045929

British Library Cataloguing-in-Publication Data
A catalogue record for this book is available from the British Library.

In-house Editor: Darilyn Yap

Typeset by Stallion Press
Email: enquiries@stallionpress.com

Printed in Singapore

Dedication

Fredric M. Pieracci

To my wife, Antonia, and my children, Emma, Luca, and Gia, for their unwavering support.

Ernest E. Moore

To my physician wife, Sarah, and physician boys, Hunter and Peter, for their enduring belief in my endeavors.

Table of Contents

Foreword

Critically ill patients encountered in the practice of acute care surgery are a diverse lot. They may have widely divergent patterns of injury, or profound immunosuppression from injury, massive transfusion, neoplastic disease, or therapy, as after solid organ transplantation. Moreover, they may present at the extremes of age, with diverse physiology and responsiveness to stress, particularly among elderly patients, who have senescent immunity and impaired wound healing, and may have multiple medical co-morbidities — such as cardiovascular disease or diabetes mellitus — that may impair responsiveness to injury-related stress, whether it be due to multiple injuries or major surgery, or both.

Despite this diversity, there are crucial aspects of their disease states and the care that critically ill surgical patients receive have much in common. The practice of acute care surgery is inherently invasive. Incisions, percutaneous interventions, and indwelling monitoring catheters breach natural epithelial barriers to invasion of the host by pathogens, posing incremental risk to a vulnerable population. The risk of nosocomial infectionis increased by about one-third compared with comparably ill medical intensive care patients. In turn, such infections have been associated with increased risk of mortality and other types of morbidity related to multiple organ dysfunctions syndrome. The financial cost is enormous, and survivors of complicated ICU courses may need months or years to achieve full functional recovery.

The great paradox of critical surgical illness is that the most unstable, at-risk patients often need the most aggressive, invasive care to achieve favorable outcomes. The experienced acute care surgeon combines detailed knowledge of anatomy, physiology, biochemistry, pharmacology, immunology, medical imaging, ethics, rehabilitation medicine, communication skills, team building, monitors, devices, and biomaterials with consummate technical skill to integrate pathophysiology and balance risk and benefit. Complex decision-making must occur continuously and in parallel for multiple issues in several patients, and must often be followed by decisive interventions. There is no substitute for experience; computerized decision support systems and artificial intelligence engines have yet to prove that they are equal to the task.

This procedure-oriented volume is directed appropriately and suited especially to medical students, surgery residents, and fellows in acute care surgery or surgical critical care. Described herein are all of the common procedures that may be indicated in daily practice in the surgical intensive care unit or the trauma bay. Experienced practitioners will recognize that the descriptions in these pages represent "a way" of doing things, not necessarily "the way." There is indeed, as the saying goes (with apologies to all animal-lovers), "more than one way to skin a cat." These procedure descriptions represent the collective wisdom and experience of the skilled, dedicated practitioners at Denver Health Medical Center (DHMC), an institution of renown that is recognized for expertise and compassionate care for an underserved patient population. In their hands, these interventions are effective and rendered as safe as they can be. Doctors Pieracci and Moore and the group at DHMC are to be commended for this valuable contribution. It is hoped that the readership will be guided and inspired to master these techniques and develop their own technical refinements to incorporate into their own practices.

More than just a "how-to" manual, disease-state information is provided to orient the reader to the appropriate use of these interventions. This contextual information is fundamental by design, so the reader is reminded and encouraged to look elsewhere for the detailed knowledge of critical illness and critical care described above, which is mandatory and essential. Early command of these techniques will provide the readership the opportunity to devote maximal effort to mastery of the vast body of knowledge needed to practice acute care surgery effectively and safely. Experience will accrue with time and effort.

Philip S. Barie, MD, MBA, Master CCM, FIDSA, FACS
Professor of Surgery
Professor of Public Health in Medicine
Joan and Sanford I. Weill Medical College of Cornell University

Attending Surgeon
Chief, Preston A. (Pep) Wade Acute Care Surgery Service
New York-Presbyterian Hospital/Weill Cornell Medical Center
New York, New York
USA

Contributing Authors

Ashok Babu, MD

Assistant Professor of Surgery
University of Colorado School of Medicine
12505 E. 16th Ave.
Aurora, CO 80045
Email: Ashok.babu@ucdenver.edu

CARDIOTHORACIC

James R. Bailey, MD

Orthopaedic Surgery Fellow
University of Colorado School of Medicine
777 Bannock St. MC 0188
Denver, CO 80204
Email: James.Bailey@dhha.org

ORTHOPAEDICS

Carlton C. Barnett, MD

Professor of Surgery
University of Colorado School of Medicine
777 Bannock Street, MC0206
Denver, CO 80204
Email: Carlton.barnett@dhha.org

HEPATOPANCREATICOBILIARY
INTRA-ABDOMINAL INFECTIONS

Kathryn Beauchamp, MD

Chief of Neurosurgery
Denver Health Medical Center
University of Colorado Health Sciences Center
777 Bannock Street, MC0206
Denver, CO 80204
Email: kathryn.beauchamp@dhha.org

CEREBRAL BLOW FLOW
INTRA-CRANIAL HYPERTENSION
LUMBAR PUNCTURE

Marshall T. Bell, MD

Surgical Resident
University of Colorado School of Medicine
12631 E. 17th Ave, C-305
Aurora, CO 80045
Email: Marshall.bell@ucdenver.edu

BLOODSTREAM/CENTRAL VENOUS CATHETER-ASSOCIATED
INFECTIONS

Bethany Benish, MD

Assistant Professor of Anesthesiology
University of Colorado School of Medicine
777 Bannock Street
Denver, CO 80204
Email: Bethany.benish@dhha.org

ARTERIAL CANNULATION

Daine T. Bennett, MD

Surgical Resident
University of Colorado School of Medicine
12631 East 17th Ave MS 302
Aurora, CO 80045
Email: daine.bennett@ucdenver.edu

PLEURAL SPACE AND MEDIASTINUM

Denis Bensard, MD

Professor of Surgery
University of Colorado School of Medicine
777 Bannock Street, MC0206
Denver, CO 80204
Email: denis.bensard@dhha.org

PEDIATRIC

Clay Cothren Burlew, MD

Director of Surgical Intensive Care Unit
Denver Health Medical Center
Professor of Surgery, University of Colorado School of Medicine
777 Bannock Street, MC 0206
Denver, CO 80204
Email: clay.cothren@dhha.org

ABDOMINAL COMPARTMENT SYNDROME
PERCUTANEOUS TRACHEOSTOMY
BEDSIDE LAPAROTOMY

Dominykas Burneikis, MD

Surgical Resident
University of Colorado School of Medicine
12631 East 17th Ave, MS C313, Aurora CO 80045
Email: Dominylas.Burneikis@ucdenver.edu

ACID-BASE PHYSIOLOGY

Walter L. Biffl, MD

Associate Director of Surgery, Denver Health Medical Center
Professor of Surgery, University of Colorado School of Medicine
777 Bannock St., MC 0206
Denver, CO 80204
Email: walter.biffl@dhha.org

RECOGNITION AND CHARACTERIZATION OF SHOCK
TUBE FEED INTOLERANCE

Brandon C. Chapman, MD

Surgical Resident
University of Colorado School of Medicine
777 Bannock Street, MC0206
Denver, CO 80204
Email: Brandon.Chapman@ucdenver.edu

HEPATOPANCREATICOBILIARY

Shea Cheney, MD

Emergency Department Resident
Denver Health Medical Center
Department of Emergency Medicine
777 Bannock Street
Denver, CO 80204
Email: sheajcheney@gmail.com

CENTRAL VENOUS CANNULATION

Theresa L. Chin, MD, MPH

Surgical Resident
University of Colorado School of Medicine
12631 East 17th Ave, C313
Email: Theresa.chin@ucdenver.edu

GLYCEMIC CONTROL

Daniel Craig, MD

Neurosurgical Resident
University of Colorado School of Medicine
777 Bannock St, MC 0206
Denver, CO 80204
Email: daniel.craig@ucdenver.edu

LUMBAR PUNCTURE

Maria Albuja Cruz, MD

Assistant Professor of Surgery
University of Colorado School of Medicine
12631 East 17th Ave, MS C313
Aurora, CO 80045
Email: Maria.albujacruz@ucdenver.edu

ENDOCRINE EMERGENCIES

Thomas M. Dunn, PhD

Associate Professor of Psychological Science
University of Northern Colorado, Greeley
Greeley Clinical Instructor of Psychiatry University of Colorado School
of Medicine
Email: Thomas.Dunn@dhha.org

SURGICAL CRITICAL CARE AND BEHAVIORAL HEALTH
ETHICS OF SURGICAL CRITICAL CARE

C.N. Eisenhauer, MD

Surgical Resident, University of Colorado School of Medicine
12631 East 17th Ave, MS C313
Aurora, CO 80045
Email: Charles.Eisenhauer@ucdenver.eud

INITIAL APPROACH TO THE TRAUMA PATIENT

Charles J. Fox, MD

Chief of Vascular Surgery
Denver Health Medical Center
University of Colorado Health Sciences Center
777 Bannock Street, MC0206
Denver, CO 80204
Email: Charles.fox@dhha.org

VASCULAR EMERGENCIES
INFERIOR VENA CAVA FILTER

Lisa S. Foley, MD

Surgical Resident
University of Colorado School of Medicine
Division of Cardiothoracic Surgery
12361 East 17th Avenue, MS C302
Aurora, CO 80045
Email: lisa.foley@ucdenver.edu

TUBE THORACOSTOMY

Eduardo Gonzalez, MD

Surgical Resident
University of Colorado School of Medicine
777 Bannock St. MC 0206
Denver, CO 80204
Email: Eduardo.Gonzalez@dhha.org

PREVENTION AND MANAGEMENT OF COAGULOPATHY
DIAGNOSIS AND MANAGEMENT OF VENOUS THROMBOEMBOLISM

Raffi Gurunluoglu, MD, PhD

Professor of Surgery
University of Colorado School of Medicine
777 Bannock St, MC 0206
Denver, CO 80204
Email: Raffi.Gurunluoglu@dhha.org

FREE FLAP MONITORING

Michelle K. Haas, MD

Assistant Professor of Medicine
University of Colorado School of Medicine
777 Bannock Street, MC0206
Denver, CO 80204
Email: Michelle.Haas@dhha.org

ANTIMICROBIAL STEWARDSHIP

James Haenel, RRT

Surgical Critical Care Specialist
Denver Health Medical Center
777 Bannock St, MC 0206
Denver, CO 80204
Email: James.Haenel@dhha.org

MECHANICAL VENTILATION
LIBERATION FROM MECHANICAL VENTILATION
CENTRAL VENOUS CANNULATION
PERCUTANEOUS ENDOSCOPIC GASTROSTOMY

Yasuaki Harasaki, MD

Assistant Professor of Neurosurgery
University of Colorado School of Medicine
777 Bannock Street, MC0206
Denver, CO 80204
Email: Yasuaki.Harasaki@dhha.org

CEREBRAL BLOW FLOW

Paulo E. Jaworski, MD

Urology Fellow
Denver Health Medical Center
777 Bannock St, MC 0206
Denver, CO 80204
Email: Paulo.Jaworski@dhha.org

PRINCIPALS OF ULTRASOUND
DIFFICULT URINARY CATHETERIZATION

Timothy Jenkins, MD

Assistant Professor of Medicine
University of Colorado School of Medicine
777 Bannock Street, MC0206
Denver, CO 80204
Email: Timothy.Jenkins@dhha.org

ANTIMICROBIAL STEWARDSHIP

Jeffrey L. Johnson, MD

Associate Professor of Surgery, University of Colorado School of Medicine
MC0206, 777 Bannock St
Denver, CO 80204
Email: Jeffrey.Johnson@dhha.org

ACUTE RESPIRATORY DISTRESS SYNDROME
BARIATRIC

Edward L. Jones, MD

Surgical Resident, University of Colorado School of Medicine
12631 East 17th Ave, C313
Aurora, CO 80045
Email: edward.jones@ucdenver.edu

RHABDOMYOLYSIS
HEPATOPANCREATICOBILIARY
INTRA-ABDOMINAL INFECTIONS
NECROTIZING SOFT TISSUE INFECTION

Teresa Jones, MD

Surgical Resident, University of Colorado School of Medicine
12631 East 17th Ave, C313
Aurora, CO 80045
Email: Teresa.jones@ucdenver.edu

FUNDAMENTALS OF OXYGEN TRANSPORT AND CELLULAR METABOLISM
RHABDOMYOLYSIS
NECROTIZING SOFT TISSUE INFECTION

Gregory J. Jurkovich, MD

Chief of Surgery and Trauma Services, Denver Health Medical Center
777 Bannock St, MC 0206
Denver, CO 80204
Email: Jerryj@dhha.org

INITIAL APPROACH TO THE TRAUMA PATIENT

Fernando J. Kim, MD, FACS

Professor of Surgery
University of Colorado School of Medicine
777 Bannock St. MC 0206
Denver, CO 80204
Email: fernando.Kim@dhha.org

PRINCIPALS OF ULTRASOUND
DIFFICULT URINARY CATHETERIZATION

Claudia Kunrath, MD

Assistant Professor of Pediatrics
University of Colorado School of Medicine
777 Bannock Street, MC0206
Denver, CO 80204
Email: claudia.kunrath@dhha.org

PEDIATRIC

Gordon Lindberg, MD

Associate Professor of Surgery
University of Colorado School of Medicine
1635 Aurora Court
Aurora, CO 80045
Email: Gordon.Lindberg@ucdenver.edu

BURN

Daniel Lollar, MD

Fellow, Trauma and Acute Care Surgery
Denver Health Medical Center
University of Colorado Health Sciences Center
777 Bannock Street, MC0206
Denver, CO 80204
Email: daniel.lollar@ucdenver.edu

VASOACTIVE MEDICATIONS
ELECTROLYTES
ADRENAL INSUFFICIENCY

Michael A. Maccini, MD

Surgical Resident
University of Colorado School of Medicine
777 Bannock St, MC 0206
Denver, CO 80204
Email: Michael.Maccini@dhha.org

NUTRITIONAL IN THE CRITICALLY ILL

Sara Mazzoni, MD, MPH

Assistant Professor of Obstetrics and Gynecology
University of Colorado School of Medicine
777 Bannock Street, MC0660
Denver, CO 80204
Email: Sara.mazzoni@dhha.org

OBSTETRICS

Cyril Mauffrey, MD

Associate Professor of Surgery
University of Colorado School of Medicine
777 Bannock St. MC 0188
Denver, CO 80204
Email: Cyril.Mauffrey@dhha.org

ORTHOPAEDICS

Robert McIntyre, Jr., MD

Professor of Surgery
University of Colorado School of Medicine
12631 East 17th Ave, C313
Aurora, CO 80045
Email: Robert.mcintyre@ucdenver.edu

FUNDAMENTALS OF OXYGEN TRANSPORT AND CELLULAR METABOLISM
ENDOCRINE EMERGENCIES

Anna Kristina Melvin, PA-C

Physician Assistant
Boulder Community Hospital
1100 Balsam Ave, Boulder, CO 80304
Email: Anna.Kristina@bch.org

RECOGNITION AND CHARACTERIZATION OF SHOCK
TUBE FEED INTOLERANCE

Robert A. Meguid, MD, MPH

Assistant Professor of Surgery
University of Colorado School of Medicine
12631 East 17th Ave, MS 310
Aurora, CO 80045
Email: robert.meguid@ucdenver.edu

PLEURAL SPACE AND MEDIASTINUM
TUBE THORACOSTOMY

John D. Mitchell, MD

Professor of Surgery
University of Colorado School of Medicine
12631 East 17th Ave, MS 310
Aurora, CO 80045
Email: john.mitchell@ucdenver.edu

PLEURAL SPACE AND MEDIASTINUM
TUBE THORACOSTOMY

Wilson R. Molina, MD

Assistant Professor of Surgery
University of Colorado School of Medicine
777 Bannock St. MC 0206
Denver, CO 80204
Email: Wilson.Molina@dhha.org

PRINCIPALS OF ULTRASOUND

Ernest E. Moore, MD

Professor of Surgery, Vice-Chair of Surgical Research, Department of Surgery,
University of Colorado School of Medicine
Editor, Journal of Trauma and Acute Care Surgery
655 Broadway, Ste. 365
Denver, CO. 80203
Email: Ernest.moore@dhha.org

CRITICAL CARE RESPONSIBILITY IN HEALTH CARE REFORM
NUTRITIONAL IN THE CRITICALLY ILL
DIAGNOSIS AND MANAGEMENT OF COAGULOPATHY
PERVENTION AND MANAGEMENT OF VENOUS THROMBOEMBOLISM
PERCUTANEOUS ENDOSCOPIC GASTROSTOMY

Hunter B. Moore, MD

Surgical Resident
University of Colorado School of Medicine
12631 E. 17th Ave. MS C313
Aurora, CO 80045
Email: Hunter.Moore@ucdenver.edu

CRITICAL CARE RESPONSIBILITY IN HEALTH CARE REFORM

Greg Myers, MD

Assistant Professor of Surgery
University of Colorado School of Medicine
777 Bannock Street
Denver, CO 80204
Email: greg.myers@dhha.org

ECHOCARDIOGRAPHY

Nicole Nadlonek, MD

Surgical Resident
University of Colorado School of Medicine
12631 E. 17th Ave. MC C302
Aurora, CO 80045
Email: Nicole.nadlonek@ucdenver.edu

URINARY TRACT INFECTION

Abraham M. Nussbaum, MD

Assistant Professor of Psychiatry
University of Colorado School of Medicine
777 Bannock St.
Denver, CO 80204
Email: Abraham.Nussbaum@dhha.org

SURGICAL CRITICAL CARE AND BEHAVIORAL HEALTH
ETHICS OF SURGICAL CRITICAL CARE

Erik Peltz, MD, DO

Assistant Professor of Surgery
University of Colorado School of Medicine
12631 East 17th Ave, C313
Aurora, CO 80045
Email: Erik.Peltz@ucdenver.edu

FUNDAMENTALS OF OXYGEN TRANSPORT AND CELLULAR METABOLISM
ENDOCRINE EMERGENCIES

Fredric M. Pieracci, MD, MPH

Acute Care Surgeon, Denver Health Medical Center
Assistant Professor of Surgery, University of Colorado School of Medicine
Denver Health Medical Center
777 Bannock Street, MC0206, A388
Denver, CO, 80206
Email: Fredric.Pieracci@dhha.org

SYSTEMS- BASED APPROACH TO THE CRITICALLY ILL SURGICAL PATIENT
RESUSCITATION STRATEGIES
MEASUREMENTS OF PRELOAD RESPONSIVENESS
ACID-BASE PHYSIOLOGY
LIBERATION FROM MECHANICAL VENTILATION

RENAL REPLACEMENT THERAPY
INTENSIVE CARE UNIT ANEMIA AND PACKED RED BLOOD CELL TRANSFUSION
VENTILATOR ASSOCIATED PNEUMONIA
PERCUTANEOUS ENDOSCOPIC GASTROSTOMY
BARIATRIC

Clifford A. Porter, MD

Assistant Professor of Surgery
University of Colorado School of Medicine
1055 Clermont St
Denver, CO 80220
Email: Clifford.Porter3@VA.gov

RHABDOMYOLYSIS

Candine R. Preslaski, PharmD

Clinical Pharmacy Specialist
Denver Health Medical Center
777 Bannock St, MC
Denver, CO 80204
Email: candice.preslaski@dhha.org

PHARMACOLOGY

Connie Savor Price, MD

Associate Professor of Medicine
University of Colorado School of Medicine
777 Bannock Street, MC4000
Denver, CO 80204
Email: Connie.Price@dhha.org

SEPSIS

M. Dustin Richardson, MD

Neurosurgical Resident
University of Colorado School of Medicine
12631 E. 17th Ave., C307
Aurora CO 80045
Email: Dustin.Richardson@ucdenver.edu

INTRA-CRANIAL HYPERTENSION

Thomas N. Robinson, MD

Professor of Surgery, University of Colorado School of Medicine
12631 East 17th Ave, MS C313, Aurora CO 80045
Email: Thomas.Robinson@ucdenver.edu

GERIATRIC

Jennifer A. Salotto, MD

Fellow, Trauma and Acute Care Surgery
Denver Health Medical Center
University of Colorado Health Sciences Center
777 Bannock Street, MC0206
Denver, CO 80204
Email: Jennifer.salotto@ucdenver.edu

DYSRHYTHMIAS
ACUTE CORONARY SYNDROMES
GASTROINTESTINAL ISCHEMIA

Janis Sandlin, PA-C

Physician Assistant
Boulder Community Hospital
1100 Balsam Ave, Boulder, CO 80304 (303) 440-2273
Email: Janis.Sandlin@bch.org

TUBE FEED INTOLERANCE

Michael M. Sawyer, MD

Associate Professor of Anaesthesia
University of Colorado School of Medicine
777 Bannock St, MC 0206
Denver, CO 80204
Email: Michael.Sawyer@dhha.org

AIRWAY MANAGEMENT
LIBERATION FROM MECHANICAL VENTILATION

Michael J. Schurr, MD

Professor of Surgery
University of Colorado School of Medicine
12631 E 17'th Avenue
Aurora, CO 80045
Email: Michael.j.schurr@ucdenver.edu

HYPOTHERMIA

Ryan Shelstad, MD

Cardiothoracic Surgery Fellow
University of Colorado School of Medicine
12605 E. 16th Avenue
Aurora, CO 80045
Email: ryan.shelstad@ucdenver.edu

CARDIOTHORACIC

Samuel E. Smith, MD

Orthopaedic Spine Surgeon
Denver Health Medical Center
777 Bannock St. MC 0188
Denver, CO 80204
Email: Samuel.Smith@dhha.org

SPINE TRAUMA: DIAGNOSIS, CLEARANCE, MOBILITY

Talia Sorrentino, MD

Surgical Resident
General Medical Student
University of Colorado School of Medicine
12631 E. 17th Ave. MC C302
Aurora, CO 80045
Email: Talia.sorrentino@ucdenver.edu

RENAL REPLACEMENT THERAPY

Philip F. Stahel, MD

Director of Orthopaedics,
Denver Health Medical Center
777 Bannock Street, MC 0188
Denver, CO 80204
Email: philip.stahel@dhha.org

SPINE TRAUMA: DIAGNOSIS, CLEARANCE, MOBILITY

Robert T. Stovall, MD

Assistant Professor of Surgery
University of Colorado School of Medicine
777 Bannock Street, MC0206
Denver, CO 80204
Email: robert.stovall@dhha.org

APPROACH TO THE OLIGURIC/ANURIC CRITICALLY ILL SURGICAL PATIENT COLORECTAL
EVALUATION OF FEVER
URINARY TRACT INFECTION
BLOODSTREAM/CENTRAL VENOUS CATHETER-ASSOCIATED INFECTIONS
NECROTIZING SOFT TISSUE INFECTION

Molly E.W. Thiessen, MD

Assistant Professor of Emergency Medicine
University of Colorado School of Medicine
777 Bannock Street
Denver, CO 80204
Email: molly.thiessen@dhha.org

CENTRAL VENOUS CANNULATION

Nicole T. Townsend, MD

Surgical Resident
University of Colorado School of Medicine
12631 East 17th Ave, MS C313, Aurora CO 80045
Email: Nicole.Townsend@ucdenver.edu

GERIATRIC

Todd F. VanderHeiden, MD

Chief of Orthopaedic Spine Surgery
Denver Health Medical Center
777 Bannock St, MC 0188
Denver, CO 80204, USA
Email: Todd.VanderHeiden@DHHA.org

SPINE TRAUMA: DIAGNOSIS, CLEARANCE, MOBILITY

Michael J. Weyant, MD

Associate Professor of Surgery
University of Colorado School of Medicine
12631 East 17th Ave, MS 310
Aurora, CO 80045
Email: michael.weyant@ucdenver.edu

*PLEURAL SPACE AND MEDIASTINUM
TUBE THORACOSTOMY*

Cole A. Wiedel, MD

Urology Resident
University of Colorado School of Medicine
12631 East 17th Ave, MS C313, Aurora CO 80045
Email: Cole.Wiedel@ucdenver.edu

DIFFICULT URINARY CATHETERIZATION

Max Wohlauer, MD

Surgical Resident
University of Colorado School of Medicine
777 Bannock St
Denver, CO 80204
Email: Max.Wohlauer@dhha.org

ACUTE RENAL INSUFFICIENCY AND FAILURE

Heather Young, MD

Assistant Professor of Medicine
University of Colorado School of Medicine
777 Bannock Street, MC4000
Denver, CO 80204
Email: Heather.Young2@dhha.org

SEPSIS

I: Background

Chapter 1

Critical Care Responsibility in Healthcare Reform

Ernest E. Moore, MD* and Hunter B. Moore, MD†

*Professor of Surgery and Vice-Chair of Surgical Research, University of Colorado School of Medicine

†Surgical Resident, University of Colorado School of Medicine

Take Home Points

- Intensivists have a unique opportunity, and fundamental responsibility, in healthcare reform in the United States (U.S.) The objective of this overview is provide the rationale and mechanisms to provide cost-effective care in the surgical intensive care unit (SICU).

Contact information: (Ernest E. Moore) 655 Broadway St. 365, Denver, CO 80203; (Hunter B. Moore) 12631 E. 17th Ave. MS C313, Aurora, CO 80045; Email: Ernest.moore@dhha.org; Hunter.Moore@ucdenver.edu

Background

The U.S. healthcare crisis (Fig. 1)

Annual spending:[1]

- 18% Gross domestic product
- $ 2.7 trillion
- $8000 Per capita

Health status ranking among 34 Organization for Economic and Development (OECD) countries:[2]

- Life expectancy: 78.2 years = 27th
- Healthy life expectancy: 68.1 years = 26th

Proposed solution: The Patient Protection and Affordable Care Act (HR 3590, Pub L 111-148).[3]

Healthcare spending in the U.S.[4] (Fig. 2)

Risk Factors for U.S. Burden of Health[5]

(1) Dietary composition
(2) Tobacco smoking
(3) Hypertension
(4) High body mass index
(5) Physical inactivity

U.S. has highest obesity (BMI > 30) rate among all OECD countries.[2]

Preventive measures are unlikely to solve the U.S. healthcare crisis in the foreseeable future.[6]

Consequently, physician's decision-making has been recognized as the key in controlling healthcare costs.[7]

National Survey of Physicians' View of Responsibility

(1) Trial lawyers
(2) Health insurance companies
(3) Hospitals and health systems
(4) Pharmaceutical and device manufacturers
(5) Patients

(6) Government
(7) Individual physicians

Only 11% of physicians strongly agreed, "Cost to society is important in my decision to use or not use an intervention."[8]

U.S. healthcare system waste (Fig. 3)

It is estimated that more than $\frac{1}{3}$ of U.S. health care expenditure is wasted.[9]

Main Body

Balancing limited resources and care of the individual patient

- The emerging philosophy in confronting the inevitable limited resources and care of the individual patient is generally referred to as value-based care.[10]
- Academic health centers, charged with educating the next generation of physicians, will face the greatest challenge. On the other hand, inculcating this social obligation in these trainees is an undeniable responsibility.[11]
- This is not a new concept. In 1977, Dr. Ben Eiseman admonished "The science and technology of surgical care has clearly outgrown society's ability to afford it. Yet, like the financially irresponsible teenage son of a rich family, we as a profession continue to spend as though our rich uncle will never tire of providing us cash. Clearly, this is not so, and the day of reckoning will soon be on us."[12]

Intensivists have a unique opportunity (Fig. 4)

- 10% of the sickest patients consume 65% of the annual healthcare expenditure.[13]
- Use of the ICU in the last month of life is estimated at 30%.[14]
- 20% of Americans die during an ICU stay or immediately thereafter.[15]

As our understanding of the basic mechanisms of disease and related organ dysfunction have matured enormously, so have the sophistication and related costs of diagnostic and treatment modalities. Evidence-based medicine (EBM) with associated management guidelines and algorithms are an important process for cost-effective care. But this represents only the surface, and we must achieve more with appropriate point-of-care decision-making.

Reducing waste in the ICU

- Cost-effectiveness should be an integral component of our daily patient management decisions.
- Critically analyze the necessity for diagnostic tests; i.e., how will the results of this test change patient management?
- Uninformative MR studies and CT scans are conspicuous examples of wasted resources but collectively "routine" CXRs and blood chemistry measurements are an enormous potential source of unnecessary healthcare expenditure.
- Critically evaluate the cost: benefit of therapeutic interventions. The intensity of critical care is not generally maintained outside the SICU.
- Employ low cost technology for diagnosis and therapeutic interventions in the ICU; e.g., ultrasound (US) evaluation of pericardial, pleural and peritoneal fluid collections; US-assisted placement of vascular cannulae, pleural catheters, peritoneal drains, and IVC filters; and US-assessment of cardiovascular performance. The availability of contrast enhanced US may further the ability to identify organ specific disease and determine response to therapy. Endoscopic-guided percutaneous tracheotomy and gastrostomy should now be routine.
- Perhaps most contentious, is when to transfer to palliative care in the debilitated or terminally ill ICU patient. As intensivists, we know what to anticipate with advanced, prolonged organ support and should sensitively introduce the concept of futile care to the family, and alleviate their sense of guilt when there is a decision to desist with heroic efforts. We should treat our patients as how we would treat our families.

Practical Algorithms/Diagram

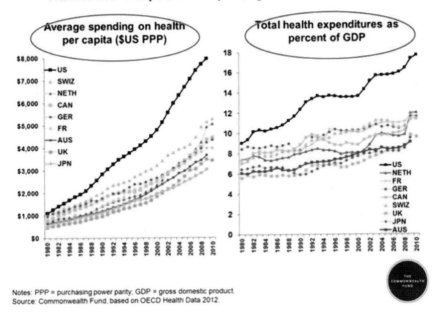

Fig. 1.   U.S. healthcare crisis.

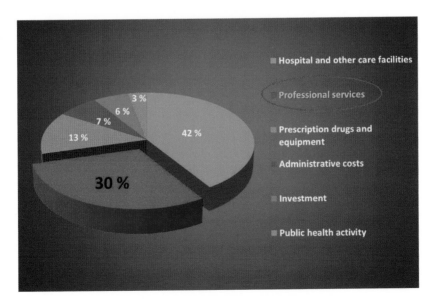

Fig. 2.   U.S. healthcare expenditure by category.

E. E. Moore and H. B. Moore

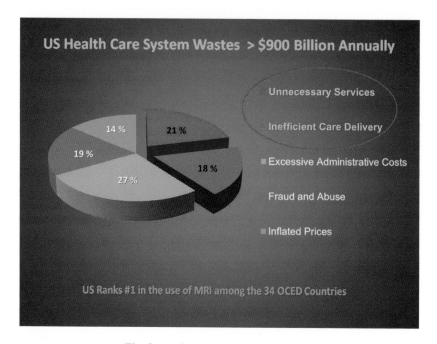

Fig. 3. U.S. healthcare system wastes.

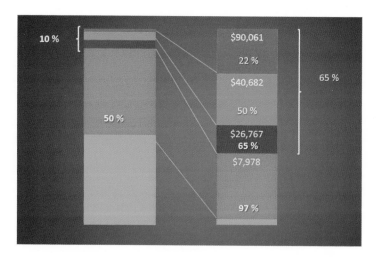

Fig. 4. U.S. population health expenditures.

Review of Current Literature with References

1) The Commonwealth Fund, accessed from: www.commonwealthfund.org
2) OECD, accessed data from: www.oecd.org/health/health
3) GovTrack, accessed from: www.govtrack.us/congress/bills/111/hr3590
4) Moses, H, Matheson, DH, Dorsey, ER, George, BP, Sadoff, D and Yoshimura, S, The anatomy of health care in the United States. *JAMA* 2013; **310**: 1947–1963.
5) US Burden of Disease Collaborators: The state of US health, 1990–2010 — Burden of diseases, injuries, and risk factors.
6) Joynt, KE, Gawards, AA, Orav, EJ, and Sha, AK, Contributors of preventable acute care spending to total spending for high cost Medicare patients. *JAMA* **309**: 2572–2578.
7) Relman, AS, Doctors as the key to health care reform. *N Engl J Med* 2009; **361**: 1225–1227.
8) Tilburt, JC, Wynia, MK, Sheeler, RD *et al.*, Views of US physician's about controlling health care costs. *JAMA* 2013; **310**: 380–388.
9) Berwick, DM, and Hackbarth, AD, Eliminating waste in US health care. *JAMA* 2012; **307**: 1513–1516.
10) Sox, HC, Resolving the tension between population health and individual health care. *JAMA* 2013; **310**: 1933–1934.
11) Fuchs, VR, Current challenges to academic health centers. *JAMA* 2013; **310**: 1021–1022.
12) Eiseman, B, Surgery's greatest challenge. *Arch Surg* 1977; **112**: 1029–1030.
13) Blumenthal, D, Performance improvement in health care — Seizing the moment. *N Eng J Med* 2012; **366**: 1953–1955.
14) Teno, JM, Gozalo, PL, Bynum, JP *et al.*, Change in end of life care for Medicare beneficiaries — Site of death, place of death, and health care transitions in 2000, 2005, and 2009. *JAMA* 2013; **309**: 470–477.
15) Angus, DC, Barnnato, AE, Linde-Zwirble, WT, Watson, RS, Richert, T, and Rubenfeld, GB, Use of intensive care at the end of life in the United States — An Epidemiologic study. *Crit Care Med* 2004; **32**: 638–643.

Chapter 2

Initial Approach to the Trauma Patient

C. N. Eisenhauer, MD* and Gregory J. Jurkovich, MD[†]

*Surgical Resident, University of Colorado School of Medicine
[†]Chief of Surgery and Trauma Services, Denver Health Medical Center

Take Home Points

- The initial evaluation of trauma patients should happen in an organized, systematic approach by a coordinated team of healthcare providers. This should include surgeons, emergency medicine physicians, nurses, respiratory therapists, and a variety of specialized technicians.
- Pre-arrival planning is essential for effective care.
- Communication, team work, and a calm and assured disposition among all healthcare providers is essential during this period of care for the acutely injured patients.
- The initial goal of care in the Emergency Department should be completion of the primary survey, recognition of life- or limb-threatening injuries, and a determination of appropriately diagnostic imaging and/or procedures.
- Procedures or tests that will not immediately provide diagnostic data that are critical to the care of the patient should not interfere with necessary care (i.e. do not stop cardiopulmonary resuscitation to place an arterial line).

Contact information: (C. N. Eisenhauer) 12631 East 17th Ave, MSC313, Aurora, CO 80045; (Gregory J. Jurkovich) 777 Bannock St., MC 0206, Denver, CO 80204; Email: Charles.Eisenhauer@ucdenver.edu; Jerry@dhha.org

- Always remember the ABC's (airway, breathing, circulation). This is the foundation of the primary survey and providers should re-evaluate these points if at any time the patient becomes unstable.
- NEVER leave an unstable patient unsupervised, even if they are on cardiopulmonary monitoring. This is true regardless of the patient's location (i.e. ED, radiology, transport, etc.).

Background

- Trauma is the leading cause of death globally, accounting for 5.8 million deaths per year. Each year there are over 31 million trauma patients evaluated by hospitals in the U.S. It is the leading cause of death among Americans under the age of 45 years, the fifth leading cause of death among the elderly, and accounts for 10% of all mortality in this country.
- In 2010, 180,811 people died from trauma. Originally described by Donald Trunkey in 1983, trauma-related deaths usually occur in a trimodal distribution.
  - Death within minutes of an accident is caused by fatal injuries with the only effective intervention being injury prevention.
  - Death within hours of an accident is usually from severe injuries, and their survival is dependent on access to a medical facility and the quality of care received.
  - Death occurring weeks after an accident is usually caused by sepsis and multisystem organ failure. Recent data have shown a marked decrease in mortality among patients admitted to the hospital for >24 hours, which is likely a result of improved critical care management.
- The CDC estimates that in 2005, over $63 billion was spent on the care of trauma patients.
  - Patients that were evaluated in the ED and release accounted for $21.4 billion with an average cost of $800 per patient.
  - Patients that were hospitalized and survived to discharge accounted for $40.4 billion with an average cost of $20,162 per patient.
  - Trauma related deaths accounted for $1.6 billion with an average cost of $9,323 per patient.

Main Body

- The American College of Surgeons Advanced Trauma Life Support is the internationally recognized and standard of practice guide to management of patients with traumatic injuries. This highly organized algorithmic approach to a trauma patient has been designed to: (1) maximize the survival of patients who have been critically injured through early recognition and treatment of life-threatening conditions and (2) ensure a thorough evaluation that minimizes missed injuries in patients who can undergo a full workup. The fundamental aspects of this approach include the primary survey, resuscitation, and secondary survey.

o While it is possible to complete the ATLS approach in a controlled stepwise manner in most trauma patients, it is absolutely critical to recognize the following:

   ▪ If at any time a patient deteriorates for an unknown reason, the algorithm of primary survey, resuscitation, and secondary survey should be stopped and healthcare providers should restart the entire evaluation from the beginning.

   ▪ Emergent operative intervention for treatment of life- or limb-threatening injuries should take precedence over completing the entire evaluation. When a patient is dying from a condition that can only be corrected surgically, the place for that patient to be is in the operating room and not the trauma bay. The only notable exception to this is the case of a resuscitative thoracotomy, where surgical intervention must be undertaken in the Emergency Department in order to stabilize the patient for transport to the operating room. This is, arguably, just a part of the "C" of the primary survey of stopping the bleeding.

   ▪ It is fundamentally important to recognize that the primary survey requires that life-threatening problems identified within each step must be corrected before moving on to the next step. It is not appropriate to do the steps of the primary survey as such: identify a series of life-threatening issues, catalogue them, and go on with the survey with plans to return to each problem. Solve them as you find them.

• Primary Survey

   o Airway Management and Cervical Spine Protection

      ▪ Being the first issue that must be addressed in any trauma patient, a secure and protected airway is of utmost importance.

      ▪ Patients can usually protect their own airway if they are awake and talking.

      ▪ Indications for immediate intubation include Glasgow Coma Score ≤ 8 or non-purposeful motor activity, obvious respiratory distress, and cardiopulmonary arrest. The importance of airway control with significant head injury is to prevent hypoxia, hyper- and hypocarbia, and aspiration.

- If prehospital personnel performed an intubation, its position should always be verified. The gold standard for this is to do so by direct laryngoscopy but end tidal capnography, moisture inside the ET tube, and bronchoscopy can all be used as well. Familiarity of the different airway devices used by prehospital personnel is essential, as several of these devices are adequate for emergency transport to the hospital but do not ensure a definitive, protected airway.
- Cervical spine collars or another immobilizing device should be placed on all patients whose mechanism of injury could cause damage to bony and ligamentous structures of the spine. Always assume that victims of multisystem trauma, especially if the patient's neurological status is altered or if there has been blunt injury above the torso.

o Breathing and Ventilation

- Once a patent and protected airway has been verified or established, assurance of oxygenation and ventilation is the next crucial step.
- Look at the patient's chest to make sure that it symmetrically rises. If a color changing capnography device is used after an intubation, look at it to ensure good color change for at least five consecutive breaths. Always remember that if an esophageal intubation has been performed on a patient that has recently consumed carbonated beverages, capnography may be falsely positive on the first few breaths.
- Listen to breath sounds on both sides to ensure adequate gas exchange. The absence of breath sounds unilaterally suggests a main-stem intubation or a pneumothorax. Absence of breath sounds bilaterally suggests an esophageal intubation. If an esophageal intubation is suspected, auscultate the epigastric area to detect gas flow into the stomach.
- Feel both sides of the chest for gaseous or bony crepitus. Gaseous crepitus over either side of the thorax suggests a pneumothorax. Gaseous crepitus over the neck suggest an aerodigestive injury. Bony crepitus suggest underlying fractures. In a conscious patient, gaseous crepitus is painless while bony crepitus is usually very painful.
- Remember that pulse oximiter devices have a 30 second delay in reporting oxygen saturations. Falsely elevated readings can be caused by carbon monoxide poisoning. Hypoperfusion, hypothermia, and

the presence of nail polish may render the device unable to determine the oxygen saturation. Methemoglobinemia, whether genetic or the result of chemical exposure, also make pulse oximeter readings inaccurate.

o Circulation and Hemorrhage Control

- The key components of "C" in the ATLS protocol are: Stop the bleeding; Assess circulation; IV-IO Access; Resuscitation fluids.
- Stop all obvious bleeding with manual pressure, a tourniquet, or a clamp.
- A manual blood pressure should be checked once before an automated blood pressure cuff is applied because automated cuffs can be inaccurate in the setting of hypotension.
- Always remember that in trauma patients, the etiology of hypotension is hemorrhage until proven otherwise. Adult patients must lose 30% of their total circulatory volume (~2L depending on body size) before hypotension occurs; Children become hypotensive only from more severe blood loss and at a near terminal event time.
- Hypotension from hemorrhage is usually associated with tachycardia. However, elderly patients who are heavily beta-blocked or whose cardiac rhythm is pacemaker dependent may not become so. Also, neurogenic shock will produce hypotension without tachycardia so this scenario should prompt attention to the exam of the cervical and high thoracic spines.
- After determination of the patient's blood pressure, all extremities should be checked for palpable pulses. The lack of a pulse in an extremity should prompt a thorough evaluation for arterial injury. Equally diminished or absent pulses in all extremities is a sign of profound hypoperfusion or cardiac arrest.
- External hemorrhage should be controlled during the primary survey and the most effective way to do so is manual compression. If a tourniquet was applied by prehospital personnel, it should be taken down in a controlled manner after all necessary physicians are present in order to determine the nature and severity of the hemorrhage.
- If external hemorrhage is not obvious in a hypotensive trauma patient, sources of occult bleeding include the thorax (hemothorax, great vessel injury), abdomen (solid organ injury, mesenteric injury), retroperitoneum (pelvic fracture, renal injury, penetrating wound), and long bone fractures.

o   Disability

- A brief neurological exam should be performed on every patient during the primary survey and should include level of consciousness, pupil size and re-activity, and movement of all extremities.
- Ideally these can be examined before the administration of sedative or paralytic medications. If these medications were administered by prehospital personnel, always remember to ask what the results of their physical exam were en route to the hospital.
- While intoxication is a frequent cause of altered mental stats, more serious etiologies include hypoperfusion of the brain, hypoxemia, and traumatic intracranial injuries. Deterioration of a patient's level of consciousness first demands re-evaluation of the ABCs but should also raise awareness of a potential head injury.

o   Exposure and Environmental Control

- In order to properly evaluate a trauma patient, all of their clothes and belongings should be removed. Hospital personnel should then securely store these for the patient.
- Environmental exposure, large volume hemorrhage, and both colloid and crystalloid resuscitation can cause hypothermia in a trauma patient. Consequences of hypothermia include cardiac arrhythmias, alterations in blood flow, decreased delivery of oxygen to tissues through increased affinity for hemoglobin, and an increased susceptibility to infection.
- At the completion of the primary survey, the patient should quickly be covered with warm blankets. Other steps to correct or prevent hypothermia include increasing the ambient temperature of the trauma bay, administration of warmed IV fluids (maximum temperature of 40°C), and using active warming devices.

- Initial Resuscitation

o   Remember: life-threatening problems identified during the steps of the primary survey must be solved before moving on to the next step. With enough expert assistance these can be done in parallel, but do not forget the principle of step-wise management.

o   Airway

- Adjunctive devices such as nasal trumpets and oral airways, along with maneuvers such as the jaw thrust may suffice in establishing an airway for a patient. Never perform a chin tilt maneuver on a patient with a possible cervical spine injury. If there is any doubt about a patient's ability to maintain or protect their airway, the patient should be intubated.

- When dealing with a patient whose cervical spine requires immobilization that needs to be intubated, there has not been any significant difference shown between direct laryngoscopy and videoscopic approaches in achieving oral intubation. The physician's experience and comfort level with each of these techniques should dictate which is chosen.

- Patients with obvious oropharyngeal, laryngeal, or tracheal injuries should be intubated with extreme caution. Never hesitate to involve other providers who have additional experience in these circumstances (i.e. anesthesiologists, CRNAs, etc.).

- Emergency surgical airways should not be considered a failure of airway management but should be reserved only for the most extreme of circumstances (direct contraindication to or inability to achieve oral or nasal intubation).

- If a patient is going to require intubation in the immediate future for an emergent procedure, it is not mandatory to do so in the ED before transport. Often times, this will delay the emergent procedure and can easily be addressed in the operating room.

o Ventilation and Oxygenation

- As a general rule, all trauma patients should receive supplemental oxygen. The route of delivery should be determined based on the patient's overall condition and oxygenation status.

- A tension pneumothorax may produce profound respiratory distress and hypotension from mediastinal shift. It must be urgently alleviated during the primary survey by immediate chest decompression. If attempting needle decompression, remember to account for the thickness of the patient's chest wall when selecting a needle for use. Tube thoracostomy is definitive.

- Massive hemothorax should be recognized during the primary survey and tube thoracostomy performed to evacuate, monitor blood loss, and get the lung inflated.

- After endotracheal intubation or establishment of a surgical airway, bag ventilation of the patient is effective at rapid correction of hypoxia and hypercapnia. However, once improved and stable, the patient should be placed on a mechanical ventilator to ensure consistent oxygenation and ventilation.

o Circulation

- Stop the bleeding; Assess circulation; IV or IO access; Resuscitate.
- As mentioned previously, manual compression is the most effective treatment of external hemorrhage and should be initiated upon recognition of the source of bleeding.
- A minimum of two large bore peripheral IV catheters (14–18 gauge) should be established in every trauma patient. If there are obvious fractures of an extremity then it should not be used for access.
- If peripheral IVs cannot be established in a patient, intraosseous catheters are safe and effective for resuscitation. They are relatively easy to establish but should not be placed in extremities with obvious fractures. Primary sites in an adult are the tibial plateau (antero-medial aspect) and the proximal (head) humerus. Sternal IO and iliac crest IO are alternatives. Some reports suggest IO to be a superior site for rapidity of access in children.
- Central venous catheters should be placed by experienced personnel if peripheral IVs and intraosseous catheters cannot be established. Good sterile technique should be practiced. The default placement location should be the femoral vein, as insertion here is not associated with the risk of carotid artery puncture or iatrogenic pneumothorax. Remember though that large bore single lumen catheters are preferred to triple lumen catheters, as triple lumen catheters have small diameters and relatively high resistance owing to their length. These lines should be removed as early as possible during the hospital course as they are often times placed under less than ideal circumstances in terms of sterility.
- Initial fluid boluses should be proportionate to the patient's estimated volume deficiency based on vital signs. Response to initial fluid bolus of 10–20 cc per kg should direct further fluid resuscitation needs. For example, adults (70–80 kg) should be treated with 1–1.5 L crystalloid for initial volume resuscitation. If tachycardia and or hypotension do not resolve, a second bolus of similar volume should be administered, and blood transfusion initiated for subsequent transfusion, while a diligent search for ongoing blood loss continues. Remember: volume is the treatment of bleeding — occluding the open blood vessel is the treatment.
- Lactated Ringer's Solution should be considered the preferred fluid for initial boluses given its chemical similarity to serum, but normal saline is also acceptable. Remember that in patients with severe liver failure,

LR will produce a lactic acidosis that may confound your clinical picture. Excessive administration of NS (>10L) over a short time can cause a metabolic acidosis that can be very difficult to correct.

- Patients presenting with hemorrhagic shock should be transfused blood products as quickly as possible. All Level 1 trauma centers are required to have a massive transfusion protocol that is reserved for such scenarios. These products should be utilized initially, until a crossmatch for the patient can be completed. It is generally agreed upon that packed red blood cells, fresh frozen plasma, and platelets should all be administered to a patient in this situation, although there is ongoing debate as to the ideal ratio of these products (i.e. 1:1:1, 1:2:1, etc.).

- Vasopressive medications should never be used until the patient is adequately volume resuscitated. Failure to do so can result in catastrophic ischemic sequelae such as myocardial infarction, intestinal necrosis, and renal failure.

- The primary method of operative hemorrhage control is surgical repair or ligation performed in the operating room, hybrid room or intervention radiology suite. Volume resuscitation is temporizing, and can be harmful if overdone.

- Adjuncts to the Primary Survey and Resuscitation

  o Pulse Oximetry

  - Pulse oximetry monitor should be attached to an ear lobe or fingertip, but without polish or tattoos. A pair of small light-emitting diodes (LEDs) emit two waveforms: one LED is red, with wavelength of 660 nm, and the other is infrared with a wavelength of 940 nm. Absorption of light at these wavelengths differs significantly between blood loaded with oxygen and blood lacking oxygen. The ratio of the red light measurement to the infrared light measurement is then calculated by the processor (which represents the ratio of oxygenated hemoglobin to deoxygenated hemoglobin), and this ratio is then converted to SpO_2 by the processor via a lookup table.

  - Remember that pulse oximeter devices have a 30 second delay in reporting oxygen saturations. Carbon monoxide poisoning can cause falsely elevated readings. Hypoperfusion, hypothermia, and the presence of nail polish may render the device unable to determine the oxygen saturation. Methemoglobinemia, whether genetic or the result of chemical exposure, also make pulse oximeter readings inaccurate.

o ECG Monitoring

- As quickly as possible, all trauma patients should be placed on an ECG monitor. This provides a real-time monitor of both heart rate and cardiac rhythm.
- Cardiac arrhythmias can be signs of underlying traumatic injuries.

  ⇨ Cardiac contusion caused by blunt trauma most frequently manifests as sinus tachycardia, but can also cause atrial fibrillation, premature ventricular contractions, and ST segment elevation indicative of ongoing ischemia.

  ⇨ Conditions causing inadequate preload (tension pneumothorax, extreme hypovolemia, cardiac tamponade) can manifest as pulseless electrical activity, or PEA.

  ⇨ Sinus bradycardia and hypertension can be a sign of cerebral herniation (Cushing's reflex).

o FAST Exam

- The focused assessment with sonography for trauma (FAST) exam is a useful adjunct to the primary survey to detect internal hemorrhage.
- The four "windows" that are routinely imaged are the hepatorenal recess (Morrison's pouch), the bladder and surrounding pelvic space, the perisplenic space, and the pericardium.
- The reported sensitivity and specificity of the FAST exam in detecting intraabdominal free fluid after blunt trauma are ~30% and ~99%, respectively. As the sensitivity is so low, a FAST exam should never be referred to as "negative." A more appropriate term would be "indeterminate," "inconclusive," or "useless" if it is not positive for blood. Repeating the exam within 24 hours of admission increases the sensitivity to ~70%, although most occult injuries are detected before this time period (Blackbourne LH *et al.*, *J Trauma* 2004;**57**:934–938). Secondary ultrasound examination within an hour increases the sensitivity of the FAST exam in blunt trauma, and should be considered best practice.
- The sensitivity and specificity of FAST in penetrating abdominal trauma are about the same as that for blunt trauma, although the indications for laparotomy or thoracotomy are uniquely different based on mechanism.
- Recently, the exam has been extended to include examination of the anterior thorax bilateral to detect the presence of pneumothorax. This is referred to as an extended FAST or eFAST. The reported sensitivity

and specficicty in detecting the presence of a pneumothorax are ~60% and ~99%, respectively (Kirkpatrick AW, Sirois M, Laupland KB *et al.*, *J Trauma* 2004; **57**: 288–295).

- Drawbacks to the FAST exam is that its accuracy is dependent on the body habitus of the patient, the experience level of the healthcare professional performing the exam, and low accuracy in patients who are severely injured due to the higher incidence of ultrasound-occult injuries among these patients. Pelvic fracture-related hematomas also make interpretation difficult.

o Urinary and Gastric Catheters

- Urinary catheters are necessary during resuscitation to have real-time data about urine production. It also facilitates uncontaminated collection of urine for a urinalysis, which should be a routine lab sent on all trauma patients. If there is any sign of urethral trauma (blood at the meatus, a high riding prostate, perineal or scrotal ecchymosis, or fractures of the pubic ramii), a retrograde urethrogram should be obtained before placing a urinary catheter.

- Gastric catheters allow for quick decompression of stomach contents and help to decrease the chance of aspiration. They do not, however, prevent aspiration and should be used with caution in patients with head and neck trauma. Never place a nasogastric tube in a patient with a suspected skull base fracture.

o Plain Films

- While X-rays obtained in the trauma bay can afford valuable diagnostic information, they should never delay the primary survey or resuscitation of a patient.

- The typical X-ray workup in the trauma bay consists of a chest film (portable AP) and a pelvic film (portable AP). Together, these are commonly referred to as "The Big Two."

- Chest X-ray provides valuable diagnostic information about the presence of a pneumothorax, hemothorax, fractured ribs, and positioning of an endotracheal tube and gastric catheter. It can also be helpful in locating missiles and other foreign bodies in penetrating trauma, which can sometimes influence operative approaches when emergency surgery is indicated. Since the chest X-ray is obtained with the patient supine, its sensitivity in detecting pneumothoraces is less than an upright film and hence is inadequate in making the diagnosis of an occult pneumothorax. If there is any question of a possible pneumothorax, never transport a patient without first viewing the portable XR — a large pneumothorax should be treated with tube thoracostomy prior to leaving the trauma bay to prevent the development of tension physiology.

- The utility of pelvic X-rays is less straightforward. In conscious patients, there is less than 10% chance of missing a pelvic fracture when complaints of pelvic pain are absent and the physical exam is negative; furthermore these missed fractures are usually clinically insignificant. Conversely, routine pelvic X-ray is advocated in patients with severe blunt trauma who are unconscious or neurologically altered given the higher incidence of pelvic fractures in these patients and inability to obtain an accurate exam.

o Diagnostic Peritoneal Lavage/Diagnostic Peritoneal Aspirate
- Once a common diagnostic procedure in the evaluation of critically injured trauma patients, diagnostic peritoneal lavage has become relatively uncommon due to the increased use of FAST examination and the accessibility of quality CT scanners.
- DPL is a lavage technique, where 1 liter of fluid is instilled into the abdomen, and as much fluid as possible withdrawn and analyzed for red blood cells, white blood cells, amylase, bacteria and food fibers. Generally, >300 ml needs to be returned to be considered adequate sampling. DPA is a simple aspirate, whereby 10 cc of blood or succus entericus aspirated is positive for injury requiring laparotomy.
- The most common use of DPL/DPA today is in the hemodynamically unstable blunt trauma patient who has an indeterminate (not clearly positive) FAST exam. In this scenario, it is not safe to transport the patient to the CT scanner and a grossly positive result would mandate emergent surgical exploration. A good example is the blunt trauma/ pelvic fracture patient who is unstable, and help is needed with the decision to go to the operating room for laparotomy, or to the angio suite for pelvic arterial embolization. In this scenario, a supra-pubic DPA will quickly assess for intra-peritoneal bleeding vs. retroperitoneal/pelvic bleeding as the source.
- DPL also has a role in the stable patient with a penetrating abdominal wound. In this circumstance, a local wound exploration that shows peritoneal violation and a DPL result of >100,000 RBCs has a high predictive value in detecting an injury that will eventually lead to peritonitis or shock and should warrant emergent exploration. If there is question of peritoneal violation or a diaphragmatic injury, many

authors advocate for using >10,000 RBCs as indicating a positive result.

- The drawbacks of DPL are that many physicians lack familiarity with the technique and supplies are often not readily available in the trauma bay. The only direct contraindication to DPL is previous abdominal surgery, as adhesions may prevent total peritoneal content sampling, in addition the risk of injury during insertion is higher.

- Consideration of the Need for Patient Transfer
  - In the U.S., there are 400 designated trauma centers that are verified by the American College of Surgeons Committee on Trauma. They are designated by different levels (I–IV) based on availability of clinical and academic resources. One hundred fifty-four of these centers carry the highest designation (Level I), having the personnel and resources to care for any aspect of a trauma patient 24 hours a day.
  - There is a growing body of evidence that shows lower in-hospital as well as one-year mortality for trauma patients that are treated at Level I centers when compared to patients cared for at hospitals lacking a trauma center designation.
  - If a trauma patient is being cared for at a hospital that lacks a trauma center designation, consideration should always be given to the necessity for transfer to a trauma center. This is especially true if a patient presents with injuries that would require resources that are unavailable at the initial hospital, or if caring for the patient would overwhelm the hospital's resources.

- Secondary Survey
  - Once the primary survey is complete, life- or limb-threatening injuries have been identified, and reasonable resuscitation has been delivered, it is appropriate to do a more comprehensive evaluation of the patient.
  - Remember that if at any time the patient's condition deteriorates and becomes unstable, return immediately to the primary survey and resuscitation.
  - The history obtained from the patient should start with the AMPLE template — allergies, medications, past history (medical, surgical, and obstetrical), last meal, and the events of the injury. The last point is especially important as the mechanism of injury defines the likelihood of related injuries.
    - For penetrating injuries, the most important detail is the type of weapon used to inflict the injury. In the case of stab wounds, details of

the knife can help determine the potential for intracavitary injuries. For gunshot wounds, low velocity missiles have a much more localized pattern of tissue destruction whereas high powered missiles cause much more injury related to blast effect.

- Most blunt injuries are the result of either motor vehicle or motor cycle crashes. Important details in these cases include the type of vehicle involved, the mechanism of the crash, the speed at which the patient was traveling, and any use of safety devices such as helmets or restraints. Many recreational and sporting activities can also result in blunt injuries, and the same details of these injuries should be documented as well. The prehospital triage criteria advocated by the ACS COT and the CDC provide important mechanisms with higher probability of significant injury.
- Remember that many details of a trauma are conveyed to providers by the prehospital personnel upon arrival to the trauma bay. This information should be documented early on so that if a patient is noncommunicative, there will be at least some data regarding what happened to the patient.

○ A more thorough examination of the patient should be performed once their history has been recorded. The purpose of this secondary survey is to detect any injuries that were not readily apparent on arrival to the trauma bay or revealed by the primary survey or patient history. It is important to remember that this examination is not definitive — up to 50% of non-life-threatening injuries are not detected during the secondary survey, especially in unconscious blunt trauma patient. However, every effort should be made at this stage to detect damage to internal organs and musculoskeletal structures to avoid delays in diagnosis.

- Head — External examination of the head should focus on detection of lacerations, hematomae, and bony crepitus. The presence of these findings should raise awareness for the possibility of a potential traumatic brain injury. Remember that due to the abundant vascular supply to the scalp, large lacerations can be the source of significant hemorrhage and should be washed out and closed as quickly as it is appropriate to do so. The preferred method of closure of a scalp laceration that is the source of significant bleeding is not stapling; instead, these wounds should be closed with a running locked stitch using monofilament suture in order to assure hemostasis.
- Maxillofacial — It is important to identify any injuries to the eyes, ears, nose, facial structures, and oropharynx. When examining the

eyes, look for conjunctival hemorrhage and abnormalities of move-ment. A pupillary exam should always be performed to detect asymmetry or nonreactivity. Otoscopic examination should be per-formed to evaluate for otorrhea or blood in the ear canal as these can be signs of a skull base fracture. The nose should be examined for obvious deformity or rhinorrhea. The mouth should be examined for blood, debris, or damaged teeth as all these things pose significant aspiration risk.

- Neck and Cervical Spine — In general, only patients who are alert, cooperative, and lack distracting injuries should have their cervical spine examined at this point. More importantly, ensure that patients have a properly positioned cervical spine immobilization device in place and defer the examination until the above criteria are met. If a patient is appropriate to undergo examination of their cervical spine, look for midline tenderness to palpation and pain with range of motion; the presence of these findings should prompt radiographic workup and re-examination. The neck should always be inspected for any external signs of trauma as well. Blunt injury to the neck can cause not only skeletal damage but also injury to neck vessels and penetrating injuries should be worked up and treated according to an organized algorithm.

- Chest — The examination of the chest at this point should be the same as done during the primary survey: look for equal chest rise bilaterally, listen for breath sounds, and feel for bony or gaseous crepitus. Also auscultate the heart to detect any possibly undiagnosed structural abnormalities of the heart. The management of chest trauma is too expansive to be covered here but physicians should be well-versed in the potential life-threatening nature of many of these injuries and what injuries warrant operative treatment.

- Back and Thoracic/Lumbar Spine — The examination of a patient's back is incredibly important but can sometimes be overlooked in the busy environment of a trauma bay. After log-rolling the patient onto their side, the entirety of the thoracic, lumbar, and sacral spine should be inspected for tenderness to palpation, bony crepitus, or step off deformities. The presence of these findings should raise awareness for a spine injury and spinal precautions should be strictly observed. Note should also be made of any evidence of blunt or penetrating trauma just as it is with the anterior structures. A rectal exam should also be performed at this point, paying specific attention to the location of the patient's prostate, the presence of blood, and strength of rectal tone.

- Abdomen — As mentioned above, the sensitivity of a FAST exam is not high enough to rely upon solely to exclude abdominal trauma. Any penetrating injury should be thoroughly explored under local anesthesia to rule evaluate fascial penetration. Notes should be made of any signs of blunt trauma, such as an ecchymosis across the lower abdomen in a seat belt distribution, as these give clues to the force of the traumatic mechanism and raise the possibility of occult intraabdominal injury. The presence of tenderness to palpation or peritoneal signs should prompt further workup of intraabdominal injury.

- Pelvis — A thorough but gentle pelvic examination of the bony pelvis should be performed in every blunt trauma patient. The anterior superior iliac spine, pubic symphysis, and lateral femoral trochanters should all be examined for crepitus and tenderness to palpation. If any of these structures are unusually mobile, the examination should be stopped as excessive force or movement can cause further injury to the patient. One important note to remember is that if you suspect a pelvic fracture based on mechanism or physical exam and the patient is hemodynamically unstable, immediately apply some form of pelvic binder in order to reduce the pelvic volume and limit further hemorrhage.

- Genitourinary — This portion of the exam is often accomplished during the placement of a urinary catheter but can be deferred until the secondary survey if that procedure was not performed. However, all patients should have at a minimum the external orifices of their genitourinary structures evaluated for ecchymoses or frank blood. Also, examine the perineum for signs of injury as well. Finding signs of injury to these structures should raise suspicion for damage to the urethra, pelvis, testicles, and vagina.

- Extremities — Examination of a patient's extremities after trauma should start with visual inspection for obvious deformities, swelling, ecchymosis, or bleeding. All extremities should be palpated in an organized fashion so as to detect any points of tenderness or crepitus. All joints should also be flexed and/or extended to examine for tenderness or crepitus. Any abnormalities should be worked up radiographically to evaluate for a fracture. Joints should also be examined for instability as a traumatic dislocation often will cause injury to surrounding neurovascular structures. If a displaced fracture of an extremity is detected, a manual BP cuff and a Doppler ultrasound device should be used to compare the systolic blood pressure in the extremity's terminal artery (i.e. radial, dorsalis pedis, or posterior tibial) to the contralateral limb as this has been shown to predict arterial injury.

- Neurologic — In addition to examination of the pupils and spine, a detailed neurologic exam should be performed. Detection of either sensory or motor deficits should raise the possibility of injury to either the central or peripheral nervous system, especially the spinal cord. Carefully document these findings so that the progression of symptoms can be monitored closely during the patient's care.

- Diagnostic Imaging
  - CT Head
    - When evaluating for traumatic injury, CT of the head should be performed without IV contrast. It can be rapidly obtained once the patient is positioned in the CT scanner and will provide invaluable data about the presence, type, and severity of intracranial hemorrhage, the presence of skull fractures and pneumocephaly, and can show signs of elevated intracranial pressure or herniation.
    - Any patient who presents with signs of hard signs of neurological deficits, has significant alterations of consciousness, or who is intubated should undergo CT scan of the head. In addition, findings on physical examination that suggest the presence of a skull fracture or traumatic brain injury should also undergo a head CT.
    - In the setting of minor head trauma, there are two tools that have been developed to determine the need for head CT — the Canadian CT Head Rule and the New Orleans Criteria. Both of these tools have been shown to reduce the need for head CT among these patients and are reported to have 100% sensitivity in detecting patients with injuries requiring neurosurgical intervention. When compared to one another, the CCHR has been shown to be less sensitive in detecting non-operative traumatic head injuries but has a greater reduction in the need for CT scans.
  - Cervical Spine — X-rays, CT, and MRI
    - Bony elements of the cervical spine can be imaged by both CT scan and plain X-ray. Despite the lack of a randomized controlled trial comparing the two directly, most experts agree that CT scan is far more sensitive and specific for identification of fractures than are plain films.

- Any patient that has sustained blunt trauma who cannot be examined because of their level of consciousness, has obvious neurological deficits or concerning physical exam findings, or has significant distracting injuries that prohibit a thorough examination should undergo cervical spine CT. Notice that these guidelines are similar to those pertaining to head CT, and often times a blunt trauma patient should undergo both tests.
- Two predictive tools have been designed to predict which patients should undergo cervical spine CT — the Canadian C-Spine Rule and the NEXUS Criteria. Prospective data has shown that the CCSR has higher sensitivity and specificity in predicting cervical spine fractures and has been accepted as the standard tool at most trauma centers.
- Unfortunately, cervical spine CT is limited in its ability to detect ligamentous injury or damage to the spinal cord. Remember that ligamentous injury alone can produce an unstable cervical spine so a negative CT cervical spine is not a definitive test. In patients who have a suspected ligamentous or spinal cord injury, an MRI is warranted to determine the presence and severity of such injuries.

- CT Chest
  - Portable chest X-rays that are obtained in the trauma bay are usually of such low quality that they should be regarded as a screening tool. While formal chest radiography with PA and lateral chest X-rays is very useful for detecting the presence of a pneumothorax, pleural effusion/hemothorax, rib fractures, or widened mediastinum, the portable trauma bay films are not sensitive enough to definitively rule out these conditions in most patients.
  - For this reason, a trauma patient should undergo chest CT if there is any question of thoracic trauma after the completion of the primary and secondary surveys. This study should always be performed with IV contrast so that the great vessels can also be evaluated for injury.
  - For patients who have been in a motor vehicle collision, it is important to remember that a velocity of 30 mph imparts enough kinetic injury to potentially cause blunt aortic injury if the rate of deceleration is significant enough. These injuries cannot be reliably excluded with plain films alone and these patients should have a chest CT for definitive diagnosis.
  - The diagnosis of an occult pneumothorax, which is a pneumothorax that is present on chest CT but not chest X-ray and does not need to be treated with immediate tube thoracostomy, is that the comparison

X-ray must be an upright film. A pneumothorax usually rises to the highest area of the chest and as such can move depending on a patient's position. A relatively large pneumothorax can be missed on a portable supine chest X-ray since they are often located anterior to the lung parenchyma, but will be easily detected on an upright film.

o CT Abdomen/Pelvis

- The early detection of intraabdominal injuries is incredibly important for both operative and nonoperative conditions, and in some instances has been related to the overall mortality of trauma patients. This is especially true of hemodynamically stable patients with hollow viscous injuries.

- Although the FAST exam is reliable in diagnosis of intraabdominal injury when it detects free fluid, the sensitivity is low enough that it should not be relied upon solely to rule out intraabdominal injury. Instead, patients who have injury mechanisms or physical exam findings that are suggestive of abdominal trauma should undergo CT of the abdomen and pelvis with IV contrast.

- While abdomen/pelvis CT has nearly 100% sensitivity for solid organ injury, it has been well-documented that the sensitivity for hollow organ injury is poor. Thus, the finding of intraabdominal fluid in the absence of a solid organ injury should give rise to a high suspicion of bowel injury and the patient should be followed closely with serial abdominal exams.

o CT Arteriogram

- As mentioned above, the finding of a displaced extremity fracture warrants a comparison of the terminal blood pressure of that limb to the contralateral limb (A:A). A ratio of <0.9 has high sensitivity in detecting acute arterial injury and should undergo imaging to diagnose this.

- Before the advent of CT scanners, arteriograms were both time and labor intensive and carried the risk of iatrogenic vascular injury. However, CT arteriogram has been widely accepted as the gold standard for detection of acute arterial injury in trauma patients.

- Given the need for urgent intervention in acute arterial injuries, CT arteriograms are often obtained at the same time as other trauma-related CT scans. Two things must be kept in mind when this is the case — the first is that the CTA is an additional contrast load in addition to the other scans requiring IV contrast, and the second is that it can be difficult to synchronize the timing of the contrast load and image acquisition when other images protocols are being obtained.

- If there is ever a question as to the accuracy of a CT arteriogram, the patient should undergo formal angiography. It is preferable to perform this in a hybrid style operating room, where open or endovascular intervention can immediately be performed after definitive diagnosis has been established.

Review of Current Literature with References

- Stiell IG *et al.* "The Canadian C-spine rule versus the NEXUS low-risk criteria in patients with trauma." *N Engl J Med* 2003; **349**: 2510–2518.

This prospective cohort study was designed to evaluate the accuracy of the Canadian C-spine rule (CCR) and the National Emergency X-Radiography Utilization Study (NEXUS) algorithms in predicting significant cervical spine injury in alert trauma patients. The data showed that the CCR was both more sensitive and specific than NEXUS in predicting significant injuries. The authors concluded that the widespread use of CCR would lead to a decreased need for cervical spine radiographs in trauma evaluations.

- Smits M *et al.* "External validation of the Canadian CT Head Rule and the New Orleans Criteria for CT scanning in patients with minor head injury." *JAMA* 2005; **294**: 1519–1525.

This prospective multicenter study conducted in the Netherlands was designed to validate and compare the Canadian CT Head Rule (CCHR) and the New Orleans Criteria (NOC), two algorithms designed to predict the need for head CT among trauma patients. Only patients with a GCS ≥13 were included in the study. The data showed that both algorithms identified every patient with an intracranial injury severe enough to warrant neurosurgical intervention, although the NOC had a higher sensitivity for clinically important findings. The authors concluded that the CCHR was the superior tool given that it would not miss any injuries requiring surgical intervention and that its widespread use would reduce the need for head CT in these patients by 37.3%, although they did not speculate as to the repercussions of the potential for increased incidence of missed clinically-important findings.

- Johansen K *et al.* "Objective criteria accurately predict amputation following lower extremity trauma." *J Trauma* 1990; **30**: 568–572.

The mangled extremity severity score (MESS) is a tool used to evaluate the severity of lower extremity trauma based on skeletal and soft tissue damage, limb ischemia, shock, and age. This review of early data for the MESS showed that there was indeed a correlation between MESS value and the need for amputation of traumatic limbs. Salvaged limbs had an average MESS of 4–5 and doomed limbs had an average MESS of 8–9 on initial assessment. A MESS value >7 was found to be 100% sensitive for predicting the need for amputation.

- Kortbeek JB *et al.* "Advanced trauma life support, 8th edition, the evidence for change." *J Trauma* 2008; **64**: 1638–1650.

In 1976, Dr. Jim Styner came to the realization that the care for trauma patients in the U.S. needed systematic improvements after he and his family were involved in an airplane crash in rural Nebraska. That tragedy led to the development of the Advanced Trauma and Life Support course in 1978. Since then, the ATLS has been the quintessential tool for the education and training of surgeons in the initial assessment and management of trauma victims. The most recent update to this course, the 8th edition, has made many evidence based changes to the longstanding course and uses graded levels of evidence to evaluate and approve course material.

- MacKenzie EJ *et al.* "A national evaluation of the effect of trauma-center care on mortality." *N Engl J Med* 2006; **354**: 366–378.

The purpose of this retrospective review was to determine the impact of hospitals with a Level 1 trauma designation in lowering mortality after trauma. To do so, the authors examined survival data from 18 Level 1 hospitals and 51 non-trauma hospitals in 14 states and included 5,191 patients aged 18 to 84 years with moderate to severe injuries. Data analysis showed a significant difference favoring patients treated at Level 1 facilities for both in-house mortality (7.6% vs. 9.5%, 95% CI 0.66–0.98) and 1 year mortality (10.4% vs. 13.8%, 96% CI 0.60–0.95), with the greatest differences seen among patients with more severe injuries. Accordingly, the authors recommended further efforts directed at regionalization of trauma care.

- Baker SP *et al.* "The injury severity score: a method for describing patients with multiple injuries and evaluating emergency care." *J Trauma* 1974; **14**: 187–196.

Now a common tool in trauma care, the injury severity score was first developed and documented in this paper by Dr. Susan P Baker as a method of determining the impact of multiple injuries on the overall survival of trauma patients. The tool is based on assessment of injury to six body regions (head & neck, face, chest, abdomen, extremity, and external) and utilizes the three most significant injuries to calculate an overall score. This scoring system has proven itself as being an accurate predictor of trauma-related mortality and is one of the most invaluable variables that can be collected and analyzed in trauma research.

Chapter 3

Systems-based Approach to the Critically Ill Surgical Patient

*Fredric M. Pieracci, MD, MPH**

*Acute Care Surgeon, Denver Health Medical Center

Take Home Points

- Most critically ill surgical patients present with complex, multi-system pathology.
- Using a standardized, systems-based approach to data collection, data presentation, assessment, and plans will minimize confusion, omission of important information, and medical errors.
- Using this approach entails creation and implementation of a standardized data collection tool, or "progress note," that is organized by systems (Fig. 1).
- This daily progress note can be supplemented with a "problem list" that is included in the front of the chart (or electronic medical record), which is continually updated as problems both arise and are solved.
- Adoption of the aforementioned approach has been associated with improved patient outcomes, as well as physician and nurse satisfaction.

Contact information: Denver Health Medical Center, 777 Bannock Street, MC 0206, A388, Denver, CO 80206; Email: Fredric.Pieracci@dhha.org

- Modern surgical critical care benefits from a multi-disciplinary approach, involving physicians, nurses, respiratory therapists, pharmacists, physical and occupational therapists, registered dieticians, and social workers. Representatives from these disciplines should be involved in daily rounds whenever possible.

Main Body

- The complex pathophysiology observed in critically ill surgical patients is simplified by using a "systems-based approach." Whenever the patient is considered, data are organized "by system," or presented "from head to toe." There are multiple ways to group information; the important point is that all relevant systems are included, and that the form is standardized such that each system is discussed every time. Our system grouping is discussed below.
- General (overnight events): *Major* interval events since the last presentation are disclosed. One should avoid summarizing relatively mundane information that will otherwise be discussed in other systems (e.g., the patient had a fever overnight and a lower respiratory tract culture was obtained). Rather, major changes in clinical status are discussed, such as new shock, new pressor requirement, return to the operating room, and major bedside procedures (e.g., laparotomy).
- Neurologic: Neurologic diagnoses are reviewed. For trauma patients, the Glasgow Coma Score is reported. The RASS and CAM scores are also reported. The remainder of the neurologic exam is reviewed, including movement, cognition, and alertness. For severely injured patients, brainstem reflexes are reviewed. Any intracranial pressure monitors and their values are reported, including ventriculostomy, bolt, and other operative drains. Strategies for elevated intracranial pressures are discussed [Chapter 4-(ii)]. Current medications, including anaglesics, sedatives, anti-pyschotics, and anti-epileptics are reviewed. A daily assessment of the ability to decrease the medications, or at least attempt a sedation holiday, is made [Chapter 5-(vi)]. Spine clearance and mobility status is reviewed [Chapter 5-(v)].
- Respiratory: Pulmonary diagnoses are reviewed. Ventilator settings are listed, including discussions of (1) appropriateness for ventilator liberation and (2) appropriateness for extubation. For patients with either acute lung injury or acute respiratory distress syndrome, additional ventilator variables are reported, such as the peak and plateau airway pressures, compliance, and P:F ratio. Presence and character of tracheal secretions are noted (this is often

a good time to touch base with the patient's respiratory therapist). The arterial blood gas is interpreted. Presence of pleural drains is noted, including type, drainage mode (water seal, suction at 20 cm H_2O, etc.), drainage amount, respiratory variation (tidal), and air leakage. If available, the daily chest X-ray is reviewed.

- Cardiovascular: The heart rate, rhythm, and blood pressure are reported. For patients in shock, secondary markers of preload responsiveness, cardiac output, oxygen delivery and oxygen consumption are reported. The diagnosis of shock, its etiologies, and use of vasoactive medications are noted. Markers of end organ perfusion and resuscitative progress are addressed (pH, base deficit, lactate). Other cardiac medications are reviewed. For patients with active vascular pathology (e.g., blunt carotid or vertebral artery injuries), the relevant physical exam findings, radiographic findings, and medications are reviewed. Assessment for compartment syndrome is included in this portion of the presentation.

- Gastrointestinal: Intra-abdominal injuries and their management are reviewed. The route, formulation, and caloric amounts of nutrition is reported. Patients who are intolerant of enteral medications should have the workup presented, including physical exam, laboratory values, and radiology studies [Chapter 8-(iii)]. Intra-abdominal pathology, including liver, biliary, and pancreatic disease [Chapter 8-(v)] are discussed.

- Renal: The urine output, as well as the total inputs and outputs over the last predetermined period, are reported. Laboratory values such as the blood urea nitrogen and creatinine are reviewed. The workup for oliguria and/or rising creatinine is reported [Chapter 7-(iii)]. Any urinary drains, their output amount and character, are presented.

- Hematologic: Anemia is reported and characterized. Indication for pRBCs transfusions are addressed [Chapter 9-(i)]. Coagulation status is reported, including platelet count, coagulations markers, and thromboelastograms. Anti-coagulant medications, their indications, and therapeutic ranges are reviewed.

- Infectious Disease: Each infection site, microbiology, and therapy is reviewed in turn. Some standard verbiage for reporting antibiotics is shown in the examples below. Note that each has (1) the infection site; (2) the microbiology; (3) the indication for therapy (i.e. prophylactic, empiric, or definitive); (4) the duration of therapy; and (5) drug dosage:

  o "The patient is on cefazolin 1 gram IV q8H, day one of one of prophylactic therapy for an open femur fracture."

- o "The patient is on vancomycin 1 gram IV q12H and cefepime 2 grams IV q12H, day 2 of empiric therapy for ventilator associated pneumonia. Cultures are pending."
- o "The patient is on cefepime 2 grams IV q12H, day 4 of 8 of definitive therapy for pseudomonas ventilator-associated pneumonia."

Workup for new infections (usually in the setting of a fever) is reported in terms of site investigated, tests performed, and cultures drawn, including pulmonary [Chapter 10-(iv)], blood [Chapter 10-(viii)], urine [Chapter 10-(v)], abdominal [Chapter 10-(vi)], central nervous system [Chapter 10-(vii)], central venous catheter [Chapter 10-(viii)], and wounds.

- Electrolytes/Metabolism: Electrolyte disturbances, their workup, etiologies, and treatments are reviewed. Glycemic control is assessed [Chapter 11-(iii)]. Total parenteral nutrition formulation and contents are reviewed.
- Prophylaxis: Indications for venous thromboembolism, stress ulcer, antimicrobial prophylaxis are reviewed, and prophylactic agents specified. For patients in whom VTE prophylaxis is current being withheld, the plan for beginning such prophylaxis is discussed (e.g., 72 hours from craniotomy) [Chapters 9-(ii) and 9-(iii)]. Duration of indwelling central venous catheters is reported.

Practical Algorithm(s)/Diagrams

ASSESSMENT/PLAN: (Add substantive information unique to this patient encounter)

Neuro RASS: _____ GCS: _____ □ ICU Delirium **PLAN:**

□ SDH □ EDH □ SAH □ IPH □ DAI □ Encephalopathy

□ Spine injury □ Other: _____

Respiratory FiO_2: _____

PEEP: _____ □ Hemothorax

□ Compromised Airway □ Pneumothorax

□ Acute Respiratory Failure □ Contusion

□ Weaning _____ □ ARDS

□ Acute respiratory insufficiency on NC at _____ L/O_2 □ COPD/Asthma

CV HR: _____ □ Pleural effusion

□ Unstable – Shock □ BP stable □ HTN   □ Afib

□ Hemorrhagic □ Neurogenic

□ Septic □ Cardiogenic □ Pressors: □ YES □ NO

GI □ Open □ Closed

□ Ileus □ Enteral TF at: _____

□ Wound _____

GU BUN / Cr: _____

□ Acute Renal Failure

Hematology Hb: _____

□ Acute Blood Loss Anemia □ Coagulopathy

ID WBC: _____ Temp: _____

□ No Issues □ Pneumonia □ Bacteremia □ Other: _____

FEN/Endo □ TPN □ Hyperglycemia

□ Hyper _____ □ Hypo _____

Skin/Wounds □ Wound care/mobility/skin breakdown/spine clearance

VTE Prophylaxis □ SCDs □ IVC filter □ LMWH/SQ heparin □ Heparin gtt □ None per Nsurg

Fig. 1. Denver health medical center surgical intensive care unit daily progress note.

Review of Current Literature with References

- Thornton *et al.* documented the high frequency of copied, redundant information throughout the medical record of critically ill patients (*Crit Care Med* 2013; **41**: 382).
- Dodek and Raboud reported improved communication and provider satisfaction after implementing a standardized, systems-based approach to patient presentation on ICU rounds (*Intensive Care Med* 2003; **29**: 1584).

II: System-Based Management

4. Central Nervous System

Chapter 4-(i)

Cerebral Blood Flow

Yasuaki Harasaki, MD* and Kathryn Beauchamp, MD†

*Assistant Professor of Neurosurgery, University of Colorado School of Medicine
† Chief of Neurosurgery, Denver Health Medical Center

Take Home Points

- The brain is a unique organ in the body due to its susceptibility to lack of oxygen and high metabolic requirements.
- The brain is supplied by four main arteries that form a circular interior artery to help maintain consistent blood flow to the brain in times of occlusion and hypoxia.
- Serious loss of blood flow to the brain can be caused by ischemic and hemorrhagic stroke. Prolonged blood loss to the brain can result in tissue death and altered mental status.
- Clinical signs of strokes should be assessed and a timely response can lessen the long term effects of blood loss.
- Functional magnetic resonance imaging (fMRI) is used to measure cerebral blood flow clinically. With improvement of this technology, physicians can accurately track changes in rate of oxygen saturation in the cerebral blood.

Contact information: Denver Health Medical Center, University of Colorado Health Sciences Center, 777 Bannock Street, MC 0206, Denver, CO 80204; Tel.: 303-436-5842 (Kathryn Beauchamp), email: Yasuaki.Harasaki@dhha.org; kathryn.beauchamp@dhha.org

- The manner in which drugs and other toxins interact with the brain is not found in the body due to the blood brain barrier.

Background

- The brain uses 25% of the oxygen while only consisting 2.5% of the body's weight. Cerebral blood flow (CBF) is defined by cerebral perfusion pressure (CPP)/Resistance (R). Blood for the brain is supplied by two internal carotid arteries as well as two vertebral arteries.
- The brain stores little oxygen in its tissues compared to how much it requires. The blood oxygenation level dependent (BOLD) effect is a dynamic change in blood flow to the active parts of the brain.
- BOLD results in a 5–10% increase in regional blood flow to the brain.
- The amount of oxygen the brain receives can vary between patients due to cardiovascular issues such as high blood pressure and blockages in the vessel. These can also lead to a cerebral vascular accident (or stroke).

  o Ischemic strokes are caused by an occlusion of blood to the brain. The body can break some of these blockages up naturally and quickly which results in a transient ischemic attack (TIA).

  o Symptoms of a TIA include partial paralysis or numbness to the face, trouble in speaking or thinking clearly.

  o Hemorrhagic strokes can be caused by the rupture of weakened vessel walls resulting in blood in the brain. High blood pressure and smoking significantly increases your risk of this type of stroke.

- The blood brain barrier allows protection for the cerebrospinal fluid, of the brain and spinal cord, from harmful drugs or toxins that may be present in the blood.

  o This is a highly coordinated exchange of limited molecules that limits which molecules can enter the brain based on size and permeability.

  o Not all substances are toxic to the body. Some of these molecules are useful for other organs; however they can be toxic to the neurons of the brain.

  o Certain circumstances, including ischmic stroke, can alter the selectivity of the blood brain barrier and result in larger substances entering the space.

Main Body

- Classically, Lassen *et al.* (1959) described a range of autoregulation in which cerebral blood flow remained constant through a range of cerebral perfusion pressure between 50–150 mmHg.

- More contemporary data in healthy volunteers (Tan, 2012) suggests that the autoregulatory cerebral blood flow plateau exists for a far narrower range of MAP fluctuation across approximately 10 mmHg, and that CBF is more passively determined by CPP.
- Normal white matter CBF 18–25 ml/100 g/min.
- Normal gray matter CBF 67–80 ml/100 g/min.
- The pressure gradient driving cerebral blood flow is determined by the mean arterial pressure (MAP) and the intracranial pressure (ICP). The actual regional cerebral blood flow is under further control of autoregulatory mechanisms which respond to variables such as $PaCO_2$ and autonomic inputs.
- Cerebral perfusion pressure (CPP) = mean arterial pressure (MAP) — intracranial pressure (ICP)
- Hypotension consisting of systolic blood pressure <90 mmHg should be avoided.
- In the setting of elevated ICP, both ICP directed and CPP directed management have been described, with no clear superiority of either strategy.
- In CPP directed management, goal CPP is 50–70 mmHg.
- Cerebral perfusion pressure (CPP) provides the main pressure gradient driving cerebral blood flow, and is defined as the difference between the mean arterial pressure (MAP) and the intracranial pressure (ICP). This may be calculated in real-time in the presence of a fiber optic coupled intracranial pressure monitor (see next chapter for ICP monitoring and management).
- Episodes of hypotension defined as systolic blood pressure <= 90 mmHg have been associated with poor outcomes (Bratton, Chestnut *et al.*, 2007).
- Cerebral blood flow is further modified by autoregulatory mechanisms which act via local vasoconstriction/vasodilation (Willie, Tseng *et al.*, 2014).
  - o Increase in $PaCO_2$ leads to local vasodilation.
  - o Increase in sympathetic input leads to vasoconstriction.
- Management strategies targeting ICP and CPP in the setting of elevated ICP are both utilized. Current guidelines for management of severe traumatic brain injury (Bratton, Chestnut *et al.*, 2007) support goal CPP of 50–70 mmHg.
  - o CPP <50 mmHg associated with poor functional outcomes.
- CPP >70 mmHg associated with five-fold increased risk of adult respiratory distress syndrome (ARDS).

Chapter 4-(ii)

Intracranial Hypertension

M. Dustin Richardson, MD* and Kathryn Beauchamp, MD†

* Neurosurgical Resident, University of Colorado School of Medicine
†Chief of Neurosurgery, Denver Health Medical Center

Take Home Points

- Intracranial hypertension is the pathologic elevation of pressure in the intracranial space, which is defined as an intracranial pressure (ICP) greater than 15–20 mmHg.
- Intracranial hypertension follows the Monroe-Kellie doctrine, which states that within a rigidly fixed volume of space the intracranial pressure will increase or decrease if the volume of the one or more of the intracranial contents changes or if additional contents are added or subtracted.
- Brain function is determined by adequate cerebral blood flow to meet the cerebral metabolic rate of oxygen consumption ($CMRO_2$). The cerebral blood flow is influenced by cerebral perfusion pressure, which is calculated by subtracting the ICP from the mean arterial pressure.

Contact information: (M. Dustin Richardson) University of Colorado at Denver and Health Sciences Center, 12631 E. 17th Ave., C307, Aurora CO 80045; (Kathryn Beauchamp) 777 Bannock Street, MC 0206, Debnver, CO 80204; Tel.: 303-724-2305. Email: Dustin. Richardson@ucdenver.edu; kathryn.beauchamp@dhha.org

- Clinical symptoms of acute intracranial hypertension may include headache, nausea, vomiting, Cushing's triad, coma, signs of herniation, cerebral ischemia, and ultimately death.
- Treatment of intracranial hypertension depends on a variety of factors including etiology of intracranial hypertension, clinical neurologic examination, clinical comorbidities.
- The ultimate goal in treating intracranial hypertension is both the reduction of pressure (which may have an independent effect on the central nervous system independent of its effect on cerebral perfusion) and the maintenance of cerebral perfusion.
- The normal value of ICP is less than 20 mmHg in adult patients.
- Pathological elevation of ICP can result from many different intracranial processes (hydrocephalus, intracranial bleeding, cerebral edema).
- Treatment of intracranial hypertension is determined by the pathophysiologic process underlying the etiology of the intracranial hypertension.
- The neurologic examination is currently the best known measure of neurologic function. Maintenance of the neurologic exam is preferred (when possible) to measurement of intracranial pressure, which is an adjunct to neurologic exam and a very indirect surrogate for neurologic function — ultimately, maintaining function is the goal of treatment regardless of intracranial pressure.

Main Body

- Normal value of ICP
  - The Monro-Kellie hypothesis asserts that the intracranial contents are contained within a rigid bony calvarium and that the brain is relatively non-compressible. Therefore, the volume of blood and cerebrospinal fluid within the intracranial space is directly proportional to the intracranial pressure. If the intracranial pressure is to remain constant, an increase in the volume of one of the intracranial contents must lead to a decrease in the volume of another of the intracranial contents. The addition of a foreign body or lesion (e.g., subdural hematoma) that occupies intracranial space will therefore result in an increase in the ICP if there is no concurrent decrease in the volume of one or more of the normal intracranial contents.
  - Normal ICP has been suggested to be less than 15–20 mmHg, though several studies have produced different threshold pressures.

- Pathological elevation of ICP
  - o In practice, any lesion which causes and expansion of the intracranial contents can lead to intracranial hypertension.
    - An increase in the intracranial volume of cerebrospinal fluid is defined as hydrocephalus.
    - An increase in cerebral intravascular blood volume is defined as hyperemia.
      - ⇨ In general, cerebral autoregulation maintains the intravascular volume of the cerebral vasculature, but in severe TBI, cerebral autoregulation can be lost allowing a direct correlation between ICP and blood pressure.
  - o Extravascular intracranial bleeding
    - Epidural hematoma — a hematoma resulting from bleeding in the potential space between the skull and the dura mater.
    - Subdural hematoma — a hematoma resulting from bleeding in the potential space between the dura propria and the arachnoid membrane.
    - Subarachnoid hemorrhage — a hematoma resulting from bleeding into the subarachnoid space.
    - Intracerebral hematoma — a hematoma that forms within the brain parenchyma; it can be spontaneous or traumatic.
    - Intraventricular hemorrhage — a hematoma that is the result of bleeding within the ventricular system of the brain.
    - In addition to forming a mass lesion, intraventricular bleeding may also result in obstruction of CSF flow pathways resulting in obstructive hydrocephalus.
  - o Mass lesions — a mass lesion in any form (tumor, vascular malformation, etc.) will result in increased ICP unless a concomitant decrease in another intracranial content has occurred.
  - o Cerebral edema
    - Vasogenic edema — the result of disruption of the blood brain barrier. Intravascular proteins extravasate into the extracellular space in the brain which results in expansion of the extracellular space.
    - Cytotoxic edema — the result of disruption of cellular metabolism which leads to a decrease in the ability of a cell to maintain its ionic equilibrium potential and a consequent increase in intracellular volume.
    - In traumatic brain injury, both mechanisms are present in most cases.

- Clinical signs and symptoms of elevated ICP

  o Elevation of ICP can produce a variety of symptoms ranging from headache to coma. In the awake patient, elevated ICP produces headache, nausea, and vomiting in the setting of intracranial trauma. The association between these clinical indicators after traumatic brain injury has been found to correlate with increased odds of requiring neurosurgical intervention after a minor head injury and should prompt CT scanning when being evaluated in the emergency department.

  o Intracranial hypertension is also classically associated with Cushing's triad, which is the clinical syndrome of hypertension, bradycardia, and respiratory irregularity. In practice, the full Cushing's triad is only observed in approximately 33% of cases of elevated ICP.

  o Elevated ICP may result in brain herniation. The brain herniation syndromes include:

    ▪ Subfalcine herniation — the cerebral hemisphere is forced under the inferior edge of the falx cerebri, which is rigidly attached. The anterior cerebral arteries course parallel with the falx and can be occluded with subfalcine herniation resulting in cerebral infarction in an anterior cerebral artery distribution.

    ▪ Transtentorial herniation — the medial temporal lobe (uncus) is forced medially and inferiorly through the tentorium cerebelli. The third nerve courses just medial to the medial temporal lobe, so when the medial temporal lobe is forced medially, it compresses the third nerve resulting in its dysfunction. This is most commonly seen as a unilateral mydriasis.

    ▪ Central herniation — Generally this occurs in a superior to inferior direction and is the result of a supratentorial force that causes the diencephalon and supratentorial contents through the tentorial notch. The posterior cerebral arteries (PCA) are at risk for compression thus resulting in an ischemic stroke risk for the cerebral PCA distribution. Downward central herniation may also result in stretch being applied to the paramedian pontine perforating vessels, which can result in duret hemorrhages in the ventral pons.

    ▪ Tonsillar herniation — lesions of the posterior fossa may result in upward herniation of posterior fossa contents through the tentorium into the middle fossa or, more commonly, result in downward herniation of the cerebellar tonsils through the foramen magnum.

- Treatment of intracranial hypertension
  - o In accordance with the most recent brain trauma foundation guidelines, we recommend initiation of treatment for intracranial hypertension above a threshold of 20–25 mmHg.
  - o Treatment options for intracranial hypertension should proceed in a stepwise fashion as listed below:
    - Patient positioning — patients suspected of intracranial hypertension should be positioned with the head elevated 30–45° with the head in a neutral position without compression of the major draining veins of the neck. Other injuries should be noted and positioning of the patient should be determined accordingly (e.g., spine fractures).
    - Normalize vital signs and metabolic factors — patients should be maintained with normal blood pressure to prevent both cerebral ischemia and hyperemia/expansion of hemorrhage following traumatic brain injury. Patients with an indication should be intubated and mechanically ventilated. $PaCO_2$ should be maintained at the lower limit of normal (35 mmHg). Hyperglycemia should be corrected. Normothermia should be maintained.
    - Sedation
      - ⇨ Fast-acting agents such as propofol in combination with a fast-acting synthetic narcotic agent such as fentanyl are preferred for neurologically injured patients as they can be rapidly titrated to allow for neurologic examination.
      - ⇨ In situations where patients will require maintenance of sedation for long periods of time and propofol is not feasible, a continuous benzodiazepine infusion is initiated.
    - Hyperosmolar therapy
      - ⇨ Mannitol — 0.25–1 g/kg bolus. This treatment likely improves rheological properties of blood which results in reduced hematocrit, decreased viscocity and increases in cerebral blood flow. There is also an osmotic effect which may draw fluids from the brain into the intravascular space. Caution should be exercised because mannitol may ultimately result in arterial hypotension. Additionally, mannitol opens the blood brain barrier and may result in rebound intracranial hypertension.
      - ⇨ Hypertonic saline — increases serum sodium and promotes a redistribution of fluids from the brain into the intravascular space.

We currently recommend maintaining normonatremia and do not recommend driving serum sodium higher than 150 as it may result in rebound intracranial hypertension over time.

⇨ Furosemide — may be used as an adjunct therapy along with mannitol — may result in decreases in cerebral edema and decrease in CSF production (see Greenberg for references).

- CSF diversion

  ⇨ External ventricular drainage should be considered in patients not otherwise requiring neurosurgical intervention if the above therapies have not resulted in control of intracranial pressure. At the discretion of the clinician, an external ventricular drain (EVD) may be inserted at the initiation of the process of treatment of intracranial hypertension both as a diagnostic and therapeutic measure.

- Pharmacologic paralysis

  ⇨ Initiation of a paralytic drip may be considered following the initiation of the above measures if intracranial hypertension persists.

- Barbiturate coma

  ⇨ Barbiturate coma can be instituted if the patient has persistent intracranial hypertension following initiation of the above measures. In general, dosage is titrated to EEG findings consistent with burst suppression and blood levels are measured to ensure that therapeutic/non-toxic levels are maintained.

- Hypothermia

  ⇨ There is some evidence that hypothermia initiated prophylactically may reduce mortality. Currently, the evidence supporting its use is insufficient to make strong recommendations.

- Decompressive surgery

  ⇨ This maximally invasive approach results in removal of the calvarium and duraplasty to allow for expansion of the brain through a cranial defect. This may be performed as the initial step in management of a traumatic brain injury at the discretion of the neurosurgeon. Indications for decompressive craniectomy range from the presence of a mass lesion to post-ischemia edema with brain shift. Though a recent trial of decompressive surgery did not demonstrate a benefit for this procedure compared with maximal medical therapy, its methodology does not permit broad application.

Practical Algorithm(s)/Diagrams

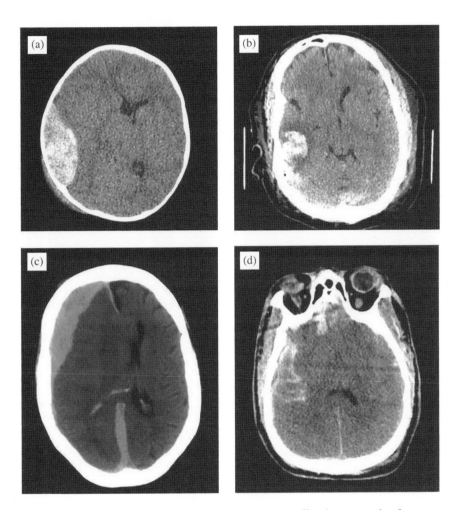

Fig. 1. Example of different intracranial pathologies suffered as a result of trauma. (a) is an epidural hematoma, (b) is a subdural hematoma, (c) is a cerebral contusion/ intraparenchymal hemorrhage, (d) is a traumatic subarachnoid hemorrhage. Note how the blood tracks the gyri and sulci into the sylvian fissure and along the insular cortex. All forms of traumatic hemorrhage occupy intracranial space, thereby displacing other intracranial contents and/or causing an elevcation of intracranial pressure.

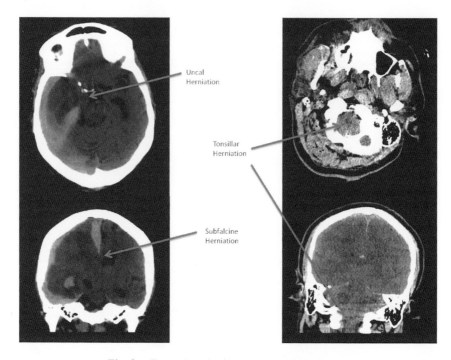

Fig. 2. Examples of different types of herniation.

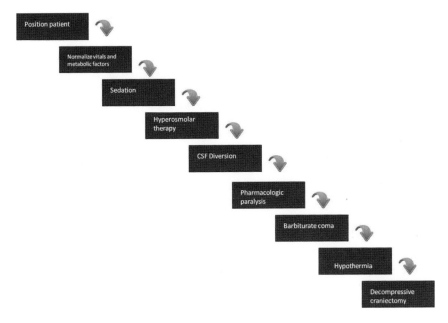

Fig. 3. Generalized stepwise algorithm for treatment of intracranial hypertension. Note that this represnts a generalized approch, but depending on the clinical situation and etiology of intracranial hypertension, one or more steps may be omitted or left out entirely.

Review of Current Literature with References

- Guidelines for the management of severe traumatic brain injury. VIII. Intracranial pressure thresholds. Brain Trauma Foundation; American Association of Neurological Surgeons; Congress of Neurological Surgeons; Joint Section on Neurotrauma and Critical Care, AANS/CNS, Bratton SL, Chestnut RM, Ghajar J, McConnell Hammond FF, Harris OA, Hartl R, Manley GT, Nemecek A, Newell DW, Rosenthal G, Schouten J, Shutter L, Timmons SD, Ullman JS, Videtta W, Wilberger JE, Wright DW. J Neurotrauma. 2007; **24** Suppl 1:S55–58. PMID: 17511546.

  o Review of most current literature regarding the threshold at which treatment for intracranial hypertension is indicated.
  o Consensus among this group of experts based on the literature review performed indicate that treatment for intracranial hypertension should be initiated at values of 20–25 mmHg.

- Guidelines for the management of severe traumatic brain injury. IX. Cerebral perfusion thresholds. Brain Trauma Foundation; American Association of Neurological Surgeons; Congress of Neurological Surgeons; Joint Section on Neurotrauma and Critical Care, AANS/CNS, Bratton SL, Chestnut RM, Ghajar J, McConnell Hammond FF, Harris OA, Hartl R, Manley GT, Nemecek A, Newell DW, Rosenthal G, Schouten J, Shutter L, Timmons SD, Ullman JS, Videtta W, Wilberger JE, Wright DW. *J Neurotrauma.* 2007; **24** Suppl 1: S59–64.

  o Review of the most current literature regarding the goal cerebral perfusion pressure which should be maintained following severe traumatic brain injury.
  o Cerebral ischemia likely begins at cerebral perfusion pressures less than 50–60 mmHg
  o Maintaining a goal cerebral perfusion pressure of 60 mmHg is likely ideal for most patients.
  o Artificially elevating cerebral perfusion pressure above 70 mmHg may be toxic and does not lead to improved outcomes.
  o Ancillary monitoring of brain tissue oxygenation may aid in tailoring treatment to individual patients' needs.

Spine Trauma: Diagnosis, Clearance, and Mobility

Todd F. VanderHeiden, MD* Samuel E. Smith, MD†
and Philip F. Stahel, MD‡

* Chief, Orthopaedic Spine Surgery, Denver Health Medical Center
† Orthopaedic Spine Surgeon, Denver Health Medical Center
‡ Director of Orthopaedics, Denver Health Medical Center

Take Home Points

- Assume a serious spinal injury exists until proven otherwise.
- Maintain strict log-roll precautions and cervical rigid-collar immobilization until spinal injury can be confirmed absent or definitive spinal treatment is provided.
- Critically injured patients need total spinal evaluation: occiput to coccyx. This includes physical examination and advanced imaging studies. Computed

Contact information: (Todd F. VanderHeiden), Department of Orthopaedic Surgery, Spine Surgery Division, Rocky Mountain Regional Trauma Center, Denver Health Medical Center, 777 Bannock Street, Mail-Code 0188, Denver, CO 80204, USA; Tel.: 303-602-1848, Fax: 303-436-3123, email: Todd.VanderHeiden@DHHA.Org

tomography (CT) is required in most cases. Magnetic resonance imaging (MRI) of injured spinal regions should be considered after formal Spine Surgery consultation.

- Complete and thorough neurological examination is mandatory.
- Classification of spinal injuries helps guide treatment. Early and accurate diagnosis of spinal injuries is essential.
- Spinal surgeons work to accomplish three goals within 24-hours of injury:

  (1) Obtain proper spinal **Alignment**.
  (2) Provide spinal **Stability**.
  (3) **Decompress** neurological structures when indicated.

- Early mobilization of critically injured patients is absolutely essential. This requires either spinal clearance or spinal stabilization — surgical and/or nonsurgical means may be employed.
- If possible, **"Spinal Clearance"** should be provided early in critical care management to enable removal of unnecessary braces and immobilizers, thereby minimizing complications.
- Spinal cord injured patients benefit from standardized institutional practice protocols to facilitate quality care. An example is DHMC's Spinal Cord Injury Clinical Practice Guideline.
- The uncritical use of steroids is considered obsolete in the management of acute, traumatic spinal cord injury except in selected circumstances.
- A multidisciplinary approach is needed to ensure proper care of critically injured patients with concomitant spinal injury. Timely transparent communication is paramount for the successful multidisciplinary management of this highly vulnerable patient cohort.

Background

- Spinal injury amongst multiply injured patients is very common. Spinal cord injury is a devastating occurrence that has far-reaching implications on the patient, family and loved ones, care providers, and the medical community. Cost is high. Preservation of function is the task bestowed upon all of the care providers tending to these severely injured patients.
- Critically injured patients with concomitant spinal injury can suffer from hemodynamic collapse and respiratory compromise that lead to hypotension and hypoxemia which can further exacerbate the spinal injury. Most specifically, this pertains to spinal injuries with associated spinal cord insult. As such, early recognition and treatment is mandatory.

- Critically ill patients with spinal injuries that experience hemodynamic instability and end-organ hypo-perfusion need to be closely assessed for neurogenic shock. Intensive care specialists need to recognize and appropriately treat this entity and also understand the difference between this problem and its often confused counterpart — spinal shock. **Spinal Shock** is a transient syndrome of sensorimotor dysfunction. It is characterized by flaccid areflexic paralysis and anesthesia below the level of a spinal cord injury. The syndrome typically lasts between 24–72 hours and has ended when reflex activity returns below the injury. **Neurogenic Shock** results from impaired sympathetic outflow tracts as a result of spinal cord injury and is accompanied by hypotension and bradycardia. It is diagnosed only after ruling out hemodynamic shock in poly-trauma patients and is typically associated with more cephalad levels of spinal injury.
- **"Spine Clearance"** continues to be a topic of debate. Multiple concepts for spinal clearance exist. Multiple algorithms attempt to "clear" the spine in critically injured patients. The ultimate goal of spinal clearance should be to confirm the absence of an injury to the spine. Once this is accomplished, the diagnostic phase of spinal assessment is complete and providers can allow immediate mobilization of patients and removal of unnecessary braces.
- Early mobilization of critically ill patients is paramount. The spine should either be "cleared" or the spine surgeon should stabilize unstable injuries to allow early patient mobility — both surgical and/or nonsurgical methods can be employed. This will allow prevention of dreaded complications associated with recumbency: pneumonia, urinary tract infections, thromboembolic events, and pressure sores to name a few.
- Spinal surgery treatment concepts involve upholding the **"Holy Trinity of Spine."**
  (1) Provide and maintain **Alignment** of spinal segments.
  (2) Provide immediate, rock-solid **Stability** to the unstable spine.
  (3) **Decompress** neurological structures (brain stem, spinal cord, spinal nerve-rootlets, cauda equina, conus medullaris, nerve-roots) if indicated and clinically relevant.
- Defining **"Spinal Stability"** is a difficult task. The working definition of stability should consider that under physiological loads (the influence of gravity on body mass), the spine does not experience increasing deformity, onset of neurological insult, or drastic increase in patient's pain. If spinal stability can be confirmed without the need for surgical intervention, then immediate mobilization of patients with or without bracing may be appropriate.

If the spine is deemed unstable, then early surgical treatment is necessary to enable safe mobilization.

- **"Spine-Damage-Control"** is a concept focused on providing immediate spinal stability within 24-hours of injury (posterior surgical approach) followed by delayed secondary surgery to complete 360° of spinal stabilization (anterior surgical approach). Much like external fixation of long-bone fractures, "spine-damage-control" enables early mobilization while facilitating patient recovery and delaying more invasive spinal procedures that may be needed for completion of spinal injury reconstruction.

- Once spinal injuries are stabilized, whether through surgical or nonsurgical means, patients often require ongoing **"Spinal Precautions."** These can create confusion amongst care providers and therefore must be clarified to ensure proper and safe mobilization of critically ill patients. If spinal precautions are significantly prohibitive, then the spine surgeon must consider surgical fixation and stabilization to enable removal of restrictions and thus facilitate the proper care by intensivists, therapists, and nurses.

- A multidisciplinary approach to critically injured patients that also suffer from spinal injury is mandatory. Explicit communication is required between care providers to ensure all body systems are appropriately managed with specific attention paid to the impact that serious spinal injury can have on each of these areas.

Main Body

- **"Spinal Clearance"**
  - o A thorough spinal evaluation has occurred to ensure that no spinal injury exists that requires treatment. Spinal injury is confirmed absent. Evaluation includes thorough history, physical examination, and radiographic analysis of advanced imaging studies. Immobilizers are thus immediately removed and patients are mobilized with nursing staff and therapists.
  - o Patients should be divided into distinct *groups* for coherent spinal clearance algorithms:
    - ▪ Asymptomatic
    - ▪ Symptomatic
    - ▪ Temporarily Non-Assessable
    - ▪ Obtunded

  - o **Asymptomatic Patients** without distracting injuries that are examinable and not intoxicated are usually clinically assessable and potentially cleared.

Assessment involves range-of-motion analysis, full neurological exam, and potentially radiographic interpretation. If any symptoms present during evaluation, patients are immediately placed into the symptomatic group.

o **Symptomatic Patients** require further radiographic analysis to determine diagnosis. Swift delivery of treatment options must then follow. Spine Surgery consultation is typically appropriate in this patient cohort.

o **Temporarily Non-Assessable Patients** require temporary rigid cervical immobilization until clearance of intoxicating substances, return of normal mentation, and/or stabilization of distracting injuries before they can be reliably assessed and potentially cleared. This entails a 24–48 hour "holding-period" and also serves to distinguish this distinct patient group from "obtunded patients."

o **Obtunded Patients** require imaging to rule out spinal injuries. Critically ill, multiply injured, poly-trauma patients typically fit into this category.

o Prolonged obtundation can present a dilemma regarding "spinal clearance." If an injury is identified, then a definitive treatment plan is determined and executed. If no injury is identified on CT scan, then the care providers must decide whether to remove the rigid cervical collar. Some providers believe an MRI scan is mandatory in this situation. Other providers feel that monitored flexion and extension radiographs (or fluoroscopic analysis) are warranted. However, the incidence of occult unstable spinal injuries occurring in the presence of a normal CT scan is extremely low. Therefore, DHMC chooses to remove the cervical collar in obtunded patients without neurological deficits that have no identified spinal injury on CT scan.

o Once allocated to a group, a patient's "spinal clearance" analysis should entail a logical, step-wise, algorithmic approach.

   ▪ **Asymptomatic Patients** are placed into the *Clinical Pathway* (Fig. 1).
   ▪ **Symptomatic Patients** are placed into the *Imaging Pathway* (Fig. 2).
   ▪ **Obtunded Patients** and **Temporarily Non-Assessable Patients** are placed into the *Obtunded Pathway* (Fig. 3).

o Completing the spinal clearance pathways should always result in accurate spinal diagnoses, appropriate treatment delivery, and insurance of preserving the **"Holy Trinity of Spine"** with the end-goal of early mobilization and facilitation of streamlined critical care.

- **"Spinal Precautions"**

   o **"Spinal Precautions"** are the restrictions placed on patient mobility to ensure safe movement and care of spine-injured patients. Precautions are upheld by all members of the care team and should therefore be simple, explicit, and easily followed.

o   Critically injured patients are initially treated as if serious spinal injuries have occurred. **"Log-Roll Precautions"** are followed until accurate diagnoses are made, treatments delivered, or the spine is "cleared." Log-Roll Precautions include supine positioning of the patient, maintaining a rigid cervical immobilizer, and moving patients with a team of care providers. Back boards should also be removed as early as possible upon arrival to the treating institution.

o   **"Routine Spinal Precautions"** are common-sense precautions that patients should follow once definitive treatment has been applied to the spinal injury. This holds true whether surgical or nonsurgical solutions have been provided. Care providers should remember "B.L.T." Common-sense limitations call for precautions in "bending," "lifting," and "twisting." Although very specific restrictions cannot be applied, the general rule is that patients should avoid painful positions and activities. Patients should not "bend too much," "lift too much," or "twist too much" so as to enact extremes of range-of-motion that may result in pain. If spinal precautions are instituted that result in restrictions above and beyond these routine limitations, then the spinal stability is in question. Therefore, spinal surgeons should rethink treatment options and act to provide adequate stability so that only routine spinal precautions are necessary for mobilizing these critically ill patients.

o   **"Spinal Precautions"** that also need to be communicated to care providers are:

   ▪   *Head-of-Bed Restrictions*: Care providers must know the safe limits of sitting patients up in bed. Head-of-bed restrictions are reasonable upon patient's arrival to the institution, but spine treatments must always result in elimination of these restrictions so as to insure proper and early mobilization.

   ▪   *Don/Doff Criteria*: Care providers must know the safe location of brace application and brace removal. Ideally, "edge-of-bed" is the preferred location for placing and removing orthoses. This is an easy position in which to manipulate a patient's brace. Alternatively, "brace only when ambulating" restrictions can allow the delivery of the most effective intensive and nursing care. Some situations, however, require application of braces in the supine position. If braces are to be applied in bed, in the supine position, then the spine's stability is in question and the spine surgeon should consider internal fixation and stabilization to eliminate reliance on brace treatment. One should consider, however, that significant force is applied to the spine when patient's move from supine to seated to standing positions and vice versa. As such, patient comfort and improved stability can be achieved when applying braces in bed in the supine position. This requires more focused effort on the part of the nurses and therapist caring for the patient.

- *Nursing and Activity Orders*: Care providers must know the appropriate precautions to take with regard to patient care, activities, and mobilization. Nurses and intensive care specialists need to know the types of braces that are required, how to appropriately administer them, when and where to place them, whether they are needed for showers or cleaning activities, and the duration of treatment. The prosthetics and orthotics specialist can be a valuable member of the care team in communicating these instructions.

- *Halo-Fixators and Gardner-Wells Tongs*: If due to a patient's compromised physiological status early surgical fixation cannot be employed, then alternative methods can be used. These methods include application of Gardner-Wells tongs traction, halo-ring traction, or halo-fixator application to reduce subluxations/dislocations in a closed manner. Halo-vest fixator application can also temporarily reduce and stabilize unstable occipitocervical and cervical injuries until internal fixation strategies can be utilized. Occasionally, halo-fixators are used as definitive treatment devices. This can present challenges to nursing and intensive care specialists. Halo-fixators should be applied early in the course of treatment so as to enable early patient mobilization. Vest and pin-site care should also be administered routinely.

o **Spinal Surgical Intervention**

- The **"Holy Trinity of Spine"** must be upheld:
  ⇨ **Alignment**.
  ⇨ **Stability**.
  ⇨ **Decompression**.

- **"Spinal Stability"** must be provided:
  ⇨ *Definition*: Under normal loading patterns, the spine must be protected against increasing deformity, onset of neurological insult, and significant increase in pain.

- If spinal alignment, spinal stability, or spinal neurological status is in question, then Critical Care Specialists are encouraged to call a formal Spine Surgery consultation.
- If and when "spinal clearance" cannot be provided and/or when even the strictest precautions cannot ensure spinal stability, then spinal surgical intervention is required.
- **"Spine-Damage-Control"** is a strategy often employed to provide rigid stabilization of spinal injuries within the first 24-hours. The associated fixation enables immediate mobilization and nursing care for patients. Once patients have been further resuscitated and compromised physiology corrected, then patients can better tolerate anterior spinal procedures for completion of total 360° spinal reconstruction. The spine surgery team at DHMC strives to fixate spinal injuries within the first 24-hours of arrival so that further intensive care is more easily delivered.
- Although spine surgical techniques are many and variable, the goals of providing and maintaining proper spinal alignment, ensuring immediate and rock-solid stabilization, and decompressing impinged neurological structures remain constant. Spine surgeons may employ anterior approaches, posterior approaches, lateral approaches, or a combination of approaches to ensure that the principles of spinal surgery and stabilization are upheld. This can frequently necessitate the expertise of general surgeons to assist with spinal exposure. As such, proper communication and teamwork are indicated to deliver proper treatment modalities.
- Accurate diagnosis and injury classification can assist spinal surgeons in clinical decision making processes as it relates to choosing operative versus non-operative management as well as choosing treatment approach and fixation methods when it comes to surgical intervention. Several classification schemes exists, but all rely upon determination of the injury mechanism and morphology, the neurological status of the patient, and the integrity of the intervertebral disk and supporting posterior ligamentous complex. Regardless of the classification system chosen, the **"Holy Trinity of Spine"** is honored.

Practical Algorithm

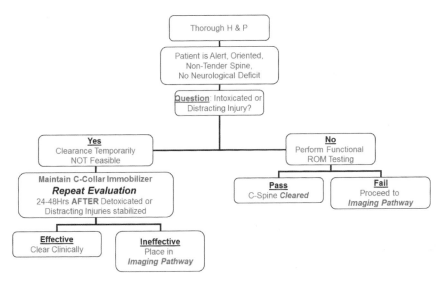

Fig. 1. Spinal Clearance: *Clinical Pathway*. With an "Asymptomatic Patient" that is awake, alert and oriented, non-painful, non-tender, and neurologically intact, the physician can usually rely on clinical findings. If any questions remain, the patient should be placed into the *Imaging Pathway*.

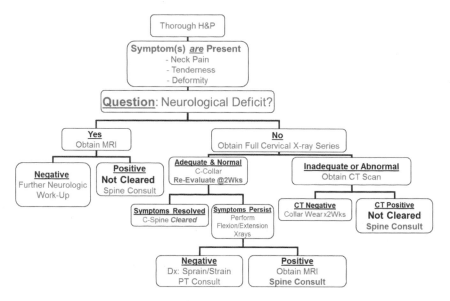

Fig. 2.   Spinal Clearance: *Imaging Pathway*. With a "Symptomatic Patient" that has spinal pain and/or tenderness on examination, a visible deformity, an abnormal neurological finding, or a combination of these problems, the physician requires imaging data in addition to clinical information to support decision-making.

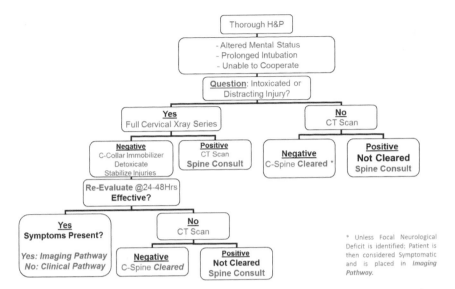

Fig. 3. Spinal Clearance: *Obtunded Pathway*. With a "Temporarily non-Assessable Patient" or "Obtunded Patient," the physician typically relies upon the imaging data to inform clinical decision-making. The distinction between these two groups is typically present after a 24–48 hour holding period where the "Temporarily non-Assessable Patient" has declared themselves assessable and can now be categorized as either a "Symptomatic Patient" or an "Asymptomatic Patient."

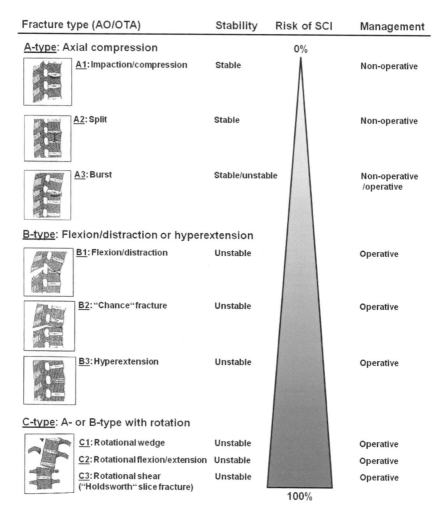

Fracture type (AO/OTA)	Stability	Risk of SCI	Management
A-type: Axial compression		0%	
A1: Impaction/compression	Stable		Non-operative
A2: Split	Stable		Non-operative
A3: Burst	Stable/unstable		Non-operative /operative
B-type: Flexion/distraction or hyperextension			
B1: Flexion/distraction	Unstable		Operative
B2: "Chance" fracture	Unstable		Operative
B3: Hyperextension	Unstable		Operative
C-type: A- or B-type with rotation			
C1: Rotational wedge	Unstable		Operative
C2: Rotational flexion/extension	Unstable		Operative
C3: Rotational shear ("Holdsworth" slice fracture)	Unstable	100%	Operative

Fig. 4. Injury Classification. Modified AO classification of spine fractures. This worksheet includes determination of the fracture type, assessment of stability, neurological status, and treatment recommendation. A-type injuries result from mainly axial forces applied to the spinal column and produce anterior and middle column injuries ("A" = axial). B-type injuries involve bending forces that can couple both compression and tension depending on the location of the center-of-rotation ("B" = bending). The posterior ligamentous complex (PLC) is typically ruptured in these injuries. C-type injuries involve multidirectional forces and produce highly unstable injuries involving 360° of the spinal column ("C" = circle), including rupture of the PLC. When spine surgeons couple these fracture mechanisms, the morphology of the injury, along with the neurological status of the patient, it can become straight-forward to determine stability and incorporate a surgical treatment strategy.

Table 1. Injury scoring system. The thoracolumbar injury classification and severity score (TLICSS) can help the spine surgeon determine the need for surgical intervention.

	Score
Fracture Morphology	
Compression Injury	1
Burst Fracture	+1 = 2
Translational/Rotational Injury	3
Distraction Injury	4
Neurological Injury	
Intact	0
Nerve-root Injury	2
Complete Injury	2
Incomplete Injury	3
Cauda Equina Injury	3
Posterior Ligamentous Complex	
Intact PLC	0
Injury Suspected in PLC	2
Injured PLC	3
Summation	Total score
NonOperative Zone	<4
"Grey" Zone	=4
Operative Zone	>4

Review of Current Literature with References

- A meta-analysis of almost 15,000 patients done by Pancyzkowski *et al.*, published in the *Journal of Neurosurgery*, determined that removing the rigid cervical immobilizer in obtunded patients is reasonable and safe so long as the CT scan of the cervical spine was negative for acute injury. MRI was deemed unnecessary in this situation [Panczykowski DM, Tomycz ND, Okonkwo DO, "Comparative effectiveness of using computed tomography alone to exclude cervical spine injuries in obtunded or intubated patients: meta-analysis of 14,327 patients with blunt trauma." *J Neurosurg* (2011); **115**: 541–549].

- A retrospective cohort study of nearly 400 patients at a single institution showed that CT scan of the cervical spine identified all unstable spinal injuries. Furthermore, the investigators concluded that clearing the spine does not require further radiographs once a CT scan is determined to exclude acute injury. In fact, obtaining upright X-rays delayed spinal clearance in a large proportion of patients [Harris TJ, Blackmore CC, Mirza SK, Jurkovich GJ, "Clearing the cervical spine in obtunded patients." *Spine (Phila Pa 1976)* (2008); **15**; 33: 1547–1553].

- A retrospective cohort study at a single institution analyzing data from nearly 700 patients showed that MRI scan was not necessary to clear the cervical spine in patients with normal trauma cervical CT scans using modern imaging protocols. In reviewing data from patients that had an MRI scan of the cervical spine contemporaneously, 21% of patients had injuries diagnosed by MRI that were not identified on the CT scan. However, none of those patients had unstable injuries, none of those patient required surgical treatment, and none of those patients developed instability [Tomycz ND, Chew BG, Chang YF, Darby JM, Gunn SR, Nicholas DH, Ochoa JB, Peitzman AB, Schwartz E, Pape HC, Spiro RM, Okonkwo DO, "MRI is unnecessary to clear the cervical spine in obtunded/comatose trauma patients: the four-year experience of a level I trauma center." *J Trauma* (2008); **64**: 1258–1263].

- A very recent cross-sectional, observational study evaluating the concept of cervical "spinal clearance" protocols at United States Level 1 Trauma Centers showed that this idea is still a highly-debated, controversial, and challenging topic with immense variability. The paper does show the importance of dividing trauma patients into groups and utilizing a step-wise, algorithmic approach to spinal clearance. It also addresses the interesting topic of evaluating patients with ongoing neck pain despite negative imaging [Theologis AA, Dionisio R, Mackersie R, McClellan RT, Pekmezci M, "Cervical spine clearance protocols in level I trauma centers in the United States." *Spine (Phila Pa 1976)* (2013) (Epub ahead of print)].

- Early spinal fixation and stabilization is the rule for managing unstable spinal trauma in critically injured patients. The DHMC spine team recommends surgery within 24-hours of injury (**"<u>Spine-Damage-Control</u>"**) to enable the best results for avoiding complications in these highly injured patients. A prospective cohort study shows that this treatment approach significantly decreases length of hospitalization, ventilator dependent days, and other complications [Stahel PF, VanderHeiden TF, Flierl MA, Matava B, Gerhardt DC, Bolles G, Beauchamp K, Burlew CC, Johnson JL, Moore EE, "The impact of a standardized 'spine-damage-control' protocol for unstable thoracic and lumbar spine fractures in severely injured patients: a prospective cohort study." *J Trauma Acute Care Surg* (2013); **74**: 590–596].

- Accurate diagnosis and classification of spinal injuries helps to guide treatment of critically injured patients. As such, the impact of utilizing classification systems is widely appreciated amongst spinal surgeons. The Thoracolumbar Injury Classification and Severity Scale (TLICSS Score) has proven to be a valid instrument with which to help guide treatment. A retrospective cohort study confirmed the efficacy and validity of this tool as it helped provide successful treatment decisions for spinal trauma patients as well as diminished the need to convert to surgical management in patients initially treated non-operatively [Joaquim AF, Lawrence B, Daubs M, Brodke D, Tedeschi H, Vaccaro AR, Patel AA, "Measuring the impact of the Thoracolumbar Injury Classification and Severity Score among 458 consecutively treated patients." *J Spinal Cord Med* (2014); **37**: 101–106].

- The use of steroid protocols after acute spinal cord injury was long considered the standard of care in view that there was a perceived benefit from methylprednisolone on neurological recovery. However, more recent data suggest that there is in fact no significant benefit in neurological recovery for patients suffering acute spinal cord injury that receive steroids [Ito Y, Sugimoto Y, Tomioka M, Kai N, Tanaka M, "Does high-dose methylprednisolone sodium succinate really improve neurological status in patient with acute cervical cord injury?: A prospective study about neurological recovery and early complications." *Spine (Phila Pa 1976)* (2009); **34**: 2121–2124]. Furthermore, it appears that patients receiving steroid infusions after acute spinal cord injury suffer from more complications. These include infections, gastrointestinal complications, and most significantly, pulmonary compromise [Matsumoto T, Tamaki T, Kawakami M, Yoshida M, Ando M, Yamada H, "Early complications of high-dose methylprednisolone sodium succinate treatment in the follow-up of acute cervical spinal cord injury." *Spine (Phila Pa 1976)* (2001); **26**: 426–430]. As such, DHMC Critical Care providers and Spinal Surgeons avoid the use of steroid administration protocols for acute spinal cord injury. In place of these protocols, early surgical intervention is employed.

Chapter 4-(iv)

Surgical Critical Care and Behavioral Health

Thomas M. Dunn, PhD* and Abraham M. Nussbaum, MD†

* Greeley Clinical Instructor of Psychiatry, University of Colorado School of Medicine
† Assistant Professor of Psychiatry, University of Colorado School of Medicine

Take Home Points

- Mental illness and psychological distress commonly occur in surgical patients.
  - With high base rates of mental illness in the general population, it is inevitable that such patients will develop a co-occurring condition requiring surgical intervention.
  - Patients who have harmed themselves as a result of a mental illness often have surgical needs.

Contact information: Denver Health, 777 Bannock Street, MC 0490, Denver, CO 80204; Email: Thomas.Dunn@dhha.org; Abraham.Nussbaum@dhha.org

- Often, the need for surgery is precipitated by a traumatic event, leaving surgical patients particularly vulnerable to stress responses and mood disruption.
  - o Both mental illness and psychological stress are treatable in the critical surgical patient.
- The most commonly occurring acute psychiatric presentation in surgical patients is delirium.
  - o Delirium is a life-threatening condition associated with prolonged hospital stays and poorer outcomes.
  - o It is commonly overlooked due to its waxing and waning nature.
- While the surgical team can manage many preexisting psychiatric conditions, in some instances a formal psychiatric consult may be indicated.
  - o If a patient with a serious mental illness is not currently receiving adequate treatment.
  - o If a patient requires surgical intervention because of behavior related to his or her mental illness.
    - Suicide attempts
    - Self-mutilation
    - Lack of self-care leading to surgical emergency
  - o Those patients, or their families, spouses or partners, who request consultation from a psychiatrist or psychologist.
  - o Patients currently enrolled in a methadone treatment program for opioid addiction.

Background

- Mental illness is quite prevalent in the U.S.; the National Institute of Mental Health estimates that in a given year, 1 in 4 adults suffers from symptoms meeting criteria for a mental disorder.
  - o There are often co-occurring mental disorders; nearly half of all persons with mental illness cope with two or more conditions.
  - o Severity of these conditions is often directly related to the degree of stress the patient is experiencing.
    - Severe medical problems can worsen some mental disorders.
    - Exacerbation of preexisting mental illness, particularly depression, can impair a patient's ability to follow a postoperative regimen.

o Rarely, however, does mental illness present for the first time during a surgical admission. The surgeon should be wary of the patient who acutely develops severe symptoms of mental illness after surgery.

  ▪ Sudden psychosis and agitation is likely delirium or the effect of a psychoactive substance. Delirium is often secondary to post-surgical complication, such as infection. Organic causes should be ruled out before attributing psychosis to a primary psychiatric condition.

  ▪ Depression symptoms may be an acute stress response.

  ▪ Nightmares and anxiety may suggest acute stress.

- Substance use disorders are also quite common and likely to be minimized by the patient.

  o Withdrawal from alcohol can be quite severe and seriously complicate a surgical course.

  o Some patients may continue to use drugs of abuse while admitted.

  o The latest (5ᵗʰ) edition of the Diagnostic and Statistical Manual of the American Psychiatric Association, the DSM, no longer distinguishes between substance abuse and substance dependence.

  ▪ Collectively known as "substance use disorders."

- While self-harm behavior makes up only a small percentage of overall psychiatric patients, they are over-represented in surgical settings.

  o Nearly a third of individuals attempting suicide will do so using an injurious mechanism, most often cutting or stabbing, firearms, hanging, or jumps from heights.

  o Individuals suffering from self-inflicted trauma are believed to be incapable of refusing surgical care.

  o All states have specific laws addressing the involuntary psychiatric treatment of suicidal patients.

  ▪ Many of these laws specify a very short period of time (in many states, 72 hours) that an individual can be hospitalized involuntarily.

Main Body

- Delirium

  o May occur in up to 80% of intensive care unit patients, with postoperative patients particularly susceptible.

  o The most common acute psychiatric condition in the surgical setting.

- Associated with increased mortality and length of stay.
- Significant burden on nursing staff.
- Less than half of those who become delirious will return to their base-line cognitive functioning and the one-year mortality rate is approximately 35%.
- Delirium is often misidentified early in its course.
- Although typically lasting a few days, some cases may take up to eight weeks to resolve.
- Early identification and intervention is critical.

o Defining features

- Abrupt disturbance in attention and awareness developing in hours to days.
- An accompanying cognitive deficit (often in language, memory or perception, sleep/wake functioning).
- A waxing and waning presentation.

o Classically, delirium will present in one of three states:

- Hyperactive: Agitation, restlessness, over-activity.
- Hypoactive: Lethargy, somnolence, under-activity.
- Mixed State: Features of both.

o Hyperactive delirium may present with combativeness, hallucinations, restlessness, pressured speech/shouting, singing, anger/irritability, wandering, distractibility, etc.

- Often confused with psychosis, or being irritable at baseline.

o Hypoactive delirium may present as poverty of speech, staring for long periods of time, decreased activity, and significant apathy.

- Often confused with depression or negativity.

o The pathophysiology of delirium is very complicated, but likely due to a poverty of acetylcholine and/or an excess of dopamine.

- Usually secondary to multiple etiologies (including disease states and neural insults).

o Identifying delirium

- There are commercially available screening instruments; the richmond agitation sedation scale (RASS) and the confusion assessment method intensive care unit (CAM-ICU) are commonly in use.

- Because of its sudden onset, as well as its tendency to wax and wane, the surgeon is unlikely to be the first to become aware that the patient is having trouble.
  - ⇨ Typically nursing or family members are the first to notice.
- o Risk factors for delirium (acronym is I WATCH DEATH)
  - Infection
  - Withdrawal from alcohol and benzodiazepines
  - Acute metabolic abnormalities
  - Trauma — particularly brain injury, factures and burns
  - CNS pathology, including seizures, intracranial bleeding, space occupying lesions
  - Hypoxia
  - Deficiencies, particularly thiamine
  - Endocrinopathies
  - Acute vascular disturbances, such as hypertensive encephalopathy
  - Toxins/drugs, including drugs of abuse, opioids, benzodiazepines, and drugs with anticholinergic properties
  - Heavy metals, such as lead poisoning
- o Additional risk factors for delirium
  - Multiple indwelling catheters
  - Immobility
  - Age ≥65
  - Sensory impairment (e.g. blindness or deafness)
  - Premorbid neural insults, including severe mental illness, developmental delay, severe substance use, traumatic brain injury.
  - Severity of illness: Those with APACHE II scores of 18 and higher often transition to delirium.
- o Treatment of delirium tends to be broken down into nonpharmacological and pharmacological approaches.
- o Nonpharmacological treatment of delirium:
  - Be vigilant for delirium, SICU nurses should be specifically trained to be aware of this condition.
    - ⇨ There are several screening instruments available to identify and rate severity of delirium, including CAM and CAM-ICU.

- ▪ Reverse possible causes.
  - ⇨ Have low index of suspicion for alcohol withdrawal.
  - ⇨ Treat infection, remove indwelling catheters, discontinue medicines that are highly anticholinergic, etc.
- ▪ Encourage being out of bed during the day and allow for as much sleep as possible at night.
  - ⇨ During the day, room lights are on and shades are open.
  - ⇨ Television should be on, encourage family/friends to interact with the patient.
  - ⇨ Intercom turned down at night.
  - ⇨ Minimize night-time interruptions, perhaps gathering vital signs and administered medicine can be combined at the same time.
  - ⇨ Patient should be wearing their hearing aids and glasses during the day.

- o Pharmacological treatment of delirium
  - ▪ Sedation may be required, particularly in a highly agitated patient.
  - ▪ Ideally, the level of sedation should be sufficient to ameliorate agitation and other hyperactive symptoms, but only to the point where the patient will rouse with stimulation.
  - ▪ Avoid benzodiazepines, particularly lorazepam (which is known to precipitate delirium), unless treating alcohol withdrawal.
  - ▪ Avoid sleep aids that resemble benzodiazepines, especially zolpidem. A safer treatment for insomnia is trazodone 50–200 mg prn insomnia.
  - ▪ Avoid polypharmacy.
  - ▪ Antipsychotics are commonly used to treat the behavioral disturbances associated with delirium.
    - ⇨ Haloperidol is an inexpensive dopamine antagonist available in multiple formulations that has an excellent safety profile. It is widely used for the treatment of delirium.
    - ⇨ Haloperidol is less anticholinergic activity than most antipsychotics.
    - ⇨ However, its use is associated with the prolongation of the QT interval in a dose-dependent fashion.
    - ⇨ Consider starting haldol at 0.5mg PO/IM and increasing the dose in half milligram increments until agitation is controlled.
      - — Take 50% of this loading dose and divide into q6 hour increments.

— Taper down as patient improves.

— IV dosing of haloperidol should only occur with careful cardiac monitoring.

⇨ Generally, scheduled medication is more effective and better tolerated than as needed dosing.

- Patients with hypoactive delirium may still benefit from very low doses (0.25 mg to 0.5 mg) of haloperidol.

• Substance Use Disorders

  o A person exhibiting signs (or reporting symptoms) of a mental illness may be experiencing the effects of psychoactive substance use.

  - The variety of psychoactive substances that people use and misuse is remarkable, so when seeking the cause of a patient's distress, always consider drugs of abuse, as well as prescription, over-the-counter, sleeping aids, and herbal medicines.

  - Psychoactive substance use is common among persons admitted to surgical services. In addition, surgical teams often prescribe psycho-active substances. People can experience mental distress during substance use, intoxication, and withdrawal.

  o Consider these possibilities:

  - Substance Intoxication:

    ⇨ People often underreport substance use. Urine and serum lab tests include common substances, but do not include many psychoactive substances like synthetic cannabinoids and club drugs, so a "negative utox" does not rule out intoxication.

    ⇨ Many states have online registries to track controlled substance administration, to help confirm or deny suspicions about a patient's substance use.

    ⇨ To prevent intoxication, we recommend judicious prescription of psychoactive substances only when necessary.

  - Substance Withdrawal:

    ⇨ Most psychoactive substances have a characteristic withdrawal syndrome.

    ⇨ Treatment protocols exist to treat most withdrawal syndromes, usually focusing on symptomatic treatment.

— We caution against using these protocols automatically as they often include substances that can mask dangerous clinical signs.

— For example, in many hospitals it is common to place persons with opiate use disorders on a clinical opiate withdrawal scale (COWS) protocol.

— The COWS protocol includes clonidine, which reduces autonomic hyperactivity, but does not prevent withdrawal seizures.

— Instead, we advise that treatment should be focused on those substances for which withdrawal can be lethal.

⇨ Alcohol withdrawal

— Early treatment can prevent complicated withdrawal. Multiple withdrawal protocols (CIWA, SEWS, etc.) are available and many hospitals will have a preferred protocol.

— While we generally recommend judicious use of benzodiazepines in the surgical critical care setting to reduce the risk of delirium, benzodiazepines (especially diazepam or lorazepam) are the cornerstone of treatment for alcohol treatment.

⇨ Benzodiazepine withdrawal

— No standard protocol exists for treating benzodiazepine withdrawal, which is typically prolonged because of the comparatively long half-life of many benzodiazepines, especially clonazepam.

— The first step is to determine the daily dose of benzodiazepines, the duration of benzodiazepine use, and the presence or absence of physiological dependence.

— For a person who is physiologically dependent on benzodiazepine, it is preferable to decrease daily benzodiazepine dose gradually, by 20% per week, to avoid withdrawal seizures.

— In an acute setting, a loading dose of a long-acting benzodiazepine like diazepam (initial doses are typically 30–50 mg) can be given and then transition to schedule doses.

— Avoid the use of as needed benzodiazepines.

— Avoid the use of the short-acting benzodiazepine alprazolam, which is frequently abused and diverted.

⇨ Barbiturate withdrawal:

— While barbiturate use has markedly decreased over the past two decades, barbiturate withdrawal can be lethal.

— The treatment is essentially the same as benzodiazepine withdrawal.

✓ However, if a patient has epilepsy (as opposed to a history of withdrawal seizures), consulting a neurologist is recommended.

o Substance Use

- Substance use and misuse complicates surgical treatment and recovery.
- Screening for substance use, encouraging cessation, and referring patients to substance use treatment is critical.

⇨ Many hospitals will have substance abuse counselors who can speak to patients as they near discharge.

⇨ At discharge, careful medication reconciliation to minimize the availability of drugs of abuse is advised.

o The Methadone Patient

- Methadone maintenance programs are subsidized treatment programs for those with Opioid Use Disorder.
- There are strict laws about dispensing methadone as part of an addiction treatment regimen.
- It is prudent to continue to treat these patients who will withdraw while admitted if their regimen is not followed.

• Self-harm

o In the U.S., more people die each year from suicide than from motor vehicle collisions.

- Surgeons frequently treat people who have either survived suicide attempts or have engaged in self-injurious behavior without intent to die.

o More than half of all suicide attempts involve intentional ingestions, which have low rates of mortality.

- Attempts using firearms have the highest rates of morbidity and mortality, followed by hanging and jumping from heights.
- While cutting is very common, its overall mortality rate is about 1%.

o The demographic most highly associated with completed suicide is older white men, living alone, unemployed, abusing substances, with a chronic medical condition, who are not participating in a faith community. Further,

- 90% of people who complete suicide have a diagnosed mental disorder.
- Depression, hopelessness, and despondence are correlated with suicide.

- Psychotic individuals may also engage in self-harm because of delusions.
- Men tend to use lethal means of harming themselves and have higher rates of completed suicide.
- Suicide attempts often follow a significant life stressor, such as job loss or a relationship ending.
- Involving a firearm in a suicide attempt has a fatality rate above 80%.
- The military has noticed very high rates of suicide among veterans of the Afghanistan and Iraq wars, particularly those serving in the army.

  o Surgeons should be wary of individuals from high-risk groups who have suspicious injuries, such as patients:
    - With *any* self-inflicted gunshot wound, despite claims that it was accidental.
    - Involved in single vehicle motor vehicle collisions.
    - With unexplained falls from heights.

  o Despite severe self-inflicted injuries and a patient who may intubated, involving a consulting psychiatrist or psychologist early in the patient's course is prudent.
    - Collateral information identifying the particular circumstances of the injury can be ascertained.
    - Disposition of mental health holds are time sensitive.
    - Continuity of care is increased.

- Involuntary detention of the mentally ill who are dangerous.
  o In the North America, it is generally believed that thoughts of suicide or suicidal behavior are pathological.
    - It is also widely accepted that those who are mentally ill and potentially dangerous lose their capacity to refuse evaluation and treatment.
    - Some cultures, however, may accept ritualized suicide.

  o All states have mechanisms to detain individuals who are believed to be mentally ill and dangerous.
    - Some states allow detaining individuals who may be dangerous to property (such as fire setting).
    - Substance use disorders may also meet criteria.
    - Many states also allow the involuntary treatment of individuals whose mental illness is so severe, it makes them gravely disabled and unable to take care of themselves.

o While the specifics change from state to state, most jurisdictions allow for an emergency detention of a mentally ill person who is believed to be a danger to self or others and is refusing voluntary treatment.

- Emergency detention lasts a short period of time and permits evaluation of the patient.
- The evaluation is time limited to serve as a check against unlawful detention.

⇨ In many states, this time limit is 72 hours; however this period of time ranges from 24 hours (Texas) to 15 days (Connecticut).

- During the emergency detention, the patient is evaluated and a determination is made if longer involuntary detention is required.

⇨ If longer detention is required, then judicial review is invoked and evidence presented in a court of law regarding whether the patient should be committed.

o Involuntary treatment of a person with mental illness also varies widely from state to state.

- Even involuntary detained mentally ill persons retain the right to refuse psychotropic medication unless they are a danger to self or others.
- Many states allow the pharmacological treatment of treatment of individuals over their objections, by force if necessary, but only after a court order.
- Some jurisdictions allow the involuntary treatment of psychiatric patients accused of a crime to restore their competency to stand trial.
- Other states have very strict regulations about forcibly treating the mentally ill to a very narrow set of circumstances and only under extraordinary conditions.

⇨ This includes physical restraint.

o Typically, such mental health holds are unnecessary with patients who are voluntarily seeking treatment.

- Further, involuntary detention is not necessary in instances where the patient is incapable of making informed medical decisions.

⇨ The intubated and sedated patient does not need to be on a mental health hold.

⇨ Children typically do not need to be held involuntarily.

⇨ The patient impaired by intoxication or substance withdrawal, shock, or delirium.

o Recall that many states forbid the involuntary medication of patients being detained unless approved by a court.

- The delirious patient who is so confused that he cannot make medical decisions technically cannot receive an antipsychotic like haloperidol (in some states) without a court order.

  ⇨ Despite this being the treatment of choice and done in the perceived best interests of the patient.

o Acute surgical patients whose injuries are due to self-harm may often be best managed by considering them as having impaired medical decision-making capacity.

- This allows the surgeon to make a life- or limb-saving intervention despite the patient objecting to the procedure.

  ⇨ It is presumed that if the patient were not impaired by their suicidal wishes, he or she would consent to the treatment.

- It permits using standard patient restraint protocols in surgical settings, such as those designed to prevent accidental extubations, or removing indwelling catheters.

- Initiating a mental health hold starts a clock on how long the individual can be detained over his or her objections.

  ⇨ It does no good to have the clock running when the patient is intubated.

- Protocols and state laws about the treatment of a patient lacking medical decision-making capacity permits keeping patients safe by not permitting AMA discharge.

  ⇨ Be certain to include proxy decision-makers when treating patients who lack decision-making capacity to refuse treatment.

- Mental Illness and the Surgery Patient

o The vast majority of persons with mental illness suffering a co-occurring surgical condition will require only standard surgical care.

- It is prudent to continue home psychiatric medications, unless medically contraindicated.

o Patients with preexisting depression or anxiety may experience relapses with the added stress of surgical condition.

- Changes in psychiatric medication regimen should be coordinated with a patient's outpatient mental health practitioner.

- The Traumatized Surgical Patient
  - o Psychological trauma often co-occurs with physical trauma.
    - While it is widely recognized that individuals injured in violent confrontations (such as combat or violent crime) may have an untoward psychological reaction to their injury, those with more mundane mechanisms of injury (such as a motor vehicle collision), may also experience problems.
    - Having suffered physical trauma sufficient to require surgery predisposes patients to suffering from a trauma- or stressor-related disorder.
    - Severe illness and surgery may be sufficiently traumatizing to precipitate a trauma-related psychiatric condition.
  - o It should be noted that there are a range of presentations that may occur following a traumatic event that are not, necessarily, pathological.
    - It is not unusual for injured individuals to report nightmares, restlessness, fear, and depressed mood (among other symptoms).
    - Typically, however, these symptoms are short-lived and not severely impairing.
    - Severely impairing symptoms are those that
      - ⇨ Are the source of considerable personal distress.
      - ⇨ Persist beyond a few days.
      - ⇨ Impair patients' ability to participate in their treatment.
      - ⇨ Cause impairment in the patient's ability to interact with others.
      - ⇨ Present as being grossly out of proportion with extent of injury suffered.
  - o When patient's psychological reaction becomes severely impairing, it may meet the criteria for either acute stress disorder (ASD) or posttraumatic stress disorder (PTSD).
    - Both ASD and PTSD are psychiatric conditions which follow a traumatic event where an individual is exposed to threat of death, severe injury, or sexual violation. Their major difference is when symptoms appear.
      - ⇨ The onset of ASD is from three days after the traumatic event to one month.
      - ⇨ Symptoms that continue past one month, or impairment that does not start until a month after the event is PTSD.

- While ASD and PTSD have separate diagnostic criteria beyond time of onset, generally, both share the following symptoms:
    ⇨ Symptoms of intrusion, such as nightmares, flashbacks, intruding thoughts about the event.
    ⇨ Negative mood, such as depression, irritability, etc.
    ⇨ Dissociative symptoms, such as having trouble remembering important features of the traumatic event.
    ⇨ Avoidance of things that remind the individual of the trauma.
    ⇨ Hyperarousal, such as difficulty sleeping, restlessness, exaggerated startle response, angry outbursts, problems with attention and concentration.

  o Treatment of ASD/PTSD in the surgical critical care setting.
    - As many surgical patients report sub-clinical symptoms of ASD/PTSD, a prudent surgeon can warn his or her patients that these distressing symptoms are common responses.
    - The treatment literature for ASD/PTSD is most germane to the outpatient behavioral health setting.
    - Treatment of ASD/PTSD in the surgical critical care setting may be best directed at short-term management of the most severe symptoms.
        ⇨ Nightmares, hyperarousal, and sleep disturbance may subside with prazosin.
        ⇨ Extreme anxiety may respond to a short-course of a sedating medicine, such as hydroxyzine 50 mg po q6 prn anxiety, trazodone 50–200 mg po q6 prn insomnia, which can be continued at discharge if necessary.
        ⇨ If these prove insufficient, judicious use of a benzodiazepine like lorazepam or clonazepam, or even a sedating antipsychotic like haloperidol, quetiapine, or olanzapine may be indicated. These medications should usually be discontinued at discharge.
        ⇨ Patients who require intervention during their acute surgical care for severe stress reactions should be referred for outpatient treatment of ASD/PTSD.

- Psychiatric Conditions Presenting with a Surgical Complaint
  o DSM-5 renames somatoform disorders "Somatic Symptom and Related Disorders."
    - Hypochondriasis has been replaced by "Somatic Symptom Disorder" for a person with significant somatic symptoms and significant health

anxiety. The diagnosis of Pain Disorder is now a subtype of Somatic Symptom Disorder.

- For a person with minimal somatic symptoms, but significant health anxiety, DSM-5 replaces hypochondriasis with "Illness Anxiety Disorder."

o Factitious Disorder

- Individuals with Factitious Disorder are known to deceptively induce illness or injury to themselves for reasons other than secondary gain (e.g., financial settlement, narcotic pain relievers, coping with home-lessness).

- Such individuals are clearly making themselves ill or creating a condition requiring surgical intervention, but hiding this fact from care providers.

  ⇨ Precisely why individuals engage in this behavior is debated in the literature.

  ⇨ Generally, if a satisfying explanation for the behavior can be identified, then the condition is not likely Factitious Disorder.

  ⇨ Less likely are patients with this condition who feign particular symptoms.

- While there are varying presentations of Factious Disorder, these individuals have some unifying features.

  ⇨ A tendency to go from hospital to hospital with dramatic complaints, telling fantastic stories.

    — Likely to have lengthy medical records.
    — Often reluctant to allow providers to request medical records.
    — May have a "gridiron gut."

  ⇨ They often have an unusual understanding of medical terminology and jargon for a layperson.

    — Although, often these individuals may have worked in healthcare at an entry level position (such as a medical assistant or technician).

  ⇨ Women in their 20s and 30s are over-represented.

  ⇨ Often present as hostile, controlling, and angry during admission.

  ⇨ May have a history of substance use disorder.

o Often, those with Factitious Disorder:

  ⇨ Are eager for a medical test or procedure that would make other people worried or uncomfortable.

⇨ Have symptoms that cannot be directly observed, or are not present, when a physician is present.

⇨ Have sudden and unexplained setbacks during their hospital course.

- Treating this condition is very difficult.

    ⇨ Individual psychotherapy is indicated, but rarely do these individuals have enough insight into their situation to participate.

    ⇨ Despite suspecting that the patient may suffer from Factitious Disorder, the patient often engages in behavior that requires surgical intervention.

    ⇨ Certainly it is prudent to involve a psychiatrist or psychologist in the case, but these individuals will often move on to another hospital once they are challenged.

o Illness Anxiety Disorder (formerly hypochondriasis)

- Some people are preoccupied with the fear that they have, or are going to acquire, a serious medical condition.
- Despite assurances that they are well, they continue to have irrational fear about their health.
- Typically, somatic complaints are minimal or absent.
- These individuals do well with individual psychotherapy and other traditional treatments for anxiety.

    ⇨ Unfortunately, they may see referral to a mental health specialist by a surgeon as being dismissive.

o Somatic Symptom Disorder (formerly somatoform disorder, hypochondriasis, pain disorder)

- Individuals with somatic symptoms (often pain, but does not need to be) whose thoughts, feelings or worry about their complaints are out of proportion and are disrupting their daily life.
- This could manifest itself by:

    ⇨ Having excessive anxiety or stress about symptoms.
    ⇨ Obsessing about their symptoms.
    ⇨ Spending an excessive amount of time and energy devoted to their symptoms or health concerns.

- These individuals tend to be unhappy with explanations by medical providers and are often deaf to assurances by physicians that their symptoms are not indicative of a major illness or surgical emergency.

- While resistant to treatment by a mental health provider, these individuals tend to suffer from co-occurring depression.
  - ⇨ There is an elevated risk of suicide with such patients, making referrals to an outpatient mental health provider very important.
- o Delusions of Somatic Nature
  - Delusions of grandeur or of persecution are not uncommon in patients suffering from psychosis.
  - Less common are somatic delusions, but do occur with some frequency in those suffering from Delusional Disorder.
    - ⇨ Some may believe that they have a foul odor emanating from their body.
    - ⇨ Others may believe that somatic sensations indicate the presence of animals in their body or insects under their skin.
    - ⇨ Infrequently, some people believe that they are missing vital organs, or organ systems are missing.
  - Antipsychotic medications are effective in treating such delusions.
- Patients Requesting Amputation
  - o Infrequently, patients may present to the surgeon asking that a healthy limb be removed.
  - o Generally, patients without a surgical problem asking that a limb be removed fall into one of three categories:
    - Body Integrity Identity Disorder
      - ⇨ The sense that a portion of an individual's body (usually a limb) foreign.
      - ⇨ A paradoxical perception then sets in: in order to feel complete, an individual must have part of their body amputated.
      - ⇨ There are reports in the literature of individuals with this condition amputating their own limbs.
        - — And on occasion, amputating a limb that had already been surgically re-attached.
    - Apotemnophilia
      - ⇨ These are individuals who have an erotic association with losing a limb.
      - ⇨ Their drive for sexual satisfaction may be sufficient to deliberately injure the limb in hopes that it will need to be amputated.

- Severe Psychosis
  - ⇨ There are numerous case reports of patients suffering severe psychosis and having the delusional belief that an end can be achieved by undergoing an amputation.
  - ⇨ We have treated a patient who believed world peace could be achieved by amputation of his dominant hand.
    - — When rebuffed by a surgeon, he mangled his hand in a garbage disposal.
- o Obviously, patients requesting amputation are often suffering from severe mental illness.
  - In many cases, these individuals may benefit from psychiatric intervention, particularly those who are psychotic.
- The Psych Consult
  - o There are some surgical patients that require consultation by a psychologist or a psychiatrist.
    - Those whose surgical admission is secondary to self-harm.
    - Patients who have been placed on mental health holds.
    - Psychotic patients whose delusional beliefs have resulted in hospital admission.
    - Individuals who have clozapine (Clozaril) as a home medication.
  - o Strongly consider consultation for these patients:
    - Psychotic patients.
    - Patients with severe mental illness that is untreated.
    - Ongoing questions about a patient's capacity to make medical decisions.
    - Any patient who has become threatening and/or assaultive while not intoxicated, withdrawing, or confused.
    - For any patient who requests it (or whose family, spouse, or partner makes such a request).
  - o Before placing a psych consult
    - Request necessary medical records from existing prescribers, or notes from recent psychiatric admission.
    - Inform the patient that a behavioral health provider will visit and assess them.
    - Verify that outpatient psych medications have been restarted or there is a rationale for deferring their administration.

Practical Algorithm(s)/Diagram

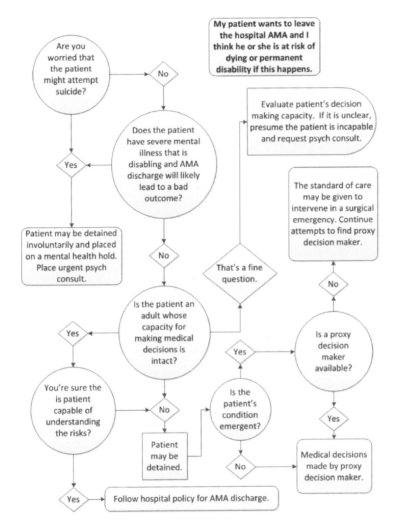

Fig. 1. Danger if patient leaves AMA algorithm.

Review of Current Literature with References

- Prazosin for PTSD Symptoms and Nightmares in Active-Duty Combat (*Am J Psychiatry* 2013; **170**: 1003–1010).

  o Both Acute Stress Disorder and PTSD are associated with nightmares and hyperarousal, such as irritability, insomnia, and hypervigilance.

  o The use of the antihypertensive prazosin, a CNS alpha-1 antagonist, has been associated with reducing nightmares.

    ▪ Typically, 1 mg is started at hs for three nights, followed by 2 mg through day 7.

    ▪ If nightmares continue, and hypotension/orthostasis is not significant, the dose may be increased to 4 mg. Some patients may require titration to a maximum daily dose of 15 mg over four weeks.

    ▪ There may be an increased risk of priapism if trazadone and prazosin are given together.

  o A recent study evaluated the reduction of hyperarousal using higher doses (and twice daily dosing) of prazosin in a randomized, placebo controlled experiment involving soldiers with PTSD.

    ▪ Sixty-seven soldiers (10 women) meeting criteria for PTSD and combat related nightmares at least twice a week comprised the sample.

      ⇨ Exclusion criteria included:

        — Supine systolic blood pressure < 110 mmHg
        — Orthostatic hypotension
        — Acute or unstable medical condition
        — Severe psychiatric illness or suicidality
        — Substance use disorders

    ▪ The prazosin group showed clear reduction in both nightmares and symptoms of hyperarousal, with improved sleep and daily functioning.

    ▪ Mean first dose (given mid-morning) for men was 4 mg, and 2 mg for women. Mean hs dose was 16 mg for men and 7 mg for women.

    ▪ Three individuals in the prazosin group had a remittance of their PTSD, no members of the placebo condition did.

    ▪ Blood pressures did not differ between groups; there were no adverse effects associated with prazosin.

  o While an impressive study, it should be noted that its participants were physically fit and were not injured.

- ▪ Obviously, a drug that may cause hypotension is contraindicated in some surgical patients.

- Dexmedetomidine [Precedex] and the reduction of postoperative delirium after cardiac surgery (*Psychosomatics* 2009; **50**: 206–217).

  - o This study observed the occurrence of delirium in patients managed on one of three different agents used for postoperative sedation: dexmedetomidine, midazolam, or propofol.

  - o The design was a prospective, randomized controlled (but not double blinded) study of elective cardiac valve replacement patients.

  - o Exclusion criteria included:

    - ▪ Children and adults over age 90.

    - ▪ A preexisting diagnosis of dementia, schizophrenia, or substance use disorder.

    - ▪ CVA in the last six months.

    - ▪ Evidence of a heart block.

    - ▪ Anticipated intraoperative deep hypothermic circulatory arrest.

  - o A total of 90 patients completed the study, 30 in each treatment arm:

    - ▪ Dexmedetomidine patients received a loading dose of 0.4 µg/kg followed by a maintenance infusion of 0.2–0.7 µg/kg/hr.

    - ▪ Those in the propofol arm were dosed at 25–50 µg/kg/hr.

    - ▪ Midazolam patients were given 0.5–2 mg/hr.

    - ▪ Randomized assignment into one of the three conditions resulted in roughly equivalent groups based on age, baseline cognitive functioning, length of procedure, time on bypass, and period of time under anesthesia.

  - o In the first 24 hours postoperatively, only fentanyl was used for pain management.

    - ▪ After 24 hours, ketorolac, hydrocodone, and oxycodone were all used for analgesia.

  - o Whether delirium developed in the first three days postoperatively was assessed using the Delirium Rating Scale.

  - o The incidence of delirium was then compared between the three groups and the results were striking and statistically significant:

    - ▪ Incidence of delirium for dexmedetomidine: 3%

    - ▪ Incidence of delirium for midazolam: 50%

    - ▪ Incidence of delirium for propofol: 50%

o The dexmedetomidine group also had significantly shorter ICU length of stay, briefer hospital course, and reduced financial costs.
o In this study, dexmedetomidine was associated with significantly reduced occurrence of delirium.

5. Cardiovascular

Fundamentals of Oxygen Transport and Cellular Metabolism

Teresa Jones, MD* Robert McIntyre, Jr., MD[†] and Erik Peltz, DO[‡]

*Surgical Resident, University of Colorado School of Medicine
[†]Professor of Surgery, University of Colorado School of Medicine
[‡]Assistant Professor of Surgery, University of Colorado School of Medicine

Take Home Points

- The principal goal of "resuscitation" is to provide optimal/adequate oxygen at the tissue level.
- Oxygen balance is dependent on: arterial oxygen delivery (oxygen content and cardiac output), patient metabolic demand and cellular oxygen consumption (VO_2).
- Oxygen delivery (DO_2) is more readily modified by augmenting arterial oxygen content and cardiac output than patient metabolic demand or cellular VO_2.
- Oxygen content is dependent on arterial hemoglobin oxygen saturation (SaO_2) and hemoglobin.

Contact information: Department of Surgery, 12631 East 17th Ave, C313, Aurora, CO 80045. Email: Teresa.jones@ucdenver.edu; Robert.mcintyre@ucdenver.edu; Erik.peltz@ucdenver.edu

- Cardiac output is dependent on heart rate and stroke volume ($CO = HR \times SV$).
- Stroke volume is dependent on rate, rhythm, preload, afterload and contractility.
  - Oxygen content consists primarily of hemoglobin bound oxygen. Goal SaO_2 and hemoglobin levels are necessary to optimize oxygen content.
  - Anemia has a much greater influence on arterial oxygenation than hypoxemia.
  - Oxygen uptake/consumption is difficult to measure without specialized equipment (indirect calorimetry). Surrogates for oxygen uptake are mixed venous hemoglobin oxygen saturation (SvO_2) and central venous hemoglobin oxygen saturation ($ScvO_2$).
  - SvO_2 or $ScvO_2$ are dependent on SaO_2, hemoglobin, CO and VO_2.
  - Oxygen extraction is measured via invasive methods but can assess the relative adequacy of oxygen delivery and impaired oxygen extraction.
  - States that increased metabolic demand and oxygen consumption include sepsis, fever, shivering, seizures or excess work of breathing.
  - Beyond maximizing VO_2, there are few interventions to correct mitochondria oxidative dysfunction in both septic and trauma patients.

Background

A fundamental element of aerobic life is a combustion reaction utilizing oxygen to release stored energy in foods while carbon dioxide (CO_2) is produced as a byproduct. In healthy individuals, oxygen is often in excess and aerobic metabolism is possible even with moderate amounts of stress.

However, the critically ill oxygen delivery can be the rate limiting step creating a delicate balance of sufficient DO_2 to meet the patients increased metabolic requirements and cellular VO_2.

An imbalance in adequate oxygen supply to meet cellular metabolic demand leads to anaerobic metabolism for energy production and is commonly referred to as SHOCK (inadequate tissue perfusion with oxygen). This anaerobic metabolism becomes clinically apparent with increased lactate levels and metabolic acidosis.

Thus a fundamental goal of resuscitation in the critically ill or injured patient must be directed at the restoration of this balance between DO_2, oxygen demand (metabolic state of the patient) and VO_2.

DO_2 is the most readily modifiable factor in this process while altering patient metabolic state or VO_2 are more difficult to achieve.

Main Body

Cellular metabolism

Cellular respiration — combustion of nutrient fuels to produce energy in the form of ATP occurs by two principle means:

- o Aerobic metabolism — When adequate oxygen is present for the complete oxidation of glucose the result is the production of 36 moles of ATP (673 Kcal).
- o Anaerobic metabolism — With inadequate oxygen delivery to tissues or inadequate oxygen uptake by cells the result is a precipitous decline in the production of ATP (2 moles ATP/glucose via anaerobic glycolysis) and an associated production of pyruvate which is converted to lactate as a byproduct (1 glucose molecule produces 2 lactate molecules).
- o This production of lactate leads to an anion gap metabolic acidosis and is often followed clinically to assess adequacy of resuscitation.
- o In both septic and trauma patients, there can be defects in O_2 utilization in mitochondria, limiting metabolism despite adequate DO_2.

Assessment of cellular metabolism

- o Lactate is an end product of anaerobic glycolysis.
- o The normal serum lactate concentration is <2 mM/L.
- o Serum lactate production increases with tissue hypoxia (shock, organ ischemia) aka type A lactic acidosis and with conditions unrelated to hypoxia, aka type B, i.e. increased protein catabolism, decreased hepatic clearance, and hematologic malignancy.
- o Serum lactate clearance is decreased with liver failure and shock.
- o In sepsis, defects in O_2 utilization in mitochondria increases serum lactate. Components of the bacterial cell wall including endotoxin have been implicated.
- o Base deficit is determined by arterial blood gas and is defined as the amount of base that must be added to one liter of blood to raise pH to 7.4.
- o The normal base deficit is <2 mmol/L.
- o Elevation in base deficit is a non-specific marker for impaired tissue oxygenation and is a surrogate for serum lactate.

Oxygen delivery

- Oxygen delivery (DO_2) is described by two clinical parameters; the amount of oxygen within the blood [**arterial oxygen content (CaO_2)**] and the flow which delivers this to tissues [**cardiac output (CO)**].

$$DO_2 = CO \times CaO_2 \qquad \textbf{Normal } DO_2 \approx 1000 \, ml/min$$

Normalizing for patient size/habitus

Often more important than the absolute amount of blood pumped per minute (CO) is the amount of blood pumped per minute in relation to the patient's overall size which can be approximated by total body surface area.

In clinical practice, our patients vary significantly in body habitus and to assess the adequacy of cardiac output providing blood flow in relation to the smaller or larger total tissue beds for a given patient (i.e. normal weight vs. morbidly obese patients), the CO in relation to total body surface area in m^2 is calculated as the cardiac index (CI).

$$\textbf{CI} = \textbf{CO/m}^2 \textbf{ total body surface area} \qquad \textbf{Normal CO} = \textbf{4–8 L/min/m}^2$$

$$\textbf{Normal CI} = \textbf{2.4–4 L/min/m}^2$$

Similarly using CI in place of cardiac output (CO) to determine DO_2 will provide the oxygen delivery index (DO_2I) in relation to total body surface area.

$$\textbf{DO}_2\textbf{I} = \textbf{CI} \times \textbf{CaO}_2 \textbf{ in ml/min/m}^2$$

$$\textbf{Normal DO}_2\textbf{I} = \textbf{520–570 ml/min}$$

We will now evaluate specific factors contributing to CaO_2 and CO/CI which in turn determine DO_2/DO_2I.

1) **Arterial oxygen content (CaO_2)** is composed of hemoglobin (Hgb) bound O_2 and dissolved O_2.

$$(CaO_2) = (Hgb \times SaO_2 \times 1.34) + PaO_2 \times 0.003 \qquad \textbf{Normal CaO}_2 = \textbf{20 ml/dl}$$

Hemoglobin bound oxygen is the predominate portion of blood oxygen

- o **Hgb bound O_2 = 1.34 (ml/g) × Hgb (g/dL) × SO_2 = ml's O_2/100 mL**
    - SO_2 = % of hemoglobin molecules that are saturated with O_2
    - Provided as a percent = Oxygenated Hgb/Total Hgb.

o   Example:

  ▪ Trauma patient with Hgb of 7 g/dL and SO_2 95%

  ⇨ $1.34 \times 7 \times 0.95 = 8.9$ ml $O_2/100$ mL

Dissolved oxygen is a minor portion of blood oxygen content

  ▪ **Dissolved O_2 = 0.003 mL/100 mL/mm Hg × PaO_2 mm Hg**
  ▪ Oxygen does NOT dissolve readily in blood, thus need Hgb (i.e. PaO_2 = 100, 1L of blood only contains 3 mL of dissolved O_2)

o   Example:

  ▪ Trauma patient with PaO_2 100 mm Hg on ABG

  ⇨ 0.003 (mL/100 mL/mm Hg) × 100 mm Hg = 0.3 mL $O_2/100$ mL of dissolved O_2 in pt's blood

o   Given the relatively small contribution of dissolved oxygen, clinically CaO_2 content can be simplified to **CaO_2 = 1.34 × Hgb × SaO_2**

o   Example:

  ▪ Trauma patient with Hgb 7 g/dL, SO_2 95% and PaO_2 100

  ⇨ $(1.34 \times 7 \times 0.95) + (0.003 \times 100) = 9.21$ ml $O_2/100$ mL

  ▪ Increasing Hgb by 2 g/dl (Hbg 9, SO_2 95% and PaO_2 100)

  ⇨ $(1.34 \times 9 \times 0.95) + (0.003 \times 100) = 11.76$ $O_2/100$ mL

  ⇨ **22% increase in blood oxygen content**

  ▪ While increasing PaO_2 to 300 mm Hg (Hgb 7 g/dL, SO_2 95% and PaO_2 300)

  ⇨ $(1.34 \times 7 \times 0.95) + (0.003 \times 300) = 10.1$ ml $O_2/100$ mL

  ⇨ **Only 9.6% increase in blood oxygen content.**

Assessment of Oxygen Content

o SaO_2 — Pulse oximetry
o   Hgb — Hematology
o PaO_2 — ABG

2) Cardiac Output

As previously described oxygen delivery is dependent on CaO_2 and CO. To optimize DO_2, we have previously evaluated and augmented arterial oxygen content. We must now assess and optimize the rate oxygen is carried to the vital organs by CO to deliver the oxygen to tissues.

Cardiac output = Heart Rate × Stroke Volume

- **CO is dependent on rate, rhythm, preload, afterload and contractility**
  - Rate:
    - ⇨ Tachycardia decreases diastolic ventricular filling time resulting in a decrement in ventricular preload and sub-optimal Frank-Starling forces impairing both stroke volume (SV) and contractile force.
      - — slow the rate
    - ⇨ Bradycardia: If SV is relatively fixed secondary to age (pediatric physiology) or in certain cardiomyopathies then bradycardia may be the limiting factor in cardiac output.
      - — increase the rate
  - Rhythm:
    - ⇨ Ineffective rhythm: (i.e. atrial fibrillation) this can result in impaired preload. Up to 20% of ventricular filling, and supplemental preload and ventricular wall tension are, in part, reliant on atrial contraction [Chapter 5-(vi)].
  - Treat the specific rhythm disturbance
    - ⇨ Tachy-dysrrythmias adversely impact as above under rate.
      - — Treat the specific rhythm disturbance
  - Pre-load: The goal is to optimize the cardiac myocyte overlap and the Starling curve [Chapters 5-(iii) and 5-(iv)].
    - ⇨ Hypovolemia: In addition to impaired preload secondary to tachycardia and dysrhythmias inadequate central venous pressure from hypovolemia or distributive shock (i.e. sepsis/adrenal insufficiency) impairs ventricular filling and preload.
      - — Treatment in this setting is directed towards fluid resuscitation followed by reassessment [Chapter 5-(iv)].
    - ⇨ Hypervolemia: Over distension of the ventricle as can occur with congestive heart failure, myocardial infarction, cardiac contusion can lead to impaired stroke volume and cardiac output.
      - — Treatment goals are aimed at reducing circulating volume, or the addition of inotropic agents to augment contractile force and stroke volume. Treatment may include diuretics, dialysis [Chapter 7-(iv)] or inotropic agents.

- Afterload:
  - ⇨ Increased afterload in the setting of myocardial strain from severe illness or injury can precipitate heart failure and impair CO. This is analogous to a strained heart attempting to pump against a relatively closed circuit.
    - — Treatment directed at afterload reduction (vasodilators, diuretics).
  - ⇨ Low afterload may have less direct impact on cardiac — maintaining mean arterial pressure such that forward flow continues to the peripheral tissue beds is essential for delivery of oxygen (i.e. distributive shock associated with sepsis, burns, adrenal insufficiency may require agents with α-adrenergic activity for support of MAP and oxygen delivery).
    - — Treatment directed at the underlying cause and hemodynamic support with volume resuscitation and vasopressors.
- Contractility:
  - ⇨ Impaired by pre-existing cardiac defects (i.e. wall motion abnormalities, history of MI, CHF, etc.), cardiac injury, medication side effect (i.e. anesthetics/sedation), electrolyte abnormalities (i.e. hypocalcemia) and by acidosis.
    - — Treatment directed at the underlying cause or precipitating factor and hemodynamic support of the patient with inotropes and vasopressors.

o Rate, rhythm, preload, afterload and contractility are patient specific. As an example; a 75-year-old patient with history of MI and pre-injury/illness ejection fraction of 40% may be significantly more sensitive to diminished preload due to atrial fibrillation or SVT. This patient may also require a significantly increased central venous pressure/preload to develop adequate contractility and SV as compared with a healthy 30-year-old patient.

o In healthy patients without pre-existing CV comorbidities, the approach can often be to clinically challenge the patient with resuscitation and increased preload while this may require invasive monitoring in the patient with previous CV dysfunction.

Assessment of CO

o Severe blood loss affects both oxygen content (via Hgb) and cardiac output (via stroke volume).

o Rate/Rhythm: telemetry, EKG.
o Preload: Central venous pressure via central venous catheter, ultrasound evaluation of respiratory variability in the infra-hepatic vena cava diameter, stroke volume variability via continuous arterial catheter cardiac output monitoring or approximated by "delta-down" (systolic pulse pressure variability) in the arterial line tracing.
o Contractility/Stroke Volume: echocardiography, pulmonary artery catheter.
o Cardiac Index/Cardiac Output: pulmonary artery catheter. Other devices are available to indirectly estimate cardiac output by assessing thoracic bio-electric impedance or pulse volume waveform associated with arterial lines.

Assessing oxygen balance and cellular metabolism

After optimizing oxygen content and cardiac output, it becomes necessary to assess overall oxygen balance and effect on metabolism. Oxygen uptake is the rate at which oxygen dissociates from hemoglobin and moves into tissues — it can be thought of as VO_2.

o When VO_2I is low, it means there is either inadequate DO_2, inadequate oxygen uptake or increased cellular metabolism.
o When VO_2 is less than the metabolic rate, anaerobic metabolism occurs, producing lactate.
o VO_2 itself is **difficult** to assess.

Assessments of VO_2

o Calculated uptake $VO_2 = Q \times (CaO_2 - CvO_2) \times 10$ (mL/Min)
  ▪ This reverse Fick method of calculating VO_2 does not include the O_2 consumption of the lung, which can be highly variable in septic/trauma patients.

o Indirect Calorimetry: assessment of the rate of oxygen disappearance and carbon dioxide production by monitoring of gas exchange during respiration through a ventilator circuit or "metabolic hood" placed over the patients head. This requires specialized personnel and equipment and is often not clinically applicable during acute resuscitation but may help to provide a measure of metabolic rate and oxygen consumption after initial stabilization.

o Oxygen uptake (VO_2) is also proportional to the oxygen extraction ratio (O_2ER), the ratio of oxygen consumption to oxygen delivery, and can be estimated by the difference between arterial and venous oxygen content ($O_2ER \approx (CaO_2 - CvO_2)/CaO_2$). **Normal O_2ER = 20–30%**

- **$VO_2 = DO_2 \times O_2ER$** and $O_2ER \approx (CaO_2 - CvO_2)/CaO_2$
- **$VO_2 = DO_2 \times (CaO_2 - CvO_2)$**

o CaO_2 and CvO_2 share the equation for hemoglobin binding ($1.34 \times Hb$) and subsequently the equation can be isolated as such:

- $VO_2 = DO_2 \times 1.34 \times Hgb \times (SaO_2 - SvO_2)$

o Like CI and DO_2I, VO_2 is often calculated using DO_2I to provide oxygen uptake in relation to body surface area in m^2 as VO_2I.

Normal VO_2 = 180–280 ml/min
Normal VO_2I = 110–160 ml/min/m^2

Central and Mixed Venous Oxygen Saturations ($ScvO_2$ and SvO_2)

o As stated above, oxygen uptake can be estimated by the difference between arterial and venous oxygen content and a normal Oxygen Extraction Ratio is 20–30% of the oxygen delivered to peripheral tissues. Estimation of adequate oxygen delivery can then be made by evaluating the saturation of venous blood returned to the heart.

- Arterial oxygen saturation in blood delivered peripherally is normally 90–100% (SaO_2).
- If O_2ER = 20–30% then saturation of blood returning to the heart should be approximately 60–80%.

Mixed venous and central venous saturations are followed clinically to assess efficacy of resuscitation and adequacy of oxygen delivery

Assessment of SvO_2 and $ScvO_2$

o Mixed venous saturation: SvO_2 can be measured via venous blood gas drawn from the distal channel of a pulmonary artery catheter and represents a true mixed venous O_2 from all peripheral blood return to the heart.

o SvO_2 can also be continuously monitored with fiberoptic venous oximetry available with pulmonary artery catheters.

Normal SvO_2 is 60–80%

T. Jones, R. McIntyre and E. Peltz

o Central venous saturation: $ScvO_2$ is assessed by venous blood gas drawn from central venous catheters and represents O_2 saturation in the superior vena cava. Assessment of oxygenation at this location will not reflect lower body oxygen extraction and on average can be <u>10–15% higher</u> than SvO_2 in critically ill patients. One must consider this "over-estimation" of mixed venous saturation (SvO_2) during evaluation and assessment of $ScvO_2$.

o $ScvO_2$ can additionally be followed continuously with fiberoptic venous oximetry available with some specialized central venous catheters.

Normal SvO_2 is 65–85%

A decrease in SvO_2 (< 70%) can be due to:

o Hypoxemia (overall decrease in SaO_2 leading to decrease oxygen delivery)
o Anemia (decrease Hgb leading to decrease oxygen delivery)
o Decreased cardiac output
o Increased VO_2 (increased oxygen consumption)

Unfortunately, an increase in SvO_2 (>75%) may indicate defect in oxygen utilization at a mitochondria (decreased oxygen uptake) which may indicate septic shock, as opposed to improvement in clinical condition.

Practical Algorithm(s)/Diagrams

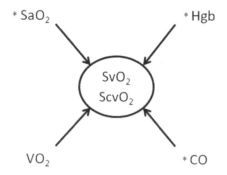

Fig. 1. Factors affecting SvO_2 and $ScvO_2$.

*Changes in SvO_2 and $ScvO_2$ are directly proportional to changes SaO_2, Hgb, and CO while they are inversely proportional to changes in VO_2.

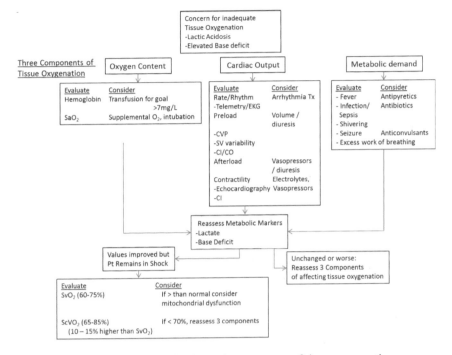

Fig. 2.   Protocol for evaluation and management of tissue oxygenation.

Review of Current Literature with References

- McKinley *et al.* found there was no difference in outcomes between trauma patients who were resuscitated to a DO$_2$I of 500 vs 600. DO$_2$I was increased via a computerized protocol of volume resuscitation and inotropes. Less volume and transfusion requirements were required for similar outcomes. (*J Trauma* 2002; **53**: 825–832).

- To determine the value of early goal-directed therapy in the resuscitation of critically ill patients, Rivers *et al.* randomized 263 patients diagnosed with sepsis to standard resuscitation vs. early goal directed therapy. Therapy was directed at optimizing the balance between systemic oxygen delivery and oxygen demand in this critically ill population. Clinical endpoints for early goal directed therapy included CVP, MAP and ScvO$_s$. This early goal-directed group received crystalloid to achieve central venous pressure of 8–12 mm HG. If MAP remained <65 mmHG vasopressors were started. As a surrogate for adequate oxygen delivery an $ScVO_2$ goal of $\geq 70\%$ was chosen. After CVP, MAP and HCT (≥ 30) were optimized then dopamine was started and titrated to improve oxygen delivery and achieve this $ScvO_s$ goal. Overall, 28 and 60 day mortality and overall length of stay were significantly lower in the early goal directed therapy patients as compared with patients receiving standard therapy. Indicators of perfusion including base deficit, lactate and pH were also significantly improved with goal directed therapy. With goal directed resuscitation to improve oxygen delivery including preload, after-load, contractility, and inotropic support to achieve a goal $ScvO_s$ $\geq 70\%$ patient outcomes were improved. (*N Engl J Med* 2001; **345**: 1368–1377).

- In a multicenter, randomized controlled trial of 300 patients in septic shock, Jones *et al.* found there was no difference in mortality between patients who were resuscitated based on improving lactate clearance vs SvO_2. Both goals were achieved by a combination of transfusion and inotropes, however no difference between patient groups was achieved after reaching an initial goal MAP and CVP (*JAMA* 2010; **303**(8): 739–746).

- In addition to sepsis, early mitochondrial oxidative dysfunction occurs in trauma patients. By measuring decoupling of tissue oxyhemoglobin and cytochorome a,a_3 redox, Cairns *et al.* found that trauma patients in multiorgan failure displayed early evidence of mitochondrial oxidative dysfunction (*J Trauma* 1997; **42**(3): 532–536) In both trauma and septic patients, despite resuscitation to goal, it is difficult to correct O_2 utilization deficits at the cellular level.

Chapter 5-(ii)

Recognition and Characterization of Shock

Anna Kristina Melvin, PA-C* and Walter L. Biffl, MD†

*Physician Assistant, Boulder Community Hospital

†Associate Director of Surgery, Denver Health Medical Center,
Professor of Surgery, University of Colorado School of Medicine

Take Home Points

- Shock represents inadequate perfusion of tissues with oxygenated blood.
- The characterization of shock is of practical importance in that it impacts definitive treatment.
- Characterization of the type of shock is based on history and physical examination along with a few basic diagnostic maneuvers.

Background

- Shock represents inadequate perfusion of tissues with oxygenated blood, resulting in cellular hypoxia.
- Shock may be manifested by alterations in physiology (hypotension, tachycardia, tachypnea), alterations in physical exam (decreased level of

Contact information: (Anna Kristina Melvin) Boulder Community Hospital, 1100 Balsam Ave, Boulder, CO 80304; (Walter L. Biffl) Dept. of Surgery, DHMC, 777 Bannock St., MC 0206, Denver, CO 80204; Tel.: 303-602-1861, email: walter.biffl@dhha.org; Anna. kristina@bch.org

consciousness, delayed capillary refill, cool or mottled extremities), or alterations in laboratory values/organ function (metabolic acidosis, oliguria, azotemia).

- The etiology of shock is of practical importance in that it impacts the overall treatment plan.
- There are seven fundamental types of shock which differ in both pathophysiology and treatment:

  - o Obstructive
  - o Cardiac compressive
  - o Cardiogenic
  - o Neurogenic
  - o Septic
  - o Hypovolemic

    - Hemorrhagic

  - o Anaphylactic

Main Body

Recognition of shock

- Shock may be recognized based on manifestations of the shock state, or the response to the shock state.
- Manifestations of shock result from hypoperfusion, and include alterations in physiology (hypotension), alterations in physical exam (decreased level of consciousness, delayed capillary refill, cool or mottled extremities), or alterations in laboratory values/organ function (metabolic acidosis, oliguria, azotemia).
- The compensatory response to hypoperfusion may include alterations in physiology (tachycardia, tachypnea), or alterations in physical exam (delayed capillary refill, cool extremities).

Characterization of shock (Fig. 1)

- Obstructive shock, generally due to tension pneumothorax or other cause of mediastinal shift, narrows the vena cavae and obstructs venous return to the point of cardiovascular collapse. Evaluation of physical exam for jugular venous distension, tracheal deviation, and breath sounds should make the diagnosis; ultrasound can reveal a pneumothorax. Chest X-ray should not be necessary.

- Cardiac compressive shock is generally due to pericardial tamponade, in which fluid accumulates in the nondistensable pericardium and restricts cardiac diastolic filling. Evaluation of physical exam for jugular venous distension and heart tones; electrocardiogram for low voltage; and echocardiogram for pericardial effusion and cardiac contractility, will aid in characterization.
- Cardiogenic shock represents inadequate cardiac output due to heart failure, dysrhythmia, or acute coronary syndrome. Evaluation of physical exam for jugular venous distension and heart tones; electrocardiogram for rhythm and ischemic changes; and echocardiogram for cardiac contractility, will aid in characterization.
- Neurogenic shock is caused by disruption of sympathetic pathways causing loss of vasomotor tone. Tachycardia is often absent, and skin is often pink and warm. The clinical context of a spinal cord injury and loss of distal sensorimotor function will aid in characterization.
- Septic shock is a severe systemic inflammatory response to infection. In the context of a source of infection, leukocytosis or leukopenia, and fever or hypothermia will aid in characterization.
- Hypovolemic shock is the most common type in the surgical patient. Hypovolemia may result from hemorrhage (traumatic, gastrointestinal, post-operative, etc.), fluid sequestration (due to infectious or inflammatory processes, bowel obstruction, etc.) or dehydration (due to insensible/wound losses, lack of intravenous or enteral intake). Evaluation of hydration status (by physical exam, ultrasonography, or central venous pressure monitoring) and measurement of hemoglobin concentration, in the appropriate clinical context, will aid in characterization. The amount of intravascular fluid loss corresponds to the clinical manifestations (Table 1).
- Anaphylactic shock must be considered if there is no other explanation. It may be due to drug or blood transfusion reaction, or allergic reaction to food, latex or other substance.

Practical Algorithm(s)/Diagrams

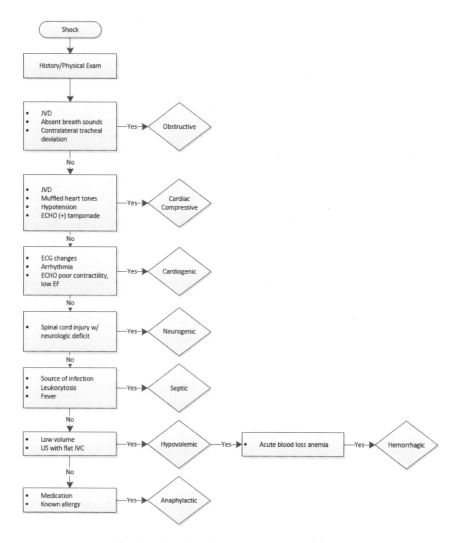

Fig. 1.   Algorithm for characterization of shock.

Table 1. Physiologic manifestations of fluid loss by categories.

	Class I	Class II	Class III	Class IV
Blood Loss, %	<15	15–30	30–40	>40
Blood Loss, mL	<750	750–1500	1500–2000	>2000
Heart Rate, bpm	<100	>100	>120	>140
Systolic Blood Pressure	Normal	Normal	Decreased	Decreased
Respiratory Rate/min	<20	20–25	25–35	>35
Mental Status	Normal/Anxious	Anxious	Agitated/Confused	Lethargic
Urine Output mL/hr	>30	20–30	<20	Nil

Review of Current Literature with References

- *Advanced Trauma Life Support for Doctors student Manual*, 8th Ed. Chicago, IL: American College of Surgeons, 2008.

  o This represents the gold standard for trauma evaluation and resuscitation.

- Boffard KD (ed): *Manual of Definitive Surgical Trauma Care*, 3rd Ed. London, UK: Hodder Arnold, 2011.

  o Developed for International Association for Trauma Surgery and Intensive Care, this course emphasizes rapid diagnosis and intereventions.

- Ferrada P, Anand RJ, Whelan J, *et al.* Limited transthoracic echocardiogram: So easy any trauma attending can do it. *J Trauma* 2011; **71**: 1327–1332.

  o Outlines the utility of echocardiography to assess cardiac contractility, pericardial fluid, and overall fluid status.

- Dellinger RP, Levy MM, Rhodes A, *et al.* Surviving sepsis campaign: International guidelines for management of severe sepsis and septic shock: 2012. *Crit Care Med* 2013; **41**: 580–637.

  o The latest evidence-based guidelines for identification and management of septic shock.

Chapter $5\text{-}(iii)$

Resuscitation Strategies

Fredric M. Pieracci, MD, MPH*

*Acute Care Surgeon, Denver Health Medical Center

Take Home Points

- Obey the four main principals of resuscitation:

  (1) Only resuscitate patients in shock.
  (2) Resuscitate based on shock etiology; multiple etiologies frequently co-exist.
  (3) Re-evaluate frequently with pre-determined markers.
  (4) Stop resuscitation once pre-determined markers are reached.

- There is no consensus on the benefit of volume expansion with crystalloid vs. colloid. Colloid is more expensive.
- Hypotensive resuscitation should be reserved for highly selected trauma patients in hemorrhagic shock in the field. There is no place for it in the ICU.
- Volume expansion with hypertonic saline may be beneficial in two very specific clinical scenarios: (1) remote locations and (2) severe traumatic brain injury.

Contact information: Denver Health Medical Center, 777 Bannock Street, MC 0206, A388, Denver, CO 80206; Email: Fredric.pieracci@dhha.org

- Patients in hemorrhagic shock should be transfused until (1) the bleeding is stopped and (2) end organ perfusion is restored. Avoid using arbitrary hemoglobin transfusion triggers.
- Resuscitation to supra-normal tissue perfusion does not improve outcomes and leads to massive volume expansion and its complications, most notably cerebral edema and abdominal compartment syndrome [Chapter 8-(vi)].
- The use of pulmonary artery (PA) catheters in guiding resuscitation has fallen out of favor because (1) several large series have failed to document an outcome benefit and (2) less invasive, dynamic measurements of preload responsiveness are now available [Chapter 5-(iv)].

Background

- Resuscitation is defined as the reversal of shock. Resuscitation is commonly equated with volume expansion, which is only true if the etiology of shock is hypovolemia. Rather, vasopressors for vasodilatory shock, inotropic support for cardiogenic shock, and decompressive laparotomy for abdominal compartment syndrome (obstructive shock) are all considered "resuscitation."
- Shock is defined as inadequate energy production to meet metabolic needs. Most cases of shock are secondary to impaired oxygen delivery.
- Oxygen delivery is dependent upon six fundamental variables (listed below). Derangement of one or more of these variables leads to the six types of shock [Chapter 5-(ii)]. Resuscitation involves assessing and optimizing these six variables (in order).
  - o Hemoglobin concentration
  - o Arterial hemoglobin oxygen saturation
  - o Heart rate
  - o Preload
  - o Contractility
  - o Afterload
- Oxygen supply-demand mismatch manifests by either organ specific or global markers of tissue hypoperfusion.
- Organ-specific markers include altered mental status (central nervous system) and oliguria (renal system). These markers are not specific for shock.
- Global markers are more specific for shock and include (1) venous hemoglobin oxygen saturation, (2) serum lactate concentration and (3) serum hydrogen concentration (or its surrogates, pH, serum bicarbonate concentration, and base deficit).

Main Body

Resuscitation strategies

- <u>Timing of resuscitation</u>: Animal models of hemorrhagic shock have concluded that tissue damage becomes irreversible beyond a critical period of hypoperfusion, after which restoration of tissue perfusion is superfluous. This period is termed the "resuscitation window" and appears to be on the order of 2 hours. *Begin resuscitation immediately after recognizing shock.*

- <u>Resuscitation by protocol</u>: This strategy refers generally to a standardized, algorithm-based approach, which uses specific endpoints of resuscitation and guides interventions until a prespecified endpoint is reached. Such algorithms consist usually of a series of binary steps (e.g., transfuse for hemoglobin concentration <7 g/dL) that simplify the resuscitative process. Strict adherence to resuscitation protocols has been criticized for resulting in oversimplification of the complex, evolving the nature of shock. A standardized resuscitation protocol that limits variability in care yet allows room for individualized interpretation of clinical circumstances represents a practical compromise.

- <u>Crystalloid vs. Colloid</u>: The ideal fluid for volume expansion during resuscitation remains debated. There are no convincing data to support one over the other. However, because colloid as compared to crystalloid involves increased cost in the absence of a survival benefit, it is not recommended preferentially for volume resuscitation.

- <u>Hypertonic Saline</u>: There are many potential benefits of using hypertonic saline as a resuscitative fluid. Due to an increase in oncotic pressure, administration of hypertonic saline acts as a transient "auto transfusion" of fluid from the interstitium to the vascular space. Similar to colloid, endpoints of resuscitation may thus be achieved using less volume relative to crystalloid. This benefit may be particularly important for patients with head injury, for which cellular dehydration results in decreased intracranial pressure. The relatively lower weight and volume. Clinical trials of hypertonic saline, with or without the addition of dextran, have not substantiated the aforementioned theoretical benefits, and the routine use of hypertonic saline as a resuscitative fluid is not currently advocated.

- <u>Blood product transfusion</u>: See Chapter 9-(i).

- <u>Blood substitutes</u>: Hemoglobin-based oxygen carriers are currently not approved for use in either North America or Europe.

- <u>Resuscitation to Supranormal tissue perfusion</u>: Survivors of shock demonstrate increases in oxygen delivery to "supranormal" levels (>600 mL/min/m^2).

However, artificial attainment of this level of oxygen delivery (1) is extremely difficult and (2) requires excessive volume expansion. Results of clinical trials randomizing critically ill patients to supra-normal oxygen delivery have not demonstrated improved outcomes, and have observed an increased risk of pulmonary edema, intestinal ischemia, and ambominal compartment syndrome.

- Corticosteroids for septic shock: See Chapter 11-(ii).

Resuscitation markers

- No one marker is superior to the other; use multiple markers when possible; be aware of the limitations of each marker; follow trends, not isolated values.
- SvO_2: Advantages include potentially earlier recognition of shock (prior to initiation of anaerobic metabolism). Disadvantages include (1) invasive and (2) false negatives seen with septic shock and cell death.
- Lactate: Advantages include specificity for tissue hypoperfusion (as compared to the base deficit). Disadvantages include the need to differentiate type A lactic acidosis (over-production) from Type B lactic acidosis (impaired clearance). This distinction can be made by calculating the lactate to pyruvate ratio, which is high in Type A lactic acidosis and normal in Type B lactic acidosis.
- Base deficit: Advantages include rapidity and unaffected by hepatic and renal clearance. Disadvantages include lack of specificity. One common problem is that of non-anion gap, hyperchloremic metabolic acidosis. Specifically, volume expansion with chloride rich fluid results in hyperchloremia and, to maintain electroneutrality, excretion of bicarbonate. A non-anion gap metabolic acidosis ensues, which can be misinterpreted as worsening shock. The incorrect reaction is to give more chloride-rich fluid, exacerbating the problem. Avoid this trap by obtaining a serum chloride concentration and calculating an anion gap on every patient with a metabolic acidosis [see also Chapter 7-(v)].

Practical Algorithm(s)/Diagrams

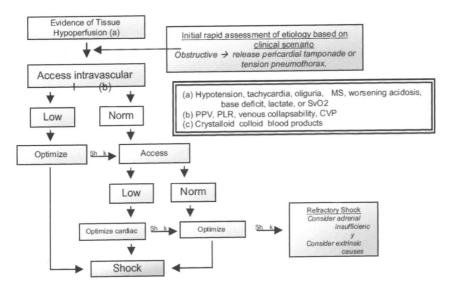

Fig. 1. Algorithm for the management of shock. ACS indicates abdominal compartment syndrome; CVP, central venous pressure; PAOP, pulmonary artery occlusion pressure; PEEP, positive end expiratory pressure; PLR, passive leg raise; PPV, pulse pressure variation; SPV, systolic pressure variation (Reproduced with permission from Pieracci and Biffl).

Review of Current Literature with References

- Kern *et al.* conducted a meta-analysis of 21 randomized trials comparing goal-directed therapy to conventional management of patients in shock. The majority of studies involved optimization of PAOP, cardiac output, and DO_2 to either normal or supranormal levels. A benefit to such therapy was observed only among those studies that maximized DO_2 either before or early after the onset of organ dysfunction (*Crit Care Med* 2002; **30**: 1686).
- The largest individual trial of crystalloid vs. colloid is the Saline versus Albumin Fluid Evaluation (SAFE) study, which randomized nearly 7,000 critically ill patients to resuscitation with either 4% albumin or saline. Mortality, organ failure, and length of stay were equivalent between groups.

F. M. Pieracci

A priori subgroup analyses revealed a trend toward an increased mortality for the albumin as compared to the saline group among trauma patients (13.6% vs 10.0%, respectively, P ¼ .06) and a decreased mortality among patients with severe sepsis (30.7% vs 35.3%, respectively, P ¼ .09). However, reduced statistical power in these subgroup analyses precluded meaningful interpretation (*New Engl J Med* 2004; **305**: 2247).

Chapter 5-(iv)

Measurements of Preload Responsiveness

Fredric M. Pieracci, MD, MPH*

*Acute Care Surgeon, Denver Health Medical Center

Take Home Points

- The relationship between left ventricular end diastolic volume (LVEDV), commonly termed preload, and stroke volume (SV) is described by the Starling Curve (Fig. 1).
- Preload responsiveness refers to the ability of an increase in LVEDV to result in a clinically meaningful increase in SV. A clinically meaningful increase in generally considered to be ≥10%.
- Achievement of a clinically meaningful increase in SV is the fundamental intention of volume expansion of critically ill patients in shock. Volume administration that does not result in a clinically meaningful increase in SV provides no benefit in terms of increasing cardiac output (and ultimately oxygen delivery), and exposes the patient to the deleterious effects of overzealous fluid administration.

Contact information: Denver Health Medical Center, 777 Bannock Street, MC 0206, A388, Denver, CO 80206. Email: Fredric.pieracci@dhha.org

- Many ICU variables are routinely misused as measurements of preload responsiveness, when in fact they provide no such information. These include heart rate, blood pressure, and urine output.
- Measurements of preload responsiveness may be divided into static and dynamic.
- Static measurements of preload responsiveness provide a point-in-time estimation of LVEDV. These measurements are then used to predict if volume expansion will result in a clinically meaningful increase in SV. Although most static variables measure pressure as a surrogate for volume, it is possible to measure LVEDV directly using echocardiography (Chapter 13). Commonly used static measurements of preload responsiveness include the central venous pressure (CVP) and pulmonary capillary wedge pressure (PCWP).
- Whereas static measurements predict preload responsiveness, dynamic measurements actually measure it. This measurement is done by exploiting natural changes in LVEDV that occur during respiration (either spontaneous or while ventilated), and their corresponding effects on SV or its surrogates. Commonly used examples of dynamic measurements of preload responsiveness include stroke volume variation (SVV), systolic blood pressure variation (SPV), and pulse pressure variation (PPV). For any of these variables, respiratory variation of $\geq 12\%$ predicts preload responsiveness with a high degree of accuracy.
- Multiple comparative studies have documented the superiority of dynamic measurements over static measurements of preload responsiveness. A basic understanding of Starling Curve physiology explains this discrepancy. In addition to improved accuracy, dynamic measurements are also generally less invasive, and able to predict preload responsiveness prior to fluid administration.
- Clinical situations in which the accuracy of dynamic measurements of preload responsiveness may be compromised include cardiac dysrhythmias and ventilator dysynchrony. In these cases, a modified "preload challenge," achieved by either passive leg raise (PLR) or exogenous fluid administration, may be employed to determine an accurate measurement of preload responsiveness.
- Despite strong evidence documenting superiority, dynamic measurements of preload responsiveness are still employed infrequently in ICUs, mostly because of unfamiliarity. However, the prevalence of these techniques has increased, and they are now included in several professional organizations' recommendations, including the most recent Surviving Sepsis Campaign Guidelines.

Background

- The extremes of intravascular volume are equally deleterious. Hypovolemia results in impaired tissue perfusion due to decreased cardiac output. However, hypervolemia also results in decreased tissue perfusion due to increased hydrostatic pressures within tissues (resulting in increased afterload), and organ dysfunction from tissue edema.
- Volume expansion of critically ill patients is exceedingly common. The average critically ill patient is 2–4 L positive each day.
- A positive fluid balance correlates linearly with mortality among ICU patients.
- Common, organ-specific sequellea of overzealous volume expansion include worsening intra-cranial hypertension in patients with traumatic brain injury [Chapter 4-(ii)], worsening gas exchange in mechanically ventilated patients with acute lung injury [Chapter 6-(v)], and intra-abdominal hypertension [Chapter 8-(vii)].
- On the most fundamental level, the purpose of volume expansion is to improve oxygen delivery to tissues by increasing cardiac output, which is in turn increased by increasing stroke volume, that is then increased by increasing preload (assuming preload responsiveness) [Chapter 5-(i)].
- It may be extrapolated from the previous point that volume expansion will be useful only if (1) there is evidence of impaired tissue perfusion and (2) an increase in preload will result in a clinically meaningful increase in SV.
- Unfortunately, many studies have reported that only about 50% of patients who are considered to be preload responsive, and therefore receive a fluid bolus, actually realize a clinically meaningful increase in SV. Therefore, the other half of patients was exposed to the risks of volume expansion without any benefit.
- As a result of the deleterious effects of overzealous volume expansion, it is imperative to utilize tests that estimate preload responsiveness with a high degree of accuracy, thereby minimizing the likelihood of unnecessary fluid administration.

Main Body

- According to the Starling Curve (Fig. 1), increases in preload have variable effects on SV depending on the baseline preload; whereas a low baseline preload corresponds to a large increase in SV following volume expansion, a high baseline preload results in no increase in SV following volume expansion.

- Every patient's Starling Curve is different. Furthermore, multiple Starling Curves exist within any individual patient; both the slope and position of the curve are affected by changes in cardiac dynamics, vasopressor requirements, and afterload, among other variables.
- Most static measurements of preload responsiveness attempt to estimate baseline preload by using pressure as a surrogate for volume. This strategy is problematic for several reasons:
  - Intravascular pressure is affected by multiple other variables besides preload, including intra-thoracic pressure, intra-abdominal pressure, and intra-cranial pressure.
  - The intravascular pressure within more proximal structures is used to estimate left ventricular end diastolic pressure; superior vena caval/right atrial pressure in the case of CVP and pulmonary capillary pressure in the case of PCWP. This accuracy of this estimation is decreased in the setting of any mechanical abnormality between the two structures (e.g., valvular disease).
  - Even when pressure is a reliable surrogate for volume, a static measurement provides no information about (1) the patient's current Starling Curve and (2) the baseline preload location on that curve. ***This is the fundamental limitation of static measurements***. For example, a CVP of two may correspond to any baseline preload location on any of the curves shown in Fig. 1. Furthermore, as shown in Fig. 1, the same baseline preload (A) results in a markedly different response in SV following volume expansion depending on the underlying Starling Curve (a to b vs. a' to b'). This limitation holds true even at the extremes of preload estimation (e.g., CVP of 1 or CVP of 20), as well as when using trends as opposed to absolute values.
  - Static measurements typically are invasive, requiring a central venous catheter in the case of CVP, and a pulmonary artery catheter in the case of PCWP.
- These theoretical limitations of static measurements have been borne out by outcomes data (see *Review of Current Literature* section): multiple publications have documented the inability of both the CVP and PCWP to predict preload responsiveness in a variety of clinic scenarios, even when accounting specifically for both extreme values and trends.
- In contrast to static measurements, dynamic measurements of preload responsiveness estimate on which portion of the Starling Curve a patient is

currently operating. They are therefore able to predict preload responsiveness with a high degree of accuracy.

- All variations of dynamic measurements exploit inherent respiratory-mediated changes in both preload and corresponding SV. These natural variations are summarized in Fig. 2.
- Patients who are operating on the steep (preload responsive) portion of the Starling Curve demonstrate exaggerated respiratory variation in SV, and thus both cardiac output and blood pressure.
- A respiratory variation in stroke volume (SVV), systolic blood pressure (SPV), and pulse pressure (PPV) of $\geq 12\%$ has been found to be highly accurate for predicting a clinically meaningful increase in SV following volume expansion.
- The value of 12% corresponds to the maximum value minus the minimum value, and divided by their average. In the case of SPV:

$$SPV = (SPV_{max} - SPV_{min})/(SPV_{max} + SPV_{min}/2)$$

For example, inputting SPV_{max} of 130 and SPV_{min} of 127 would result in SPV of 2.3%. This value would not suggest preload responsiveness. By contrast, inputting SPV_{max} of 130 and SPV_{min} of 115 would result in SPV of 12.2%. This value would not suggest preload responsiveness.

- Both the SPV and PPV can be measured accurately in mechanically ventilated patients with a functional arterial catheter in place (Chapter 15).
- Measurement of SVV requires a specialized catheter that uses arterial pulse contour analysis to provide both SVV and continuous cardiac output. This is advantageous as (1) measurement of cardiac output helps differentiate the various etiologies of shock [Chapter 5-(ii)] and (2) the effect of volume expansion on cardiac output may be assessed real time. These devices are commercially available from multiple vendors.
- In addition to improved accuracy for predicting preload responsiveness, dynamic measurements have the following advantages over static measurements:
  - They are less invasive, requiring only a functional arterial line as opposed to a central venous catheter.
  - They predict preload responsiveness prior to giving a fluid bolus, such that unnecessary volume expansion is avoided.
  - The measurement is continuous, such that a response to volume expansion may be accessed real-time.

- Multiple publications have demonstrated high accuracy for predicting preload responsiveness for SPV, PPV, and SVV, with a receiver operator characteristic area under the curve in the 0.85 range.
- The accuracy of dynamic measurements of preload responsiveness is limited in the presence of either cardiac arrhythmias or ventilator dysynchrony. In these cases, either the systolic blood pressure (SBP) or SV (most commercially available devices also provide continuous measurement of SV) may be exploited to determine preload responsiveness. First, the baseline SV is noted. Volume expansion using 10 cc/kg is then given. The SV measurement is again noted. A change in SV of ≥10% is considered preload responsive, and the volume expansion is repeated until either (1) the patient is no longer in shock or (2) the change in SV is <10%.
- A PLR may be used in place of the exogenous fluid bolus in order to avoid a potentially unnecessary volume expansion. This maneuver, shown in Fig. 3, involves tilting the patient in order to return venous blood pooled in the lower extremities into the cardiac circulation. Studies have shown that a PLR results in approximately 250–500 mL of venous blood return in a 70 kg patient. Thus, in order to determine preload responsiveness in a patient with either cardiac arrhythmia or ventilator dysynchrony, the SV or SBP is noted, a PLR is performed, and the SV or SBP is repeated. A change of ≥10% suggests preload responsiveness. Note that in this example, no fluid bolus is necessary to determine preload responsiveness.
- These relatively non-invasive measurements should be performed in all critically ill patients when volume expansion is being considered (e.g., hypotension, oliguria, tachycardia). Current data suggest that only one half of these patients will demonstrate evidence of preload responsiveness. In this case, utilization of dynamic measurements not only avoids unnecessary volume expansion, but also expedites the search for other sources of the original derangement (e.g., blunt cardiac injury as a cause of tachycardia, or acute tubular necrosis as a cause of oliguria).

Practical Algorithm(s)/Diagrams

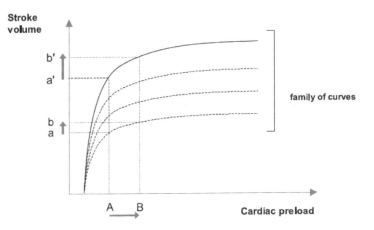

Fig. 1. The starling curve.

The Starling Curve depicts the relationship between cardiac preload (*x* axis) and stroke volume (SV, *y* axis). The curve begins at its steepest, wherein small changes in preload corresponding to large changes in SV. It then begins to flatten exponentially, such that further increases in preload achieve smaller corresponding increases in SV. Finally, the curve becomes flat; over this range, further increases in preload result in no increase in SV. In this graph, a family of Starling Curves is shown, reflecting the heterogeneity of curves both between and among critically ill patients. As can be seen in the graph, an identical volume expansion (from A to B) results in a drastically different effect on SV depending on the curve (from a to b on the bottom curve, as opposed to from a' to b' on the top curve). In this case, the static measurement A would be unable to predict the effect of volume expansion without knowing under which Starling Curve the patient is operating.

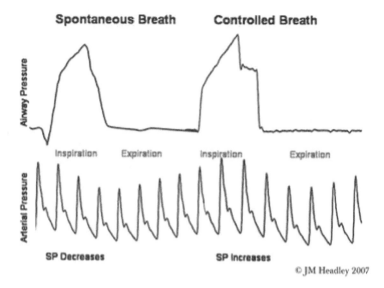

Fig. 2.   Respiratory variation in systolic pressure.

During spontaneous respiration, inspiration results in a decrease in preload, as blood is drawn from the left atrium into the pulmonary vasculature by negative intra-thoracic pressure. This corresponds to a decrease in stroke volume, the magnitude of which is dependent upon the position on the Starling Curve. The opposite effect is seen during expiration, as positive intra-thoracic pressure pushes blood from the pulmonary vasculature into the left atrium, resulting in an increase in preload. During positive pressure ventilation [Chapter 6-(iii)], these phenomena are reversed. The magnitude of the change in stroke volume depends on the baseline position on the Starling Curve.

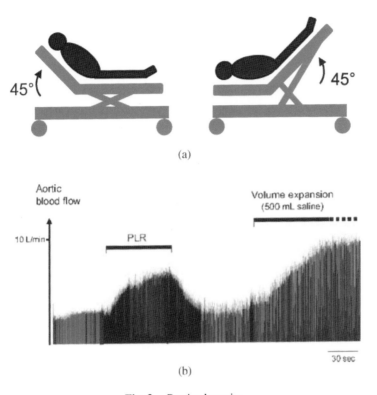

(a)

(b)

Fig. 3. Passive leg raise.

(a) For patients in the semi-recumbent position, a passive leg raise (PLR) is achieved by manipulating the bed such that the torso is flat and the legs are raised to a 45° angle. (b) The effect of a PLR on aortic blood flow, as compared to volume expansion with 500 mL of normal saline, on a patient who is preload responsive.

Review of Current Literature with References

- Shippy *et al.* compiled 1,500 simultaneous measurements of blood volume (using nuclear spectroscopy) and central venous pressure (CVP) among 180 critically ill patients. There was no correlation between these two variables ($r^2 = 0.27$). In this sample, there were patients with a very low CVP and volume overload, as well as patients with a very high CVP and volume depletion (*Crit Care Med* 1984; **12**: 107–112).
- A meta-analysis of the ability of the CVP to predict preload responsiveness included 43 studies. The receiver operator characteristic area under the curve was 0.56, suggesting a predictive ability no different than chance alone.

This association did not change when specifically examining the change in CVP after volume expansion [*Crit Care Med* 2013: **41**(7): 1774–1781].

- A systematic review of dynamic measurements of preload responsiveness included 29 studies and 685 critically ill patients. The receiver operator characteristic area under the curve for the pulse pressure variation, systolic pressure variation, and stroke volume variation were 0.94, 0.86, and 0.84, respectively (*Crit Care Med* 2009; **37**: 2642–2647).

Chapter **5-(v)**

Vasoactive Medications

Daniel Lollar, MD*

* Fellow, Trauma and Acute Care Surgery, Denver Health Medical Center

Take Home Points

- All patients undergoing infusions for blood pressure management in the ICU should be monitored with an arterial line. Because of the risk for tissue necrosis with extravenous extravasation, vasopressors should be administered via a central venous catheter as soon as the clinical situation allows.
- Norepinephrine is the first-line vasopressor for fluid-resuscitated patients in septic shock. It should be started at a dose of 0.10 mcg/kg/min and titrated up to a maximum dose of 0.60 mcg/kg/min. Vasopressin infusion at 0.03 units/hr should be administered for hormonal replacement after the norepinephrine dose passes 0.15 mcg/kg/min.
- Epinephrine should be added to norepinephrine as a second agent in septic shock unless continued hypotension is thought to be secondary to myocardial dysfunction as opposed to vasodilation. For refractory septic shock with significant myocardial dysfunction, dobutamine is the preferred second agent.

Contact information: Denver Health Medical Center, University of Colorado Health Sciences Center, 777 Bannock Street, MC 0206, Denver, CO 80204; Tel.: 303-436-6024, email: daniel.lollar@ucdenver.edu

- Epinephrine is first-line vasopressor choice in cardiac arrest and anaphylactic shock (both IgE-dependent and IgE-independent types). Note that the dosing for anaphylaxis is 1 mg/mL of 1:1000 solution either subcutaneously or intramuscularly or in 100 mL normal saline given over 5–10 minutes, versus the dose for cardiac arrest which is 1mg intravenous (IV) push, repeated every 3–5 minutes. A vasopressin bolus of 40 units can also be used to improve outcomes in cardiac arrest.
- Patients in cardiogenic shock due to intrinsic cardiac dysfunction may be started on an inotrope such as dopamine, dobutamine or milrinone. There is no consensus on which agent is preferred. Afterload reduction with vasodilators such as nitroglycerin or nicardipine may also be beneficial in patients with heart failure or acute coronary syndromes who are maintaining acceptable blood pressures.
- Neurogenic shock due to spinal cord injury and loss of vasomotor tone is initially treated with fluid resuscitation. In resuscitated patients without ongoing hemorrhage, debate exists about the best vasopressor. Sympathomimetics such as phenylephrine or norepinephrine can cause α adrenergic hyper-responsiveness with difficulty in controlling hypertension. Vasopressin, as a non-sympathomimetic agent, may be safer. However, it can theoretically exacerbate vasospasm associated with subarachnoid hemorrhage though this effect has not been demonstrated.
- An uncommon condition, Takasubo's cardiomyopathy should be approached similar to patients with cardiogenic shock. In patients thought to have hypertrophic cardiomyopathy, inotropes such as dobutamine, epinephrine and milrinone should be assiduously avoided in lieu of peripheral vasoconstrictors such as norepinephrine and vasopressin.
- Blood pressure control of patients in a hypertensive emergency should begin with nitroprusside while patients with aortic aneurysms should receive esmolol as the first-line agent.

Background

- Blood pressure is a product of the systemic vascular resistance and the cardiac output which, in turn, is the product of the heart rate and the stroke volume. Before starting agents to increase cardiac output, it is important to ensure that adequate preload is available by assessing volume status and giving fluid or blood products as appropriate.

- Within the cell, free calcium binds to troponin inducing conformational changes. Intracellular calcium is regulated through sympathetic receptors via two mechanisms. Binding of agents to β1 receptors increases cyclic adenosine monophosphate (cAMP), which improves actin/ myosin binding via Troponin C and thus, increases the force of cardiac muscle contraction (inotropy.)
- α1 receptors mediate vasoconstriction by increasing calcium release into the cytosol of vascular smooth muscle cells via diacylglycerol/ inositol triphosphate second messenger system in the postsynaptic membrane. Higher arterial resistance increases afterload while elevating venous resistance increases preload, resulting in increased blood pressure.
- β1 receptors are primarily located in cardiac muscle. Activation of these receptors increases myocardial calcium via the adenylate cyclase/cAMP second messenger system. Stimulation of β1 receptors leads to increased heart rate (chronotropy), cardiac contractility (inotropy), diastolic filling (lusitropy) and conductivity (dromotropy.) Ultimately, these effects also increase cardiac myocyte oxygen utilization.
- Similar to β1 receptors, β2 receptors also utilize the adenylate cyclase/cAMP second messenger system. However, stimulation primarily affects peripheral tissues and increased intracellular calcium results in vasodilation of vascular and bronchiolar smooth muscle, in contrast to α1 receptors.
- Vasopressin, also known as anti-diuretic hormone (ADH) produces vasoconstriction by acting on V1 receptors in vascular smooth muscle. Vasoconstriction is most pronounced in the skin, muscle and splanchnic circulation.
- Nitric oxide is a potent vasodilator of smooth muscle cells. Nitric oxide is produced from arginine, oxygen and NADPH by nitric oxide syntheses in vascular endothelium. Nitroglycerin increases the amount of nitric oxide available to the vasculature by releasing inorganic nitrite, which is converted to nitric oxide also by endothelial cells. Nitroprusside releases a nitric oxide group directly into the circulation after administration. Because of this, its effects are felt on both arteries and veins.
- Calcium channel blockers inhibit the influx of calcium into to cells, lowering intracellular calcium levels. Dihydropyridine medications such as amlodipine, nicardipine and nifedipine preferentially target vascular smooth muscle while non-dihydropyridine agents such as verapamil and diltiazem have a greater preference for cardiac myocytes. Phenylalkylamine agents such as verapamil are particularly selective of myocardium.

Main Body

Cardiac support

- Dobutamine exerts primarily β1 receptor stimulation thus supporting right and left heart function with increased contractility, chronotropy and ventricular filling. However, administration can result in increased myocardial oxygen consumption and induce arrhythmias. It also possesses clinically relevant β2 activity resulting in peripheral vasodilation. Dobutamine should be started at 1.0 mcg/kg/min and titrated to effect.
- Milrinone inhibits phosphodiesterase, increasing calcium in myocytes. Similar to dobutamine, milrinone increases cardiac contractility, heart rate and ventricular filling. The starting dose of milrinone 0.375 mcg/kg/min after a loading dose of 50 mcg/kg over 10 minutes.
- Levosimendan acts uniquely as a calcium sensitizer to cardiac myocytes causing similar effects of increased contractility, rate and filing. However, levosimendan does not cause vasodilation or increased myocardial oxygen demand. The dose of levosimendan typically utilized in clinical trials is 6–12 mcg/kg over 10 minutes followed by an infusion of 0.05–0.2 mcg/kg/min. Initial response is seen within 5 minutes and peak effects are reached after 15–30 minutes of administration.
- Dopamine has significant direct β1 agonist effects at doses between 5–15 mcg/kg/min. Dopamine has emerged as a frequent initial choice for cardiac support in decompensated heart failure, as it produces both increased chonotropy and inotropy while also causing vasoconstriction.
- Epinephrine has significant α and β effects. The β1 effects are substan-tial, however peripheral vasoconstriction is prominent, as is bronchodi-lation. Epinephrine is frequently used in the initial management of patients with cardiogenic shock due to decompensated heart failure. Because epinephrine's effects are partially indirect, tachyphylaxis can develop after 36 hours.

Vasoconstrictors

- Phenylephrine is a pure α1 agonist causing isolated vasoconstriction. This can cause bradycardia and decreased perfusion to the splanchnic and renal circulations. Phenylephrine is typically used in the operating room to counteract anesthesia induced vasoplegia and it is not recommended for the treatment of septic shock.

- Norepinephrine has significant $\alpha 1$ agonist activity while also possessing some mild $\beta 1$ agonism. Because septic shock causes significant vasodilation, norepinephrine has emerged as the first-line choice for septic shock due its receptor profile and relatively lower rate of arrhythmias versus dopamine. Norepinephrine's $\beta 1$ activity also helps counteract the direct cardiac dysfunction seen in septic shock.
- Dopamine possesses splanchnic vasoconstrictive α activity at lower levels, β activity at moderate levels and peripheral vasoconstrictive α activity at higher levels. While lower doses are felt to be renoprotective, dopamine does not prevent or treat acute renal insufficiency. While dopamine is no longer considered an important therapy in septic shock, it is considered an initial option in patients with shock from decompensated heart failure.
- Vasopressin is frequently used as an adjunct to norepinephrine in septic shock. Vasopressin has also been found to decrease vasopressor requirements by enhancing their action *in vivo*, however this effect is not associated with a survival benefit.

Vasodilators and sympathetic antagonists

- Nitroprusside is the agent of choice for hypertensive emergencies starting at a dose of 0.2 mcg/kg/min and titrating to a maximum dose of 3 mcg/kg/min. It is also a useful adjunct in patients with acute aortic insufficiency in conjunction with diuretics and inotropes and in decompensated aortic stenosis. Nitroprusside should not be used in patients with hepatic or renal impairment as both organs are needed for metabolism and clearance. Cyanide toxicity must become a concern at doses above 3 mcg/kg/min and in distinction to nitroglycerin, nitroprusside does not increase coronary artery perfusion.
- Nitroglycerin at 5–10 mcg/min should be used to relieve chest pain in patients with unstable angina and to decrease afterload in patients with decompensated heart failure and normal blood pressures. Moreover, nitroglycerin is useful in valvular diseases such as mitral regurgitation. In addition to peripheral venodilation, nitroglycerin dilates coronary arteries and improves coronary perfusion. Nitroglycerin can be increased as needed by 5–10 mcg/min every 5 minutes to a maximum dosing of 100 mcg/min. At levels above 50 mcg/min, nitroglycerin exhibits arterial dilation in addition to venodilation. Tachyphylaxis frequently develops after 18–24 hours of administration.

- Esmolol is a selective β1 antagonist with a half life of 9 minutes. Due to the short half-life, esmolol is administered as a continuous infusion. The loading dose is 500 mcg/ kg followed by an infusion of 50 mcg/kg/min, titrated by 25 mcg/kg/min every 5 minutes to reach goal heart rate or blood pressure. Esmolol is the agent of choice in patients with aortic dissections or aneurysms and can be useful in patients with mitral valve stenosis by increasing diastolic filling.
- The combined α and β blocker labetolol is frequently used for blood pressure control in a number of disease states including aortic dissection. Initial dosing is 20 mg IV over 2 minutes followed by either an infusion at 1–2 mg/min or 20 mg boluses every 10 minute to therapeutic endpoints. Maximum cumulative dose is 300 mg.
- Nicardipine is a calcium channel blocker that reduces systemic vascular resistance and can reduce anginal symptoms. Additionally, nicardipine can be administered as a continuous infusion at 5 mg/hr and titrated by 2.5 mg/hr every 5–15 minutes to hemodynamic endpoints. This drug should be used with caution in patients with threatened renal function as it can precipitate decline in renal function. This medication is often used in patients with aortic aneurysms, pseudo-aneurysms or dissections.

Practical Algorithm(s)/ Diagrams

Table 1. Receptor stimulation of vasoactive medications.

Agent	α1	β1	β2	D1
Dopamine (low dose)	−	−	−	++
Dopamine (moderate dose)	−	+++	+++	++
Dopamine (high dose)	+++	+++	+++	++
Norepinephrine	+++	+	−	−
Epinephrine	+++	++++	+++	−
Dobutamine	−	++	+	−
Phenylephrine	+++	−	−	−
Isoproteronol	+	++++	−	−

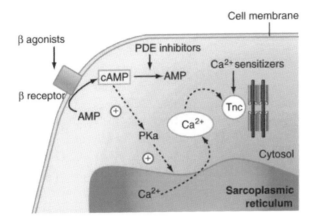

Fig. 1. Mechanism of inotropes at the cellular level.

Review of Current Literature with References

- The Surviving Sepsis Guidelines revised in 2012 [*Crit Care Med 2013*; **41**(2): 580–637] recommend norepinephrine as a first-line therapy for patients in shock due to sepsis. The strongest evidence in support of this recommendation was published by De Backer (*N Eng J Med* 2010; **362**: 779–789) in a multicenter, randomized control trial comparing dopamine to norepinephrine as first-line therapy for patients in shock. While there was no mortality difference demonstrated (52.5% with dopamine versus 48.5% with norepinephrine), there was a statistically significant difference in adverse events demonstrated. Patients treated with dopamine experienced a 24.1% rate of arrhythmia compared with 12.4% in patients treated with norepinphrine. These results were confirmed in a meta-analysis (*Crit Care Med* 2012; **40**: 725–740) demonstrating an increased relative risk of arrhythmia of 2.34 and an increased risk of mortality of approximately 1.1.

- The surviving sepsis guidelines also recommend the use of low dose vasopressin for septic shock. In the VASST trial (*N Eng J Med* 2008; **358**: 877–887), patients with shock resistant to fluids and norepinephrine at 5 mcg/min were randomized to vasopressin at 0.03 units/min versus norepinephrine at 15 mcg/min. Those who required additional open-label vasopressors above the blinded treatment drug were defined as more severe sepsis while those without additional pressors were deemed less severe. Though there was no mortality benefit found overall, (35% versus 39%), there was a trend for survival benefit in the less severe group (mortality 26.5% with vasopressin versus 35.7% in norepinephrine group).

- In patients with shock secondary to heart failure, inotropes to support cardiac functions should only be used when blood pressure is insufficient. In this case, inotropes should only be started in patients with signs of volume overload and inadequate cardiac function. Guidelines from the American College of Cardiology and the American Heart Association [*J Am College Cardiology* 2009; **53**(15) e1–e90] do not advise use of any one agent or combination of agents for this purpose. However, Levy *et al.* (*Crit Care Med* 2011; **39**: 450–455) published a randomized controlled trial of 30 patients comparing epinephrine to norepinephrine plus dobutamine in patients with non-ischemic heart failure (cardiac index <2.2 L/min and mean arterial pressure < 60 mmHg) resistant to dopamine plus dobutamine. While both groups were able to attain goal hemodynamics (MAP >65 mmHg), the epinephrine group had higher rates of arrhythmias and higher lactate levels. Additionally, the epinephrine group demonstrated decreased microcircular perfusion based on tonometry of the gastric mucosa.

Chapter 5-(vi)

Dysrhythmias

Jennifer A. Salotto, MD*

* Fellow, Trauma and Acute Care Surgery, Denver Health Medical Center

Take Home Points

- Cardiac arrhythmias occur due to a derangement in electrical impulse initiation, conduction, or both within the heart.
- In surgical patients, factors including volume overload, manipulation of the heart, intra-atrial catheters, electrolyte imbalances, and excess sympathetic tone can predispose to arrhythmia. Underlying structural abnormalities of the heart, congestive heart failure, and coronary artery disease may also promote arrhythmia.
- History and electrocardiography are essential in the evaluation of arrhythmia.
- Bradycardias result when impulses fail to generate at the sinoatrial node or when these impulses are blocked along their path to the ventricles. Common bradycardias include sinus bradycardia, sinus node dysfunction, and atrioventricular heart block.
- Tachycardias are categorized by the location of the origin of the irregular impulse — above the atrioventricular node (supraventricular tachycardia) or

Contact information: Denver Health Medical Center, University of Colorado Health Sciences Center, 777 Bannock Street, MC 0206, Denver, CO 80204; Tel.: 857-928-4766, email: Jennifer.salotto@ucdenver.edu

below the atrioventricular node (ventricular tachycardia). Common supraventricular tachycardias include atrial fibrillation, atrial flutter, and ectopic supraventricular tachycardia. Ventricular tachycardias include premature ventricular beats, ventricular tachycardia, and ventricular fibrillation. When sustained or hemodynamically significant, these entities require urgent intervention as they may lead to sudden death.

- The impact of an arrhythmia will depend upon the ventricular response to the arrhythmia, the ability to preserve cardiac output, and the degree of underlying structural or ischemic disease.
- The foundation of therapy for arrhythmias includes antiarrhythmic drugs, cardioversion, defibrillation, and permanent implantable pacemaker/defibrillator devices.

Background

The conduction system of the heart

- The sinoatrial node (SA node) is the physiologic pacemaker of the heart. It generates the cardiac impulse and displays automaticity.

  o The sinus node lies at the junction of the superior vena cava and the right atrium.
  o The artery supplying the sinus node branches from the right circumflex coronary artery in 60% of people, and from the left circumflex coronary artery in 40% of people.

- After conduction through the atria, electrical signals are transmitted to the atrioventricular node (AV node). Transmission continues through the interventricular septum via the Bundle of His, the right and left bundle branches, and then to the Purkinje fibers, which activate the ventricles.

  o The AV node and the His-Purkinje system are both capable of pacemaker activity. They can override the SA node if it is suppressed.
  o The main function of the AV node is to control atrial impulse transmission to the ventricles, thus regulating the speed of atrial and ventricular contraction.

- The cardiac conduction system is heavily innervated by the parasympathetic and sympathetic nervous system. Heart rate and speed of conduction are determined by the relative degree of input from parasympathetic and sympathetic stimuli.

○ Parasympathetic innervation is supplied by the vagus nerve, which releases acetylcholine. This neurotransmitter acts on muscarinic receptors to slow sinus node impulse generation and conduction through the AV node.

○ Sympathetic stimulation causes epinephrine and norepinephrine to act on adrenergic receptors. The result is faster conduction and increased impulse generation by the SA node.

Cardiac electrophysiology and understanding the electrocardiogram

- The P wave on an electrocardiogram (EKG) represents atrial depolarization.
- The PR interval is the time from the beginning of the P wave to the beginning of the Q wave, the length of which depends on the conduction velocity through the AV node. A slower conduction means a lengthened interval.
- The QRS complex represents the depolarization of the ventricle.
- The QT interval is the interval from the beginning of the Q wave to the end of the T wave. The QT interval represents depolarization and repolarization of the ventricle.
- The ST segment is the end of the S wave to the beginning of the T wave. The T wave represents ventricular repolarization, when the ventricle relaxes and prepares for another contraction.

Main Body

Arrhythmia in the postoperative period

- Postoperative arrhythmias are very common after both cardiac and non-cardiac surgery.
- Baseline patient characteristics which can contribute to arrhythmia include structural abnormalities of the heart (for example, prior scarring after myocardial ischemia), cardiomyopathy, congestive heart failure, and coronary artery disease.
- Iatrogenic factors which promote arrhythmia include cardiopulmonary bypass, manipulation or direct injury of the heart, certain drugs, and intra-atrial catheters.
- Characteristics of the postoperative state including metabolic and electrolyte imbalances, hypoxemia, excess sympathetic tone from pain or stress, and volume overload all predispose the postoperative patient to arrhythmia.

The evaluation of a patient with an arrhythmia

- Begin with a thorough history and physical exam.

  - Ask about family history of arrhythmias or sudden cardiac death, ischemic or valvular heart disease, and recent medications.
  - A review of systems should include questions regarding chest pain, shortness of breath, a feeling of skipped heartbeats or palpitations, presyncope (dizziness, lightheadedness, feeling faint), or syncope. These symptoms may accompany any of the arrhythmias.
  - Try to determine factors which may precipitate or terminate the symptoms. For example, are symptoms relieved with breath-holding or the Valsalva maneuver? This would indicate a problem at or above the AV node (a supraventricular tachycardia).

- Physical exam

  - Begin by assessing if the patient is hemodynamically stable or unstable, and address the fundamentals of airway, breathing and circulation. Ensure adequate intravenous access.
  - Assess mentation, ability to protect the airway, pulse rate, blood pressure, distal perfusion, and consider any underlying ischemia or congestive heart failure. Ensure that the patient is monitored with telemetry and continuous pulse oximetry.

    - The urgency of therapy depends on hemodynamic stability.
    - If the patient is symptomatic from a bradycardia, call for a transcutaneous pacer.
    - If the patient has lost consciousness and the monitor demonstrates a wide QRS complex, call for an electrical defibrillator.

  - If the patient is stable and the monitor demonstrates a rapid, narrow QRS complex with P waves, consider supraventricular tachycardia as the diagnosis. In this situation, vagal maneuvers should be attempted (see below).

- Progress from simple, less invasive testing to more complex testing. The first-line in diagnosis is electrocardiography (EKG).

  - Look for the presence of P waves. If P waves are not visible, suspect atrial fibrillation. An atrial rate around 300 beats per minute suggests atrial flutter. In atrioventricular block, there are more P waves than QRS complexes — the sinoatrial node is firing but the signal is not conducting to the ventricles.

- o A wide QRS complex is seen with ventricular tachycardias and also with supraventricular tachycardias with a bundle-branch block or an accessory pathway.
- Early in the evaluation of an arrhythmia, be sure to address any underlying abnormalities which may be triggering the arrhythmia, including ischemia, hypercarbia, proarrhythmic drugs, electrolyte imbalances, volume overload, or a catheter which is placed too far into the right atrium.
- Another tool used in the evaluation of an arrhythmia is an echocardiogram. This will evaluate for functional and structural abnormalities which may predispose to arrhythmia, and is especially recommended for those with ventricular arrhythmias.
- Finally, invasive electrophysiological testing can give more information. Cardiologists usually recommend this for those with a history of myocardial infarction and ventricular tachyarrhythmia prior to ablation, for those with syncope and impaired LV function or for those with structural heart disease.

Bradyarrhythmias

- Bradyarrhythmias are usually due to SA node dysfunction (failure to initiate an impulse) or an AV conduction block (failure of conduction) which results in a heart rate less than 60 beats per minute. Bradyarrhythmia can represent a response to a medication, or it may be physiologic and present at baseline.
- Common bradyarrhythmias in the postoperative period include sinus bradycardia, bradycardia from sinus node dysfunction, and the AV nodal heart blocks.
- Bradyarrhythmias are commonly asymptomatic, but if cardiac output fails to meet physiologic demands, symptoms can result. Despite a low heart rate, cardiac output and oxygen delivery can be preserved if the heart is able to compensate with an increase in stroke volume.
- Physiologic sinus bradycardia is caused by depressed automaticity in the SA node. Sinus pauses up to 3 seconds or a heart rate as low as 30 beats per minute can be considered in the normal range if the patient is asymptomatic. Sinus bradycardia is common in healthy athletes and during sleep. Bradycardia may be present during periods of hypoxia in patients with obstructive sleep apnea.

    - o Symptoms include syncope, pre-syncope, fatigue, hypotension, and weakness.

- Bradycardia from sinus node dysfunction is often referred to as "sick sinus syndrome." This entity is caused by abnormalities in the sinus node which lead to disorders in atrial impulse formation and conduction. It may be caused by fibrosis of the SA node, most commonly from inflammation, infection, aging, surgical trauma, or infarction. Less commonly, sick sinus syndrome may be caused by infiltrative diseases, increased vagal tone, or collagen vascular diseases.

  o Extrinsic causes of sick sinus syndrome include medications like beta-blockers, calcium channel blockers, and digoxin, electrolyte abnormalities, excess intracranial pressure, hypothermia, and hypothyroidism.
  o An EKG demonstrates bradycardia, sinus pauses, or transient sinus arrest.
  o Sick sinus syndrome is a common cause for pacemaker implantation.

- Bradycardia from atrioventricular conduction disturbances are commonly known as atrioventricular block. AV block results from delayed conduction through the atrioventricular node or through the His bundles. It may be secondary to fibrosis of the pathway, an electrolyte imbalance, an endocrine disorder, or drugs. The etiology is similar to that causing sinus node dysfunction (fibrosis, inflammation, aging, etc.) A myocardial infarct in the distribution of the right coronary artery may cause transient AV block.

  o First degree AV block is slowed conduction through the AV junction. The PR value is greater than 0.2 seconds, with every P wave followed by a QRS complex. The ratio of atrial to ventricular contractions is maintained at 1:1.
  o Second degree AV block occurs when the atrial rhythm fails to conduct in a 1:1 ratio, but some transmission is maintained.

    ▪ Mobitz type I (Wenckebach) will demonstrate a stable PP interval, a shortening of the RR interval, and progressive prolongation of the PR interval until one P wave fails to conduct on an EKG.
    ▪ Mobitz type II will demonstrate a stable PR interval with no predictable prolongation of the PR interval and random failure of P wave conduction on EKG.
    ▪ Second degree, high grade AV block is any conduction ratio of over 3:1.

  o Third degree AV block is known as complete heart block, and represents a complete dissociation between atrial and ventricular activity.

- The treatment of symptomatic bradycardia depends on the presence or absence of symptoms and hemodynamic stability.

o No treatment is needed for asymptomatic bradycardia, unless the etiology is third degree heart block.

o Correct electrolytes and withhold any medications which block the AV node.

o For symptomatic bradycardia leading to hypotension, altered mentation, chest pain, or shock, give atropine 0.5 mg intravenously every 3–5 minutes up to a total does of 0.04 mg/kg. This should be done in a monitored setting.

o Initiate transcutaneous pacing if the arrhythmia is refractory to atropine.

  ▪ Place pads anteriorly over the apex of the heart and posteriorly between the spine and the scapula.

  ▪ Transcutaneous pacing is effective but uncomfortable to the patient.

o Initiate transvenous temporary pacing if the patient requires pacing for longer than a few minutes.

o A permanent pacemaker is indicated for ongoing symptomatic SA dysfunction, severe symptoms related to bradycardia, Mobitz type II second degree or any third degree heart block, and symptomatic bradycardia with atrial fibrillation. After myocardial infarction, a persistent second or third degree heart block (especially if symptomatic) or any AV block associated with a bundle branch block should be treated with pacemaker.

Tachyarrhythmias

• Tachycardias are categorized by where the irregular impulse originates, either above the atrioventricular node (supraventricular tachycardia) or below the atrioventricular node (ventricular tachycardia). Tachyarrhythmia implies a rhythm that produces a heart rate greater than 100 beats per minute.

• Symptoms may include dyspnea, palpitations, dizziness, chest pain, or syncope. Hemodynamic compromise may result.

• Supraventricular Tachycardia

o In supraventricular tachycardia, an impulse arises above the bundle of His and leads to a heart rate greater than 100 beats per minute. In postoperative patients, the most common of these arrhythmias include atrial fibrillation, atrial flutter, and ectopic supraventricular tachycardia.

o Atrial Fibrillation

- Atrial fibrillation occurs when an impulse arises above the bundle of His which results in disorganized atrial activity and a dyssynchrony of contraction of the atrium and the ventricle. Because contraction is not coordinated, this causes loss of the "atrial kick" which in turn reduces cardiac output. In those with poor heart function or little reserve, this may lead to unstable hemodynamics. Stasis of blood in the heart can lead to thromboembolic events.
- Atrial fibrillation is the most common postoperative arrhythmia. Onset usually occurs within 4 days of surgery.
- The hallmark of atrial fibrillation on EKG is a loss of P-waves. Atrial activity is rapid and disorganized, with an unpredictable ventricular response.
- Complications of atrial fibrillation include increased costs, longer hospital stays, and an increased risk of thromboembolic events after 24 to 48 hours.
- The most important risk factor for the development of atrial fibrillation after surgery is age over 60 years old. Other risk factors include male gender, congestive heart failure, and valvular disease. Surgeries including esophagectomy, pulmonary resection, intra-abdominal surgery, and vascular surgery all carry an increased risk of postoperative atrial fibrillation.
- Most postoperative atrial fibrillation is transient and often requires no therapy. Of those who do not resolve spontaneously, the majority will resolve with pharmacologic rate or rhythm control during hospitalization.
- Therapeutic intervention should be initiated for those with heart failure, atrial fibrillation lasting over 48 hours, uncontrolled ventricular rates, and a history of prior stroke. Before initiating therapy, ensure correctable etiologies such as electrolyte imbalance or volume overload have been addressed.
- The pillars of treatment for atrial fibrillation are rate control and rhythm control.
- Rate control slows the ventricular response to atrial fibrillation, allowing for improved ventricular and coronary filling and improved cardiac output. This is a good choice for early (<24 hours) postoperative atrial fibrillation.

- Beta-blockers
  - Beta-blockers are safe and effective agents which have direct antiarrhythmic activity on conduction cells and myocardial cells. They counteract the

hyperadrenergic state of the postoperative period and have been shown to accelerate conversion to sinus rhythm in comparison to calcium channel blockers.

o Recommended agents:

- Esmolol (500 mcg/kg IV over 1 minute loading dose, then 50 mcg/kg/minute IV drip).
- Metoprolol (5 mg over 3–5 minutes, up to 3 doses, followed by 5 mg IV every 6 hours).

o Contraindications: hypotension, bradycardia, heart block, decompensated heart failure, asthma.

- Calcium channel blockers (CCBs)

o CCBs are recommended as second-line therapy for rate control, or as first-line in patients who cannot tolerate beta-blockers. They provide a strong blockade of the calcium channel in the AV node which leads to slowed impulse conduction.

o One study by Siu *et al.* showed superior time to ventricular rate control and symptom control with diltiazem when compared to amiodarone or digoxin.

o Recommended agents:

- Verapamil (5–10 mg over 3-5 minutes, followed by 2.5–10 mg maintenance dose)
- Diltiazem (0.25 mg/kg over 3–5 minutes for maximum of 20 mg, followed by 5–15 mg/hour maintenance dose).

o May result in hypotension.

- Amiodarone

o A good choice for ventricular rate control in atrial fibrillation in those with heart failure and in those who are hemodynamically unstable.

o Must be used under monitoring as side effects may include sinus bradycardia, AV block, respiratory dysfunction, and hypotension. For these reasons, not a great first-line agent in stable patients.

o Dose: 15 mg/min for 10 minutes, then 1 mg/min for 6 hours; follow with maintenance dose of 0.5 to 1 mg/minute.

- Digoxin works indirectly by increasing parasympathetic stimulation to the heart. This may not be enough to counteract the excess sympathetic stimulation found in a surgical patient. It is a good agent to use in heart failure.

- o Dose: 0.25 mg IV over 3 minutes, followed by 0.25 mg every six hours to a total dose of 10 mcg/kg lean body weight. It will begin to act within 30 minutes. Follow with 0.125–0.25 mg/ day.

- Rhythm control re-synchronizes the atrium and the ventricle back to normal sinus rhythm. It may be accomplished through pharmacological or electrical means, via direct current cardioversion.

  - o The physician can use one of the following in a single oral dose to convert back to sinus rhythm:

    - Flecanide 300 mg PO
    - Propafenone 600 mg PO

      ⇨ These agents may increase risk of ventricular tachycardias and sinus bradycardia. They are contraindicated in coronary artery disease.

  - o Ibutilide is a safe and effective agent for rhythm control. It may be used for unstable hemodynamics. Side effects include nausea.

    - Ibutilide 1 mg over 10 minutes, then maintain with 1–4 mg/minute.

  - o Amiodarone is a good choice for those patients in atrial fibrillation with heart failure or structural heart disease (see above for dose).
  - o Direct current (DC) cardioversion can be used for ongoing stable atrial fibrillation after 48 hours, atrial fibrillation refractory to medical therapy, early atrial fibrillation in patients who cannot tolerate decreased coronary or ventricular filling, or unstable hemodynamics. It is not indicated for asymptomatic arrhythmias.

    - 120–200 joule biphasic or 200 joule monophasic shock should be performed in synchrony with the QRS complex after sedation has been given.
    - If AF has been present over 48 hours, exclude intracardiac thrombus with TEE before cardioversion.
    - The success rate of DC cardioversion for atrial fibrillation in postoperative patients has been shown to be as low as 35% (see below).

  - o Agents used for maintenance of sinus rhythm after rhythm conversion:

    - Amiodarone: load with 150 mg/minute for 10 minutes, then 1 mg/ minute for 6 hours. Follow with an IV infusion at 0.5–1mg/minute.
    - Sotalol 80 mg PO twice daily, monitor QT interval.

- o Begin anticoagulation with intravenous heparin in the absence of contraindications after 12–24 hours.

  - ▪ Can use lepirudin as an alternative to heparin in patients with heparin-induced thrombocytopenia.

- Atrial flutter

  - o Atrial flutter is a reentrant arrhythmia in which an alternate circuit rotates around the tricuspid valve annulus. It is characterized by a regular sawtooth pattern of P waves on EKG in leads II, III, avF. The usual rate of atrial flutter is 240–320 beats per minute.

    - ▪ A rate of exactly 150 beats per minute should cause the clinician to suspect atrial flutter with 2:1 AV block.

  - o Ventricular rate control can be attempted with diltiazem, verapamil, or beta-blockade. Digoxin is a good choice in congestive heart failure (see above for dosage information).
  - o Ibutilide, dofetilide, and sotalol are the pharmacological agents typically used to terminate atrial flutter. These drugs are proarrhythmic in that they may prolong the QT interval and lead to torsades de pointes (see below).

    - ▪ Ibutilide: 1 mg over 10 minutes, then maintain with 1–4 mg/minute.
    - ▪ Dofetilide: 500 mcg orally every 12 hours; must adjust dose with impaired creatinine clearance.
    - ▪ Sotalol: 80 mg orally every 12 hours.

  - o Patients are frequently treated with DC cardioversion starting with a 50 joule biphasic shock with sedation. Often a 100 joule shock is effective.
  - o Recurrent atrial flutter is often treated with catheter ablation.

- Supraventricular tachycardia (SVT)

  - o Common subtypes include atrioventricular nodal reentrant tachycardia, atrioventricular reciprocating tachycardia, and focal atrial tachycardia.
  - o SVT frequently has a sudden onset and termination, and is not necessarily associated with any underlying cardiac disease.
  - o Most types of SVT have narrow QRS complexes <120 milliseconds.

    - ▪ A wide QRS complex can be seen if SVT is present in conjunction with a bundle-branch block, an accessory pathway, or a ventricular tachycardia.

- The P wave may be buried within the QRS complex if both atrium and ventricle are simultaneously activated.

o Vagal maneuvers including carotid massage and the Valsalva maneuver are effective first-line therapy for SVT in hemodynamically stable patients. These maneuvers stimulate baroreceptors which trigger an increase in vagal nerve activity, and this slows impulse conduction through the AV node. To perform carotid massage, apply pressure to one carotid artery at the level of the cricoid in a circular motion for 10 seconds, and follow with the other side as needed. Carotid massage should not be performed in the presence of known carotid plaque or a bruit on auscultation.

o If vagal maneuvers fail, intravenous adenosine or verapamil is safe and effective to terminate SVT.

- Adenosine is an AV nodal blocking agent with a half life of about 10 seconds. It is the first-line drug for converting narrow complex SVT and can also be useful in diagnosis and treatment of wide-complex SVT. Administration of adenosine should be done under cardiac monitoring with defibrillation pads in place, as transient asystole or ventricular fibrillation may result.

  ⇨ Adenosine 6 mg IV push, repeat with 12 mg IV after 1–2 minutes as needed.

  ⇨ Common side effects include facial flushing, chest pain and hypotension.

  ⇨ Contraindications include: atrial fibrillation, those with a heart transplant, obstructive lung disease, wide QRS complex tachycardias (unless certain it is SVT with aberrancy) and Wolff-Parkinson-White syndrome.

- Verapamil (5 mg IV every 3–5 minutes, up to 15 mg) and diltiazem (0.25 mg/kg IV bolus) are calcium channel blockers used in patients with recurrent SVT after adenosine. CCBs may result in vasodilation or bradycardia; use with caution in patients with low cardiac output. Do not use in Wolff-Parkinson-White syndrome or wide complex tachycardia.

- Esmolol (500 mcg/kg IV loading dose over 1 minute, followed by 50–200 mcg/kg/min drip), a beta-blocker, is useful to terminate SVT. Avoid use in patients with renal disease, bradycardia, and asthma.

○ SVT refractory to the agents listed may be treated with antiarrhythmics. These agents prolong the QT interval and may increase the risk of torsades de pointes (see below).

■ Procainamide 15 mg/kg IV over 60 minutes follow with 1–4 mg/ minute IV drip.

■ Ibutilide 1 mg over 10 minutes, then maintain with 1–4 mg/minute.

○ Recurrent, symptomatic SVT should be treated with prophylactic beta-blockade or calcium channel blockade.

○ If hemodynamically unstable, perform R-wave synchronous DC conversion with 100–200 joules.

• Ventricular tachyarrhythmias

○ Premature ventricular contractions (PVCs)

■ On EKG, PVC is noted as an aberrant wide QRS complex which may occur in a pattern of bigeminy, where every sinus beat is followed by a PVC, or trigeminy, where two sinus beats are followed by one PVC.

■ Often asymptomatic and incidental on telemetry, these PVCs increase with age and with the presence of structural cardiac abnormalities.

■ Three or more consecutive PVCs are termed ventricular tachycardia (VT).

■ In the absence of heart disease, PVCs are benign and require no treatment. In those with underlying heart disease, PVC runs of greater than 10 beats may indicate an increased risk of adverse events.

○ Nonsustained ventricular tachycardia (NSVT)

■ NSVT is the occurrence of three or more PVCs which terminate spontaneously in less than 30 seconds.

■ In a patient with prior myocardial infarction and depressed ejection fraction, NSVT should trigger further workup and evaluation for an implantable defibrillator.

○ Sustained ventricular tachycardia (VT) and ventricular fibrillation (VF)

■ VT and VF are accelerated heart rhythms in which an impulse originates below the bundle of His at a rate >100 beats per minute. In most cases, hemodynamic instability results which can lead to inadequate cardiac output, poor end organ perfusion, hypotension, and cardiac arrest if untreated.

- Hemodynamic stability depends on the rate, underlying heart disease and function, ability to compensate, and the presence of retrograde conduction.
- In sustained VT, the wide (>120 millisecond) QRS complex may be monomorphic or polymorphic.

  ⇨ Monomorphic VT demonstrates a uniform morphology of the QRS complex. It is usually secondary to an underlying cardiac structural abnormality such as scarring of the myocardium after an infarction.

  ⇨ Polymorphic VT demonstrates a changing shape of the QRS complex and suggests underlying ischemia or inflammation of the heart.

  ⇨ One example of polymorphic VT is torsades de pointes.

    — Torsades de pointes is VT associated with a long QT and twisting of the peaks of the QRS complexes around an isoelectric line on EKG.

    — Drugs which can lengthen the QT interval and lead to torsades include dofetilide, ibutilide, procainamide, quinidine, sotalol, amiodarone, clarithromycin, erythromycin, haloperidol, and methadone.

  ⇨ Any form of polymorphic VT should prompt an ECHO to evaluate cardiac size and function. If a new wall motion abnormality or depressed systolic function is identified, the patient should be further evaluated for ischemic heart disease. If right ventricular dilation is identified, this could be the structural abnormality underlying arrhythmia.

- "VT storm" is the term for more than two episodes of VT in one day. It is often secondary to underlying ischemia.
- Ventricular fibrillation is caused by discharge from an ectopic ventricular pacemaker other than the sinus node, and is usually more than 300 beats per minute. It is an irregular rhythm with variable QRS complex durations, morphologies and amplitudes. Ventricular fibrillation indicates an electrically unstable heart.
- Treatment of ventricular tachycardias

  ⇨ Monomorphic VT

    — Use direct current (DC) synchronized cardioversion with 100 joules if hemodynamically unstable. This is rapidly effective, but requires sedation. Defibrillation does not prevent recurrence.

— A procainamide infusion is first-line treatment in stable monomorphic VT. Dose: 20–50 mg/minute until arrhythmia is suppressed with a maximum dose of 17 mg/kg; follow with a maintenance infusion of 1–4 mg/kg.

— An amiodarone infusion can be utilized for unstable, refractory, or recurrent monomorphic VT. Use a loading dose of 150 mg/minute for 10 minutes, then 1 mg/minute for 6 hours. Follow with an IV infusion at 0.5–1mg/minute.

— If VT is suspected to be from underlying ischemia, use lidocaine 1–3 mg/kg IV at 20–50 mcg/minute, follow with an IV infusion of 1–4 mg/minute.

— If cardiac function is poor, lidocaine or amiodarone is acceptable.

⇨ Torsades de Pointes

— Stop any drugs which prolong the QT interval.
— Treat with IV magnesium sulfate 25–50 mg/kg up to 2 g.

— Use temporary pacing if torsades is refractory or secondary to heart block.

⇨ Polymorphic VT or VF

— In unstable VT/VF, perform synchronous defibrillation at 360 joules if using a monophasic shock, and 200 joules if a biphasic shock.

— Infusions of lidocaine, procainamide, or amiodarone can be used in stable VT/VF. Amiodarone is especially useful in patients with a low ejection fraction. See recommended doses under the treatment of monomorphic VT.

— Correct underlying acidosis and electrolyte abnormalities.

— Use IV beta-blockers for recurrent polymorphic VT, especially if ischemia is the suspected etiology.

⇨ VT Storm

— Use IV Beta-blockade if polymorphic VT, and defibrillation for unstable hemodynamics.

— Perform urgent revascularization if ischemia is present.

○ Calcium channel blockers should not be used to terminate wide-complex tachycardias.

○ Consider ischemia as an underlying mechanism and treat accordingly.

   ▪ CABG is recommended in patients resuscitated from sudden cardiac death or for sustained ventricular tachycardia believed to be caused by significant coronary artery disease.

○ Evaluate for an internal cardiac defibrillator (ICD)

   ▪ An ICD should be considered for patients with an ejection fraction <35%, with a history of non-sustained ventricular tachycardia, and for those with inducible VT on electrophysiological testing.

   ▪ An ICD is recommended for patients after cardiac arrest from VT/VF, for those with structural heart disease and spontaneous sustained VT, for those with VT leading to hemodynamic compromise, and for those with VT and depressed systolic function.

Practical Algorithm(s)/Diagrams

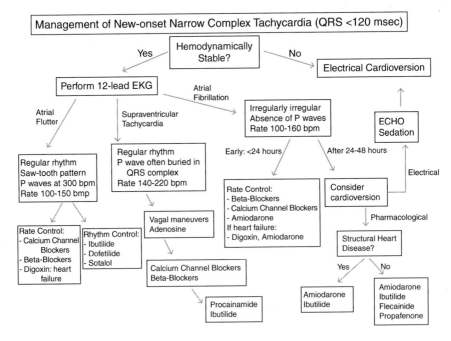

Fig. 1.   Management of new-onset narrow complex tachycardia.

Review of Current Literature with References

- A prospective database was used to study patients undergoing major non-cardiac thoracic surgery at a single institution from 1998 to 2002. They studied 2,588 patient records to identify risk factors associated with the onset of atrial fibrillation after thoracic surgery. The rate of atrial fibrillation was 12.3%. They found statistically significant risk factors to include male sex, age over 50 (with incremental increase in risk each decade above 50), a history of congestive heart failure, a history of arrhythmias, intraoperative transfusions, and increasing risk with increasing amounts of lung resected (lobectomy, relative risk 3.89; pneumonectomy relative risk 8.91). The development of atrial fibrillation significantly increased mortality rates (from 2.0% to 7.5%), length of stay, and cost of stay (*J Thorac Cardiovasc Surg* 2004; **127**: 779–786).

- Siu *et al.* performed an open-label, randomized control trial of 150 patients with symptomatic, new-onset atrial fibrillation in order to compare the effectiveness of diltiazem, digoxin, and amiodarone for rate control and symptom improvement. Time to rate control, percentage rate controlled, and symptom improvement was best achieved with diltiazem. There was no difference noted in rhythm conversion. Excluded patients with hypotension, congestive heart failure, recent myocardial infarction, or unstable angina, and they used lower doses of digoxin and amiodarone than the maximal recommended doses [*Crit Care Med* 2009; **75**(11): 1653–1654].

- One non-blinded, randomized trial looked at the rate of conversion to sinus rhythm in 64 non-cardiac surgery ICU patients with supraventricular tachycardias at 2 and 12 hours after treatment. A majority of patients were in atrial fibrillation. All patients were initially given adenosine, and those who remained in SVT were then randomized to receive IV diltiazem or IV esmolol for rate control. None of the patients converted to sinus rhythm with adenosine. In the patients getting esmolol, 59% of patients converted in 2 hours, after 12 hours 85% had converted. In those randomized to diltiazem, 33% converted by 2 hours, and 62% had converted at 12 hours. Although there was no significant difference in rates of conversion at 12 hours, the time to conversion was significantly shorter with esmolol (*Anesthesiology* 1998; **89**: 1052–1059).

- A prospective study was performed to examine the primary success rate of direct-current cardioversion in postoperative ICU patients with new-onset supraventricular tachycardias. Of 37 patients, 31 presented in atrial fibrillation. Sinus rhythm restored in 35% after 1 shock, with 100% converted after

4 shocks. At 48 hours, only 13.5% remained in sinus rhythm. They speculate that different pathophysiologic mechanisms may exist in surgical patients, making them less responsive to direct current cardioversion (*Crit Care Med* 2003; **31**: 401–405).

- One retrospective review examined rates of ventricular tachycardia and fibrillation (VT/VF) in 9211 patients with acute coronary syndromes. They found risk factors for VT/VF to include prior heart failure, an ejection fraction <30%, and triple vessel coronary artery disease. In this high-risk patient population, VT/VF was as likely to occur after 48 hours of infarction as within the first 48 hours, and median time to arrhythmia was 5 days. They recommend telemetry monitoring to continue beyond 48 hours after infarct (*Circulation* 2012; **126**: 41–49).

- A multicenter, retrospective, observational study examined 197 patients with wide QRS complex tachycardias. Of those patients, a response to adenosine was noted in 90% with supraventricular tachycardia and 2% in patients with ventricular tachycardia. They noted no adverse events in either of the patient groups. A response to adenosine increased the odds of SVT by 36 times, and a nonresponse increased the odds of ventricular tachycardia by 9 times. They conclude that adenosine can be safely used in patients with a wide-complex tachycardia as both a diagnostic measure and as a treatment (*Crit Care Med* 2009; **37**: 2512–2518).

Chapter 5-(vii)

Acute Coronary Syndromes

Jennifer A. Salotto, MD*

* Fellow, Trauma and Acute Care Surgery, Denver Health Medical Center

Take Home Points

- The term 'acute coronary syndrome' includes three clinical entities: unstable angina, non-ST-segment elevation myocardial ischemia (NSTEMI), and ST-segment elevation myocardial ischemia (STEMI).
- The three diagnoses included under ACS often share a common etiology: coronary plaque disruption with subsequent thrombosis. If a thrombus causes significant obstruction to coronary blood flow, myocardial ischemia can result.
- Coronary atherosclerosis is the predominant feature underlying acute coronary events.
- The majority of postoperative deaths after surgery are traced to cardiovascular etiologies.
- Myocardial infarction (MI) in the postoperative period may be asymptomatic and clinically dissimilar to myocardial infarction in the non-operative population.

Contact information: Denver Health Medical Center, University of Colorado Health Sciences Center, 777 Bannock Street, MC 0206, Denver, CO 80204; Tel.: 857-928-4766, email: Jennifer.salotto@ucdenver.edu

- A careful history and physical, risk stratification, electrocardiography, echocardiography, and cardiac biomarkers are fundamental to the diagnosis of ACS.
- Patients with suspected ACS should be managed promptly with antiplatelet agents, anti-anginal medications, and anti-coagulants in the absence of contraindications.
- In UA/NSTEMI, the goal of therapy is to prevent further thrombosis and to allow innate fibrinolysis to dissolve thrombus and reduce the degree of stenosis. Revascularization therapies are employed in high-risk patients to increase blood flow and prevent recurrent ischemia.
- STEMI represents a complete coronary vessel occlusion. Treatment modalities focus on pharmacological thrombolysis or catheter-based reperfusions. Urgent/emergent coronary artery bypass is indicated in certain populations.
- Important sequelae of acute myocardial infarctions include: heart failure, cardiogenic shock, right ventricular infarct, new-onset mitral regurgitation, cardiac rupture, ventricular aneurysm, pericardial effusion, pericarditis, and arrhythmia. The surgical intensivist must be aware of the diagnosis and treatment of these potential complications.

Background

- Cardiac physiology
  - The cardiac cycle consists of systole (contraction of cardiac muscle) and diastole (relaxation of cardiac muscle). The coronary arteries fill during diastole.
  - Cardiac output is the product of stroke volume and heart rate.
    - Heart rate is influenced by sympathetic and parasympathetic input to the sinoatrial node, drugs, hormones, age, gender, and physical condition.
      - ⇨ Sympathetic neurotransmitters (epinephrine and norepineprhine) increase heart rate, electrical conduction velocity, and contractility.
      - ⇨ The parasympathetic neurotransmitter acetylcholine slows the heart rate, reduces electrical conduction velocity, and decreases contractility.
    - The determinants of stroke volume include preload, afterload, and contractility.
      - ⇨ Preload is mainly determined by the pressure and volume of blood within the left ventricle at the end of diastole [See the Starling Curve, Chapter 5-(iv)].

⇨ Afterload is the pressure that the left ventricle must work against to push blood forward into circulation. Key determinants include systemic blood pressure, aortic stenosis, and peripheral vascular resistance.

⇨ Contractility is the ability of the heart to squeeze. Contractility depends on the degree of stretch of cardiac myocytes at the end of diastole.

⇨ Factors which influence contractility include heart rate, sympathetic or parasympathetic stimulation, and cardiac glycosides such as digitalis.

o Cardiac oxygen supply and demand

■ Cardiac oxygen consumption is directly related to the amount of tension generated by the ventricles. Factors influencing this include heart rate, cardiac contractility, size of the heart, and afterload.

⇨ During tachycardia, diastole is shortened and coronary blood flow is decreased. Contraction of the ventricle narrows the coronary arteries and this also impedes flow.

⇨ Wall stress is proportional to ventricular pressure and volume, and inversely proportional to wall thickness.

■ The coronary circulation can increase blood flow to the heart up to five times during exercise. Factors which influence coronary vasodilation include neural input, adenosine, and nitric oxide.

■ Coronary oxygen extraction at rest is nearly maximal. In times of maximal demand, increasing oxygen supply depends on increasing coronary blood flow.

• Pathophysiology of myocardial infarction

o In the majority of patients, obstruction of coronary blood flow is caused by the rupture of an unstable atherosclerotic plaque, leading to local thrombus formation. This may lead to partial (NSTEMI) or complete (STEMI) occlusion of the coronary artery. Plaques may rupture multiple times before causing a clinically significant stenosis.

o In surgical patients, perioperative MIs may also be caused from an increase in oxygen demand with a fixed supply secondary to baseline coronary stenosis.

o Rare causes of acute myocardial infarction include coronary artery dissection, coronary arteritis, coronary emboli, and coronary spasm.

o After cardiac ischemia, cell death begins within 30 minutes and is complete in 3–6 hours.

- o There is a key window of time in which restoration of blood flow will reverse ischemic changes and restore cardiac function.
- o Severity of myocardial ischemia depends on the location of flow obstruction, metabolic activity of the threatened myocardium, and degree of preexisting collateralization.
- o In surgical patients, contributors to post-operative myocardial infarction may include:
  - ▪ Baseline atherosclerosis.
  - ▪ An imbalance of myocardial oxygen supply and demand.
    - ⇨ Increased demand: tachycardia, hypertension
    - ⇨ Decreased supply: blood loss, hypothermia, hypoxia
  - ▪ Physical and emotional stress.
  - ▪ The hypercoagulable state of surgery as well as platelet hyper-reactivity.
  - ▪ A heightened inflammatory state.
- o Most post-operative myocardial infarctions will occur within four days of surgery and are ST-segment depression in nature.

Main Body

Defining the acute coronary syndromes

- Unstable angina
  - o Unstable angina is a syndrome of myocardial ischemia without bio-chemical evidence of cell death (no troponin elevation). It is caused by an atherosclerotic plaque with exposed mural thrombus. Forward flow through the vessel is maintained, preventing infarction.
  - o Clinical features of unstable angina include pain at rest, usually lasting >20 minutes and located in the chest, shoulder, back, jaw or arm, or new-onset severe angina.
  - o In unstable angina, episodes are unpredictable and worsen over time.
- Non-ST-segment elevation myocardial infarction (NSTEMI)
  - o In the case of NSTEMI, a ruptured atherosclerotic coronary plaque leads to thrombosis. When this thrombus causes partial occlusion of a cardiac vessel, insufficient blood supply will lead to cardiac ischemia and cell death.
  - o The clinical picture is that of chest pain, biochemical evidence of myocardial necrosis, and ST-segment depressions on electrocardiogram.

- ST-segment elevation myocardial infarction (STEMI)

  o A STEMI results when the rupture of an atherosclerotic plaque with thrombus formation leads to complete occlusion of a major coronary artery.

  o The clinical picture includes cardiac chest pain, serologic evidence of myonecrosis, and ST-segment elevations on electrocardiogram.

  o The loss of coronary blood flow leads to myocardial ischemia and necrosis unless urgent revascularization is undertaken.

  o New left bundle branch block (LBBB) is considered a STEMI equivalent.

- Defining acute myocardial infarction

  o Myocardial infarction is cardiac cellular injury caused by prolonged, inadequate oxygen supply of any etiology.

  o The following is the American College of Cardiology and the European Society of Cardiology's consensus definition of myocardial infarction from 2012:

    ▪ Detection of a rise and/or fall of cardiac biomarker values, preferably cardiac troponin, with at least one value above the 99th percentile upper limit and one of the following:

      ⇨ Ischemic symptoms, new or presumed new ST-segment T-wave changes or new left bundle branch block, development of pathological Q waves on EKG, imaging evidence of new loss of viable myocardium or new regional wall motion abnormality, or intracoronary thrombus by angiography or autopsy.

  o In the setting of recent coronary artery bypass, MI is defined by both:

    ▪ Elevation of cardiac biomarkers in setting of a normal baseline troponin.

    ▪ Evidence of new pathological q waves or LBBB, angiographic evidence of graft or coronary artery occlusion, or imaging evidence of new loss of viable myocardium or new regional wall motion abnormalities.

Evaluation of a patient with a suspected acute coronary syndrome

- History:

  o Anginal pain is often localized to the substernal, epigastric, and interscapular regions.

    ▪ It is not positional or not reproducible with palpation and may be described as dull, a pressure sensation, or chest heaviness. Pain may radiate to the neck, lower jaw, left arm, or left shoulder.

- Pain usually lasts >20 minutes with an acute myocardial infarction.
- Most perioperative MIs occur within 48 hours of surgery.

o Anginal equivalents include: dyspnea, fatigue, nausea, vomiting, and dia-phoresis.

- Physical Exam:

   o Evaluate vital signs and hemodynamic stability.
   o Physical findings include diaphoresis, vomiting, syncope, new-onset bibasilar rales, or a new murmur.
   o Atypical presentations are seen especially in diabetics, women, or those on post-operative pain medications.
   o High-risk patients are commonly asymptomatic.

- Differential:

   o Chest pain: MI, pulmonary embolus, pneumothorax, pneumonia, dissec-tion, pericarditis.
   o Epigastric pain: MI, cholecystitis, gastro-esophageal reflux, peptic ulcer.

- Assess Cardiac Risk Factors

   o Use to quickly identify patients at high risk for cardiovascular events.
   o Cardiac risk factors Include:

      - Previous history of CAD, peripheral vascular disease, CABG, or stroke.
      - Hypertension, smoking or smoke exposure, diabetes, hyperlipidemia.

   o Abdominal aortic surgery, vascular surgery, surgery lasting over three hours, or emergency surgery put a patient at higher risk for adverse coro-nary events.
   o One evidence-based risk assessment model is the TIMI Risk Score (www.timi.org).

      - Identifies patients with ACS who are at risk for death, myocardial infarction or recurrent ischemia within 14 days of hospitalization.
      - Variables (1 point each):

         ⇨ Age ≥65
         ⇨ ≥3 risk factors (hypertension, DM, family history, lipids, smoking)
         ⇨ Known CAD (stenosis ≥50%)
         ⇨ Aspirin use in past 7 days
         ⇨ Severe angina (≥2 episodes within 24 hours)

⇨ ST-segment deviation ≥0.5 mm
⇨ Elevated cardiac biomarkers

- Risk of death or ischemic event through 14 days:

    ⇨ Low 0–2 points (<8.3% event rate)
    ⇨ Intermediate 3–4 points (<19.3% event rate)
    ⇨ High 5–7d (41% event rate)

    — Indicates role for early invasive therapy.

Early diagnostic measures

- Electrocardiogram (EKG)

    o Perform within 10 minutes of initial evaluation for ACS. An EKG may be non-diagnostic in early ACS, so consider serial EKGs every 30 minutes.
    o **Compare with prior EKGs on record.**
    o Ventricular tachycardia, ventricular fibrillation, or total AV block may be the first sign of myocardial infarction.
    o **What to look for on an EKG:**

        - Classic findings in UA:

            ⇨ EKG changes that correlate with symptoms.
            ⇨ Transient ST-segment elevations or depressions and T-wave inversions.

        - Classic EKG findings in NSTEMI:

            ⇨ ST-segment depressions in more than 2 contiguous leads, more than 1 mm below the baseline; persist over 20 minutes.

        - Classic EKG findings in STEMI:

            ⇨ ST-segment elevation in more than 2 contiguous leads, >2 mm in men or >1.5 mm in women; persist over 20 minutes.
            ⇨ New Q-waves.
            ⇨ New left bundle branch block.

                — Never physiologic.
                — QRS complex >0.12 seconds.

- Coronary biomarkers

    o The detection of cardiac biomarkers in the bloodstream is a common method used to detect myocardial infarction, as they are released from cells upon cell death. Cardiac biomarkers include Troponin I, T, and creatine kinase MB fraction (CKMB).

○ Cardiac troponin (T or I) is the preferred coronary biomarker due to high sensitivity and specificity.

  ▪ CKMB has limited specificity — it is also released from skeletal muscle and is often elevated after surgery.

○ Elevated biomarkers alone are insufficient to diagnose acute myocardial infarction. They are sensitive and specific to myocardial injury, but non-specific to the cause of the injury.

  ▪ Non-ACS sources of elevated troponins include:

    ⇨ Cardiac contusion, myocarditis, rhabdomyolysis, tachyarrythmias and bradyarrhythmias, acute stroke, pulmonary embolism, pulmonary hypertension, sepsis, shock, and congestive heart failure.

    ⇨ Drug toxicity may elevate troponins, responsible agents include: adriamycin, 5-flourouracil, and herceptin.

○ Blood samples to test for Troponins should be drawn at the first assessment for ACS and repeated 3–6 hours later.

  ▪ Do not wait for results to begin treatment if clinical suspicion is high.
  ▪ It may take 6–12 hours after cell death for a troponin assay to be abnormal.
  ▪ Relying on a single troponin value should be avoided: diagnostic accuracy is improved with serial measurements.
  ▪ Patients with cardiac or renal failure may have chronic elevations of cardiac troponins. It is necessary to document the trend.

○ Troponin levels remain elevated for 5–14 days after infarction. For this reason, they are not useful to detect recurrent ischemia after a myocardial infarction.

• Chest X-Ray (CXR)

○ A CXR should be obtained early in the work-up of chest pain to rule out alternative sources of pain including pneumothorax and pneumonia.

Cardiac imaging

• Echocardiogram (ECHO)

○ A sonogram of the heart, which employs 2-dimensional, 3-dimensional, and Doppler ultrasound to capture images of the heart. Low in cost and imparts no radiation.

  ▪ Evaluates size, shape, function, and structure of the heart.

- ○ ECHO may be performed trans-thoracic (TTE) or trans-esophageal (TEE).
    - ▪ TTE: non-invasive, accurate, quick.
    - ▪ TEE: invasive, requires sedation; used if TTE not sensitive enough.
- ○ ECHO is highly sensitive for myocardial ischemia in the setting of a non-diagnostic EKG.
    - ▪ In MI, ECHO will show a new wall motion abnormality or reduced myocardial contractility.
    - ▪ **The absence of wall motion abnormalities excludes major myocardial ischemia.**
    - ▪ Helpful to rule out pericardial effusion, aortic dissection, or pulmonary embolus.
- Coronary angiography
    - ○ Coronary angiography is the radiographic visualization of the coronary vessels after injection of radiopaque contrast.
    - ○ Coronary angiography allows for intervention (balloon angioplasty, stenting), determines extent and location of coronary stenoses, and provides hemodynamic measurements of cardiac pressures and function. It is expensive and invasive.
    - ○ When is coronary angiography recommended?
        - ▪ In patients with cardiogenic shock, STEMI or suspected STEMI, high-risk patients with UA/NSTEMI, or suspected ACS with new wall motion abnormality or perfusion defect on a stress imaging study.
        - ▪ In patients with a prior CABG, angiography is recommended for intermediate- or high-risk findings on noninvasive studies and/or worsening symptoms.
        - ▪ Recommended for patients resuscitated after cardiac arrest and for those with ventricular fibrillation/sustained ventricular tachycardia of unknown etiology.

Treatment of acute coronary syndrome

- Early interventions:
    - ○ Oxygen if oxygen saturations <90%, heart failure or dyspnea.
        - ▪ There is no data to support the use of oxygen to improve outcomes in ACS.
        - ▪ Use caution in COPD and in patients with carbon dioxide retention.

- ○ Telemetry monitoring for arrhythmias.
- ○ Evaluate need for blood transfusion.

  - ▪ The ideal transfusion trigger for patients with ACS is currently under debate [Chapter 9-(i)].
  - ▪ Red blood cell transfusion for hemoglobin <8 g/dL may be beneficial in patients with ACS.
  - ▪ There is no evidence that transfusing for a hemoglobin >8 g/dL improves outcomes or mortality, but there is evidence to suggest that it may be harmful. RBC transfusion promotes platelet activation and adhesion and increases blood viscosity. This promotes the thrombotic etiology of ACS. Transfusion also activates inflammatory cascades and increases infection potential.

- ○ Consider placing a pulmonary artery catheter for patients with shock and questionable right ventricular failure or pulmonary hypertension.

- • Pharmacological therapy

  - ○ Anti-ischemic therapy

    - ▪ These medications decrease myocardial oxygen demand and/or increase myocardial oxygen supply.
    - ▪ Agents include nitroglycerin, morphine, beta-blockers, and calcium channel blockers.

      - ⇨ Nitroglycerin

        - — Reduces myocardial oxygen demand by decreasing left ventricular preload and afterload through systemic vasodilation. It also dilates coronary arteries, increasing coronary blood flow.
        - — Dose: Nitroglycerin 0.4 mg sublingual tablets, up to three doses, each five minutes apart until pain subsides.
        - — A nitroglycerin drip may be indicated for persistent or recurrent chest pain or uncontrolled hypertension.

          - ✓ Start nitroglycerin drip at 5–10 mcg/min, titrate by 10 mcg/min every 5 minutes until symptom relief or systolic blood pressure <100 mmHg.

        - — Avoid in suspected right ventricular infarct, hypotension, or recent 5′-phosphodiesterase inhibitor use.

⇨ Morphine

— Pain relief and anxiolysis leads to decreased sympathetic activation, heart rate, and coronary oxygen demand. Also causes systemic vasodilation which reduces ventricular preload.
— Use for pain refractory to nitroglycerin.
— Dose: Morphine 4–8 mg IV bolus, with additional 2 mg at 5–15 minute intervals until pain is controlled.

  ✓ May result in a decrease in blood pressure, and must monitor respiratory rate.

⇨ NSAIDs (except aspirin) should be avoided or discontinued in cases of suspected ACS or in post-CABG patients, as they have been shown to increase the risk of death and re-infarction.
⇨ Beta-blockers: metoprolol.

— Inhibit beta-1 adrenergic receptors in the myocardium, which decreases heart rate, blood pressure, and cardiac contractility, and therefore cardiac oxygen demand.
— Beta-blockers have been demonstrated to reduce the risk of recurrent myocardial infarction in patients with ACS.
— Oral beta-blocker therapy should be initiated within 24 hours of the onset of ACS.

  ✓ Dose: Metoprolol, 25 mg PO twice daily, titrate to heart rate of 50–60 beats per minute.
  ✓ Use IV beta-blockers for hypertension or arrhythmias.
  ✓ Contraindications: hypotension, bradycardia, heart block, decompensated heart failure, asthma, cocaine-induced myocardial infarction.

⇨ Calcium Channel Blockers

— Inhibit contraction of the myocardium and vascular smooth muscle, leads to coronary vasodilation and decreased afterload.
— Recommended for refractory angina after nitrates and beta-blockers, or for contraindications to beta-blockade.
— Recommended agents: diltiazem or verapamil. These agents also decrease heart rate.
— Avoid in heart failure or pulmonary edema.

o   Antiplatelet agents

   ■   Purpose: prevent further platelet aggregation, thrombus propagation and any further vessel occlusion.

   ■   Initiation of at least two antiplatelet agents is recommended in the patient with suspected or confirmed ACS.

   ■   Recommended agents: aspirin, thienopyridines, or glycoprotein IIb/IIIa inhibitors.

     ⇨   Aspirin

       — Non-enteric coated chewable aspirin should be given to all patients with suspected ACS.

       — Irreversibly inhibits platelet aggregation and causes vasodilation by inhibiting thromboxane production.

       — Dose: Aspirin 325 mg orally once, then 81 mg orally daily.

       — Contraindications: active gastrointestinal bleed, aspirin hypersensitivity, hepatic disease.

     ⇨   Thienopyridines: Clopidogrel (Plavix)

       — Reduce platelet aggregation by blocking platelet adenosine diphosphate receptors. Effects are additive with aspirin.

       — Dose: Clopidogrel 300 mg PR once, then 75 mg PO daily.

       — Hold for 5 days if planning CABG.

       — Contraindicated in liver failure.

     ⇨   GPIIB/IIIA inhibitors: abciximab, eptifibatide, tirofiban.

       — Block IIB/IIIA receptor on platelets, and therefore inhibit fibrinogen-mediated platelet cross-linking.

       — Used as an alternative to clopidogrel in high-risk patients, those with ongoing ischemia, or as an adjunct to angioplasty and PCI.

   ■   Anti-coagulants

     ⇨   Purpose: inhibit the clotting cascade, prevent further clot formation.

     ⇨   Evidence supports the use of unfractionated heparin, low-molecular weight heparin, fondaparinux or bivalirudin in UA/NSTEMI.

     ⇨   In STEMI with revascularization planned, recommended agents include unfractionated heparin and bivalirudin.

       — Unfractionated heparin (UFH)

✓ Binds to antithrombin and inactivates thrombin and clotting factors IXa and Xa, XIa, and XIIa.

✓ Dose: bolus 60–70 units/kg, follow with infusion of 12–15 units/kg/hr with a goal activated partial thromboplastin time at 1.5–2 times normal.

✓ Must monitor for heparin-induced thrombocytopenia.

✓ Consider bleeding risk before initiation.

— Low-molecular weight heparin (LMWH)

✓ Recommended agent: enoxaparin (Lovenox).

✓ Dose: enoxaparin IV bolus of 40 mg, follow with 1 mg/kg subcutaneously for 5 days.

✓ In those treated invasively, LMWH has a higher bleeding risk than unfractionated heparin.

— Fondaparinux (Arixtra).

✓ A factor XA inhibitor.

✓ Dose: fondaparinux 2.5 mg subcutaneously daily.

✓ No risk of thrombocytopenia.

✓ Preferred agent in patients treated conservatively with a high bleeding risk.

✓ Contraindicated in renal impairment and in patients who weigh <50 kg.

— Bivalirudin

✓ A direct thrombin inhibitor.

✓ Acceptable for patients with heparin-induced thrombocytopenia, or for those treated with an invasive strategy and at high risk for bleeding.

■ Treatment for complicated myocardial infarctions

⇨ For MI complicated with bradycardia or high-degree AV block:

— Temporary pacing

⇨ For MI complicated by cardiogenic shock:

— Vasopressors and inotropes: see Chapter 5-(v).

— Intra-aortic balloon pump is recommended to augment cardiac output in patients who do not stabilize with maximal medical therapy.

— Revascularization.

⇨ For MI complicated by ventricular fibrillation:

— Cardiopulmonary resuscitation and early defibrillation.
— Medications according to the Advanced Cardiac Life Support protocol.

⇨ Therapeutic hypothermia is now recommended for all resuscitated patients with STEMI complicated by cardiac arrest.

Definitive therapy for ACS

- Treatment for UA/NSTEMI

  o Goal of immediate treatment is to provide relief of ischemia and to prevent the recurrence of ischemic events.
  o In addition to anti-ischemic, antiplatelet, and anticoagulant therapy, two treatment options exist for UA/NSTEMI:

    ▪ Early conservative therapy

      ⇨ Maximal medical therapy, with invasive therapy only for refractory or recurrent ischemia. This is recommended for low-risk patients without troponin elevation, hemodynamic instability, prior CABG or PCI, or heart failure.

    ▪ Early invasive strategy

      ⇨ Consists of catheterization followed by percutaneous coronary intervention or coronary artery bypass grafting, depending on anatomy (see below). Patients who benefit most from this strategy include intermediate or high-risk patients (TIMI score >3), known stenosis >70%, or those with hemodynamic instability, prior CABG, PCI, or heart failure.
      ⇨ Fibrinolysis should not be performed for NSTEMI.

- Treatment Options for STEMI

  o Reperfusion therapy should be performed in all eligible patients with persistent ST-segment elevation or new left bundle branch block within 12 hours of symptom onset. Reperfusion therapy is also accepted for symptom onset 24 hours prior.
  o Options for reperfusion therapy include percutaneous coronary intervention, fibrinolytic therapy, and coronary artery bypass surgery.

o Percutaneous coronary intervention (PCI):

- Refers to angioplasty and/or stenting.
- Indications:

  ⇨ First-line therapy for patients with one or two vessel coronary artery disease in absence of left main disease.

  ⇨ STEMI and cardiogenic shock, irrespective of time delay.

  ⇨ Contraindications or failure of fibrinolysis.

  ⇨ For three vessel or left main disease if significant delay to CABG exists or if the patient is not a surgical candidate.

- Benefits are time dependent and should be performed for STEMI within 90–120 minutes of presentation.

  ⇨ PCI should be performed in STEMI patients with symptoms <12 hours. It is acceptable for symptoms up to 24 hours.

  ⇨ PCI is not available at all hospitals, and transfer should be considered if transfer and PCI can be performed within 120 minutes of diagnosis.

- Advantages: decreased risk of vessel re-occlusion, bleeding, and re-infarction, improved overall mortality when compared with fibrinolysis.
- Complications: embolization, acute stent thrombosis, arterial dissection and perforation, stroke, and femoral access site complications.
- Adjuncts to PCI include:

  ⇨ Aspirin indefinitely.

  ⇨ Thienopyridines for one year after bare metal stenting and beyond one year for drug-eluting stents.

  ⇨ Unfractionated heparin or a GPIIb/IIIa inhibitor while inpatient.

o Fibrinolytic therapy

- An infusion of an agent which converts plasminogen to plasmin and leads to clot lysis.
- Agents include streptokinase, alteplase, reteplase, and tenecteplase.
- Recommended for patients with STEMI with onset of symptoms less than 12 hours and no access to PCI within 120 minutes of diagnosis, in the absence of contraindications. Acceptable at up to 24 hours of symptom onset.
- Not indicated for STEMI and cardiogenic shock.

- Complications: intracerebral hemorrhage, bleeding requiring transfusion, coronary vessel re-occlusion.
- Contraindications to fibrinolytic therapy:
  - ⇨ Any prior hemorrhagic stroke, head trauma, spinal trauma, or ischemic stroke within three months, cerebral neoplasm or AV malformation, active bleeding or clotting disorder, suspected aortic dissection, or severe uncontrolled hypertension.

- Relative contraindications to fibrinolytic therapy:
  - ⇨ Prior ischemic stroke in over three months, oral anticoagulants, pregnancy or within one week post-partum, refractory hypertension, advanced liver disease, active peptic ulcer, major surgery within three weeks, gastrointestinal bleeding within one month, dementia, non-compressible punctures (liver biopsy, lumbar puncture), traumatic or prolonged CPR >10 min.

- Adjuncts include:
  - ⇨ Antiplatelet and anticoagulants.
  - ⇨ Early routine catheterization.

○ Coronary artery bypass grafting (CABG)

- First-line therapy for those patients with three or more vessel disease and/or >50% left main coronary artery stenosis.
- Revascularization (PCI vs. CABG) recommended for STEMI within 24 hours of symptom onset if features of severe heart failure, persistent ischemia, or hemodynamic instability.
- Emergent CABG is indicated in patients with an acute myocardial infarction for patients with:
  - ⇨ Refractory ischemia after successful or failed PCI.
  - ⇨ Unfavorable coronary anatomy for PCI.
  - ⇨ Cardiogenic shock or life-threatening ventricular arrhythmias in the presence of left main stenosis >50% and/or 3-vessel disease.
  - ⇨ Mechanical complications of MI including acute mitral regurgitation, ventricular rupture or ventricular septal defect.
  - ⇨ Mechanical complications after PCI including perforation, dissection, stent dislodgment or fractured guidewire.

- Emergent CABG should not be performed after failed PCI in the absence of ischemia.

Sequelae of myocardial infarction

- Heart failure

  o Heart failure is associated with a poor short and long-term prognosis in the acute phase of MI. Symptoms include rales, shortness of breath, sinus tachycardia, and a third heart sound. Assess pulmonary congestion with chest X-ray. An echocardiogram is the primary diagnostic tool. Treatment includes oxygen, diuretics, inotropes as needed. Heart failure after MI is an indication for angiography with intent for revascularization.

  o ACE inhibitors should be prescribed indicated in the absence of hypotension to prevent remodeling.

- Cardiogenic shock

  o A state of systemic hypoperfusion characterized by a systolic pressure <90 mm Hg or a cardiac index <1.8 L/min/m² caused by loss of viable myocardium. Most cases occur within 24 hours of infarct. Diagnosis of cardiogenic shock is commonly made with the use of ECHO or a pulmonary artery catheter. See Chapter 5-(ii) for more details.

  o Treatment: fluids and inotropes to target a wedge pressure >15 mmHg and a cardiac index >2 L/kg/min. Agents include dobutamine, milrinone, and dopamine as needed [See Chapter 5-(v)]. IABP can be used when needed as a bridge to definitive therapy. Emergent PCI or CABG is indicated for patients with shock due to cardiac failure after STEMI regardless of time delay.

- Right ventricular (RV) infarction

  o This manifests with a clinical triad of hypotension, clear lung fields, and elevated jugular venous pressure. Treatment recommendations include maintaining RV preload and reducing afterload. Milrinone is a commonly used inotrope. Definitive treatment is reperfusion.

- Mitral regurgitation (MR)

  o Mitral regurgitation commonly develops within 2–7 days of MI due to mitral annulus dilation due to post-infarction LV remodeling or secondary to papillary muscle dysfunction or rupture after inferior MI.

  o Exam reveals a new-onset systolic murmur. Diagnosis is with ECHO.

  o Patients with acute MR should undergo mitral valve replacement promptly, as they may deteriorate suddenly. IABP is used as a bridge to definitive care.

- Cardiac rupture

  o Free wall rupture

    ▪ An acute free wall rupture presents with recurrent chest pain, ST and T-wave changes on EKG, with fast progression to hypotension, cardiovascular collapse and death. In a minority of cases, presentation is subacute, and with accurate diagnosis there is time to intervene.
    ▪ Risk factors include: first MI, anterior infarction, older age, and female sex.
    ▪ Physical exam demonstrates signs of tamponade: hypotension, jugular venous distention, and muffled heart sounds. Rupture is confirmed with ECHO.
    ▪ Those who survive require emergent surgery, with operative mortality greater than 50%.

  o Ventricular septal rupture

    ▪ Most commonly manifests in first 24 hours after fibrinolysis for STEMI with sudden severe clinical deterioration accompanied by a loud systolic murmur and cardiogenic shock.
    ▪ ECHO will show the location and size of the defect.
    ▪ Treatment includes vasodilators (nitroglycerine), and IABP if in shock in preparation for surgery. Emergent surgery is always indicated as defect may expand abruptly.

- Left ventricular aneurysm

  o Ventricular aneurysms usually form after a large, transmural myocardial infarct.
  o True aneurysms form when blood flow stretches and thins necrotic muscle, which fibroses and forms an aneurysm. These rarely rupture, but contain thrombus and may lead to embolic events. Surgery is indicated for heart failure, refractory arrhythmias or recurrent thromboembolism.
  o False aneurysms result from a small free wall rupture contained by pericardium. They require urgent surgical intervention due to rupture risk.

- Pericardial effusion

  o Effusions are common after myocardial infarction, and often asymptomatic.
  o Must exclude free-wall rupture, especially if effusion is more than 1 cm wide.

    ▪ Hold anticoagulation if effusion >1cm or enlarging.

- Pericarditis

  o Inflammation and fibrosis are usually localized to the area of infarction.

  o Include in differential for recurrent chest pain after myocardial infarction.

  o Symptoms include sharp chest pain which is pleuritic in nature and positional. Clinical findings include a new pericardial rub, an elevated neutrophil count, and fever.

  o Treat: NSAIDS or aspirin.

- Arrhythmias [Chapter 5-(vi)]

  o Arrhythmias following myocardial infarction are very common. They may be atrial, ventricular, or secondary to conduction system disturbances.

  o The most common supraventricular arrhythmia is atrial fibrillation.

  o Sinus bradycardia is common after STEMI. It is generally asymptomatic and needs no intervention other than to hold beta-blockers. For symptomatic or hemodynamically significant bradycardia treat with atropine and temporary pacing if unresponsive to medical therapy.

  o Ventricular tachyarrhythmias are a major source of sudden death after MI. They are most commonly noted within 12 hours after a myocardial infarction. Treatment is immediate defibrillation for ventricular fibrillation and ventricular tachycardia with appropriate antiarrhythmic pharmacotherapy. Use of prophylactic beta-blockers in the setting of STEMI reduces the incidence of VF. Correction of magnesium and potassium deficits also helps to minimize risk.

  o Prophylactic use of antiarrhythmics is not recommended after NSTEMI.

  o No treatment is required for ventricular ectopic beats or nonsustained ventricular tachycardia.

  o Implantable cardioverter-defibrillators are recommended prior to discharge for those patients with sustained VT/VF > 48 hours after STEMI to prevent sudden cardiac death.

Post-myocardial infarction hospital care

- Ambulate 12–24 hours after MI when possible.
- Blood pressure control, with beta-blockade, target: 140/90 mmHg.
- Blood glucose control in diabetics, target 100–180 mg/dL, avoid hypoglycemia.
- Continue antiplatelet agents:

  o Aspirin daily.

- o Clopidogrel for at least one year for all patients with bare metal or drug-eluting stents.
- Statin therapy for lipid management and plaque stabilization.
- PPI if need for dual antiplatelet therapy, especially if high-risk for gastrointestinal bleed.
- DVT/PE prophylaxis.
- Angiotensin-converting enzyme inhibitors (ACE-Is)
  - o Vasodilatory effects which reduce myocardial oxygen demand.
  - o Inhibits post-myocardial infarction remodeling.
  - o Start in first 24 hours after myocardial infarction if no contraindication.
  - o Avoid in hypotension, renal failure, or hyperkalemia.
- Angiotensin-receptor blockers are acceptable alternatives for those who cannot tolerate ACE-Is.
- Consider a repeat ECHO to assess cardiac function and rule out intraventricular thrombus.
- Discuss goals for exercise, dietary counseling, lipid management, and smoking cessation.

Practical Algorithm(s)/Diagrams

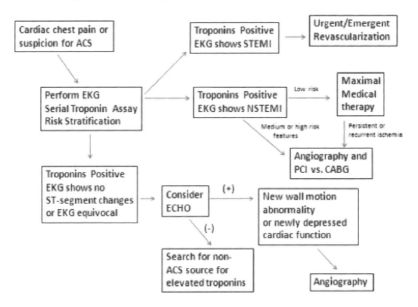

Fig. 1. Diagnostic algorithm for suspected ACS.

Review of Current Literature with References

- A prospective trial by Devereaux *et al.* looked at over 8,300 patients enrolled in a randomized prospective trail of beta-blocker therapy before and after non-cardiac surgery. They found the rate of postoperative myocardial infarction to be 5%, and of those with infarction, 74% had clinical evidence of infarct within 48 hours of operation. A majority (65%) of myocardial infarctions were asymptomatic with a diagnosis made based upon elevated cardiac enzymes. Most postoperative myocardial infarctions demonstrated ST-wave depression or T-wave inversion. The authors recommend cardiac biomarker monitoring in the early postoperative period. In this study, risk factors for MI included older age, vascular surgery, urgent or emergent surgery, postoperative bleeding, creatinine >2 mg/dl, and sustained increases in heart rate of more than 10 beats per minute (*Ann Int Med* 2011; **154**: 523–528).

- Another study examined a cohort of 377 randomized patients after elective vascular surgery and found the rate of perioperative MI in this group to be around 26.5%. This was not influenced by pre-operative coronary revascularization or extent of coronary artery disease. Predictors of MI included abdominal aortic surgery, diabetes, and baseline ST-T wave abnormalities. Patients were not randomized to therapy with beta-blockade (*Eur Heart J* 2008; **29**: 294–401).

- A prospective trial by Keller *et al.* examined the sensitivity of various cardiac biomarkers in the detection of ACS. In 1,800 patients with suspected ACS, a 3-hour troponin assay had a sensitivity of 98%, a negative predictive value of 99.4% and a positive predictive value of 96% in the presence of a serial change from baseline (*JAMA* 2011; **306**(24): 2684–2693).

- The Vascular Events in Non-cardiac Surgery Patients Cohort Evaluation (VISION) study was an international prospective study including over 15,000 surgical patients. They showed a strong association between peak troponin levels in the first three days after surgery and 30-day mortality. Time to death after peak troponin values varied between one and two weeks. They suggest the use of routine post-operative troponin monitoring to improve risk stratification and increase the opportunity for early intervention [*JAMA* 2012; **307**(21): 2295–2304].

- The use of oxygen is a therapy for ACS has been debated in the literature. One study by Mc Nulty *et al.* looked at the effect of 100% oxygen in 18 patients with stable coronary heart disease undergoing elective cardiac catheterization. They found an increase in coronary resistance of 40%, decreased coronary blood flow of 30%, and a blunted response to acetylcholine (an arterial vasodilator) as compared to those patients on room air (*Am J Physiol Heart Circ* 2005; **288**: H1057–1062). A Cochrane review later examined four trials of 430 patients with confirmed STEMI or NSTEMI. They observed a two-fold increase in mortality in those treated with oxygen, but ultimately these numbers were underpowered. They concluded that evidence in support of oxygen use in ACS is sparse, and that oxygen should be used with caution given the trend towards harm (*Cochrane Database of Systemic Reviews* 2013; Issue 8 Art No: CD007160).

- Rao *et al.* performed a retrospective review of over 24,000 patients in three trials of patients with ACS. Cohorts were divided into those who received blood transfusions or not. The group undergoing transfusion had a significantly higher rate of 30-day death (8% vs. 3%), myocardial infarction (25% vs. 8%) and death or MI (29% vs. 10%). They calculated a hazard ratio for 30-day death with transfusion at 3.94, and this was statistically significant. The risk of 30-day death was higher with transfusion hematocrit triggers above 25%. (*JAMA* 2004; **292**: 1555–1562).

Chapter 5-(viii)

Vascular Emergencies

Charles J. Fox, MD*

*Chief of Vascular Surgery, Denver Health Medical Center

Take Home Points

- Early initiation of damage control resuscitation (blood in 1:1:1 ratios and limiting crystalloid) is crucial in performing a successful simultaneous vascular reconstruction without ongoing physiologic derangements.
- A vascular assessment should begin in the admitting area using a handheld continuous wave Doppler device.
- A CT angiogram may be useful for cervical or truncal vascular injuries to plan the best approach, but rarely necessary for extremity vascular injury.
- Pre-hospital tourniquets should be exchanged for the pneumatic type and removed in the operating room if the patient is unstable or if hemorrhage is expected.
- Vascular repairs often require massive transfusion, therefore temporary shunting with delayed repair should be considered at remote community hospitals with limited blood banks.

Contact information: Denver Health Medical Center, University of Colorado Health Sciences Center, 777 Bannock Street, MC 0206, Denver, CO 80204; Tel.: 202-697-1456, email: Charles.fox@dhha.org

- A second surgical team can save time by placing external fixation, and performing saphenous vein harvests or fasciotomy.
- A vein interposition graft is durable when there is adequate muscle coverage; otherwise a longer bypass tunneled out of the zone of injury should be chosen to prevent desiccation or delayed rupture.
- Veins can be ligated but repair time permitting will improve outflow.
- Trust your repair. Remember, a patient in shock may not have a palpable pulse when leaving the operating room.

Background

- Traumatic vascular emergencies have special importance as injuries to major vessels offer unique surgical challenges, and comprise the majority of potentially preventable deaths from penetrating injury.
- In the presence of hemorrhagic shock, you will routinely perform vascular surgery in less than optimal situations.
- These situations demand early deliberate preparation to ensure successful management of vascular wounds.
- Many lessons learned during U.S. military operations continue to advance the practice of vascular trauma surgery and now, translates into the current surgical practices which are recommended.
- Common non-trauma vascular emergencies such as iatrogenic vascular access complications, vasopressor induced ischemia and acute thromboembolism are common to the ICU setting.

Main Body

- Assessment of the vascular trauma patient

  o Vascular trauma usually involves extremities and is often part of the injury complex in patients with exsanguinating hemorrhage. Optimal management requires proper planning and recognition of the essential priorities necessary to prevent immediate hemorrhagic death. Following immediate airway control, attention is directed at controlling hemorrhage and obtaining vascular access. External bleeding can often be hidden by warming blankets or transport gear. You will find that direct pressure is the most effective way to control hemorrhage. A volume depleted patient may not always manifest active arterial bleeding at the time of admission. Pre-hospital tourniquets, if used, should nonetheless be inspected and readjusted or replaced once the resuscitation restores adequate peripheral perfusion. Intravenous access may be hindered by shock, and immediate intraosseous access into the tibia or the humerus is easy and rapid. Initial laboratory studies will depict the degree of physiologic distress that is used to guide the resuscitation and early operative planning. Damage control resuscitation, a strategy of liberal blood product administration, minimal crystalloid use, should begin early in the emergency room and continue intra-operatively. The goal is to achieve hemostasis, restore normal physiology, and potentially complete a vascular reconstruction, upon arrival in the ICU. If the graft is done correctly, it should not fail because you withheld heparin or gave hemostatic agents to a coagulopathic patient. Blood products should be transfused within minutes of arrival with an emergency release of four units of type O packed red blood cells (PRBCs), and two units of thawed AB plasma sent from the blood bank. The blood products are best transfused through a rapid infuser system that is reserved in the admitting area. Unstable patients with a truncal injury or those with more than one mangled extremity are considered "in-extremis" and should trigger a massive transfusion protocol. This involves a standardized release and transfusion of PRBCs, thawed plasma, cryoprecipitate, and platelets.

o Recognizing the need for vascular reconstruction at the time of the trauma admission is crucial for success as indecision and progressive ischemic burden can result in ultimate graft failure and subsequent limb loss. Most of the extremity injuries involve fractures and large soft tissue wounds that can make the diagnosis, by physical exam alone, very accurate. Radiographs can provide early clues that extremity vascular injuries exist and you should take a close look at the plain films as you enter the admitting area. For example, supracondylar femur and tibial plateau fractures are frequently associated with injuries to the distal femoral and popliteal artery. This is among the most common lower extremity vascular injury patterns that you will encounter. Deformed extremities are straightened and the onset of additional hemorrhage is controlled with direct pressure, gauze packing, hemostatic dressings or additional tourniquets. Alternatively, in stable patients, without active bleeding, pre-hospital tourniquets should be carefully loosened to determine the degree, if any, of vascular injury. A Doppler assessment is advised to confirm the absence of pedal pulses and to perform an Ankle-Brachial Index when possible. A patient assessment done in concert with an orthopedic surgeon will facilitate the necessary discussion regarding the sequence of the operation, and preferred techniques for external fixation that best aid in the anticipated vascular exposure. Important information to relay to the entire operative team should include ideal patient positioning, the plan for vein harvesting in a contralateral extremity, and the desire for a C-arm or arteriography. Special instruments located in "peel packs" can ease the apprehension of not having the favored instruments when needed quickly. The earlier you relay this information to the OR, the easier and faster your case will be.

- Tips and strategies for success

  o For extremity injury, a two-team practice reduces ischemic time as the primary team may be preoccupied with thoracotomy, or laparotomy to control hemorrhage, or other damage control maneuvers. Do not hesitate to involve a second team as they can be used to apply external fixation, perform fasciotomies, begin a peripheral vascular exposure, or harvest vein from a non-injured or amputated extremity. It is important to take some extra "careful" time when doing the vein harvest. You should always caution your assistant on the potential for injury to the saphenous vein when performing a fasciotomy. Position the patient to enable unimpeded access to another body cavity or limb in the event of unexpected deterioration or need for additional vein harvesting.

  o Initial control of hemorrhage is often accomplished by digital occlusion using an assistants hand prepped directly into the bleeding wound bed with betadine spray. This is followed by a careful dissection proximal and distal to the site of injury. Balloon catheters may also tamponade hemorrhage when a tourniquet or manual pressure is not effective. Blind insertion of surgical instruments can be unproductive, or harmful, and is discouraged. Tourniquets are left in place until the anesthetist has sufficient time to resuscitate the patient. Proximal femoral injuries are best managed by division of the inguinal ligament or a simple retroperitoneal approach and clamp control of the external iliac artery. For proximal axillo-subclavian wounds, sternotomy or left anterior thoracotomy and clamping of the subclavian artery eliminate the error of uncontrolled dissection through an expanding hematoma of the chest. You should approach distal axillary and proximal brachial arterial injuries with infraclavicular incisions, and extend across the deltopectoral region into the upper arm as needed. The medial approach is preferred for femoropopliteal injuries. The approach in relation to the knee joint is directed by the level of the wound, however total division of muscular attachments at the knee is sometimes required to control hemorrhage of transected arteries and veins. You may find that the transected end can be difficult to identify in the destroyed tissue. Although often thrombosed at the time, these vessels must be found and ligated because they will re-bleed later after the patient is resuscitated. Retrograde advancement of a Fogarty catheter from an uninjured distal site can also be used to locate the transected artery in a horrific wound that is no longer bleeding. When making a decision to amputate or salvage an extremity, you should consider the patients' condition, extent of injury, and your willingness to commit the patient to the necessary definitive orthopedic care and physical rehabilitation. No one situation or scoring system can replace the surgical judgment developed by an experience team.

o   A primary end-to-end repair is preferred when lateral sutures cannot repair the injured vessel. Advantages of this repair include a single anastomosis, and use of autologous tissue. Dividing nearby branches may gain some length in non-calcified vessels, but this repair should be both expedient and tensionless. A complete debridement of any disrupted tissue is an essential step of the repair, and sacrifices made to avoid an interposition conduit should be keenly resisted. The complexity and additional operative time required for vein harvest and interposition grafting or bypass should be appreciated, and the final operative plan and estimated time should be communicated early to the entire operative team. The saphenous vein is the preferred conduit for vascular injuries. The poor historical results of prosthetic material when used in contaminated wounds are the justification for this approach. In my experience, prosthetic grafts placed in larger vessels with good muscle coverage have been used successfully. I have used prosthetic grafts for "clean" subclavian and carotid wounds, however inferior long term patency of prosthetic materials and the potential for infection in war wounds have restricted its widespread use in combat-related extremity wounds.

o   High energy munitions produce large cavitary wounds, with numerous disruption of the skin, and loss of underlying muscle that may prevent attempts to achieve suitable graft coverage. When you are confronted with this situation, a longer vein graft tunneled completely around the zone of injury should be chosen over a shorter poorly covered vein interposition conduit. Appropriately applied external fixation will take this issue into consideration, and this is an important subject to discuss before fasciotomy incisions are made. Devitalized tissue is excised and irrigated under low pressure, with careful evaluation of muscle tissue for viability.

A lengthy and meticulous debridement at the outset is not necessary as these wounds look much better in a few days after subsequent washouts and vacuum dressings.

○ Ballistic trauma can transmit kinetic energy and result in intimal injury well beyond the transected arterial segment. Therefore, perform your debridement with a great deal of concentration and focus on the quality of the luminal surface and strength of the arterial inflow relative to the patients' hemodyanamics. When necessary, a Fogarty catheter should be carefully advanced as pre-hospital tourniquets and incomplete heparin dosing in trauma may result in thrombus accumulation proximally. A four quadrant, heel-to-toe anastomosis that is well-spatulated is the easiest repair method to teach and perform in difficult situations. Small Heifetz clips or Bulldog clamps can also minimize the chance of a clamp injury. Special precautions are worthwhile and should in particular include routine flushing of the graft, and native artery with heparinized saline to dislodge fibrin strands, and platelet debris.

○ Upper extremity injuries should not be underestimated, and often require massive transfusions, from ongoing blood loss and resuscitation requirements. The arm swelling and wound expansion that can result highlights the importance of a wide tunnel for a saphenous vein graft. There has been a sustained interest in repair of venous injuries to avoid the potential for early limb loss from venous hypertension or long term disability from chronic edema. With combined injuries, arterial repair should precede venous repair to minimize further ischemic burden, unless the vein repair requires very little effort.

○ The temporary use of shunts for vascular trauma is a very effective damage control technique to allow for delayed reconstruction. The value of temporary shunting should be compared with the consequences of simple ligation. For example, ligation of the brachial artery after confirming distal signals and palmar blood flow, allows for elective delayed reconstruction if indicated. Surgeons at smaller remote facilities may prefer shunting when rapid evacuation to places capable of matching transfusion requirements or performing emergent complex vascular repairs is necessary.

○ While arteriography remains the gold standard for guiding surgical reconstruction, static film arteriography has largely been replaced with portable C-arm units capable of digital subtraction angiography. Contrast arteriography is very useful for locating the injured vascular bed when there are diffuse fragmentation wounds to the extremity. Hand injected contrast images using butterfly needles without special wires or catheters can be acquired quickly using the digital subtraction mode on a mobile C-arm unit. Rotating the table before the start of the case may be necessary to properly maneuver the C-arm. When all else fails, holding the feet off the end of the table may allow for the acquisition serial images to satisfactorily complete the case. The logistics of maintaining a robust inventory in a field hospital continues to limit the capability to carry out these interventions in combat. Completion assessments following open repair or endovascular interventions make use of a combination of physical exam, the handheld Doppler and selective arteriography.

- Delayed evaluation and postoperative care

  o The early postoperative period is focused on patient warming, resuscitation, and hourly vascular checks which should be performed with a hand-held continuous wave Doppler probe. Palpable pulses and, sometimes, normal ankle-brachial ratios (>0.9) may be delayed until an appropriate resuscitation period has occurred. Patients should remain in the ICU for the at least 24 hours. In addition to ensuring overall cardiopulmonary and metabolic stability, plans for evacuation out of the war zone should take the threat of early graft failure and post-operative bleeding into consideration. The vascular injured patient should not be hurried unnecessarily through the chain of evacuation. External fixators are readjusted based on the appearance of plain film radiographs, and a wound inspection is normally performed within 24 hours. The typical patient is returned to the operating room every 48–72 hours for additional washouts, debridement's, and negative pressure "vacuum" dressing changes. A careful assessment for the development of a compartment syndrome is essential, especially when the patient is transferred out of the combat zone to providers unfamiliar with the initial post-operative exam. You should always maintain a low threshold for performing a fasciotomy for patients' with extremity vascular injury.

- Non-trauma emergencies

  o **Pseudoaneurysm:** A pseudoaneurysm can develop after a traumatic arterial injury and, unlike a hematoma, will demonstrate arterial flow through a neck into a false space contained by surrounding tissue. This occurs frequently following arterial puncture and may be from inadequate compression. Pseudoaneurysms are characterized by a pulsatile mass, tenderness and in severe cases, ulceration or necrosis of the overlying skin. A Duplex ultrasound evaluation can determine the size and location. The typical pulsatile echolucent sac will have a swirling "to-and-fro" flow pattern. Compression (10–30 mins) may avoid surgery but is often too painful and may lead to embolization or thrombosis of the native artery. Ultrasound-guided thrombin injection (1000 units/mL) is generally considered a first-line therapy for anatomically favorable lesions (saccular, narrow neck). The tip of a 22 gauge spinal needle is directed away from the inflow neck to avoid distal embolization and 0.1–0.2 ml of thrombin is injected into the sac. An ultrasound performed in 24–48 hrs confirms resolution. Direct surgical repair or endovascular interventions continue to be employed for challenging lesions. Open techniques involve traditional proximal and distal control with suture or patched repair. However, directly entering the capsule and applying digital pressure is an expeditious approach. In the endovascular era, adjunctive balloon occlusion, coil embolization, or covered stents may simplify the approach in surgically inaccessible areas.

o **Arterial-Venous Fistula:** Percutaneous techniques such as central venous cannulation and arterial catheterization have led to an increased incidence in arteriovenous fistulae. When the adjacent artery and vein are simultaneously punctured, an abnormal connection can form. The local hemodynamic changes result in elongation and dilation of the proximal veins and the arterial circulation may be compromised distally by steal. In larger chronic fistulas, the systemic circulation may also be affected. A thrill may be palpated over the affected site or a bruit appreciated on auscultation. The natural history is thought to be one of gradual enlargement or thrombosis. Symptomatic patients require repair by open or endovascular techniques to restore normal perfusion and venous drainage by closing the communication. Extensive collateral circulation and friability of the artery can make the operation technically difficult when delayed. Therefore, most surgeons prefer to treat these cases when diagnosed. Open repairs involve either isolation of all four limbs, and quadruple ligation or ablation of the communication channel and restoration of flow by suture repair, patch, or interposition grafting of the two vessels. Transcatheter embolization and covered stent grafts have gained popularity particularly in surgically inaccessible areas. Endovascular interventions are particularly less morbid but the materials are expensive. Long-term follow-up is required to evaluate stent patency and monitor for stent migration.

o **Percutaneous Closure Devices:** Closure devices have permitted earlier ambulation and discharge following diagnostic and therapeutic catheterizations. The incidence of complications ranges from 0.5–5% depending on the sheath size, use of anticoagulation, and indications. Closure devices can actively or passively close the puncture site by using suture-mediated, collagen-based, or metal clip/disk-based mechanisms of action. The typical complication is device malfunction resulting in bleeding and necessitating manual compression or surgical exploration. Compression site thrombosis or vessel occlusion from the device itself may cause lower limb ischemia. It is necessary to have documentation of the baseline exam. Usually upon exploration, suture-mediated devices disrupts the back wall and dissects the artery or in the case of collagen devices, the material inadvertently advances into the lumen of the artery. Treatment options include exploration, surgical thrombectomy and primary repair.

o **Vasopressor Induced Ischemia:** Vasopressor agents such as norepinephrine, dopamine, vasopressin, and epinephrine are often used to treat shock. Intricate mechanisms exist that modulate vasomotor tone by these vasoactive substances. The vasomotor response of vascular smooth muscle depends on whether an intact endoluminal endothelial layer is present or absent. When present, the endothelium responds to blood-borne substances that influence smooth muscle contractility. Paracrine mediators such as nitric oxide modulate the response. When endothelium is absent as in advanced peripheral arterial disease, the direct effect by vasoactive substances on vascular smooth muscle is often unopposed vasoconstriction. The consequences on digital blood flow can be significant and result in gangrenous changes. Ischemic areas should be protected from additional mechanical injury which is expected given the likelihood of impaired sensation in the affected parts. Increasing ambient temperature and rewarming of any tissue not deemed to be irreversibly ischemic will improve tissue perfusion and prevent further tissue loss. Antimicrobial ointments such as silver sulfadiazine should be applied to blistered and de-epithelialized areas. Similar to a frostbite injury, the ischemic areas should be allowed to demarcate for auto-amputation in very severe cases.

o **Acute Limb Ischemia:** Arterial embolus produces acute limb ischemia characterized by pulselessness, pallor, paralysis, pain and parasthesias. In comparison, thrombotic events are more gradual and associated with atherosclerotic disease. Most embolic events are cardiac in origin or derived from the atheroemboli of peripheral aneurysms. The specific level of the arterial occlusion directs the preference for catheter-directed thrombolysis (distal small vessels) or opens surgical embolectomy (larger proximal vessels). Therapeutic unfractionated intravenous heparin should be started as soon as the diagnosis is suspected. The standard approach is a wide surgical preparation and longitudinal incisions to expose multiple arterial beds or perform a fasciotomy. The arteriotomy may be transverse if there is no suspicion for atherosclerosis and need for a bypass; otherwise a longitudinal arteriotomy is made. A balloon embolectomy catheter is inserted, carefully inflated with a volume of saline that is annotated on the hub of the catheter. A 5-6 French (Fr) catheter is used for Aorto-iliac and subclavian vessels, 3-4 French for femoropopliteal or brachioaxillary vessels, and a 2 Fr for the tibial or radioulnar vessels. Caution should be exercised such that the intimal surface is not injured yet properly aligned to the wall. Certain embolectomy catheters can be guided over wires and used in conjunction with fluoroscopy to easily pass the catheter to the desired location. Successful passage may require several attempts and should be repeated until all thromboemboli is removed. Back bleeding should be brisk and a completed angiogram should confirm restoration of flow. Intra-arterial injection of 30–60 mg of papaverine or 200–400 µg of nitroglycerin may be given along with a liberal amount of heparinized saline to relieve vasospasm. When thrombectomy is incomplete, consider using 5–10 mg of tissue plasminogen activator (TPA) in 20 cc of saline. Fasciotomy should always be considered in any patient with prolonged (>2 hrs) of ischemia.

- **Final Points**

The simultaneous management of peripheral vascular injuries in the pursuit of life and limb is very challenging. The decision to amputate or reconstruct an ischemic requires sound judgment that often comes with experience. These patients have significant transfusion requirements and the resuscitation should not be separated from the surgery. A two-team approach is an effective method that will keep speed on your side. Not all vessels have to be repaired, as brachial and tibial vessels can be ligated when a Doppler signal is obtainable in the distal limb. Systemic heparin is not necessary; however adequate intimal debridement and liberal flushing with heparinized saline vein during the repair is essential. A well-covered interposed saphenous vein graft is a durable conduit and favored over prosthetic materials. Venous reconstruction should be performed when time permits. Completion arteriography is not usually necessary, but you should confirm your pulse exam with a continuous wave Doppler. Remember, your completion assessment should be continuous over the next 24 hours. Trust yourself, give the patient time to "catch-up", and recognize that the vascular exam will improve over time with successful repairs. The following references are highly recommended for additional reading about the management of peripheral vascular injury on the front line.

Practical Algorithm(s)/Diagrams

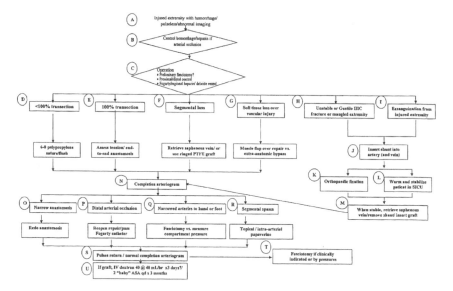

Fig. 1. Management algorithm for peripheral vascular injuries (Adapted from Feliciano *et al. J Trauma Acute Care Surg.* **75**: 3 2013).

TRIAGE CATEGORIES AND MANAGEMENT GUIDELINES FOR EXTREMITY VASCULAR INJURIES

CATEGORY I: ISOLATED VASCULAR INJURY
• One surgical team required
• Vascular injury, restoration of flow, reconstruction, and limb salvage take priority
• Extremity tourniquet may be removed in the operating room in coordination with the anesthesia team
• Venous injury should be repaired
• Complex or lengthy reconstructions acceptable

CATEGORY II: VASCULAR INJURY IN CONJUNCTION WITH OTHER NON–LIFE-THREATENING INJURIES
• Two-team approach preferable to treat vascular and other injury
• Vascular injury, restoration of flow, reconstruction, and limb salvage take priority
• Extremity tourniquet may be removed in the operating room in coordination with the anesthesia team
• Venous injury should be repaired
• Complex or lengthy reconstructions acceptable

CATEGORY III: MULTIPLE VASCULAR INJURIES
• Two-team approach preferable to treat multiple vascular injuries
• Vascular injury, restoration of flow, reconstruction, and limb salvage take priority
• Extremity tourniquet may be removed in the operating room in coordination with the anesthesia team
• Diminished role for venous injury repair
• Diminished role for complex or lengthy reconstructions

CATEGORY IV: VASCULAR INJURY IN CONJUNCTION WITH LIFE-THREATENING INJURIES
• Two-team approach optional after life-threatening injury is stabilized
• Life-threatening torso, neck, or head injury takes priority
• Extremity tourniquets should remain in place until the life-threatening injury* is stabilized
• Diminished role for venous injury repair
• Diminished role for complex or lengthy reconstructions

Fig. 2. Triage categories for severe extremity vascular injury in conjunction with other injuries. [Adapted from *Rutherford's Textbook of Vascular Surgery. 8th ed. Box 160-1, Section 26, Vascular Trauma* (eds). J. Cronenwett, W. Johnston. Elsevier. Philadelphia, PA. 2013].

Review of Current Literature with References

- A case control study of 40 patients with life-threatening hemorrhage who underwent arterial vascular reconstructions using a saphenous graft for 10 upper (25%) and 30 lower extremity (75%) wounds. The study illustrates the effectiveness of blood product resuscitation during simultaneous limb salvage and provides important emphasis on the correction of physiological derangements upon completion of the vascular reconstruction [*J Trauma.* 2008; **64**(2): S99–S107].

- Kragh *et al.* performed a large prospective survey of tourniquet use in 232 combat casualties with 428 tourniquets to describe the actual morbidity of its use. No limbs were lost because of tourniquet use and tourniquet use was not associated with increased morbidity [*J Trauma* 2008; **64**(2 Suppl): S38–S49].

- Starnes and colleagues provide an excellent summary of important technical tips for successful extremity arterial reconstruction. This publication is a very important referent for the practicing community general surgeon [*J Trauma* 2006; **60**(2): 432–442].
- This is an important synopsis of important lessons learned during U.S. combat operations that has set the standard for contemporary surgical management of military vascular injuries [*Surg Clin North Am* 2007; **87**(1): 157–184, vii].
- Gifford and colleagues published an outcome analysis study. Data was collected from the Joint theater trauma registry (JTTR), Balad vascular registry (BVR), and the Walter reed vascular registry (WRVR). It compared 64 shunted U.S. casualties sustaining extremity vascular injury from June 2003 through December 2007 to 61 not shunted. After propensity score adjustment, use of TVS suggested a reduced risk of amputation, particularly in more severely injured limbs, but was not statistically significant. The authors concluded that temporary vascular shunting used as a damage control adjunct in management of wartime extremity vascular injury does not lead to worse outcomes. The use of temporary vascular shunts has now gained popularity as a result of its use during the wars in Iraq and Afghanistan [*J Vasc Surg* 2009; **50**(3): 549–555].
- This detailed analysis of the modern combat experiences during the Global War on Terror in approximately 500 patients has characterized the improved limb salvage seen with rapid evacuation, immediate repair or reconstruction, and use of damage control principles. Also provided is important epidemiologic data to compare with the civilian experience and to highlight major differences and unique aspects of modern vascular trauma (*J Trauma Acute Care Surg* 2012; **73**: 1515–1520).

6. Respiratory

Chapter 6-(i)

Airway Management

Michael M. Sawyer, MD*

*Associate Professor of Anaesthesia, University of Colorado School of Medicine

Take Home Points

- Airway management in the ICU requires knowledge of cardio-pulmonary physiology, advanced airway practices and facile ability with a multitude of airway devices.
- A thoughtful team based approach is the most important thing when addressing the critically ill.
- The ICU patient and their therapy present numerous caveats to normal airway management, both anatomically and physiologically.
- Ability to move quickly down the difficult airway algorithm and modify that algorithm for your institution is essential in developing an Airway Care Plan.
- This care plan requires a pre packed airway cart or box and ready availability of tools to address the unforeseen difficult airway.
- The care plan also requires daily examination and long term planning around extubation.
- While anesthesia staff may not be required for all intubations and extubations in the ICU, a close communication between the ICU and the Anesthesiology service allows anesthesiology to be present when requested.

Contact information: Denver Health Medical Center, University of Colorado Health Center, 777 Bannock St., MC 0206, Denver, CO 80204; Email: Michael.Sawyer@dhha.org

- The Anesthesia department as well as the ICU department is responsible for constant review and improvements of practice.

Background

- The Advent of the Difficult Airway Algorithm in 1993 was the first step in the unified approach to the teaching of advanced airway techniques as a comprehensive measure.
- Evaluation of the Anesthesiology Closed Claims database noted the difference in outcomes after the advent of the algorithm.
- A time period before the advent of the algorithm was compared to the initial five years after the algorithm which noted a significantly decrease in the amount of death/brain death on induction of anesthesia. (Peterson *et al.* from airway grand rounds)
- This success created the birth of a whole industry dedicated strictly to airway device technology.
- Also, these improvements prompted the development of the Society for Airway management in 1995.
- The algorithm was reworked after the introduction of the LMA on 2003 into its current state today.
- The use of the supraglottic airways in routine use as well as their emergence in the emergency pathway has caused a relative inexperience with advanced airway techniques that are essential to the management of the critically ill patient. (46 in Nolan)
- Improvement of airway equipment and algorithms have improved the success rates of managing the ICU airway.
- These advances, though, still come with a learning curve and require numerous intubations before a user is facile.
- Yet, these advanced tools often create a scenario when the airway is being handled by personnel that is not comfortable with the sophisticated airway techniques.
- For these reasons, a systematic approach to the airway of the ICU patient is mandatory.

Main Body

ICU patient/physiology

- A myriad of issues are compounded in the critically ill patient needing airway manipulation. These can include rapidly worsening illness, continued hypoxia, tenuous cardiopulmonary status, aspiration risks, facial/airway swelling and injury, poor access to equipment and inexperience of those using the equipment. (NOLAN)

- Long-term intubations often lead to inadvertent extubation due to transport, self-extubation or lack of vigilance.
- The incidence of inadvertent extubations has been seen to increase as patient sedation is decreased for evaluation.
- The incidence of difficult intubation in the Emergent Non OR setting has been shown to be twice that of the patient undergoing general anesthesia (NOLAN and Ref. [18] out of NOLAN).
- Factors affecting this include, the changes in pulmonary function of the critically ill, airway changes that often accompany massive resuscitation or injury, also the less than optimal position of the patient for airway manipulation in the ICU bed.
- For this reason the need to train ICU physicians in advanced airway management, as well as creation of an ICU advanced airway team has been adopted in some institutions. (REYNOLd) And at Denver Health, we have Airway Care Plan that allows ICU personnel to realize when they are moving toward an advance airway.
- Many of the medications given in the ICU for long-term sedation are subjected to increasing Context Sensitive half times that alter the patients return to baseline. For many of the drugs used in the ICU, their metabolism and clearance are more complex than first order kinetics and requires knowledge of their individual pharmacokinetics to plan for a return to baseline.
- Many of these medications also alter the patient's own response to CO_2.
- These known sequelae of the sedative medications and the known mechanical functional change in airway anatomy in the ICU patient makes proper handling the airway of the critically ill very eloquent.
- Shunt is an area of lung that is perfused but poorly ventilated. The equation $Qs/Qt = (CcO_2 - CaO_2)(CcO_2 - CvO_2)$ represents the shunt flow as a proportion of total lung volume.

  o   Where $CaO_2 = (1.34 \times Hgbx\ O_2\ Sat) + (0.003 \times PaO_2)$.

- CcO_2 and CvO_2 are end capillary and mixed venous oxygen contents respectively. This is dependent on cardiac output, tissue O_2 consumption and lung function. Critically ill patients often suffer from poor ventilatory mechanics for many reasons that increase their closing capacity and worsen shunt. Once a shunt fraction is found to be greater than 30%, simply increasing the FiO_2 will not improve oxygenation. Hence even with appropriate preoxygenation, ICU patients often quickly desaturate as they are induced for intubation.

Airway equipment/management

- The advent of the video laryngoscope has helped to revolutionize modern airway management. While knowledge of the fiber optic bronchoscope is helpful in the ICU, when fiber optic assistance is needed, the anesthesiologist presence is mandatory.
- It is useful to be facile with the basic laryngoscope blades, the utility of the Laryngeal Mask Airway, and the percutaneous cricothyrotomy kit as well.
- The ASA difficult airway algorithm depicts a step wise approach to management of the difficult airway. At DHMC, we consider all ICU intubations difficult airway intubations for the reasons previously described.
- In our ICU each intubation plan is accompanied by the Respiratory therapy team, anesthesiology either on standby or in the room, and a uniform ICU intubation tray.
- These trays are prepackaged and checked frequently to make sure they are stocked and that batteries have been changed.
- Medications to be used are chosen based on the physiologic state of the patient, and from agreement between both the ICU and Anesthesiology services.
- After pre-oxygenation, as best as possible the patients is induced.
- The decision on the use of depolarizing versus non-depolarizing neuromuscular blockade, as well as the need for fiber optic back up requires close communication between the ICU and Anesthesiology services.
- Generally, the ICU intubation is done in a rapid sequence fashion unless contraindicated either by airway issues (requiring awake fiber optic assistance) or neurologic issues (burn injury, spinal cord injury, prolonged immobilization).
- A simple method to follow for the ICU physician is the 'Pop, Drop, and Roll' 3-step intubation.

  o (1) As much as possible, attempt to 'Pop' the mandible open while being sure to not greatly sublux or dislocate the mandible.

  o (2) 'Drop' the laryngoscope as far into the posterior pharynx as possible. Being mindful to not attempt to visualize the vocal cords at this point because, as with most any instrument used in the OR, the laryngoscope must be set up correctly to work correctly. All too often, untrained practitioners attempt to visualize the epiglottis and vocal cords before the blade is deep enough. By placing the blade in until the posterior pharynx is contacted, the blade will be assumed to be deep enough to view the epiglottis and vocal cords when the oropharangeal, laryngeal, and pharyngeal axis are aligned.

o (3) If not contraindicated, gently roll the patient's head back to align the three axis in play for intubation.

o These steps should allow the laryngoscope blade to be resting near the epiglottis, and is a simple strategy for manipulating an airway for those with limited airway experience.

- Management of the difficult airway in the ICU follows the difficult airway exam put forth by the ASA. The one caveat is swift decision and timely use of alternative measures. This includes early change from laryngoscopy to video laryngoscopy.
- The use of the LMA, while essential for airway management and a critical part of the difficult airway algorithm, can only be considered a temporizing agent in the ICU.
- Therefore, if intubation has failed and video laryngoscopy has failed, an LMA may help in the short-term but is not a long-term answer.
- The LMA will allow the ICU/Anesthesia team to create a new plan, or allow short-term management while a surgical airway is obtained.
- To that end, the decision to move towards a surgical airway should be part of every conversation and this decision should become a swift action if there is airway difficulty.
- Overall at DHMC, the key is our easy communication between services, an Airway Care Plan, access to advanced airway tools and personnel and our close approximation between the OR and ICU.
- This allows Anesthesiology to easily help in management of the difficult airway, as well as to discuss management with the ICU team.

Extubation

- Both the intensive care literature and the anesthesiology literature have exhaustive algorithims for intubation of the challenging airway. But there is very scant knowledge guidelines for the extubation of these difficult patients.
- A similar level of vigilance is required for the safe extubation of the previously ventilated patient as there has been for the safe intubation of the ICU patient.
- In fact, extubation should be considered more dangerous than intubation and studies have shown greater complications during extubation.
- The ASA guidelines for management of the difficult airway do not give any concrete guidelines for extubation.

- Traditional extubation criteria should be applied if possible and correlated to the clinical picture of the patient. These include:
  - o Following commands
  - o Clear oropharynx with intact gag reflex
  - o 5 second head lift/ hand grasp
  - o Vital capacity $>=$ 10 ml/kg
  - o NIF >20 cmH$_2$O
  - o Tidal volume >6 cc/kg
  - o Arterial Blood gas showing adequate oxygenation
- One should realize that the majority of ICU patients that are intubated are actually intubated before they are brought to the ICU, hence a review of the previous airway notes are essential before embarking on routine extubation.
- Extubation should be addressed with the plan already in place for possible failure and urgent reintubation.
- It is best done during the day shift.
- If trial extubation over an airway exchange catheter is planned. Anesthesia should be at bedside, this is a advanced technique that is not commonplace.
- Simply, extubation should include members of the ICU team, respiratory therapy team and anesthesiology should be present when there is a possibility of failure if the Airway Care Plan indicates a difficult airway.

Practical Algorithm(s)/ Diagrams

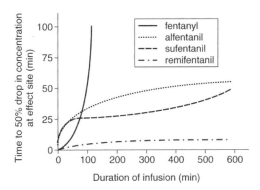

Fig. 1. Pharmacokinetic properties of commonly used anesthetics.

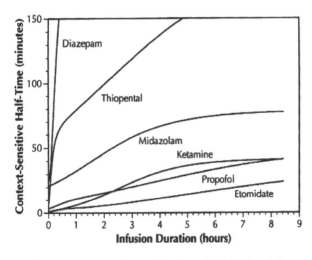

Fig. 2. Wilhelm and Kreuer, *Crit Care* 2008 **12**(Suppl 3): S5.

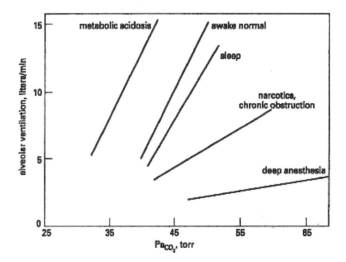

Fig. 3.   Patient responsiveness to increasing partial pressure of carbon dioxide.

- The curve is a basic CO_2 response curve, it illustrates the patient responsiveness to increasing CO_2, as sedation is administered the patient's ability to maintain respiratory drive in the face of increasing $PaCO_2$ is diminished.
- From MG Levitzky, *Pulmonary Physiology*, 5th.

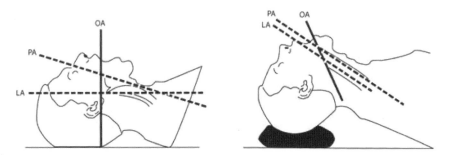

Fig. 4.   From (*Miller's Anesthesia* 6th Edition).

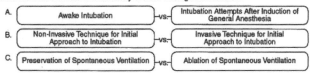

DIFFICULT AIRWAY ALGORITHM

1. Assess the likelihood and clinical impact of basic management problems:
   A. Difficult Ventilation
   B. Difficult Intubation
   C. Difficulty with Patient Cooperation or Consent
   D. Difficult Tracheostomy

2. Actively pursue opportunities to deliver supplemental oxygen throughout the process of difficult airway management

3. Consider the relative merits and feasibility of basic management choices:

   A. Awake Intubation –vs– Intubation Attempts After Induction of General Anesthesia

   B. Non-Invasive Technique for Initial Approach to Intubation –vs– Invasive Technique for Initial Approach to Intubation

   C. Preservation of Spontaneous Ventilation –vs– Ablation of Spontaneous Ventilation

4. Develop primary and alternative strategies:

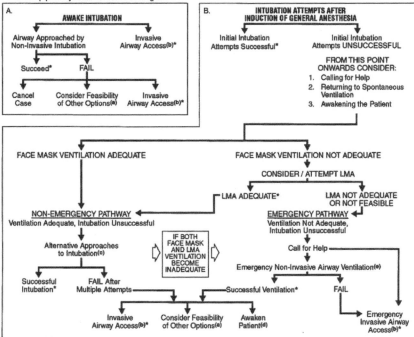

* Confirm ventilation, tracheal intubation, or LMA placement with exhaled CO₂

a. Other options include (but are not limited to): surgery utilizing face mask or LMA anesthesia, local anesthesia infiltration or regional nerve blockade. Pursuit of these options usually implies that mask ventilation will not be problematic. Therefore, these options may be of limited value if this step in the algorithm has been reached via the Emergency Pathway.

b. Invasive airway access includes surgical or percutaneous tracheostomy or cricothyrotomy.

c. Alternative non-invasive approaches to difficult intubation include (but are not limited to): use of different laryngoscope blades, LMA as an intubation conduit (with or without fiberoptic guidance), fiberoptic intubation, intubating stylet or tube changer, light wand, retrograde intubation, and blind oral or nasal intubation.

d. Consider re-preparation of the patient for awake intubation or canceling surgery.

e. Options for emergency non-invasive airway ventilation include (but are not limited to): rigid bronchoscope, esophageal-tracheal combitube ventilation, or transtracheal jet ventilation.

Fig. 5. ASA Task force 2003 difficult airway algorithm.

Review of Current Literature with References

- Current literature consists mainly of hospital specific experiences and retrospective studies.
- The addition of more user friendly advanced airway tools such as the video laryngoscopes have been helpful in the ICU.
- Most of these studies have similar plans to what is done at Denver Health. Our adoption of close communication and team approach toward the Airway Care Plan helps to ensure that less surprise airway emergencies occur.
- Some have advocated for a specific airway cart with every airway tool available. We feel that by limiting these devices, it prohibits the undertrained resident or ICU personel from inadvertanly getting into a difficult situation. This will ensure that the lines of communication remain open for these difficult patients.

Chapter 6-(ii)

Acid-Base Physiology

Dominykas Burneikis, MD* and Fredric M. Pieracci, MD, MPH[†]

* Medical Student, University of Colorado School of Medicine
[†] Acute Care Surgeon, Denver Health Medical Center

Take Home Points

- Acid-base disturbances are always a consequence of an underlying disease process or metabolic derangement.
- Correctly interpreting the arterial blood gas (ABG) aids in identifying the underlying disease process so that it can be addressed appropriately.

Background

- Acid-base physiology incorporates processes that increase or decrease [H^+] in blood.

Contact information: (Dominykas Burneikis) 12631 East 17th Ave, MSC313, Aurora, CO 80045; Tel.: 720-220-2053, (Fredric M. Pieracci) Denver Health Medical Center, 777 Bannock Street, MC 0206, A388, Denver, CO 80206; Email: dburneikis@gmail.com; Fredric.pieracci@dhha.org

- [H$^+$] in extracellular fluids is represented by the pH, which is defined by the following equation:

  o pH = $-\log_{10}$[H$^+$]

- pH is tightly regulated, and relatively small derangements have profound physiologic consequences on cardiovascular, hematologic, and endocrine homeostasis.
- In blood, the ratio of PCO$_2$ to HCO$_3$ determines [H$^+$], and thus pH. This relationship is classically defined by the Henderson-Hasselbach equation:

  o pH = 6.1 + $\log_{10}$([HCO$_3$]/0.03 × [PCO$_2$])

- Combining the above equations, a simplified relationship between [H$^+$], HCO$_3$, and PCO$_2$ can be derived:

  o [H$^+$] = 24 × ([PCO$_2$]/[HCO$_3$])

- PCO$_2$ is regulated primarily through ventilatory gas exchange at the level of the alveoli, while changes in HCO$_3$ are directed by the proximal tubules in the kidneys.
- Whereas changes in minute ventilation rapidly change PCO$_2$ (seconds to minutes), changes in HCO$_3$ reabsorption occur over the course of days.
- Normal values of pH, PCO$_2$, and HCO$_3$ are: 7.40, 40 mmHg, and 24 mEq/L respectively.
- Acidosis and alkalosis refer to the processes that lead to states of low and high blood pH (acidemia or alkalemia respectively).
- A patient is acidemic when blood pH < 7.38, and alkalemic when blood pH >7.42.
- ABG analysis yields values of pH, PCO$_2$ and HCO$_3$, which are key in identifying primary disturbances of acid-base balance and evaluating secondary compensatory responses.

Main Body

I. Common indications for ABG:

- Admission to the ICU
- New onset hypoxia, acute respiratory failure, or clinical deterioration of a mechanically ventilated patient
- Shock
- Intracranial hypertension

II. ABG interpretation

Primary acid-base disturbances

- Check the pH to determine whether the patient is acidemic (pH < 7.38) or alkalemic (pH > 7.42).
- Check PCO_2 and HCO_3 to identify the primary driver of acid-base disturbance (metabolic vs. respiratory).
- If the patient is acidemic (pH < 7.38) and PCO_2 is elevated (>40), then the primary disturbance is respiratory acidosis. Alternatively, if the patient is acidemic and HCO_3 is decreased (<24), then the primary disturbance is metabolic acidosis.
- In cases of severe acidemia, both respiratory and metabolic acidosis can be present simultaneously. Such acid-base disturbance is easily identified without accounting for compensatory response, as PCO_2 is >40 while $HCO_3 < 24$.
- If the patient is alkalemic (pH > 7.42) and PCO_2 is decreased (<40), then the primary disturbance is respiratory acidosis. Alternatively, if the patient is alkalemic and HCO_3 is increased (>24), then the primary disturbance is metabolic alkalosis.
- As with acidemia, severe alkalemia can be the result of compound respiratory and metabolic alkalosis ($PCO_2 < 40$ while $HCO_3 > 24$). There is no need to account for compensatory response in such cases.
- It is possible to see normal pH (7.38 < pH < 7.42) in the context of equal-and-opposite metabolic disturbances, as in metabolic alkalosis and concomitant respiratory acidosis.

Compensatory responses and mixed acid-base disorders

- To offset the changes in pH produced by the primary acid-base disturbance, the body mounts a secondary response by adjusting either PCO_2 or HCO_3 via lungs and kidneys, respectively.
- The degree of compensatory response can be predicted and should be calculated in order to identify any co-existing primary acid-base disturbances.
- In metabolic acidosis and metabolic alkalosis, PCO_2 should decrease and increase, respectively, by the amount predicted in Table 1. If actual PCO_2 is less than predicted, then a concomitant respiratory alkalosis may be present. Alternatively, if actual PCO_2 is greater than predicted, then a coexisting respiratory acidosis must be considered.

- For metabolic acidosis specifically, calculating the anion gap and the gap-gap ratio (Table 2) can further aid in developing a differential diagnosis and is discussed below.
- For metabolic alkalosis, measuring urine [Cl⁻] can help differentiate between potential primary drivers of the acid-base disturbance.
- Primary respiratory acid-base disturbances must be broadly classified as acute or chronic. This determination is made by clinical evaluation that takes into account patient's history (e.g. pre-existing COPD, acute lung injury, ventilatory support etc.)
- In respiratory acidosis and alkalosis, HCO_3 will increase and decrease, respectively, by the amount predicted in Table 1.
  - For primarily acute respiratory acid-base disturbance, if actual HCO_3 is less than predicted, then a concomitant metabolic acidosis may be present. Alternatively, if actual HCO_3 is greater than predicted, then a coexisting metabolic alkalosis must be considered.
  - For primarily chronic respiratory acid-base disturbance, compensatory mechanisms are slower and can take up to three days to respond fully. Thus if actual HCO_3 is less than predicted, then the compensatory response is considered to be incomplete, or a coexisting metabolic acidosis is present. Similarly, if HCO_3 is greater than predicted, the compensatory response is incomplete or a coexisting metabolic alkalosis is present.
- Mixed acid-base disturbances can make ABGs a challenge to interpret, therefore therapy should be aimed at treating the underlying disease and not chasing numbers.

Anion Gap

- Anion gap (AG) is calculated to estimate the amount of unmeasured anions (e.g. lactic acid) present in blood. AG is derived from equation in Table 2, which uses measured electrolyte concentrations obtained with a basic metabolic panel.
- AG can be used to further differentiate between "gap" and "non-gap" metabolic acidosis.
- The principal unmeasured anion that determines AG is albumin. Thus in patient's with low albumin, AG should be corrected according to equation in Table 2. Failing to correct for albumin may result in a falsely-normal AG and concealed presence of an AG acidosis.
- It is possible to have a "gap" and "non-gap" metabolic acidosis occur simultaneously. Such a scenario can be unmasked by calculating the gap-gap ratio (GGR) (Table 2).

- GGR is a ratio of change in AG to change in HCO_3. GGR less than 1 indicates that the AG does not fully account for the decrease in HCO_3, and thus a "non-gap" metabolic acidosis must be present (e.g. coexisting hyperchloremic acidosis and lactic acidosis). Alternatively, GGR greater than 1 indicates that HCO_3 is higher than would be expected for a given AG, and thus a concomitant metabolic alkalosis should be suspected.

III. Common causes of acid base disturbances in the ICU

- Metabolic acidosis

  o Anion gap

    ▪ Diabetic ketoacidosis
    ▪ Alcoholic ketoacidosis
    ▪ Lactic acidosis
    ▪ Renal failure with accumulation of organic anions
    ▪ Methanol and ethylene glycol intoxication
    ▪ Salicylate overdose

  o Non-anion gap

    ▪ Dilutional, resuscitation with HCO_3-free fluids resulting in hyperchloremia
    ▪ Diarrhea, fistulas resulting in GI loss of HCO_3
    ▪ Renal tubular acidoses (RTAs)

- Metabolic alkalosis

  o Chloride responsive

    ▪ Vomiting, gastric suctioning resulting in GI loss of H^+
    ▪ Diuretic use resulting in intravascular depletion

  o Chloride resistant

    ▪ Hyperaldosteronism
    ▪ Hypokalemia
    ▪ Excess HCO_3 administration

- Respiratory acidosis

  o Airway obstruction
  o Asthma
  o COPD
  o Ventilatory restriction (rib fractures, flail chest)

- o   Pneumonia
- o   Pulmonary edema
- o   CNS depression
- Respiratory alkalosis
  - o   Pregnancy
  - o   High-altitude residence
  - o   Salicylate overdose
  - o   Anxiety-hyperventilation syndrome

IV. Sample ABG analyses

Example 1:   7.62/20/20

1.   acidosis or alkalosis? → alkalosis
2.   primary respiratory or metabolic? → respiratory ($PCO_2 < 40$ mm Hg)
3.   secondary metabolic disturbance? → NO [predicted $\Delta HCO_3 = 0.2\ (40\text{–}20) = 4$ mEq]. So, predicted $HCO_3 = 20 =$ actual HCO_3.
4.   diagnosis = pure respiratory alkalosis

Example 2:   7.28/33/18   Na = 135 Cl = 111 HCO_3 = 18

1.   acidosis or alkalosis? → acidosis
2.   primary respiratory or metabolic? → metabolic ($HCO_3 < 24$ mm Hg)

   Anion gap? → NO $\{Na - (Cl + HCO_3) = 135 - (111 + 18) = 6\}$

3.   secondary metabolic disturbance? → NO [predicted $\Delta PCO_2 = 1.2 \times (24\text{–}18)$. So, predicted $PCO_2 = 33 =$ actual PCO_2.
4.   diagnosis = non-AG metabolic acidosis, likely hyperchloremic (Cl = 111)

Example 3:   7.26/32/14

1.   acidosis or alkalosis? → acidosis
2.   primary respiratory or metabolic? → metabolic ($HCO_3 < 24$)
3.   secondary metabolic disturbance? → YES [predicted $\Delta PCO_2 = 1.2 \times (24\text{–}10) = 12$]. So, predicted $PCO_2 = 40\text{–}12 = 28$. Because actual $PCO_2 >$ predicted PCO_2 additional respiratory acidosis must be present.
4.   diagnosis = primary metabolic acidosis with secondary respiratory acidosis

Example 4:   7.34/30/16   Na = 133 Cl = 107 HCO_3 = 16   Albumin = 1.7 g/dL

1.   acidosis or alkalosis? → acidosis

2. primary respiratory or metabolic? → metabolic ($HCO_3 < 24$)

Anion gap? → NO $(Na - (Cl + HCO_3)) = 133 - (107 + 16) = 10$

Corrected AG? → $AG + 2.5 \times (4.5 - Albumin) = 10 + 2.5 \times (4.5 - 1.7)$

AGc = 17

3. secondary metabolic disturbance? → NO [predicted ΔPCO_2 = $1.2 \times (24 - 16) = 9.6$]. So, predicted $PCO_2 = 30$ = actual PCO_2.

4. diagnosis = pure AG acidosis

Example 5: 7.34/30/16 Na = 145 Cl = 115 HCO_3 = 16

1. acidosis or alkalosis? → acidosis

2. primary respiratory or metabolic? → metabolic ($HCO_3 < 24$)

Anion gap? → YES $(Na - (Cl + HCO_3)) = 145 - (115 + 16) = 14$

GGR? → $(AG - 12)/(\Delta HCO_3) = (14 - 12)/(24 - 16) = 0.25$. Since GGR < 1, a concomitant non-AG metabolic acidosis should be suspected

3. secondary metabolic disturbance? → NO [predicted ΔPCO_2 = $1.2 \times (24 - 16) = 9.6$]. So, predicted $PCO_2 = 30$ = actual PCO_2.

4. diagnosis = combined AG metabolic acidosis and non-AG metabolic acidosis

Practical Algorithm(s)/Diagrams

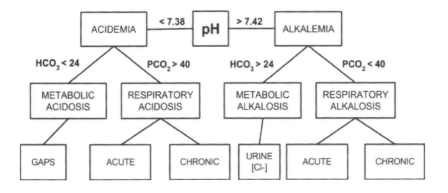

Table 1. Equtions for calculating expected compensation to acute acid-base disturbances.

Metabolic Acidosis	$\Delta PCO_2 = 1.2 \times \Delta HCO_3$	$PCO_2 <$ predicated = resp. alkalosis
Metabolic Alkalosis	$\Delta PCO_2 = 0.7 \times \Delta HCO_3$	$PCO_2 >$ predicated = resp. acidosis
Acute Respiratory Acidosis	$\Delta HCO_3 = 0.1 \times \Delta PCO_2$	$HCO_3 <$ predicated = metab. acidosis
Acute Respiratory Alkalosis	$\Delta HCO_3 = 0.2 \times \Delta PCO_2$	$HCO_3 >$ predicated = metab. alkalosis
Chronic Respiratory Acidosis	$\Delta HCO_3 = 0.4 \times \Delta PCO_2$	$HCO_3 <$ predicated = incomp. response
		$HCO_3 >$ predicated = metab. alkalosis
Chronic Respiratory Alkalosis	$\Delta HCO_3 = 0.4 \times \Delta PCO_2$	$HCO_3 <$ predicated = metab. acidosis
		$HCO_3 >$ predicated = incomp. response

Table 2. Equations used to calculate the Gap-Gap Ratio.

$AG = Na - (Cl + HCO_3)$ [nl = 12 +/- 4]	$AG > 12 =$ gap acidosis
$AGc = AG + 2.5 \times (4.5 - albumin)$	for pts w/ hypoalbuminemia
Gap-Gap Ratio = $(AG - 12) / \Delta HCO_3$	GGR < 1 = nl AG metab. acidosis
	GGR > 1 = metab. alkalosis

Review of Current Literature with References

- An alternative, physiochemical approach to examine acid-base homeostasis was proposed by Stewart in 1983 [Stewart *et al. Can J Physiol Pharmacol* 1983; **61**(12): 1444–61]. The "Stewart Method" addressed many of the criticisms of the physiological approach. Specifically, it redefined H^+ and HCO_3 as dependent variables that change in response to acid-base derangements rather than cause them. Stewart identified three independent variables responsible for acid-base homeostasis in the human body: PCO_2, total weak acid concentration (ATOT), and the strong ion difference (SID). SID is central to the physiochemical approach and is defined as follows:

  o   SID = (Na + K + Ca + Mg) – (Cl + Lactate)   normal = 40–42 mEq/L

  Because of the principle of electric neutrality, SID will change in the same direction as pH. While the "Stewart Method" is more aligned with the laws of physical chemistry, the physiological approach described in this chapter is still the most commonly utilized approach clinically.

Mechanical Ventilation

James Haenel, RRT*

*Surgical Critical Care Specialist, Denver Health Medical Center

Take Home Points

- The decision to provide mechanical ventilation should be based on the clinical examination and assessment of gas exchange.
- The decision must be individualized because arbitrary cutoff values for PO_2, PCO_2 or pH as indicators of respiratory failure may not be appropriate to all patients.
- Simplistically, a mechanical ventilator can be considered to be a pump that functions to replace the patient's intrinsic pump and as a supportive tool during lung failure.
- Classification of mechanical ventilators is based on modes which consist of a combination of control, phase, and a variety of conditional variables that permit either mandatory or spontaneous breaths.
- Selection of initial ventilator mode for acute respiratory failure is dependent on diagnosis, gas exchange abnormalities, hemodynamic status and various extrinsic factors such as patient position and body habitus.
- Current evidence supports the use of lower tidal volumes to reduce mortality when acute lung injury is present.

Contact information: Denver Health Medical Center, 777 Bannock St., MC 0206, Denver, CO 80204; Email: James.Haenel@dhha.org

- There is currently insufficient evidence for determining the optimal setting of positive end expiratory pressure (PEEP), the value of recruitment maneuvers or use of rescue modes of ventilation.
- Avoidance of ventilator asynchrony is a complex interplay between the patient's intrinsic pump (Pmus) and that of the mechanical ventilator pump (Pvent). Additional patient factors that come into play include mechanical, chemical, neuroreflexes and behavioral components that will alter demand for ventilation.
- Acute hypoxic events occur in upwards to 20% of ventilated patients and necessitates an immediate and thorough evaluation to discriminate between an emergent airway event versus an acute pulmonary decomposition.
- Since the introduction of mechanical ventilation, the primary goal in the setting of respiratory failure is to minimize the potential for side effects, mainly hemodynamic compromise and ventilator-induce lung injury while supporting gas exchange thus allowing the underlying disease process to reverse.

Background

- The decision to intubate a patient and provide mechanical ventilation is frequently not a "blood gas" decision. Assessment of vital signs in conjunction with evidence of tachypnea, use of accessory muscles, ability to protect the airway, and worsening hypoxemia based on noninvasive monitoring all validate the need for early intubation and mechanical support.
- There are three conditions for which mechanical ventilation (MV) may be required:

   (1) Inadequate respiratory drive i.e. immediate post-operative period, drug overdose, brain injury.
   (2) Inability to maintain adequate alveolar ventilation i.e. neuromuscular disease, high cervical injury, chronic ventilatory failure.
   (3) Hypoxia i.e. Acute lung injury, acute respiratory distress syndrome, COPD.

- MV when properly applied offers support of gas exchange and maintenance of lung volumes.

   At no time should MV be considered curative and in fact, it may potentially be responsible for ventilator induced lung injury (VILI). Pragmatically, in the absence of an appropriate pressure generated by the patient's own respiratory muscles (Pmus), the conveyance of an external pressure by the

MV (Pvent) will provide air flow and tidal volume according to the equation of motion: Pvent + Pmus = RV$'$ + EV + Pi where RV$'$ is the resistive load defined as the pressure required to deliver the flow of gas (resistance times flow) and EV + Pi is the elastic load or the pressure required to deliver the tidal volume (elastance or compliance times tidal volume). Simplistically, the MV may be seen as a pump when the patient's own intrinsic pump fails. Conversely, during respiratory (lung) failure, the MV is utilized purely as a supportive tool to enhance gas exchange.

- Manufacturers frequently make available the nomenclature used to describe modes of mechanical ventilation and this often contributes to the confusion and unfamiliarity of clinicians when prescribing mechanical ventilation. Compounding this, a significant amount of the published literature and by far the most contentious debates surrounding mechanical ventilation apply to only a small subset of patients intubated and ventilated in the ICU, i.e. patients with acute respiratory distress syndrome (ARDS). The vast majority of ventilated ICU patients actually spend an average of four days or less receiving mechanical ventilation.

- Initially following intubation, the goal of mechanical ventilation is to provide Full ventilator support (FVS) in order to optimize oxygenation and to eliminate $PaCO_2$. Once hemodynamic stability has been achieved, the patient may either be extubated or converted to a partial mode of ventilation (PVS), see Fig. 1.

- A primary goal of MV is to optimize the patient-ventilator interaction and achieve ventilator synchrony. Ventilator breaths can either be controlled or assisted. A controlled breath is a machine delivered breath where the rate, the inspiratory time (I:E ratio) and tidal volume are clinician-determined so as to relieve the patient of all work. An assisted breath consists of the same input variables but it is essential that the ventilator flow as well as pressure delivery are synchronized with the patients effort during all three breath phases: initiation or *trigger*, delivery of breath or *target* and termination or *cycle*.

- Ventilator settings such as: tidal volume, respiratory rate, FiO_2, inspiratory: expiratory ratio and PEEP selection will vary in different clinical circumstances. Appropriate settings will depend upon the patients clinical and pulmonary status, i.e. does the patient have normal underlying lung function, does the patient have obstructive lung disease such as COPD or asthma or severe restrictive disease secondary to ARDS?

- Ventilation with low tidal volumes (Vt) using 6 ml/Kg/ normalized to ideal body weight (IBW) has become clinically accepted for ARDS patients after the results of the National Institutes of Health trial that compared 6–12 Ml/Kg/IBW.

Controversy still remains regarding Vt selection in the patient who does not exhibit acute lung injury but none the less remains at risk.

- To minimize the possibility for ventilator asynchrony, the ventilator's flow and pressure delivery must synchronize with the patient's effort during all three phases of breath delivery: breath initiation (trigger), peak flow delivery and breath termination (cycling).

- Acute hypoxic events during MVcan result in malignant consequences in the critically ill patient who has marginal cardiopulmonary reserves. J.S. Haldane astutely pointed out in 1921 that "Anoxemia not only stops the machine but wrecks the machinery." Adequate oxygenation is crucial for survival. As little as four minutes of cerebral hypoxia may cause irreversible brain injury. Moreover, suboptimal peripheral oxygen delivery has been recognized as a critical etiologic factor in multisystem organ injury.

Main Body

Initiation of ventilation: modes of ventilation and phase variables

- Three different types of breaths are available during mechanical ventilation. Selection is dependent upon whether the patient or ventilator performs the work and whether the ventilator or the patient initiates (triggers) the breath. Initial choice of the mode of mechanical ventilation basically comes down to choosing either a controlled or an assisted breath delivery. A controlled breath means that the clinician sets the rate, the inspiratory time and the tidal volume with the goal being that the patient will do no work of breathing. The term "control" can be confusing. It does not refer to a machine setting but infers that breath delivery is managed by either sedation or a combination of sedation and use of a neuromuscular blocking agent (NMB). Risks involved with use of controlled breaths are diaphragmatic muscle weakness and atrophy, impaired cough and secretion retention, and an array of sedation and NMB drug complications. In contrast to controlled breaths is the assisted breath, where the patient is permitted to interact with the ventilator on all or just an occasional breath. The amount of work performed during an assisted breath ideally will be shared by the ventilator; however if the patients respiratory drive is increased (sepsis, fever, agitation or increased deadspace ventilation) and the ventilators peak flow setting or set pressure is inadequate then the patient may experience significant levels of work. Spontaneous breaths are selected usually once the patient is ready to perform some or all of the work for breathing. These breaths are triggered, limited and cycled by the patient.

- Practically speaking most patients receive a short period of controlled ventilation following intubation until either gas exchange stabilizes or the NMB associated with the intubation period is no longer present. At this point, use of assisted breaths is the general rule. Since the patient is expected to interact with the ventilator, sedation must be titrated to minimize anxiety but not suppress respiratory drive. Strict attention to the ventilators flow and pressure settings is obligatory to allow the patient to synchronize their inspiratory efforts during all three breath phases: initiation (triggering), flow delivery and termination (cycling). Improper attention to any of the three phases of breath delivery can result in increased effort to initiate breath delivery, continued diaphragm contraction beyond the triggering of the breath if flow is inadequate or mismatching of timing of end inspiration to exhalation. Any one of these situations may lead to excessive work loads imposed on the patient.
- Clinicians and manufacturers offer an assortment as well as a bewildering number of ways to provide mechanical ventilation. There is a popular textbook of mechanical ventilation that describes over 62 modes! I will be using the KISS principle (keep it simple) because that is what I am capable of! Let us look at the phase variables because this incorporates 90% of what you need to master. There are three phase variables that are used to begin one of the three phrases (trigger, target and cycle) of the ventilator cycle.
  o Trigger: The trigger variable is clinician set and permits inspiration to begin.
    ▪ It may either be a preset *pressure* (generally –2 cm H_2O), a preset *volume*, a designated *flow* change (generally 3 L/M) or an elapsed time period.
  o Target: The target variable is what governs gas flow during the breath.
    ▪ The target variables may either be pressure, flow or volume and they cannot be exceeded during inspiration. Inspiration is therefore limited once a preset volume is delivered, a preset peak airway pressure is reached or when a preset peak flow is attained.
  o Cycling: Cycling refers to the factors that terminate inspiration and lead to exhalation.
    ▪ A breath may be pressure, volume or flow cycled.

The definition of what constitutes a "mode of ventilation" then is the relationship between the breath types (Mandatory, Assisted and Spontaneous) and the inspiratory phase variables just described.

o   Based on the breath types and phases used to initiate a ventilator breath conventional ventilators today offer only five basic breath types:

  ▪   Volume-Controlled: time-triggered, flow-targeted and volume-cycled
  ▪   Volume-Assisted: effort-triggered, flow-targeted and volume cycled
  ▪   Pressure-Controlled: time-triggered, pressure-targeted and time-cycled
  ▪   Pressure-Assisted: effort-triggered, pressure-targeted and time-cycled
  ▪   Pressure-Support: effort-triggered, pressure-targeted and flow-cycled

o   Once the mode, breath type, respiratory rate and FIO_2 are selected then the clinician will then set a peak inspiratory flow rate in liters/minute in Volume-Control or a % inspiratory time in seconds or fraction thereof in Pressure-Control.

  ▪   Fundamentally, the peak flow setting (in L/M) is what fine tunes the I:E ratio. In volume ventilation, the I:E ratio is generated by a combination of the Vt, RR and peak inspiratory flow setting. The flow wave selection (generally either a square wave or decelerating waveform) will also impact the I:E ratio.
  ▪   The peak inspiratory flow rate delivered in the volume modes is a fixed or flow-targeted setting. This means that if the patients demand for ventilation increases for any reason and the RR increases then the I:E ratio will decrease. Conversely, with pressure-targeted breaths, the flow will adjust to maintain the pressure target. An inadequate delivered flow of gas is a common reason for ventilator asynchrony and must be addressed.

Positive-end expiratory pressure

•   As discussed above the mode selection and manipulation of phase variables all deal with manipulation of inspiration. Conversely PEEP is the management of end-expiratory pressure above atmospheric pressure. There are two primary indications for PEEP:

o   To recruit lung volume and attempt to return the functional residual capacity (FRC) towards normal and thus improve or reverse hypoxemia.
o   To reduce or minimize the inspiratory work of breathing associated with severe acute restrictive lung disease or that associated with dynamic hyperinflation and Auto-PEEP.

By recruiting and stabilizing collapsed small airways and alveoli PEEP may increase the respiratory system compliance and thus the FRC, and therefore mitigate the effects of intrapulmonary shunting associated with acute lung injury.

- o Much controversy still exists regarding how to select the optimal PEEP/ FIO_2 levels. Whether PEEP should be titrated to optimize compliance, minimize the intrapulmonary shunt fraction, prevent dorsal alveolar collapse from hydrostatic imposed pressures or minimize ventilator induced lung injury from atelectatrauma or stretch induced over-inflation from high tidal volumes remains to be determined.

- Setting Positive End Expiratory Pressure

  - o First and foremost, there is no compelling evidence for a low versus high PEEP setting nor is there strong evidence that performance of pressure-volume curves used to identify the lower or upper inflection points is necessary to optimize an individual PEEP setting.

  The vast majority of patients have been satisfactorily managed with PEEP values of 5–15 cm H_2O.

  - o The ARDS Network titration table for determining PEEP/FIO_2 has been available for over a decade and has performed well in thousands of patients enrolled in various ARDS Network trials.
  - o Arguments against the PEEP/FIO_2 titration table are that it is "cook book" and that not all ARDS are the same. ARDS may be classified as either Pulmonary ARDS or Extrapulmonary ARDS. It has been noted that the main difference between the two types of ARDS is that chest wall compliance is normal in Pulmonary ARDS but significantly lower in Extrapulmonary ARDS thus the response to PEEP may be dramatically different.
  - o To account for the differences in types of ARDS as well as different patient's body habitus, potential for mixed obstructive defects complicating the acute restrictive defects an individual approach may be needed.
  - o Recruitment maneuver(s) to identify optimal PEEP:
    - Use Pressure-control mode
    - Set RR to 10/min
    - Adjust I"E ratio to 1:1
    - Set peak inspiratory pressure to 20 cm H_2O
    - Increase baseline PEEP to 20–40 cm H_2O for 1–2 minutes

- Generally, recruitment maneuvers are used in response to a patient who has experienced a sudden decline in oxygenation while on their baseline ventilator settings. Recruitments should be performed while closely monitoring the patient's hemodynamic response. It is not unusual to see a decrease in blood pressure or even saturation during the maneuver. Changes greater than 20% may require stopping the maneuver. Certainly any decrease in heart rate necessitates immediate discontinuation. The recruitment maneuver should be repeated in response to new or continued desaturation events and the baseline PEEP increased by 2.5–5.0 cm H_2O following each recruitment until oxygenation has improved or there is no further positive response.

o   Adverse effects of PEEP

  ▪   Elevation of PEEP levels will necessarily increase both end-inspiratory as well as the mean airway pressures. The potential exists for a fall in cardiac output as a result of decreased venous return to the right side of the heart. In lieu of a decrease in cardiac function, any increase in PaO_2 will be negated based on the principal of oxygen delivery ($DO_2 = CaO_2$ [$Hb \times 1.36 \times SPO_2$]). Strong consideration of monitoring cardiac output should be made when PEEP levels > 15 cm H_2O are used. Also, any unexplained tachycardia or the need for inotropic agents would suggest the need for monitoring of cardiac output.

Ventilator asynchrony

Ventilator synchrony requires a perfect matching of the patient's inspiratory effort to be in concert with the ventilators ability to provide both flow and pressure. There are three crucial periods where this relationship between patient and ventilator may become uncoupled: during triggering, flow delivery or at breath termination. Failure of the ventilator to respond at the appointed time may result in the patient experiencing excessive muscle loads, compromised alveolar ventilation, ventilator induced injury or excessive periods of dyspnea resulting in use of excess sedation. Evidence for asynchrony includes new respiratory distress, diaphoresis, tachycardia and anxiety.

•   Types of Asynchronies

During trigger phase

  o   Ineffective triggering — missed triggers

Auto-PEEP

  o   Autocycling
  o   Double triggering
  o   Triggering delay

During flow delivery phase
- o Inadequate set peak flow in volume mode
- o Excessive set peak flow/excessive I:E ratios

During cycling phase

- o Increased neural inspiratory demand
- o Prolonged machine inspiratory time
  - ▪ Ventilator asynchrony has been reported to occur in upwards to 25% of patients receiving positive pressure ventilation. Interestingly, the adverse effects of patient-ventilator asynchrony remain unknown in terms of duration of ventilator days or increase length of weaning times.
- o Approach to management of Ventilator Asynchrony
  - ▪ During breath triggering

Delayed or miss triggers are common in the presence of Auto-PEEP. First and foremost, treat Auto-PEEP. Try adding set PEEP to offset Auto-PEEP. Change from pressure trigger to flow trigger.

Autocycling occurs when sensitivity is set inappropriately low i.e. "Hair Trigger." Decrease sensitivity. Extra triggers may be caused by chest tube negative pressure in setting of a bronchopleural fistula (BPF) and will respond to decreasing pressure trigger sensitivity. To and fro motion from excessive water in vent circuits is not uncommon and easily addressed. Cardiac oscillations may occur in the hyperdynamic heart when sensitivity is overly low.

- o During flow delivery

Increase set peak inspiratory flow until patient appears comfortable (in volume modes).

Switch from volume mode to pressure mode for variable flow rates.

If plateau pressures are not excessive, increase set tidal volume.

Decrease flow or pressure if patient is actively making expiratory efforts to terminate breath.

- o During cycling phase

If secondary to altered neural inspiratory times are greater than machine inspiratory times, then lengthening of cycle criteria may help (volume, time, flow).

If secondary to prolonged machine inspiratory time compared to neural inspiratory time, then decreasing cycle variables may result in a better match.

Acute hypoxic events during mechanical ventilation

Nothing is more stressful for the patient's cardiopulmonary and neurologic system, not to mention the stress put on the responsible bedside staff, than having to respond to a serious life-threatening acute hypoxic event. Acute hypoxemia is a frequent ICU event and has been reported to occur in up to 25% of patients receiving mechanical ventilation, that is 1 out of every 4! As a result, it is incumbent upon all critical care personnel to be capable of an immediate and cogent response to identify and reverse this potentially life-threatening situation.

Over two decades ago, we developed a bedside algorithm that specifically addresses both the immediate response required to address life-threatening hypoxemia in the ventilated patient as well as the steps to identify the primary etiologic cause. See Fig.1.

The algorithm is divided into a primary and secondary survey. The thought behind this was that immediate threats to life must be identified and managed within minutes. Once an acute hypoxic event is identified, the patient should instantly be hand ventilated with a high flow manual resuscitator (>20 L/M of O_2 flow). The goal is to identify an airway occlusion that must be reversed immediately. Difficult bagging is suggestive and further addressed by passage of a section catheter. Inability to pass the catheter pin points to the problem which must be rectified without delay. Artificial airway leaks while problematic can usually be troubled-shot by an experienced therapist, thereby preventing unnecessary reintubation. Clearly, if the patient responds to bagging with an increase in oxygen saturation then attention should be turned to the ventilator looking for circuit or settings that are inappropriate. Once the airway is eliminated as a primary concern (this should take <60 seconds) and the patient remains unstable, tension pneumothorax must be considered. When in doubt and in the face of life-threatening hypoxemia, the chest should be vent prior to obtaining a chest X-ray. Once oxygenation has stabilized but the etiology remains unclear, performance of the secondary survey should commence. Clearly, a recent intervention i.e. new medication, transport etc. may have been responsible. Likewise, complications from procedures must be recognized as well as the possibility for progression of the underlying disease process. A common mistake is to attribute an acute hypoxic event to a pulmonary embolism when a portable chest X-ray reveals a new infiltrative or collapse. The last place you want to be is in a dark, cold radiology room at two in the morning with a hypoxic patient who more likely has a much more common problem like mucous plugging or atelectasis!

Practical Algorithm(s)/Diagrams

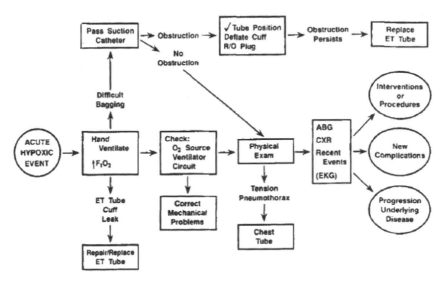

Fig. 1. Algorithm for initial management of acute hypoxic events.

Liberation from Mechanical Ventilation

Fredric M. Pieracci, MD* James Haenel, RRT[†]
and Michael Sawyer, MD[‡]

*Acute Care Surgeon, Denver Health Medical Center
†Surgical Critical Care Specialist, Denver Health Medical Center
‡Associate Professor of Anaesthesia, University of Colorado School of Medicine

Take Home Points

- Mechanical ventilation is hazardous to all organ systems and the appropriateness for liberation from it should be assessed at least daily.
- The term "weaning from the ventilator" refers to a gradual increase in patient work of breathing after a prolonged (days to weeks) period of mechanical ventilation that has resulted in both gas exchange and respiratory muscle embarrassment. This clinical scenario applies only to the minority of critically ill surgical patients. Rather, most surgical ICU patients may be rapidly liberated from mechanical ventilation without a prolonged wean. Therefore, the term "liberation from mechanical ventilation" is preferred to "weaning."

Contact information: Denver Health Medical Center, 777 Bannock Street, MC 0206, A388, Denver, CO 80206; Email: Fredric.pieracci@dhha.org; James.Haenel@dhha.org; Michael.Sawyer@dhha.org

- The surgical intensivist must distinguish appropriateness for ventilator liberation from appropriateness for extubation. The former refers specifically to the contribution of the ventilator to work of breathing. The latter includes more general issues such as mental status and upper airway patency.
- Certain predisposing factors and injury patterns can predict early the need for prolonged ventilator support via tracheostomy.
- General contraindications to transitioning a patient from a full support mode of ventilation (e.g., assist control) to a partial support mode (e.g., pressure support ventilation) include any condition that significantly either depresses or elevates minute ventilation. Recent neuromuscular paralysis is a common example of the former; shock is a common example of the latter.
- Appropriateness for extubation may be assessed using the pneumonic "SOAP"

  o Secretions
  o Oxygenation
  o Airway/Alertness
  o Parameters

- The most studied and useful parameter for predicting successful extubation is the rapid shallow breathing index (RSBI, A.K.A. the Toben Index), defined as the respiratory rate divided by the spontaneous tidal volume (L). Assuming all other aspects of the SOAP pneumonic are favorable, a RSBI < 100 suggests a high likelihood of successful extubation.
- Most patients who fail extubation do so within the first hour. Be ready to emergently re-intubate your patient before you extubate them. Identify potentially difficult airways [Chapter 6-(i)] prior to extubation and muster the appropriate resources.
- If you are unsure whether your patient needs to be re-intubated, then your patient probably needs to be re-intubated. You will regret a missed opportunity to re-intubate far more than a potentially unnecessary re-intubation.

Background

- Mechanical ventilation is a necessary evil. Although it is life-saving for patients with respiratory failure, it is fraught with complications, including atelectasis, baro and volutrauma, pneumonia, respiratory muscle atrophy, agitation, and delirium.
- Surgical ICU patients differ from medical ICU patients in several ways that are pertinent to liberation from mechanical ventilation. In general, surgical

ICU patients are younger, more likely to have a rapidly reversible pathology, and less likely to have chronic pulmonary disease. These conditions combine to make rapid liberation from mechanical ventilation more appropriate for the surgical, as compared to the medical ICU patient.

- Normal minute ventilation (V_e) is 6–10 L/min; multiple pathologies may be operating to either decrease or increase V_e in the surgical ICU patient.

Main Body

Predicting the need for prolonged mechanical ventilation early

- Early and safe extubation should be the goal for every ventilated patient.
- However, certain factors increase significantly the likelihood that a patient will require prolonged mechanical ventilation, and thus inform the decision to perform a trachesotomy early in the patient's course (Chapter 19). This strategy will allow the patient early exposure to the benefits of trachesotomy, including:

    o Ability to minimize both analgesic and sedative infusions
    o Improved pulmonary toilet
    o Improved comfort
    o Improved communication with the patient
    o Decreased risk of inadvertant extubation
    o Decreased airway resistance
    o Possible decreased risk of VAP

- These risk factors may be divided into two categories: (1) pre-existing conditions and (2) injury patterns.

    o Injury patterns

        - Severe traumatic brain injury
        - Severe facial fractures
        - Laryngotracheal trauma

    o Pre-existing conditions:

        - Age >70 years
        - Psychiatric illness
        - Substance abuse, particularly alcohol abuse
        - Chronic obstructive pulmonary disease
        - Morbid obesity
        - Prior need for trachestomy

Transitioning the work of breathing to the patient

- Ventilatory support modes vary from full support (e.g., assist control) to supplemental oxygen only (e.g., T-piece for endotrachel tube or trach collar via a tracheostomy tube) [Chapter 5-(ii)].
- Most ventilated critically ill surgical patients without underlying respiratory disease do not require prolonged weaning. Rather, the necessity for mechanical ventilation is transient and related to the underlying acute pathology. Time for substantial deconditioning of respiratory muscle/drive has not elapsed. Therefore, stable patients may be rapidly transitioned to a partial support mode and evaluated for extubation.
- Although this transition may occur quickly, it is contingent upon several fators. Broadly speaking, the patient's metabolic requirements (and thus CO_2 production and ultimately required V_e) must be low enough to be managed independently by the patient. Conversely, the patient's mental status and neuromusclar condition must be sufficient to initiate spontaneous breaths and maintain adeqaute V_e.
- A patient's ability to successfully sustain spontaneous ventilation depends upon the mechanical load on the respiratory system, including:
  o Resistance
  o Elastance
  o Intrinsic PEEP
  o Respiratory muscle fatiuge
- The following represent relative contra-indications to transitioning a patient to a partial ventilatory support mode:
  o Recent neuromuscular paralysis
  o Elevated intra-cranial pressure
  o Shock
  o $FiO_2 > 50\%$
  o Minute ventilation <5 or >15 L/min

Determining successful transitioning

- Transitioning to a partial support mode will not be successful if the patient is not able to generate sufficient respiratory effort and tidal volume to maintan a normal V_e, or if the ventilatory requirements (CO_2 elimination) of the underlying disease process are too great.
- Both hypoxemia and desaturation of arterial hemoglobin are infrequent and late finding in failed transitioning.

- In general the following are indicative of failed transitioning:
  - o Apnea
  - o Respiratory rate >30
  - o Sustained heart rate >20% baseline for >5 minutes
  - o Systolic blood pressure >180 mm Hg or <90 mm Hg
  - o Hypercapnia
  - o Anxiety/diaphoresis
  - o Abdominal paradox

The myth of "minimal ventilator settings"

- One method of predicting successful liberation from mechanical ventilation entails attempting to replicate as closely as possible the conditions that the patient will face after extubation.
- This theory has led to the concept of "minimal ventilator settings," which typically refers to both a pressure support and PEEP of 5 cm H_2O, which are purported to apply only that pressure which negates the resistence of the tube and replicates intrinsic PEEP.
- This reasoning is flawed for several reasons:
  - o Upper airway edema and inflammation that develops in response to intubation likely results in airway resistance which far exceeds that imposed by a standard endotracheal tube.
  - o The addition of as little as 5 mm H_2O of pressure support can decrease inspiratory work by as much as 40%.
  - o The concept of physiologic PEEP is not substantiated by data. The static recoil pressure of the respiratory system is zero at end-expiration in a healthy adult.
  - o Furthermore, the addition of 5 cm H_2O of PEEP can decrease inspiratory work of breathing by as much as 40%.
- Intensivists may then be lulled into a false sense of security when observing a patient breathing comfortably on "minimal ventilator settings."
- Most ventilated patients can tolerate an approximately 50% increase in respiratory load following extubation. Thus, they are able to compensate for the removal of both pressure support and PEEP.
- In the remainder of cases, and when any doubt as to the success of extubation is raised, a trial of spontaneous breathing with the artificial airway still in place (e.g., T-piece or trach collar) may be executed, thereby removing the advantages of both pressure support and PEEP.

Extubation

- Both the intensive care literature and the anesthesiology literature have exhaustive algorithims for intubation of the challenging airway. But there is very scant knowledge guidelines for the extubation of these difficult patients.
- A similar level of vigilance is required for the safe extubation of the previously ventilated patient as there has been for the safe intubation of the ICU patient.
- In fact, extubation should be considered more dangerous than intubation and studies have shown greater complications during extubation.
- The ASA guidelines for management of the difficult airway do not give any concrete guidelines for extubation.
- Traditional extubation criteria should be applied if possible and correlated to the clinical picture of the patient. These include:
  - Following commands
  - Clear oropharynx with intact gag reflex
  - 5 second head lift/hand grasp
  - Vital capacity $> = 10$ ml/kg
  - NIF > 20 cm H_2O
  - Tidal volume >6 cc/kg
  - Rapid shallow breathing index < 100
  - Arterial Blood gas showing adequate oxygenation
  - Positive "cuff leak"
- One should realize that the majority of ICU patients that are intubated are actually intubated before they are brought to the ICU, hence a review of the previous airway notes are essential before embarking on routine extubation.
- Extubation should be addressed with the plan already in place for possible failure and urgent reintubation.
- It is best done during time periods when adequate staffing is availible.
- If trial extubation over an airway exchange catheter is planned, anesthesia should be at bedside: this is an advanced technique that is not commonplace.
- Simply, extubation should include members of the ICU team, respiratory therapy team and anesthesiology should be present when there is a possibility of failure if the Airway Care Plan indicates a difficult airway.

The difficult to wean patient

A small subset of critically ill or injured surgical patients may require a formal weaning plan.

Common scenarios for when a structured weaning plan is required include:

- Cervical spine injuries resulting in tetraplegia, particularly above C-5.
- Critical illness polyneuropathy complicating the primary admission diagnosis.
- COPD associated with post-operative acute on chronic respiratory failure.
- Persistent inflammation and immunosuppression related to MOF.
- Pneumonectomy /lobectomy associated with post-operative pneumonia.

Classification of the difficult to wean patient

Time to successful ventilator discontinuation starting with the first spontaneous breathing trial (SBT) can be used to describe the degree of difficulty involved in the weaning process.

- *Simple weaning* consists of patients who after one weaning attempt go on to successful extubation. This group of patients represents ≈69% of all patients and not surprisingly has a quoted mortality rate of 5%.
- *Difficult weaning* includes patients who fail three SBT or need seven days of additional SBT to successfully discontinue ventilator support.
- *Prolonged weaning* includes patients who have failed three SBT or require >7 days of attempts after the first SBT. As many as 15% of patients fall into the prolonged category.

  Patients classified as "*prolonged* weaning" are frequently transferred to long term rehab facilities that offer formal weaning schedules over a period of weeks to months.

Why my patient will not wean

There are essentially four reasons why a patient remains ventilator dependent.

- Cardiovascular instability
- Hypoxemia
- Psychological
- Imbalance between Demand versus Capability to breath

  o **Cardiovascular instability** may first present during a spontaneous breathing trial as new onset atrial fibrillation, premature ventricular contractions or signs of acute ischemic changes on the EKG. Alternatively, patients with known chronic left heart failure may show evidence of acute pulmonary edema when switching the patient from positive pressure ventilation to spontaneous breathing.

o **Hypoxemia** is common in intubated patients and multifactorial in origin. Initiation of spontaneous breathing without positive pressure promotes posterior diaphragm movement but may result in worsening of ventilation-perfusion matching due to dependent collapse. Ineffective secretion clearance as a result of pain or weakness sets the stage for atelectasis and increase work of breathing resulting in hypoxemia.

o **Psychological** issues, while not frequent present a challenge when they do occur. Patients with neuromuscular diagnosis's (tetraplegia and myopathies), depression, delirium, or COPD may experience periods of intense dyspnea during SBT's that may result in the patient not being willing to participate further. It is imperative that the patient feels comfortable with the care providers who are performing the SBT and this combined with judicious use of anxiolytics may result in better cooperation.

o Demand versus Capability is responsible for the preponderance of all significant delays in the ventilator discontinuation process.

- *Demand* is quantitated by assessing the patient's minute ventilation. A minute volume consistently > 13 liters a minute may result from sepsis (increased CO_2 production, metabolic acidosis), pulmonary dysfunction (increased dead space ventilation, decreased compliance, or increased airway resistance), neurogenic or psychogenic causes. The weak, elderly, malnourished patient is going to have a difficult time maintaining this level of minute ventilation.
- *Capability* is reflected by the patient's drive to breath and muscle performance i.e. respiratory rate, tidal volume, forced vital capacity, negative inspiratory force and rapid shallow breathing index.

• **Weakness versus fatigue:** is your patient weak or fatigued?

Weakness is a decreased capacity of a rested muscle to perform a task.
Fatigue is a reversible decrease in the ability of a muscle (diaphragm in this case) to contract caused by over-activity and will reverse with simple rest periods.

Once a patient has been identified as "difficult to wean," it is imperative to formulate a weaning schedule. A couple of rules:

o Post the plan for everyone to see
o Do not change the plan until it is determined it is not working!
o Document the patients progress daily
o Communicate with everyone involved, especially the patient!

What are my options?

o T-Piece trials
o Pressure support trials
o SIMV/pressure support trials

Although more labor intensive, T-Piece trials have advantages over the other two options. A T-Piece trial permits periods of work and then rest, it is easy to assess if the patient is actually making progress and the patient will notice that they are actually doing better. It is imperative that the patient "rest" in between each trial and rest at night. Resting is not guaranteed with pressure support and should be done with a full ventilator support mode.

Practical Algorithm(s)/Diagrams

PRE-EXTUBATION AIRWAY ASSESSMENT RECORD

Individual Completing Pre-Extubation Airway Assessment Record: _____

Indication for intubation: _____

Location where intubation was performed: ☐ ICU   ☐ Pre-hospital   ☐ Ward   ☐ Other Facility
                                             ☐ E.D.   ☐ OR   ☐ Other

     Was intubation described as difficult: ☐ Yes   ☐ No

     Total # of intubation attempts: _____   Complication(s): _____

Modality Utilized for Intubation Technique (check all appropriate):   ☐ Laryngoscope   ☐ Bougie
     ☐ Glidescope   ☐ Fiberoptic   ☐ Surgical airway   ☐ Laryngeal Mask Airway

---

If intubated in operating room: (Preanesthetic evaluation form and Intraoperative anesthesia record)

Pre-operative Evaluation: I. Mallampati Score _____   II. Mandible _____   III. ROM/C-Spine _____

Was patient easy to Bag-Mask Ventilate? ☐ Yes   ☐ No   (2-person, use of oral airway, poor seal)

CLINICAL EXAMINATION – "LEMON" ASSESSMENT METHOD

L – Look externally for characteristics known to cause difficult laryngoscopy (check all that apply):

     Face   ☐ small jaw   ☐ edema   ☐ loose teeth   ☐ facial hair

                      ☐ promnent teeth   ☐ disfiguring of jaw   ☐ difficult bag/mask   ☐ facial fractures

     Thorax/abdomen   ☐ pregnancy   ☐ massive ascites   ☐ morbid obesity

E – Evaluate the 3-3 rule *(image at right):*

     Mouth opening – 3 finger breadths   ☐ Yes   ☐ No

     Thyro-mental distance – 3 finger breadths   ☐ Yes   ☐ No

M – Mallampati score *(image at right)*

     Mallampati Class _____ (I, II, III, IV)

O – Obstruction

     ☐ Tumor   ☐ Congenital defects (Downs, Goiter, Pierre-Robin Syndrome) ☐ Other defects _____

N – Neck mobility

     Is patient in C-Collar   ☐ Yes   ☐ No   ☐ Halo or Cervical traction   ☐ Yes   ☐ No

     Can the patient move their jaw forward   ☐ Yes   ☐ No   ☐ Unable to assess

     Can patient fully bend/extend head and neck ☐ Yes   ☐ No   ☐ Unable to assess

---

RISK FACTORS FOR DIFFICULT MASK VENTILATION (check all that apply)

"MOANS" ASSESSMENT

M – Mask Seal   ☐ beard   ☐ small mandible   ☐ facial trauma

O – Obesity/Obstruction   ☐ BMI > 26   ☐ Mallampati ≥ 3

A – Age   ☐ > 55 years

N – No teeth   ☐

S – Snores/ Stiff lungs   ☐ snoring history   ☐ stiff lungs

Fig. 1.   The Denver Health Medical Center pre-extubation airway assessment record.

Review of Current Literature with References

- Among respiratory variables, Yang and Tobin found the rapid shallow breathing index (henceforth referred to as the "Tobin" index) to be the most accurate predictor of successful extubation in an original cohort of 100 medical ICU patients (*New Engl J Med* 1991; **324**: 1445–1450).
- The most recent Cochrane Review of early vs. late tracheostomy concluded that there was still insufficient evidence to favor one strategy over the other (*Cochrane Database Syst Rev* 2012; **14**; 3: CD007271).
- Girard *et al.* reported that a protocol of daily interruption of sedation and assessment for appropriate liberation from mechanical ventilation resulting in improved outcomes as compared to standard of care (*Lancet* 2008; **371**: 126–134).
- Both the Society for Critical Care Medicine (www.sccm.org) and the American College of Chest Physicians (www.chestnet.org) maintain updated online guidelines for discontinuation of mechanical ventilation.

Chapter 6-(v)

Acute Respiratory Distress Syndrome

*Jeffrey L. Johnson, MD**

*Acute Care Surgeon, Denver Health Medical Center,
Associate Professor of Surgery, University of Colorado School of Medicine

Take Home Points

- Adult respiratory distress syndrome (ARDS) is the manifestation of an inflammatory injury to the Alveolar-Capillary interface. It has many underlying causes, and is best thought of as a spectrum of disease.
- The clinical picture of ARDS includes hypoxemia refractory to oxygen, diffuse patchy pulmonary infiltrates and decreased pulmonary compliance.
- The pathophysiology of ARDS includes noncardiogenic pulmonary edema, infiltration of alveoli by inflammatory cells, loss of type II pneumocytes, and impaired pulmonary vasomotor function.
- The injured lung in ARDS is markedly heterogeneous. Different zones of alveoli can be characterized by four types: flooded/collapsed, recruitable, open, and overdistended.
- Strategies to open alveoli and keep them participating in gas exchange are pivotal in managing patients with severe ARDS. These may include

Contact information: MC 0206, 777 Bannock Street, Denver, CO 80204; Email: Jeffrey. Johnson@dhha.org

"recruitment" maneuvers, strategic use of PEEP, optimal sedation/analgesia, and optimal positioning (including prone).

- Fluid strategies that maintain euvolemia are optimal in a patient with ARDS.
- The only therapy proven to improve mortality in ARDS is an approach to mechanical ventilation that limits stress (tidal volume) and strain (pressure) on the lung.
- Prone ventilation consistently improves gas exchange and may improve outcome in ARDS. The optimal frequency and duration of prone ventilation is not clear.
- High frequency oscillation is ineffective as a ventilator strategy in adults with ARDS.

Background

- ARDS is a life-threatening condition that affects about 5% of patients in a surgical ICU. It was originally described as a constellation of symptoms and signs, including dyspnea, hypoxia, and panlobar pulmonary infiltrates on plain radiographs.
- Common risk factors for ARDS in surgical patients include shock, transfusion, multiple trauma, infection, aspiration and pulmonary contusion.
- We now understand that ARDS represents an autotoxic injury to the pulmonary capillary/alveolar interface. This results in flooding of alveoli, recruitment of leukocytes, and loss of pulmonary epithelium. The inflammatory injury to the lung in ARDS may be an engine for systemic inflammation and multiple organ failure, promoting systemic injury, and subsequent damage to kidneys, liver and other organs.
- Injury to the lung during ARDS occurs in a predictable, progressive phases including the exudative phase (inflammation/injury/edema), proliferative phase (inflammation/repair), and finally fibrosis.
- The modern ("Berlin") definition of ARDS improves on the 1992 (AECC) definition by standardizing the concept of "acute" onset, clarifying the importance of predisposing factors and acknowledging that volume overload and ARDS can co-exist. It divides ARDS into three severities, by oxygenation, using PO_2 to FiO_2 ratio (P/F), namely <100, 100–200, and 201–300.
- While the inflammatory nature of ARDS is widely acknowledged, pharmacologic strategies to limit inflammation have been uniformly disappointing, with the possible exception of systemic corticosteroids in select patients.
- Ventilator strategies historically used in ARDS to improve gas exchange were recognized to produce barotrauma — both overt (such as pneumothorax/

pneumomediastinum) and subtle (persistent or unremitting inflammation). The existence of ventilator-induced lung injury (VILI) is now well-established. The main components are strain and stress. Strain is from overall airway pressure effects on the structure of the lung, and stress is from the repetitive opening and closing of air units that are partially flooded.

- At the same time that VILI was being elucidated, the heterogeneous nature of ARDS, with lung regions ranging from irreparably flooded to overdistended, promoted strategies that would both open collapsed alveoli ("recruitment maneuvers") and keep them open with positive end-expiratory pressure (PEEP).

- The current strategy for mechanical ventilation incorporates both the above ideas: optimize the number of alveoli participating in gas exchange, but limit the amount of damage produced by positive pressure ventilation. This low-stretch (tidal volume ≤6 cc/kg ideal body weight), limited pressure (plateau airway pressure ≤30 mm H_2O), moderate PEEP approach is the only proven way to limit the mortality from ARDS.

- High frequency oscillation (HFO) seems attractive as an approach to ARDS, since in some ways it represents an ultra-low tidal volume, limited pressure moderate PEEP approach. Clinical trials have not borne this out as an effective strategy in adults, with the most recent trial being stopped early with some evidence of harm. HFO cannot be recommended as a routine strategy in adults with ARDS.

- Prone positioning has several promising features in terms of optimizing the amount of lung participating in gas exchange. First, gravity helps to reverse dependent (dorsal) flooding of the lungs. Second, the "weight of the heart" may be taken off the basilar segments of the left lower lobe. Third, ventilation to dorsal lung regions is improved in the prone position, while perfusion is maintained, producing better matching between ventilation and perfusion.

- Since alveolar flooding is central to the pathogenesis of ARDS, it makes intuitive sense that limiting fluid administration/promoting diuresis is of benefit. That being said, it is not necessarily hydrostatic forces that underpin pulmonary edema in ARDS, and there may be some risk to hypovolemia, particularly in surgical patients. The best trial examining the benefits of limiting volume in patients with ARDS suggests there are modest benefits in terms of ventilator days and length of ICU stay, but no mortality benefit. For the surgical intensivist, this can be incorporated as yet another reason to maintain euvolemia and avoid overzealous administration of fluids.

Main Body

- The Berlin definition can be recommended as a standard way of defining whether an individual patient has ARDS. Recognition of ARDS in its early phases promotes early application of "lung-protective" ventilator strategies, a reminder to use fluids judiciously, and an expectation of a difficult course.
- It is critical to make a best determination about the cause of the ARDS; in surgical patients, in particular, one must be diligent about searching for sepsis (pneumonia? Intra-abdominal complication?). Since there is no definitive therapy — only best supportive care — reversing the underlying cause of ARDS is of utmost importance. Furthermore, since surgical patients may need secondary insults (subsequent operations including fracture fixation), optimal timing of these interventions are worthy of some discussion so as not to exacerbate the underlying condition.
- Initial patient care should include the following:

  o Analgesia and anxiolysis that promotes excellent interface with the ventilator. Since many of these patients will have prolonged courses of mechanical ventilation, the advantage of very short acting agents would appear less. Neuroleptics or atypical antipsychotics can be recommended for patients with agitated delirium. Our practice is to use standing doses of quetiapine with haloperidol for acute agitation. Medications that produce reliable effects with minimal hemodynamic compromise are preferred. For that reason, our practice is to use infusions of lorazepam and fentanyl.

  o Neuromuscular blockers should be considered for patients with severe hypoxemia (p/f <100), or who continue to interface poorly with the ventilator despite the above. Routine use of neuromuscular blockers cannot be recommended.

  o While there are advantages to sedation "holidays" in many patients, those with severe ARDS should be considered outliers in whom even transient loss of participating lung units may be undesirable. Simply put, it is hard to get back "lost" alveoli in these parts, and the approach must be individualized.

  o *Avoidance* of factors that exacerbate intraabdominal hypertension, including gastric overdistension, colonic pseudo-obstruction, volume overload, uncontrolled ascites, and Trendelenburg position. Intraabdominal hypertension increases the pressures (read "strain") needed to inflate the lungs.

  o Drainage of substantial pleural effusions. Simply put, this can quickly provide some additional functional residual capacity for the lungs. If diuresis can promote resolution of effusions, this is a reasonable initial approach to the patient with mild disease.

o Empiric administration of antimicrobials when infection is suspected as an underlying cause and after appropriate culture material is sent.

- Initial ventilator management in the patient with ARDS should approximate:

o Pick a ventilator mode that achieves full ventilator support with a predictable tidal volume, minute volume and plateau pressure, since these are the critical variables you will need to follow. In particular, modes that are machine triggered, volume cycled and flow limited tend to be quite practical; Assist/Control has many advantages in this regard and has no clinical disadvantage over other modes.

o Tidal volumes ≤6 cc/kg ideal body weight. This should be decreased in small increments if plateau pressures remain >30; increase respiratory rate to maintain minute volume. Respiratory rates >32 tend to promote auto-PEEP due to inadequate exhalation time and cannot be recommended. In these circumstances, permissive hypercapnia should be utilized.

- Remove as much dead space between the ventilator circuit and the trachea as possible (e.g. minimal length adaptor between circuit and endotracheal tube). At extremely low tidal volumes (<4 cc/kg IBW or about 300 cc), even a small amount of dead space (30 cc) can be a significant part of each breath (10%). This may get you 2–3 Torr in improved PCO_2.

- Ignore PCO_2 per se; allow it to rise.

- Shift focus to management of arterial pH. Tolerance to acidosis varies widely. Elderly patients and patients with other organ dysfunctions may be at higher risk. If pH < 7.20 OR patient exhibits organ dysfunction in association with acidemia (e.g. bradycardia, hypotension, oliguria), use the following strategies to maintain pH:

⇨ Infusion of bicarbonate (2 ampules of sodium bicarbonate in 1 liter of D5w, with initial rate of 100 cc/hr).

⇨ Infusion of THAM. This can provide excellent buffering with lower volumes and avoidance of further CO_2 production but is not universally available.

⇨ Continuous renal replacement therapy, particularly in the part with volume overload or oliguria.

o Plateau pressures ≤ 30. This is dependent on a number of other variables including ventilator modes, flow rates, flow waveforms, I:E ratios and patient factors.

- ○ PEEP ≥5. Subsequent PEEP should be adjusted either to a predetermined scale based on FiO_2 requirements (ARDS Net approach), or individualized to the physiology of a particular patient. The latter requires experience and close observation, and is practiced by our group. The overall approach is as follows:

  - Perform a recruitment maneuver. Conceptually, this is "opening up" gas exchange units that are temporarily flooded. In mild disease and with experienced hands, this might be something as simple as hand ventilation with a bag-valve, or transient ventilation at higher tidal volumes. For more advanced disease, we can recommend the following:

    - ⇨ Use a time-cycled, machine triggered mode with the frequency set at 12 and an I:E of 1:1 (often called a "pressure control" mode). Conceptually this provides long, slow breaths.
    - ⇨ Set the PEEP at 10–20 above current PEEP, and use a pressure limit that produces a tidal volume of about 12 cc/kg IBW (approaching one liter for an adult). This may be as little pressure as 10 or as much as 40, depending on the pulmonary and chest wall compliance.
    - ⇨ Keep in mind that during this maneuver, the minute volume delivered is likely to be substantially less than what the patient requires. Expect the patient to become acutely more hypercapneic and acidemic. This may be unwise in patients with intracranial hypertension or marginal hemodynamics. In any event, should the patient's heart rate or blood pressure drop substantially, it is time to stop the maneuver.
    - ⇨ Also bear in mind that the mean airway pressure being delivered is probably substantially higher than baseline. Patients who are hypovolemic may develop hypotension that requires cessation of the maneuver. A modest volume challenge followed by a repeat attempt might be in order.
    - ⇨ It is not uncommon for patients to have transient desaturation during the early part of the maneuver followed by substantial improvement. Be prepared for this by deciding what level of desaturation you are willing to tolerate in an individual patient. Patients who do not respond within three minutes are unlikely to respond.

  - Patients who respond to recruitment should be placed on baseline PEEP +2.5 additional cm H_2O. Conceptually, this is "keeping open" air units that have been recruited. Most patients with ARDS have an optimal PEEP in the range of 10–15.

- Recruitment should be repeated in patients who respond, until they no longer respond. Conceptually, this is when the lungs have been optimally recruited, and the main goal is to keep them recruited through PEEP (now higher and presumably optimal) and adjunct measures.

- For patients with severe ARDS in whom the required FIO_2 is ≥ 0.80 despite pleural drainage, neuromuscular blockade and recruitment, we would recommend ventilation in the prone position.

  o It is very possible that some patients with less severe ARDS benefit from earlier prone positioning, yet predicting who will respond to prone positioning remains difficult.

  o Whenever possible, place the patient prone BEFORE they are desaturating on 100% FIO_2. In this circumstance, it becomes a dangerous, desperation maneuver as opposed to a planned therapeutic intervention.

  o Before placing the patient in the prone position, consider the following:

    - Do I have the right equipment? (padding for torso, pillow for face/ventilator tubing, appropriate bed; table for the head if desired) ICU beds designed specifically for prone positioning are helpful but do not eliminate this step.
    - Are there any lines or tubes that should be put in or removed PRIOR to placing the patient prone?
    - Any wound care or appliance problems that can be anticipated?
    - Do I have enough people? This is a team effort. And in the unusual circumstances where patients respond poorly, it is best to have plenty of enthusiastic helpers.

  o If prone positioning seems ineffective, perform a recruitment maneuver in the prone position.

  o If the patient responds, leave them prone for 8–12 hours, then supinate. This limits facial/tongue/corneal edema which can be both unpleasant for visitors and problematic for the patient. In general, try to execute changes in position during times of high staff availability (read "daytime"), as these tend to be periods of high lability for the patient.

Review of Current Literature with References

- For an outstanding description of the rationale behind the Berlin definition of ARDS, and its advantages over the American-European Concensus Conference definition, the practitioner will want to review the paper by Ferguson *et al.*[1] In brief, it crystallizes the concept that ARDS is a spectrum of a disease, and eliminates the idea that acute lung injury is a separate entity. It clarifies the definition of acute, and provides for situations where left atrial hypertension and ARDS may coexist.

- The pathophysiology of pulmonary inflammation in ARDS is nicely described in two recent papers, that describe the interaction between endothelium, alveolar epithelium, and the leukocytes which are thought to deliver the autotoxic insult.[2,3] Understanding the four different potential zones in the lung injured by ARDS is pivotal for optimal ventilator management. With this in mind, the strategy of prone positioning may improve gas exchange by providing better aeration to dorsal regions of the lung without significantly impacting perfusion, thus improving v/q mismatch.[4]

- For an overview of the concepts of VILI, the reader is referred to a paper by Gattinoni *et al.*,[5] which outlines the concept of stress and strain, with their biomechanical underpinnings. Lastly, it is clearly worth reviewing the ARDSnet papers which solidified the survival advantage of a minimal pressure, low stretch strategy.[6]

1. Ferguson ND, Fan E, Camporota L et al. The Berlin definition of ARDS: an expanded rationale, justification, and supplementary material. *Intensive Care Med.* 2012; **38**(10): 1573–1582. doi:10.1007/s00134-012-2682-1.

2. Matthay MA, Ware LB, Zimmerman GA. The acute respiratory distress syndrome. *J Clin Invest.* 2012; **122**(8): 2731–2740. doi:10.1172/JCI60331.

3. Lucas R, Verin AD, Black SM, Catravas JD. Regulators of endothelial and epithelial barrier integrity and function in acute lung injury. *Biochem Pharmacol.* 2009; **77**(12): 1763–1772. doi:10.1016/j.bcp.2009.01.014.

4. Guérin C, Reignier J, Richard J-C et al. Prone positioning in severe acute respiratory distress syndrome. *N Engl J Med.* 2013; **368**(23): 2159–2168. doi:10.1056/NEJMoa1214103.

5. Gattinoni L, Carlesso E, Caironi P. Stress and strain within the lung. *Curr Opin Crit Care* 2012; **18**(1): 42–47. doi:10.1097/MCC.0b013e32834f17d9.

6. Kallet R. What is the legacy of the national institutes of health acute respiratory distress syndrome network? *Respir Care* 2009; **54**(7): 912–924. Available at: http://www.ingentaconnect.com/content/jrcc/rc/2009/00000054/00000007/art00010. Accessed on January 27, 2013.

Chapter 6-(vi)

Pleural Space and Mediastinum

Daine T. Bennett, MD* Robert A. Meguid, MD, MPH[†]
John D. Mitchell, MD[‡] and Michael J. Weyant, MD[§]

[*]*Surgical Resident, University of Colorado School of Medicine*
[†]*Assistant Professor of Surgery, University of Colorado School of Medicine*
[‡]*Professor of Surgery, University of Colorado School of Medicine*
[§]*Associate Professor of Surgery, University of Colorado School of Medicine*

Take Home Points

- Not all pleural effusions require drainage. Dependent effusions less than 10 mm by ultrasound frequently resolve without intervention.
- In management of a complex pleural effusion, any of the three following criteria mandate decortication: (1) Purulent fluid at the initial thoracentesis; (2) Multiloculated fluid collection with evidence of a pleural peel; or (3) Failure to improve with fibrinolytic therapy.
- Retained hemothorax after trauma, not adequately drained after initial tube thoracostomy, should be managed with thoracoscopic/video-assisted thoracic surgery (VATS) drainage in patients who can tolerate surgery.

Contact information: University of Colorado Denver, Anschutz Medical Campus, Division of Cardiothoracic Surgery, 12631 East 17th Ave, MS 310, Aurora, CO 80045; Email: daine.bennett@ucdenver.edu, robert.meguid@ucdenver.edu, john.mitchell@ucdenver.edu, michael.weyant@ucdenver.edu

245

- Early VATS drainage has been shown to reduce cost, hospital length of stay and duration of tube drainage when compared to second tube thoracostomy for retained hemothorax.
- Descending necrotizing mediastinitis is a rare entity typically presenting after oropharyngeal/cervical infections or cervical trauma. It must be considered in patients with neck swelling and elevated inflammatory markers.
- Delay in diagnosis and inadequate drainage are the main causes of mortality from descending necrotizing mediastinitis.
- Diagnosis of descending necrotizing mediastinitis is confirmed by presence of fluid collections/abscesses on computed tomography (CT) scan. Treatment is with immediate administration of broad-spectrum antibiotic coverage and surgical debridement of the neck and mediastinum. Delay in diagnosis and treatment can have disastrous effects.

Background

- Under normal physiologic conditions, each pleural space produces approximately 5–10 ml/kg of body weight per day of fluid which is easily resorbed.
- 40% of pneumonia cases are accompanied by pleural effusion with 5% of these resulting in a complex effusion or empyema frequently requiring surgical intervention.
- Complicated pleural effusion develops in three phases: (1) Sterile effusion due to inflammation; (2) Fibropurulent phase with bacterial contamination; and (3) Organizational phase with fibroblasts creating a thick lining. Once the effusion has reached the organizational phase, surgical debridement will be necessary.
- Retained hemothorax can result in empyema or fibrothorax if not evacuated promptly or adequately.
- Descending necrotizing mediastinitis is diagnosed by neck swelling, elevated inflammatory markers and radiologic evidence. The diagnosis is confirmed by necrotizing tissue identified intraoperatively.

Main Body

Complex pleural effusion/empyema

- Not all effusions require drainage. The first step in management is evaluation of the size of the pleural effusion by ultrasound. Dependent effusions <10mm by ultrasound frequently resolve spontaneously and should be managed expectantly.

- If larger than 10 mm, the effusion should be drained by thoracentesis. Pleural fluid with pH <7.2 or glucose <60 ng/dL is considered infected. If infected by these criteria, a tube thoracostomy is necessary with bacterial cultures of the effusion obtained and antibiotics started.
- If the initial thoracentesis reveals frank purulence, the patient should be taken to the operating room for decortication.
- If the effusion is not adequately drained within 24 hours of tube thoracostomy, a CT scan is obtained to evaluate the thoracic cavity. Imaging demonstrating an established pleural peel or multiloculated empyema mandates immediate decortication.
- For retained effusions less than 3 days old and without a pleural peel, fibrinolytic therapy is indicated with tPA and DNase administration twice daily for three days through the thoracostomy tube (see review of current literature below). However, failure to improve the effusion within 24 hours of starting fibrinolytic therapy necessitates decortication.
- Decortication is indicated for the following scenarios: (1) Frank purulence at the time of initial thoracentesis; (2) Evidence of a pleural peel with associated multiloculated empyema; and (3) Failure to improve with fibrinolytic therapy.
- VATS approach is preferred to open decortication when feasible. If open decortication is necessary, a posterolateral muscle-sparing thoracotomy is preferred.

Hemothorax

- Traumatic hemothorax is initially treated with tube thoracostomy at the time of presentation to the hospital. Patients with initial evacuation of >1500 mL of blood or >200 mL/hr for 4 hours should be considered for immediate thoracotomy for management of ongoing bleeding.
- Retained hemothorax in the stable patient after initial management with tube thoracostomy can result in empyema or fibrothorax, prolonging hospital stay and complicating patient management.
- Retained hemothorax can initially be treated with a second tube thoracostomy. However, the failure rate of this management strategy is high: about 50% of patients will require surgical evacuation. This management approach should be reserved for small hemothoraces and patients unfit for surgery.
- In patients with larger retained hemothoraces who are acceptable surgical candidates, evacuation of the hemothorax with VATS is preferred. VATS technique is less invasive than open thoracotomy and allows for faster recovery. Management of retained hemothorax with VATS, instead of second tube thoracostomy, has been shown to reduce drainage duration, hospital length of stay and cost.

Mediastinitis

- The most common causes of mediastinitis are infections related to sternotomy incisions or esophageal perforations. A rarer entity, descending necrotizing mediastinitis (DNM), has a more subtle presentation and devastating outcomes if not managed promptly.
- DNM carries a mortality rate of 20–40%. DNM typically arises from an oropharyngeal or cervical infection. Presentation of DNM includes neck swelling, dysphagia and pyrexia. It is generally associated with elevated WBC and CRP. The most commonly involved organisms are *streptococcus* species and anaerobes.
- Diagnosis is confirmed by presence of neck and mediastinal fluid collections or abscesses identified on computed tomography. DNM is classified as follows: (1) Type I — localization to mediastinum above the carina; (2) Type IIA — extension from neck to anterior mediastinum; and (3) Type IIB — extension from neck to anterior and posterior mediastinum.
- Immediate treatment includes prompt administration of broad-spectrum antibiotics followed by surgical debridement. Cervical debridement and drainage is achieved with parallel, horizontal collar incisions down to infected tissue, leaving passive (Penrose) drains in place. The mediastinum is generally accessed through a right-sided anterolateral thoracotomy. All necrotic tissue is aggressively debrided and the pleural space and mediastinum is copiously irrigated with saline. The left side is avoided as the aortic arch may prohibit mediastinal debridement. After debridement thoracostomy tubes are placed in the mediastinum as well as apicoposteriorly in the pleural cavities.
- Postoperatively, the mediastinal tubes are irrigated with 1–2 liters of saline twice daily with drainage allowed through the pleural thoracostomy tubes. This is continued until pleural drainage is culture-negative for three consecutive days. In several studies, duration of drainage averaged 21 days with a range of 9 to 69 days. Antibiotics should be tailored to address sensitivities of the organisms involved.
- Serial CT scans are necessary to ensure all abscesses have been adequately drained. Undrained abscesses require further operative debridement.

Practical Algorithm(s)/Diagrams

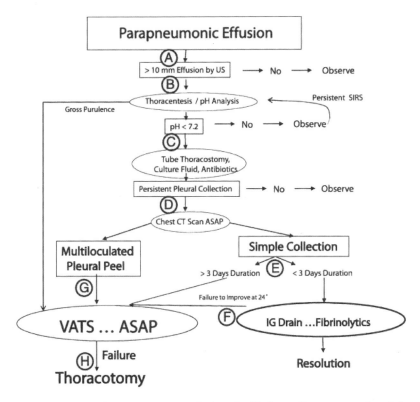

Fig. 1. Algorithm for management of pleural effusions. (Image reproduced from Moore *et al. J Trauma Acute Care Surg* 2012; **73**: 1372–1379).

Review of Current Literature with References

- The MIST2 trial was a multicenter randomized controlled trial of 210 patients published in 2011. It utilized a 2×2 factorial design where patients with an infected pleural effusion were given one of four treatments: double placebo, DNase plus placebo, t-PA plus placebo, or DNase plus t-PA. DNase (5 mg), t-PA (10 mg) or placebo were administered to the appropriate cohorts via thoracostomy tube twice daily, and the tube was clamped for 1 hour post-administration. In the DNase-t-PA group, the authors identified a statistically significant reduction in: (1) Hospital length of stay; (2) Referral for surgery; and (3)

Size of effusion relative to placebo. (Rahman *et al.* Intrapleural use of tissue plasminogen activator and DNase in pleural infection. *N Engl J Med* 2011; **365**: 518–526)

- DNM is a rare entity with mortality rates up to 40%. Iwata and colleagues describe their management of 10 patients experiencing 20% mortality. CT scan confirms diagnosis. Immediate broad-spectrum antibiotics and surgical debridement and drainage of both the neck and mediastinum are performed. Postoperatively, the mediastinum is irrigated daily with normal saline and drained via pleural thoracostomy tubes. Drainage is continued until pleural drainage is culture-negative for 3 days. (Iwata T *et al.* Early open thoracotomy and mediastinopleural irrigation for severe descending necrotizing mediastinitis. *Eur J of Cardio-thorac Surg* 2005; **28**: 384–388)

- Tong and colleagues retrospectively reviewed prospectively collected data from 420 consecutive patients undergoing VATS (326 patients) or open (94 patients) decortication. They evaluated outcomes between the groups in an intention to treat analysis with 11.4% conversion rate from VATS to open. The authors found the VATS group to have significantly shorter operative time and hospital length of stay. The VATS group also demonstrated significant reduction in prolonged air leak, ventilator dependence, number of tracheostomies, sepsis and 30-day mortality. (*Ann Thorac Surg* 2010; **89**: 220–225)

- Meyer and colleagues performed a prospective randomized trial of 39 patients comparing early VATS drainage (15 patients) to second tube thoracostomy (24 patients) in stable patients with retained hemothorax from trauma within 72 hours of initial presentation. They found a significant reduction in duration of tube drainage, hospital length of stay and hospital costs for patients undergoing early VATS drainage compared to management with second tube thoracostomy. Furthermore, 42% of patients failed management with second tube thoracostomy and ultimately required surgery. (*Ann Thorac Surg* 1997; **64**: 1396–1401)

7. Renal

Chapter 7-(i)

Acute Renal Insufficiency and Failure

Max Wohlauer, MD*

*Surgical Resident, University of Colorado School of Medicine

Take Home Points

- Although comprising 2% of the body's mass, the kidneys receive 25% of cardiac output.
- Acute renal failure (ARF), also called acute kidney injury (AKI), remains a major clinical challenge.
- AKI is characterized by the loss of the kidney's ability to eliminate waste, regulate acid base status, and regulate extracellular volume.
- Treatment is aimed at identification of high-risk patients and to treat underlying causes of renal dysfunction.

Background

- Acute kidney injury (AKI) is an abrupt decrease in renal function that leads to the buildup of nitrogenous waste and uremic toxins.
- AKI is an important complication of surgery and trauma with a high associated mortality.

Contact information: Denver Health Medical Center, 777 Bannock St., Denver, CO 80204; Email: Max.wohlauer@gmail.com

- AKI is defined as an elevation of serum creatinine of 0.5 mg/dL from baseline or need for acute renal replacement therapy.
- Glomerular filtration (GFR) is usually regulated between a wide range of systolic blood pressures (80–180 mmHg).
- GFR is used as an estimate of renal function and renal drug clearance. The Cockcroft-Gault estimates creatinine clearance and is frequently used to calculate the GFR. Patients with Stage IV CKD (estimated GFR <30 mL/min/1.73 m^2) should consider initiating hemodialysis or undergoing renal transplantation. Additionally, many medications need to be dose-adjusted with GFR <30.
- Three classifications of acute renal failure: pre-renal, renal, and post-renal.
- Despite availability of renal replacement therapy (RRT), mortality in the critically ill population exceeds 60%. Although many advocate for continuous hemofiltration, others have shown intermittent hemodialysis (HD) to be less expensive and more effective.

Main Body

- Classification of AKI:
  - Pre-renal: low cardiac output, decreased intravascular volume, renal vascular disease.
  - Renal: glomerulonephritis, acute tubular necrosis (ATN), acute interstitial nephritis (AIN), hemolytic uremic syndrome (HUS), embolism, trauma.
  - Post-renal: obstruction of ureter, bladder, or urethra.
- Other scenarios:
  - Hepatorenal syndrome (HRS): acute renal failure in the setting of liver impairment usually due to cirrhosis. Systemic vasodilation leads to profound renal vasoconstriction. HRS is multifactorial and thought to be related to activation of the renal-aldosterone-angiotensin system in response to hypotension. These patients often have severe hyponatremia, volume overload, and low urine sodium concentration (<10 mEq/L).
  - Rhabdomyolysis: When muscle is damaged, a protein pigment called myoglobin is released into the bloodstream. This compound is normally filtered out of the bloodstream by the kidneys; however, in large amounts myoglobin may block the structures of the kidney, causing damage resulting in acute tubular necrosis or kidney failure. Following injury, damaged muscle tissue may lead to an excessive amount of myoglobin and other cellular breakdown products to be released into the bloodstream.

This process is often compounded by a shock state and reduced blood flow to the kidneys. Early and aggressive hydration may prevent kidney damage by rapidly flushing myoglobin out of the kidneys. In severe cases, rhabdomyolysis may lead to acute tubular necrosis or acute renal failure and patients may need hemodialysis. Management includes fluid resuscitation to maintain adequate urine output and treatment of the underlying cause; there is no role for alkalization of the urine in treatment of rhabdomyolysis.

o   Contrast-induced nephropathy (CIN): Serum creatinine usually peaks three days post-injury and returns to baseline in seven days, although the injury is sometimes irreversible. Several techniques are in use to prevent CIN; however, there are no compelling data to support routine use of any medication in preventing contrast nephropathy. Studies suggest that N-actetylcysteine may help reduce the severity of contrast nephropathy.

o   Drug-induced AKI: Drugs are an important contributor nephrotoxicity in the surgical ICU. Patients are maintained on medications at home that may be nephrotoxic (i.e. cyclosporine, tacrolimus). Antibiotics are a common culprit. Aminoglycosides (i.e. gentamycin) are nephrotoxic and penicillins can cause AIN. Drugs with renal excretion. Vancomycin is excreted in the urine and can reach toxic concentrations in renal insufficiency. Concentrations of nephrotoxic drugs should be closely monitored and dose-adjusted according to GFR.

- Lab tests and diagnostic work-up: Serum creatinine, urinalysis, fen, creatine kinase, urine eosinophils for AIN, renal ultrasound, and renal biopsy.
- Management: Identification of high-risk patients may help the physician prevent AKI via close monitoring of volume status to prevent hypovolemia and avoiding contrast agents and other nephrotoxins. Early identification and treatment remains the hallmark of treating AKI. Treatment of prerenal causes of AKI, i.e. in trauma, stopping the hemorrhage will help restore intravascular volume, as will resuscitation from septic shock. A CT scan ordered during a trauma workup, or antibiotics ordered for treatment of sepsis can lead to intrinsic renal injury in the aforementioned patients; however, highlighting the complexities of AKI management. AKI that leads to anuria requires renal replacement therapy, which will be discussed in a separate chapter.

Practical Algorithm(s)/Diagrams

Prerenal (Hypovolemia)	Renal (Vascular)	Postrenal (Obstruction)
Diuretics	Trauma	Renal calculus
GI losses	Renal vein thrombosis	Tumor causing ureteral, urethral, or bladder obstruction
Evaporative losses (burns)	Acute tubular necrosis (ATN)	Ligation during surgery
Hemorrhage	Microangiopathy	Obstructed urinary catheter
Decreased CO (CHF, PE, MI)	Transplant rejection	Retroperitoneal fibrosis
Hepatorenal syndrome	Atheroembolism	Prostatic hypertrophy
	Acute interstitial nephritis (AIN)	

Fig. 1. Classification of AKI.

RIFLE CRITERIA

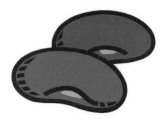

RISK: 50% INCREASE IN SERUM CREATININE
INJURY: 100% INCREASE IN SERUM CREATININE
FAILURE: 150% INCREASE IN SERUM CREATININE, OR >
12 HRS OF ANURIA
LOSS: > 4 WEEKS REQUIRING HD
END-STAGE: PERMANENT LOSS

Fig. 2. RIFLE Criteria.

Review of Current Literature with References

- A randomized controlled trial of 83 patients with chronic renal insufficiency evaluated the role of acetylcysteine in protecting against contrast nephropathy. Ten out of the 83 patients (12%) developed contrast nephropathy, 1/41 (2%) in the acetylcysteine group compared to 9/42 (21%) of patients in the saline-only control group ($p = 0.01$). The authors concluded that prophylactic oral administration of acetylcysteine (600 mg twice daily the day before and on the day of contrast agent administration, when coupled with IV saline administration) prevented contrast nephropathy, although this should be taken with a grain of salt due to the small sample size (Tepel M, van Der Giet M, Schwarzfeld C, Laufer U, Liermann D, Zidek W. Prevention of radiographic-contrast-agent-induced reductions in renal function by acetylcysteine. *N Engl J Med* 2000; **343**: 180–184).

- Role of loop diuretics in oliguric AKI: Cantarovich *et al.* performed a randomized control trial evaluating the role of furosemide in AKI. The concept of converting oliguric AKI to non-oliguric AKI is appealing because of several reasons including: (1) loop diuretics protect the loop of Henle from ischemia via inhibition of the Na^+-K^+-$2Cl^-$ pump in the loop of Henle and (2) inducing polyuria may help treat volume overload in this high-risk patient population. Although in this study, high doses of the loop diuretic helped to maintain urine output, it did not improve survival or hasten renal recovery (Cantarovich F, Rangoonwala B, Lorenz H, Verho M, Esnault VL. High-dose furosemide for established ARF: a prospective, randomized, double-blind, placebo-controlled, multicenter trial. *Am J Kidney Dis* 2004; **44**: 402–409).

- A single institution retrospective review of 2,157 trauma patients investigated the prognostic significance of early AKI. The authors showed that early AKI, with a prevalence of 2%, had a strong association with the development of MOF. The majority of the 154 renal failure cases (82%) evolved to MOF. Isolated kidney failure on day 2 (creatinine >1.8 mg/dL) was a rare event, but when it occurred, renal failure had a very high likelihood of progression to MOF (Wohlauer MV, Sauaia A, Moore EE, Burlew CC, Banerjee A, Johnson J. Acute kidney injury and posttrauma multiple organ failure: the canary in the coal mine. *J Trauma Acute Care Surg* 2012; **72**: 373–378; discussion 379–380).

- Determining the time to initiate dialysis has been a topic of considerable interest lately, and studies have shown that early initiation of dialysis is associated with improved outcomes. A multicenter prospective observational study evaluated 98 patients undergoing major abdominal surgery who developed AKI requiring renal replacement therapy (RRT) found that patients who underwent RRT earlier in their course [RIFLE 0 and R, early dialysis (ED)] had improved outcomes compared to patients initiating dialysis after the kidney injury who had progressed to injury or failure [RIFLE I-F, late dialysis (LD)]. Although serum creatinine and albumin levels were not statistically different between ED and LD groups upon ICU admission and before RRT initiation, the study is limited due to small sample size and possibly selection bias (Shiao CC, Wu VC, Li WY *et al.* Late initiation of renal replacement therapy is associated with worse outcomes in acute kidney injury after major abdominal surgery. *Crit Care* 2009; **13**: R171).

Approach to the Anuric/Oliguric Critically Ill Surgical Patient

Robert T. Stovall, MD*

*Assistant Professor of Surgery, University of Colorado School of Medicine

Take Home Points

- Oliguria should be approached in the context of the entire patient and situation — NEVER in isolation.
- Oliguria has been defined in multiple ways.
- Renal failure does not always present with oliguria.

Background

- Urine output is a commonly followed clinical parameter for information related to volume status as well as perfusion.
- Urine output may also be followed as a surrogate of kidney function.
- While a critical component of overall patient assessment, urine output must always be interpreted in the context of the overall patient situation.

Contact information: Denver Health Medical Center, University of Colorado Health Sciences Center, 777 Bannock Street, MC 0206, Denver, CO 80204; Tel.: 303-436-4029, email: robert.stovall@dhha.org

Main Body

Definition

- Anuria — virtual absence of urine output for six hours.
- Oliguria
    - <400–500 ml urine output/24 hours
    - <0.5 ml urine/kg/hour over two hours (This is usually KG of ideal body weight as its utility is lost for larger patients).

Causes of oliguria

- Categorized into three broad categories for clinical convenience:
    - pre-renal, intra-renal and post renal
- Pre-renal causes
    - Common in the SICU
    - Anything that decreases perfusion to the kidney
        - Shock — all types
        - Hypovolemic States
            - ⇨ Hemorrhage
            - ⇨ GI losses
        - Congestive Heart Failure
        - Decompensated liver cirrhosis
        - Renal artery issues
            - ⇨ Stenosis
            - ⇨ Aortic Dissection occluding renal artery
        - Hepato-renal syndrome or other drug or neuro-humeral parameters affecting normal renal auto regulation (NSAIDS, ACE-I, etc.).
- Intra-renal causes
    - Intrinsic renal pathology
        - Sequelae of shock
        - Ischemia Reperfusion
        - Contrast Nephropathy
        - Acute tubular necrosis (ATN) reportedly common in ICU patients; however this pathologic finding is not consistently found when the clinical diagnosis is given.

- Other drugs toxic to the kidney
- Acute interstitial nephritis (AIN) — often from drugs given in ICU
- Myoglobinuria
- Multiple Organ Failure
- Vasculitis
- Malignant Hypertension
- Abdominal Compartment Syndrome may affect the kidney via pre-intra or post-renal mechanisms but cannot be forgotten
- Other more chronic issues exacerbated in the ICU

- Post-renal causes (obstructed outflow)
  o Iatrogenic
    - Injured ureter or ureters intra-operatively
    - Foley occlusion
  o Renal stones causing obstruction
  o Papillary necrosis
  o Prostatic Obstruction of the urethra
  o Other Urethral/ureteral obstruction (strictures/masses)

Work-up of oliguria

- Full history and physical exam should be the first step of the evaluation as oliguria cannot be assessed in isolation.
  o Review recent events, baseline renal function, all medications administered, vitals: current and past, contrast studies, evaluate or place a Foley catheter
- Labs
  o Consider CBC, Chemistries, urine electrolytes, urinalysis with microscopy
  o CBC may suggest anemia or ongoing inflammatory process
  o Electrolytes (simultaneous serum and urine) can suggest pre-renal or not pre-renal but not perfect
    - Fractional excretion of sodium (FENa)
      ⇨ The sodium clearance divided by the creatine clearance
      ⇨ ((Urine sodium/Plasma sodium)// (Urine Cr/ Plasma Cr)) × 100
      ⇨ FENa < 1 suggests prerenal
      ⇨ Not perfect, some major limitations exist

⇨ In the setting of diuretics fractional excretion of urea (FEUrea) may be more useful.
— (FEUrea) = (SerumCr*UUrea) / (SerumUrea × UCr) %
— Has limitations but
   ✓ FEUrea <35% consistent with prerenal
   ✓ FEUrea 50–65%consistent with ATN
⇨ Other molecules that have been used similarly are lithium and uric acid.

- Suggesting Pre-renal Cause
   ⇨ FENa <1%
   ⇨ Urine Sodium <20 mEq/L
- Suggesting Intra-renal cause
   ⇨ FENa >2%
   ⇨ Urine Sodium >40 mEq/L

o Urinalysis (UA) with microscopy
   - Tubular epithelial cells and epithelial cell casts suggests ATN.
   - WBC casts suggest AIN.
   - Positive Hansel Stain (urinary eosinophils) suggests AIN but not highly sensitive; needs to be requested separately.
   - Hyaline casts suggest pre-renal cause.
   - Specific gravity is more likely to be high in pre-renal causes.
   - Pigmented casts suggests myoglobinuria.

- Imaging
   o Renal Ultrasound
      - Evaluation for dilated ureters or a very distended bladder that suggests post-renal cause of oliguria/anuria.
      - Resistive indices may support intra-renal causes.

Initial management of oliguria

- Identifying and correcting underlying cause is the most important component of management and is necessary to prevent further injury.
- Goal of fluid supplementation should be to optimize euvolemia and avoid over or under resuscitation.
- Specific treatments will depend upon the ultimate diagnosis.

Commonly used medications associated with renal injury (not a comprehensive list)

- Aminoglycosides
- Amphotericin B
- Flouroquinolones
- B-lactam antibiotics
- Sulfonamides
- Vancomycin
- Carbamazepine
- Phenobarbital
- Phenytoin
- NSAIDS
- Furosemide
- Thiazides
- Acetazolamide
- Acetaminophen
- Contrast Dyes
- Ranitidine
- Some chemotherapuetic agents
- Certain immunosuppressant medications
- Angiotensin-converting enzyme inhibitors/ARBs

Practical Algorithm(s)/Diagrams

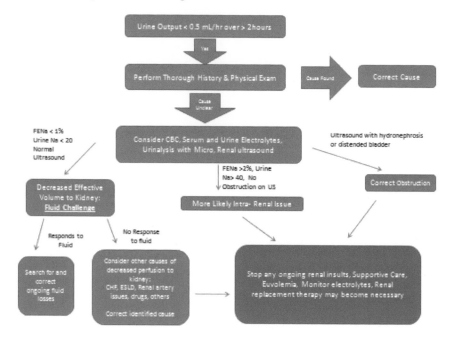

Fig.1.   Approach to oliguria.

Review of Current Literature with References

- Prowle JR, Liu YL, Licari E *et al.* Oliguria as predictive biomarker of acute kidney injury in critically ill patients. *Crit Care* 2011; **15**(4): R172.

  - Prospective review of relationship between oliguria and the development of Creatinine defined renal failure. 239 patients in multiple centers. Oliguria was significantly associated with the occurrence of new acute kidney injury but most episodes of oliguria were not followed by renal injury. They felt that the occurrence of short periods (1–6 hr) of oliguria lacked utility in discriminating patients with incipient kidney injury. They did note that oliguria accompanied by hemodynamic compromise or increasing vasopressor dose may represent a clinically useful trigger for other early biomarkers of renal injury.

- Bellomo R, Kellum JA, Ronco C. Acute kidney injury. *Lancet* 2012; **380**(9843): 756–766.

  - Review article from pathophysiology to renal replacement therapy.

- McBride WT, Gilliland H. Acute Renal Failure. *Surgery* 2009; **27**: 11.

  - Review article on perioperative renal failure.

Chapter $7-\left(\dot{\dot{\dot{i}}}\right)$

Renal Replacement Therapy

Talia Sorrentino, MD* and Fredric M. Pieracci, MD, MPH[†]

*Medical Student, University of Colorado School of Medicine
[†]Acute Care Surgeon, Denver Health Medical Center

Take Home Points

- Patients with life-threatening complications from acute kidney injury (AKI) should receive renal replacement therapy (RRT).
- Patients at high risk for these complications should also receive RRT, before signs and symptoms of AKI manifest.
- Although the decision to initiate RRT is ultimately clinical, it is generally accepted that a blood urea nitrogen (BUN) concentration of 80 to 100 mg/dL mandates initiation of RRT.
- Venovenous access is the preferred modality in any circuit.
- In deciding between continuous renal replacement therapy (CRRT) and intermittent hemodialysis (IHD), current data do not support the superiority of one over the other.

Contact information: (Talia Sorrentino) 12631 E. 17th Ave, MCC302, Aurora, Tel.: 303-902-6096, CO 80045; (Fredric M. Pieracci) 777 Bannock Street, MC 0206, A388, Denver, CO 80206; Email: taliasorrentino@gmail.com; Fredric.Pieracci@dhha.org

- Multiple factors, including resource availability, specific patient needs, and local expertise, ultimately guide the decision-making process regarding RRT.

Background

- In 1954, the Nobel Prize in Medicine was awarded to Dr. Joseph Murray, American plastic surgeon, for performing the first human kidney transplant.
- In normal physiology, the kidneys function to control fluid, electrolyte, and acid-base balance.
- In the setting of severe AKI [Chapter 7-(i)], RRT provides supportive therapy, thereby promoting renal recovery.
- AKI is a spectrum of disease ranging from subclinical injury to failure.
- On average, 7% of all hospitalized patients develop AKI.
- This number increases significantly to 36–67% in the critically ill, and is associated with in-hospital mortality rates exceeding 50%.
- Seventy percent of patients with AKI will require RRT of some form.
- Mortality of patients who require RRT is 50–70%.
- Multiple modalities of RRT exist, including IHD, CRRT, mixed therapies, and organ transplantation.
- The various modalities of RRT can be categorized based upon (1) access — arteriovenous, venovenous, or peritoneal; (2) what moves — solute versus volume; and (3) the degree of interruption — intermittent versus continuous.

Main Body

Key concepts of RRT

- The various modalities of RRT (listed below) can be simply categorized based on:
    - access — arteriovenous (AV), venovenous (VV), peritoneal dialysis (PD)
    - what moves — solute versus fluid (dialysis versus filtration)
    - the degree of interruption — intermittent versus continuous
- List of Modalities
    - Intermittent hemodialysis (IHD)
    - Continuous venovenous hemofiltration (CVVHF)
    - Continuous arteriovenous hemofiltration (CAVHF)
    - Continuous venovenous hemodialysis (CVVHD)
    - Continuous arteriovenous hemodialysis (CAVHD)

- o Slow low-efficiency dialysis (SLED)
- o Slow-continuous ultrafiltration (SCUF)
- Access
  - o Arteriovenous access is rarely used due to its reliance on the patient's vascular pressures to generate a gradient, as well as the need for arterial cannulation and the associated risks of arterial thrombosis, embolism, bleeding and limb ischemia [Chapters 5-(vii) and 15].
  - o Venovenous access is both the safest and most commonly used technique in the clinical setting. VV does not rely on the patient's pressure and instead uses an external pump to generate the pressure gradient necessary for solute and water removal.
- Solute and Fluid Removal
  - o Hemodialysis (HD) removes solutes such as urea, potassium, phosphate, creatinine, and toxins.
  - o Hemofiltration (HF) is used predominately to remove fluid in the setting of volume overload. Although fluid removal is part of the treatment goal, HF requires the patient to receive some replacement fluid.
  - o Hemodiafiltration (HDF) represents a combination of dialysis and filtration and incorporates the benefits of both. HDF will not specifically be addressed in this chapter, though it should be noted that by adjusting dialysate, and countercurrent flow rates, the degree of fluid and solute removal can be individually titrated.
- Intermittent versus Continuous Therapy
  - o Intermittent therapies such as IHD and PD have the advantage of rapidly correcting large metabolic disturbances (a few hours), and thereby freeing the patient from extracorporeal devices during the interim.
  - o The concept behind CRRT is to achieve more physiologic solute clearance over an extended time-period, thereby minimizing wide metabolic or volume shifts.
  - o CVVH is the most commonly used modality of CRRT in the acute care setting.
- Definitions: Diffusion and Convection
  - o *Diffusion* is the movement of solutes from an area of higher concentration to an area of lower concentration.
  - o *Convection* relies on a transmembrane pressure gradient to drive water across a semipermeable membrane, *dragging* both small and large molecular weight solutes dissolved in the fluid.

o *Dialysate* is a specially formulated solution containing electrolytes and minerals such as potassium, calcium, and bicarbonate. The concentrations of each solute are determined such that by diffusion of solutes across a semipermeable membrane, the patient's blood more closely resembles normal physiologic blood.

o A *flow-driven system*, such as intermittent HD, uses high dialysate flow-rates (>800 ml/min) to maximize the concentration gradient on either side of the semipermeable membrane at any given moment.

o A *pressure-driven system*, such as in HF, uses a high transmembrane pressures (hydrostatic pressure) to push large volumes across the membrane. These pressures are generated either by mechanical pumps, or the patient's blood pressure as in AV systems.

o *Solvent drag* refers to transport of solute particles small enough to pass through the filter pores in pressure-driven systems such as HF.

o *SLED* is an intermittent technique that uses faster flow-rates than continuous modalities, but is run for less than 12 hours per day.

o *SCUF*, like HF, uses convection to clear solutes but generates lower ultrafiltrate volumes than HF, which typically do not need to be replaced.

Hemodialysis versus hemofiltration: Mechanisms

- The driving force in HD is *diffusion* of solutes down their concentration gradients from higher concentration to lower concentration solutes. Thus, the limiting factor in HD is the *size* of the solute; larger molecules will diffuse across the semipermeable membrane, but only at a much slower rate than smaller molecules.

o Large: albumin, inulin, tumor necrosis factor
o Medium: glucose, uric acid, creatinine, phosphate
o Small: urea, potassium, phosphorus, sodium

- Advantages of HD include rapid solute and volume removal (per-minute solute clearance), thus it is most useful in the setting of hemodynamically stable patients with hyperkalemia, or toxin ingestion.
- The main disadvantage HD is hypotension, which occurs in 20–30% of all HD treatments, and is caused by rapid solute and volume removal. This can result in renal hypoperfusion and delayed return of function.
- In contrast to IHD, CVVH accomplishes large volume filtration without major adverse effects on hemodynamic status. HF utilizes convection, thereby mimicking the function of the glomerulus. Conceptually this means that the concentration of solute on either side of the membrane is the same, while

volume is pushed across the filter, carrying with it dissolved solutes. Due to the slow, continuous solute drag, CVVH more closely approximates physiological clearance. For the above reasons, CVVH is of considerable use in ICU patients who are often hemodynamically unstable.

- Pressure, determined by flow rate, is the determining factor of effective volume removal in HF. Because an extracorporeal pump generates the pressure necessary for HF, the risk of hypotension is considerably reduced with CVVH.
- However, CVVH is not without its disadvantages. The filter is prone to clotting, and thus requires anticoagulation.

Indications for CRRT and clinical considerations

- Indications for CRRT:
  - o oliguric renal failure with associated hemodynamic instability
  - o severe academia without a clear and quickly reversible cause
  - o electrolyte disturbances (hyperkalemia)
  - o ingestion (toxins)
  - o volume overload (iatrogenic fluid resuscitation, intravenous medication administration, congestive heart failure)
  - o uremia
  - o multiorgan failure
  - o hypercatabolism
  - o sepsis and SIRS, even in the absence of acute renal failure (removal of inflammatory cytokines may improve outcomes, though the data is limited).

- Specific Clinical Considerations and Modality of Choice
  - o Head injury or cerebral edema — CRRT due to decreased association with wide swings in cerebral perfusion pressure.
  - o The current data do not show a long-term survival benefit for CRRT over IHD. Instead, the benefits are demonstrated in short-term outcomes including renal recovery and length of stay.
  - o Data do not support the superiority of any particular mode of RRT in patients with AKI.
  - o The availability of specific resources greatly influences the practical use of the various modalities. HD requires a trained nurse. CVVH requires hourly attention from nursing staff. CRRT machines are expensive and not ubiquitously available.

   o RRT can be discontinued when renal function returns as evidenced by urine production, even if serum creatinine levels are still elevated.

Dosing

- In IHD, the "delivered dose" is equal to Kt/V, where K is the clearance of urea, t is dialysis time, and V is the volume of distribution of urea (approximated by total body water, TBW).
- With respect to dosing of RRT, IHD should be provided three times per week, alternating days, with a goal delivery of a Kt/V of ≥1.2 per treatment.
- If using CRRT, the delivered effluent rate (HF rate + dialysate flow rate) should be ≥20 ml/kg/hr.
- The Nephrology care team is a valuable resource in managing complex patients requiring CVVH. However, the primary team should understand the basic goals of therapy; for example, maintaining euvolemia verses net negative fluid balance. This can best be reported through hourly and daily goals for fluid removal (i.e. 60 ml/hr for a total of 1.5 L removed by CVVH per day).

Practical Algorithm(s)/Diagrams

Table 1. Diagnostic classification and staging of AKI: RIFLE and AKIN criteria.

RIFLE Criteria	Serum Creatinine	GFR*	Urine Output	AKIN Criteria***
Risk	1.5-fold increase	25% decrease	<0.5 ml/kg/hr for >6 hr	Stage 1
Injury	2-fold increase	50% decrease	<0.5 ml/kg/hr for >12 hr	Stage 2
Failure	3-fold increase	75% decrease	<0.5 ml/kg/hr for >24 hr; or anuria for >12 hr	Stage 3
Loss	Complete loss of kidney function for more than 4 weeks.			
ESRD**	Complete loss of kidney function for more than 3 months.			

*Glomerlar Filtration Rate
**End-Stage Renal Disease
***Acute Kidney Injury Network Criteria

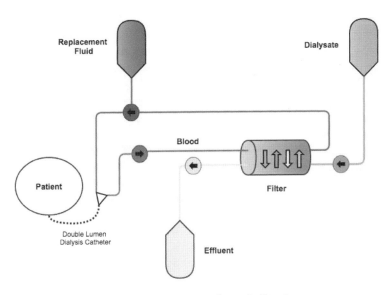

Fig. 1. Continuous venovenous hemodiafiltration set up.

Blood from the patient is run countercurrent to the dialysate. At the filter, solutes and fluids are exchanged across the membrane according to their respective concentration gradients and transmembrane hydrostatic pressure. Excess fluid and waste products are drawn off as effluent. The filtered blood mixes with a physiologic replacement fluid to account for the volume removed.

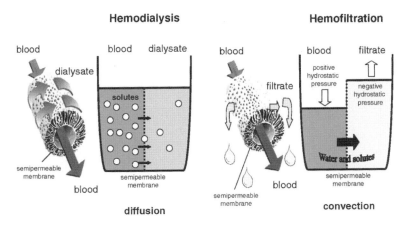

Fig. 2. Hemodialysis versus hemofiltration.

Hemodialysis and hemofiltration differ mechanistically. Hemodialysis uses diffusion, allowing high concentration solutes in the patient's blood to passively cross a semipermeable membrane into the dialysate. In contrast, hemofiltration uses positive hydrostatic pressure to drive both water and solutes across a semipermeable membrane, thereby clearing both using convection (John, Stefan and Eckardt, Kai-Uwe. CHEST 2007; 132, 4).

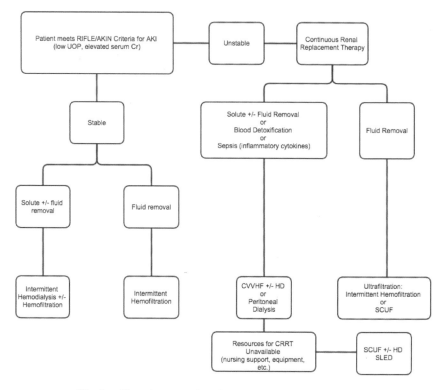

Fig. 3. Choosing a renal replacement modality decision tree.

Hemodynamically stable patients with acute kidney injury can be treated with intermittent modalities, using either hemodialysis for solute removal, or hemofiltration for fluid removal. Hemodynamically unstable patients requiring solute, toxin, or cytokine removal should receive continuous venovenous hemofiltration (CVVHF), or continuous peritoneal dialysis if access is established. If the resources for CVVH are otherwise unavailable, slow continuous ultrafiltration (SCUF) or slow low-efficiency dialysis (SLED) settings can be used instead.

Review of Current Literature with References

- The CONVINT trial is a single-center prospective randomized control trial that randomized critically ill patients with ARF to either continuous or intermittent HD (n = 252). They found no difference between study groups with respect to their primary and secondary endpoints, including 14-day, 30-day-, ICU-, and intrahospital mortality, as well as course of disease severity/biomarkers and need for organ-support therapy (Scheforld *et al. Crit Care* 2014; **18**, R11).

- On review of a 17-year trauma database, Denver Health's group noted that the develop-ment of AKI in trauma patients is significantly associated with multiorgan failure (incidence 78%) and mortality (27%). Furthermore, they noted that these data exceeded those associated with early heart, lung or liver failure (Wohlauer *et al. J Trauma* 2011; **72**, 2).
- PICARD study demonstrated an increased risk of death associated with initiation of RRT with a BUN >76 mg/dL in comparison to <76 mg/dL, showing that earlier initiation of RRT is better (Mehta *et al. Kidney International* 2004; 66).
- Suggested Reading: Liu F, Mehta R. Chapter 52. Continuous Renal Replacement Therapy. In: Lerma EV, Berns JS, Nissenson AR. eds. *CURRENT Diagnosis & Treatment: Nephrology & Hypertension.* New York, NY: McGraw-Hill; 2009. http://accessmedicine.mhmedical.com.liboff.ohsu.edu/content.aspx?bookid=372&Sectionid=39961194. Accessed October 20, 2014.

Chapter 7-(iv)

Electrolytes

Daniel Lollar, MD*

* Fellow, Trauma and Acute Care Surgery, Denver Health Medical Center

Take Home Points

- Evaluation of acid/base status begins with pH. The pCO_2 reflects the contribution of volatile acid (respiratory response). The serum bicarbonate and base deficit reflect alterations in fixed acids (metabolicresponse).
- Evaluation of metabolic acidosis begins with determination of the anion gap. Anion gap acidoses are caused by excess accumulation of acids (lactic acid, urea); non-anion gap acidoses are caused by increased production/accumulation of chloride or decreased excretion of bicarbonate.
- Evaluation of metabolic alkalosis begins with assessment of urine chloride (U_{Cl}). Chloride sensitive alkalosis ($U_{Cl} < 20\,mEq/L$) reflects chloride loss due to gastrointestinal or renal wasting and should be treated with normal saline fluid repletion. Chloride resistant alkalosis ($U_{Cl} > 40\,mEq/L$) can be caused by diverse physiology but can be categorized into normotensive versus hypertensive etiologies.

Contact information: Denver Health Medical Center, University of Colorado Health Sciences Center, 777 Bannock Street, MC 0206, Denver, CO 80204; Email: daniel.lollar@ucdenver.edu

- Calculation of the appropriate compensatory response to a given acid/base problem helps identify deviations from a predicted compensation. This practice prevents overlooking a second derangement or mixed process (Fig. 1).
- A mixed acid base disorder must be suspected with a normal pH but abnormal anion gap or bicarbonate level. For instance, salicylate toxicity is marked by a lactic acidosis combined with a respiratory alkalosis frequently resulting in a normal pH.
- Always check the anion gap and serum chloride concentration in every critically ill patient with a metabolic acidosis. This practice will avoid unnecessary and potentially dangerous volume expansion.
- A thorough evaluation of hyponatremia requires four pieces of information: the serum osmalarity, the urine osmolarity, the urine sodium, and the overall fluid status.
- Hyperkalemia can be a life-threatening disorder, as a widened QRS complex signals impending ventricular dysrhythmias. This should be recognized and treated immediately with administration of calcium chloride 1–2 g IV to stabilize cardiac myocyte membranes and 20 mg of inhaled albuterol to shift potassium out of plasma and into cells. Concomitant administration of insulin 10 units and dextrose 50 g both IV and sodium bicarbonate are also useful modalities.
- Hypercalcemia with symptoms of altered mentation or seizures should be treated with fluid resuscitation and loop diuretics such as furosemide. Severe hypocalcemia with symptoms of altered mental status or tetany should be treated with IV calcium supplementation. Calcium chloride via central venous line is the most efficient means of calcium repletion in the emergency scenario.

Background

- Homeostasis requires the excretion of acid produced by physiologic processes. Excretion of fixed acid is accomplished by the kidneys in the form of bicarbonate while volatile acids are excreted through the lungs in the form of carbon dioxide.
- Physiologic pH is accomplished by multiple buffering agents including the bicarbonate system, albumin, phosphate, hemoglobin and other weak acids.
- The Henderson-Hasselbach Equation, $pH = pKa + \log([HCO_3^-]/[pCO_2] \times 0.0301)$, describes the relationship between the metabolic and respiratory components.

- The kidney handles changes in fixed acid via three mechanisms: resorption of filtered bicarbonate, creation of bicarbonate and excretion of ammonium (NH_4^+).
- The anion gap represents the unmeasured anions in plasma, and an elevated anion gap indicates increased amounts of acid anions, produced endogenously or absorbed exogenously. Under normal situations, albumin contributes most significantly to the anion gap.
- L-lactic acid is produced from the anaerobic metabolism of pyruvate in tissue beds. Lactic acidosis accounts for 60% of anion gap acidoses in the ICU and can be of two types. Type 1 is due to increased production of lactate, most frequently from either global hypoperfusion (shock) or locally ischemic tissue beds (e.g., myonecrosis). Type 2 lactic acidosis is due to decreased clearance of lactate from the blood, typically due to impaired liver function.
- Anti-diuretic hormone (ADH) increases water reabsorption in the collecting ducts and distal convoluted tubule by increasing the number aquaporin channels thus decreasing the loss of free water. ADH is potently stimulated by dehydration and hypernatremia.
- The Na/K ATPase exchange pump moves 3 Na^+ ions outside the cell for 2 K^+ ions into the cell. This difference creates a voltage gradient in excitable tissue such as nerve and muscle.
- Potassium is exchanged for hydrogen ions via the H^+/K^+ exchanger on the cellular membrane. Thus, excess serum hydrogen ions (acidosis) will be brought into the cell in exchange for potassium ions. As a result, the body protects itself from the detrimental effects of acidosis in exchange for hyperkalemia. Conversely, alkalosis will decrease hydrogen/ potassium exchange and produce plasma hypokalemia.
- Potassium excretion is determined by flow of filtrate to the distal nephron and maintenance of the negativity of filtrate by the epithelial sodium channel (ENaC). Decreased flow of filtrate simulates the renin-angiotensin axis. Aldosterone secretion causes sodium retention and potassium wasting.

Main Body

- Acidosis
  - o The diagnosis of acidosis is made with an arterial blood gas showing a pH level less than 7.40. Respiratory acidosis is diagnosed by a low pH in conjunction with a $pCO_2 > 40$. Metabolic acidosis is diagnosed by a low pH in conjunction with a $pCO_2 < 40$. A low bicarbonate level or elevated anion gap aid in the diagnosis of a metabolic acidosis.

o Each patient is only allowed one metabolic disturbance (either acidosis or alklalosis) and one respiratory disturbance (either acidosis or alkalosis). That is, a patient cannot have both a respiratory acidosis and respiratory alkalosis at the same time. By contrast, a patient *may* have both a metabolic acidosis and respiratory alkalosis.

o Anion gap is calculated as $[Na] - ([Cl] + [HCO_3])$. A value of 9 ± 3 is considered normal. The anion gap must be corrected for the albumin level as every decrease of 1.0 (g/dL) from a normal albumin decreases the normal value for the anion gap by 2.5. Failure to do so will result in misinterpretation of an anion gap acidosis as a non-anion gap acidosis in the hypoalbumenemic patient. For example, a patient with an uncorrected anion gap of 9 and a serum albumen concentration of 2.0 (UNITS) has a corrected anion gap of 14.

o The three most common causes of non-anion gap metabolic acidosis in the surgical ICU are hyperchloremia, gastrointestinal loss of bicarbonate, and renal tubular acidosis. Hyperchloremic metabolic acidosis results from excessive administration of chloride-rich fluid, usually in the context of resuscitation. Failure to recognize this etiology of acidosis may result in misinterpretation, followed by additional administration of chloride rich-fluid, exacerbating the acidosis. This may be avoided by *always checking the anion gap and serum chloride concentration in every critically ill patient with a metabolic acidosis.*

o Simple respiratory acidosis should be compensated with an elevated bicarbonate level. In simple, acute respiratory acid-base disturbances, the pH changes by 0.08 for each change in pCO_2 of 10 mm Hg *in the opposite direction.* For example, a patient with a pH of 7.32 and a pCO_2 of 50 mm Hg has a simple respiratory acidosis. A pH < 7.32 in this situation suggests a superimposed metabolic acidosis. By contrast, a pH > 7.32 in this situation suggests a superimposed metabolic alkalosis (or chronic compensation of the respiratory acidosis). Another helpful relationship is that a normal compensation for an elevated pCO_2 is 1 mmol/L increase in bicarbonate for every 10 mmHg increase in pCO_2. For example, a patient with a pCO_2 of 60 mmHg should have a serum HCO_3^- concentration of approximately 20 mmol/L.

o Simple metabolic acidosis is initially compensated for by increasing ventilation and decreasing pCO_2 levels to create a relative respiratory alkalosis; however this compensation will never fully normalize the pH. The expected change in pCO_2 in the setting of a pure metabolic acidosis is expressed using the Winter's formula: expected $pCO_2 = 1.5(HCO_3^-) + 8 \pm 2$. Thus, a patient with a pH of 7.30 and a HCO_3^- of 10 would have an expected pCO_2 of 23 mmHg. An actual pCO_2 < mmHg would suggest a secondary respiratory alkalosis; whereas an actual pCO_2 > 23 mmHg suggests a superimposed respiratory alkalosis.

o Treatment of a metabolic acidosis involves treatment of the underlying cause. Typically this involves aggressive crystalloid resuscitation and disease specific interventions, e.g insulin administration for diabetic ketoacidosis, dialysis for severe uremia, etc.

o Respiratory acidosis up to a pH of 7.15 may be safely tolerated in order to manage plateau airway pressures in patients with Acute Respiratory Distress Syndrome and impaired ventilation. This strategy is termed permissive hypercapnea [chapter 5-(v)]. A pH below 7.15 should be managed with bicarbonate administration (typically sodium bicarbonate infusion) and vasopressors for cardiac instability.

• Alkalosis

o Alkalosis is identified by an elevated pH (>7.40). A lowered pCO_2 in the setting of a pH >7.40 indicates a respiratory etiology while an elevated bicarbonate concentration in the setting of a pH >7.40 indicates a metabolic cause.

o An elevated bicarbonate level can be caused by: (1) loss of hydrogen ions; (2) a gain of bicarbonate ions; or (3) a decrease in extracellular volume (contraction alkalosis). Metabolic alkaloses are typically asymptomatic though can be associated with other electrolyte abnormalities which may produce symptoms.

o The three most common causes of metabolic alkalosis in the surgical ICU are hypokalemia, gastrointestinal loss of acid, and volume contraction as a result of diuretic therapy.

o Initial evaluation of a metabolic alkalosis involves investigating the urine chloride level. In chloride-responsive alkaloses, a chloride deficient state (typically due to volume contraction secondary to diuretics, nasogastric tube suction or laxative abuse) impairs the resorption of bicarbonate in the distal collecting ducts.

o Chloride responsive alkalosis is best treated with fluid resuscitation with chloride-containing IVF (e.g normal saline.) To estimate chloride need, a chloride deficit is calculated by the formula 0.2 × weight (kg) × (100−[Cl]). The fluid required to meet this deficit is then calculated by the chloride deficit divided by the mEq/L of chloride in the fluid being administered (154 mEq/L in normal saline).

  o Patients with an elevated urine chloride (>40 mEq/L) have a "chloride resistant" alkalosis due to primary or secondary mineralocorticoid excess. This is typically associated with increased extracellular volume.

  o Chloride-resistant alkalosis management should initially begin with correction of associated hypokalemia. The carbonic anhydrase inhibitor acetazolamide is typically sufficient management if potassium replacement is insufficient. Very rarely, a dilute hydrochloric acid infusion is required to correct severe, refractory alkaloses.

  o The excess HCO_3 accumulated as a result of a metabolic alklalosis may serve as a helpful buffer to prevent the rapid development of a respiratory acidosis in a patient with deteriorating ventilation. For this reason, we do not routinely correct mild to moderation metabolic alkalosis (pH 7.40 – 7.60).

- Derangements of plasma sodium

  o Hyponatremia is the most common electrolyte abnormality in the surgical ICU and is caused by a relative increase in body water compared to plasma sodium concentration. Premenopausal women, children and hypoxic patients are most at risk for developing life-threatening hyponatremic encephalopathy despite sodium levels that may not be severely deranged.

  o Evaluation of hyponatremia begins by ruling out pseudohyponatremia: pseudohyponatremia exists when the absolute amount of sodium in the serum is unchanged, but there is an excess of water secondary to another osmotically active substance. The most common examples are glucose (hypergylcemia) and mannitol. In this case, the serum osmolarity will be normal. An approximate correction factor for hypergylcemia is that, for every increase in the serum glocuse level above 100 g/dL, 2.5 meQ/L can be addded to the serum sodium concentration. For example, the corrected serum sodium concentration for a patient with a serum sodium concentration of 130 mEq/L and a serum glucose concentration of 500 g/dL would be 140 mEq/L.

  o After pseudohyponatremia is ruled out, the urine osmolarity is checked; urine osmolairty < 100 mOsm/kg in the setting of hyponatremia is due to iatrogenic administration of hypotonic fluids in the surgical ICU patient (the most common cause of hyponatremia) or psychogenic polydipsia in the outpatient.

  o In patients with a low serum osmolality and normal to elevated urine osmolality, a combination of the total body volume status and urinary sodium concentration will categorize the remaining causes of hyponatremia.

    ▪ Hypervolemia indicates underlying organ dysfunction (congestive heart failure, cirrhosis or renal failure) as the causal problem.

- ▪ Euvolemic patients with a normal urine sodium (>25 mOsm/kg) have SIADH which can be caused by multiple etiologies including nausea, postoperative state, pain, or stress.
- ▪ Hypovolemic patients with a low urine sodium (<25 mOsm/kg) are dehydrated. In this case, the need to maintain volume status trumps the need to maintain eunatremia, and water is reabsorbed in response to increased ADH activity.
- ▪ Hypovolemia with a normal to high urine sodium (>25 mOsm/kg) is most commonly seen with cerebral salt wasting, a poorly understood sequellae of traumatic brain injury in which urinary reabsorption of sodium is impaired. Mineralocorticoid deficiency is another less common cause of hypovolemic hyponatremia.

o Symptoms of hyponatremia including seizures and respiratory arrest should be treated with a NaCl 3% bolus of 100 mL over 10 minutes. This can be repeated up to two times if necessary. In patients with severe symptoms such as prior seizure, lethargy, headache or nausea and vomiting or those treated with a bolus should be started on a NaCl 3% infusion at 1 mL/kg/hr. Asymptomatic patients should be treated with fluid unless felt to be hypovolemic. See Fig. 2.

o Hypernatremia is precipitated by excess free water losses in patients with impaired thirst mechanism or impaired water access. Common causes of hypernatremia include diuresis due to medications or hyperglycemia, gastrointestinal losses due to nasogastric suction or diarrhea, and insensible losses from the respiratory tract. Treatment consists of fluid resuscitation with either lactated ringers or half normal saline for serum sodium > 150 mEq/L. Free water needs are calculated by the free water deficit: $0.6 \times$ weight (kg) $\times$ ([Na] $-$ 140)/ 140. Correction should be gradual and should not exceed 1 mOsm/L/hr.

o In patients with hypernatremia, central diabetes insipidus should be ruled out as an underlying cause. This disease process is typically seen in patients with cerebral pathology including traumatic brain injury, pituitary surgery, and hemorrhagic stroke. The classic triad seen in diabetes insipidus is: (1) hypernatremia; (2) low urine osmolarity (<150 mOsm); and (3) polyuria. Treatment consists of DDAVP administration.

- Derangements of plasma potassium

o Potassium is predominantly intracellular and plasma levels represent only a small level of total body potassium. Due to the curvilinear relationship between plasma and total body potassium, twice as much total body potassium must be lost to decrease serum potassium levels for an equivalent increase in serum potassium versus increase in total body potassium.

o Serum potassium levels below 3.5 mEq/L can be due to acute shifting of potassium into cells thus decreasing plasma levels, or it may represent a true decrease in total body potassium due to renal or extrinsic causes.

o Transcellular movement of potassium into cells is precipitated by alkalosis, insulin, β2 agonists, and hypothermia. These agents are used to treat symptomatic or severe hyperkalemia. Treatment for transcellular hypokalemia involves treating the predisposing condition. Treatment for total body potassium depletion is potassium repletion typically with KCl though potassium phosphate is typically used for patients in diabetic ketoacidosis. It is important to ensure adequate magnesium stores before potassium repletion as hypomagnesemia prohibits effective repletion of potassium.

o Hyperkalemia is a much more dangerous condition than hypokalemia as it can precipitate cardiac arrhythmias. Before pursuing aggressive therapy, pseudohyperkalemia due to cell lysis in the blood sample must be excluded as it occurs in up to 20% of samples. When an unexpected, precipitous change in potassium is found, a repeat sample should be sent to confirm the finding.

o In contradistinction to transcellular hypokalemia, causes of potassium egress from cells include acidosis, β-blockers, medications (digitalis and succinylcholine) and insulin deficient states.

o Total body accumulation of potassium is due to failure to excrete potassium in the urine, typically as a result of impaired renal function. Adrenal insufficiency also causes impaired potassium excretion but hyperkalemia is only seen in chronic disease. Definitive removal of potassium involves potassium binding in the gut (kayexalate) and direct removal from the blood through hemodialysis.

- Derangements of divalent ions

o Magnesium deficiency is common in patients taking diuretics, having diarrhea, with diabetes mellitus and in chronic alcoholics. Hypomagnesemia can exacerbate cardiac irritability as it is "the body's calcium channel blocker." Magnesium should be replaced in IV form as it is poorly absorbed by the gut and precipitates diarrhea. Magnesium should be replaced in hypokalemic patients.

o Hypermagnesemia is uncommon but can be seen in renal failure and massive hemolysis. Levels above 5 mEq/L can affect cardiac conduction causing heart block and ventricular arrhythmias and should be treated with IV calcium and hemodialysis.

o Calcium is the most abundant electrolyte in the body but 99% is stored in bone. Half of plasma calcium is bound to proteins and therefore inert. Hypocalcemia may thus be due to low calcium levels or low protein (albumin) levels. Ionized hypocalcemia can be seen in sepsis, pancreatitis, renal failure, alkalosis and concomitant with blood transfusions. Calcium should be repleted orally or IV if severe. Calcium chloride is most effective for repletion but should only be used in emergency situations via a central venous catheter.

o Hypercalcemia is most commonly caused by cancer or hyperparathyroidism in non-ICU patients. Calcium levels above 12 mEq/L (or ionized calcium >3.0 mmol/L) or in symptomatic patients (altered mental status, EKG changes such as shortened QT interval) should be treated with volume expansion with normal saline and urinary calcium excretion with loop diuretics such as furosemide.

o Inorganic phosphate (PO_4) resides predominantly intracellularly and participates in glycolysis and ATP production. Dangerous hypophosphatemia can be seen in malnourished patients who receive abundant glucose administration. The movement of glucose into cells is accompanied by phosphate, thus leading to dangerously low plasma phosphate levels if total body phosphate is marginal. Treatment of this "refeeding syndrome" is aggressive phosphate repletion and gradual advancement of glucose administration (PO or IV) to goal in high-risk patients.

Practical Algorithm(s)/Diagrams

Condition	Expected Compensation/ Converison
Metabolic Acidosis	1 mmol/L ↓HCO_3 = 1 mmHg ↓pCO_2
(Winter's formula)	pCO_2 = 1.5 [HCO_3] + 8 ± 2
	pCO_2 ~ last two digits of pH
Metabolic Alkalosis	1 mmol/L ↑HCO_3 = 0.7 mmHg ↑pCO_2
Respiratory Acidosis (acute)	10 mmHg ↑pCO_2 = 1 mmol/L ↑HCO_3
Respiratory Acidosis (chronic)	10 mmHg ↑pCO_2 = 4 mmol/L ↑HCO_3
Respiratory Alkalosis (acute)	10 mmHg ↓pCO_2 = 2 mmol/L ↓HCO_3
Respiratory Alkalosis (chronic)	10 mmHg ↓pCO_2 = 4 mmol/L ↓HCO_3

Fig. 1. Work-up of acid/base derangements.

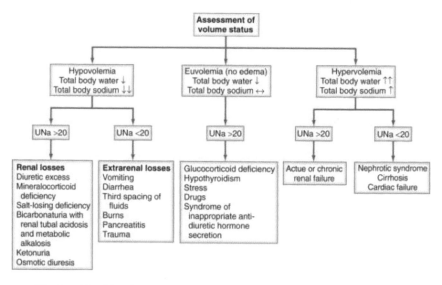

Fig. 2. Algorithm for evaluation of hyponatremia. UNa = urine sodium level.

Review of Literature

- In an observational cohort study, 209 patients were categorized based on the difference between prehospital anion gap and anion gap at ICU admission (ΔAG) by 5 point intervals. Logistic regression compared ΔAG with all cause mortality at 30, 90 and 365 days. A ΔAG of 5–10 correlated with an increased odds ratio of 30 morality of 1.56 while a ΔAG of >10 correlated with an increased odds of death of 2.18. These results indicate that an increase in anon gap of greater than 5 from prehospital to ICU admission predict the risk of all cause mortality in the critically ill.

  Lipnick MS, Braun AB, Cheung JT *et al.*, *Crit Care Med* 2013; **41**: 49–59.

- In a retrospective review of 300 critically ill ICU patients, base excess due to unmeasured anions and anion gap were compared in their ability to predict lactate levels. Logistic regression analysis showed a high degree of predictive ability in all three variables to predict a lactate level > 5 mmol/L. Confidence intervals were 0.78–0.94 for base excess, 0.78–0.93 for base excess due to unmeasured anions and 0.77–0.92 for anion gaps. However, when compared to the APACHE II score, none of these variables accurately predicted mortality.

  Rocktaeschel J, Morimatsu H, Uchino S *et al.*, *Crit Care Med* 2003; **31**: 2131–2136.

- In 2012, the relationship between pre-intensive care unit potassium levels were evaluated to see if an elevated potassium predicted mortality. Over 39,000 critically ill patients were evaluated in an observational study over a ten-year period. Patients were grouped into cohorts based on peak potassium levels the day of ICU admission. Logistic regression analysis examined mortality at multiple time points. The odds ratio for increased mortality was statistically significant at potassium levels greater than 4.5 but were highest for patients with a highest potassium level greater than 6.5 mEq/L (OR 1.72.) These data suggest that even modest elevations in a patient's potassium level at ICU admission is associated with increased mortality.

  McMahon GM, Mendu ML, Gibbons FK, Christopher KB, *Intensive Care Med* 2012; **38**: 1834–1842

- To determine if potassium repletion via continuous infusion was safe, 139 patients were enrolled in a randomized, open-label study comparing potassium repletion with a continuous infusion versus the typical bolus administration was performed in critically ill patients with serum potassium levels between 2.5 and 3.8 mmol/L. The primary outcome measured was the average difference in serum potassium levels over time. While the average serum potassium was statistically significant between the two groups by 0.22 mmol/L, this did not pre-determine level of treatment effect, calculated as 0.50 mmol/L. However, there were no adverse effects noted due to the continual infusion of potassium. This study suggests that repletion of mild to moderate hypokalemia can be safely and more effectively performed with a continuous infusion versus a standard bolus repletion practice.

Chalwin RP, Moran JL, Peake SL *et al.*, *Anesthesia Intensive Care* 2012; **40**: 433–441.

Chapter 7-(V)

Rhabdomyolysis

Edward L. Jones, MD* Teresa S. Jones, MD†
and Clifford A. Porter, MD‡

*Surgical Resident, University of Colorado School of Medicine
†Surgical Resident, University of Colorado School of Medicine
‡Assistant Professor of Surgery, University of Colorado School of Medicine

Take Home Points

- Rhabdomyolysis is injury of the skeletal muscle causing the release of intracellular components that can overwhelm elimination mechanisms. Myoglobinuria, electrolyte abnormalities and acute kidney injury (AKI) ensue.
- A high index of suspicion is required as rhabdomyolysis has numerous causes and often requires concomitant management of multisystem trauma (Table 1).
- The mainstay of treatment remains early and aggressive isotonic fluid resuscitation for a goal urine output between 2–3 cc/kg/hr to minimize renal injury.

Contact information: (Edward L. Jones and Teresa S. Jones) 12631 East 17th Ave, C313, Aurora CO 80045; (Clifford A. Porter) Denver Veterans Affairs Medical Center, Eastern Colorado Health Care System, 1055 Clermont St., Denver, CO 80220; Tel.: 303-399-8020, email: Clifford.Porter3@VA.gov; Teresa.jones@ucdenver.edu; edward.jones@ucdenver.edu

Background

- Rhabdomyolysis was originally described after crush injuries in World War II; however, in the civilian setting it can also be seen with prolong immobilization and illicit drug or alcohol use. Common examples of iatrogenic immobilization leading to rhabdomyolysis include prolonged neuromuscular paralysis during critical illness and during bariatric surgery in morbidly obese patients (Chapter 25).
- Rhabdomyolysis is diagnosed based upon history, physical exam and a serum creatine kinase (CK) level greater than five times the upper limit of normal (approximately 5000 IU/L).
- Up to 60% of patients with rhabdomyolysis will experience acute kidney injury via three major mechanisms: (1) volume depletion (hemorrhage, dehydration and necrotic skeletal muscle that can sequester up to 12L of fluid); (2) tubular obstruction by heme pigment deposition; and (3) direct tubular injury from free iron.
- Rhabdomyolysis should be considered whenever a compartment syndrome (especially in the lower extremity) is diagnosed. Alternatively, aggressive fluid resuscitation while treating rhabdomyolysis from other etiology can create a compartment syndrome.
- The mainstay of treatment is preservation of renal function which requires aggressive, isotonic fluid resuscitation for a goal urine output between 2–3 cc/kg/hr (200–300 mL/h). Urine alkalinization, forced diuresis and other adjunctive treatments have not proven beneficial in large studies unless patient presents evidence of acute kidney injury (Cr > 2.0 mg/dL).

Main Body

Pathology

- Skeletal muscle injury and necrosis results in the release of intracellular contents; including the compact heme-protein: myoglobin.
- Heme-proteins contain significant amounts of iron which is normally excreted by kidneys. However, when intra-tubule concentrations rise, they can be directly nephrotoxic and can also cause renal tubule obstruction. When combined with hypovolemia, significant renal injury can occur which often leads to associated electrolyte abnormalities (most commonly hyperkalemia, hypocalcemia and hyperphosphatemia).
- Rhabdomyolysis rarely occurs in isolation and the simultaneous management of concomitant trauma and organ dysfunction must also be done.

- High-risk populations include: morbidly obese, prolonged surgery, prolonged seizure activity, traumatic crush injuries, statin use, and illicit drug use.
- Recurrent episodes may be a sign of a defect in muscle metabolism.

Diagnosis

- History — rhabdomyolysis can often be diagnosed based upon history alone: recent trauma or exertional activity, prolonged immobilization and illicit drug or alcohol use are all possible causes of rhabdomyolysis.
    - o Common myotoxic medications may also lead to significant rhabdomyolysis: HMG-CoA reductase inhibitors (especially when used with nicotinic acid), cyclosporine, itraconazole, erythromycin, colchicine and corticosteroids.
- Common signs and symptoms:
    - o Pain, swelling, weakness or other signs of muscle injury (crush, elevated compartment pressures, etc.).
    - o Changes in urine: "tea-colored"
        - Myoglobin appears when it exceeds the renal threshold (>1.5 mg/dL on urinalysis, serum >100 mg/cL).
- Lab testing
    - o Creatine kinase (CK), (normal <100 IU/L)
        - No known threshold for increased AKI risk.
        - Rhabdomyolysis confirmed by CK > 5000 IU/L.
        - Follow every 4–6 hours until CK level peaks.
    - o Serum creatinine (Cr) — confirms renal injury but is non-specific.
    - o Myoglobinuria — often used as a qualitative test to confirm risk for rhabdomyolysis but not routinely followed. *Note: a urine dip that is positive for heme in the absence of RBCs on urinalysis is indicative of myoglobinuria (urine dip does not distinguish between hemoglobin and myoglobin).*
- Muscle biopsy — not recommended (diagnoses muscle necrosis but this is non-specific and does not change management).

Treatment

- Aggressive volume resuscitation to restore renal perfusion:
    - o Dilutes nephrotoxins.
    - o Restores renal tubule flow.

- o Treats concomitant hypovolemia which can be more injurious than the direct toxic effect of heme-proteins.
- o Isotonic fluids are recommended: normal saline or lactated ringers (LR has shown a small benefit over NS in patients with rhabdomyolysis secondary to doxylamine intoxication).
- o Goal: urine output 2–3 cc/kg/hr.

- Alkalinization of urine
  - o Myoglobin precipitates in an acidic environment; therefore bicarbonate use has theoretic benefit.
  - o Treat to goal urine pH > 6.5.
  - o Monitor arterial blood gases at least twice daily and be wary of both alkalosis and hypernatremia.
  - o Benefits of urine alkalinization have not been established in large trials but should be considered in patients presenting with, or with a history of, renal failure (Cr > 2.0 mg/dL).

- Mannitol (forced diuresis)
  - o Theoretically increases urine flow and tubule flushing.
  - o No randomized control trials: consider only in patients who are fluid replete as hypovolemia will worsen renal injury.

- Treat concomitant electrolyte abnormalities: most commonly hyperkalemia, hypocalcemia and hyperphosphatemia.

Practical Algorithm(s)/Diagrams

Table 1. Common causes of rhabdomyolysis

Hypoxic/Trauma	Exertional	Chemical	Genetic Defects	Infections
Burns/ Electrocution	Delirium Tremens	Statins/ Fibrates	Disorders of glycolysis/ glycogenolysis	Influenza A and B
Compartment			Disorders of lipid	
Syndrome	Extreme exertion	Alcohol	metabolism	Epstein-Barr virus
Prolonged	Hypo/	Heroin/	Mitochondrial	HIV
Immobilization	Hyperthemia	Cocaine	Disorders	
	Malignant	Electrolyte	Purine nucleotide	Legionella
Sickle cell trait	Hyperthemia	Derangement	disorders	
Trauma/Crush	Prolonged Seizure			Pyomuositis
Injury				
	Status asthmaticus			Clostridium
				Snake venom/ spider bites

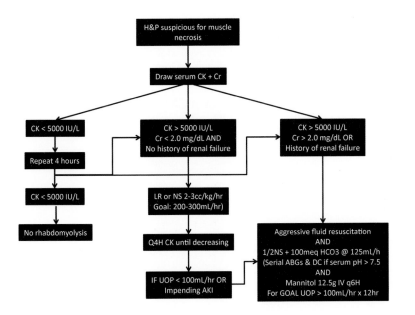

Fig. 1. Rhabdomyolysis algorithm.

Review of Current Literature with References

Review article

- Zimmerman and Shen published a review of the literate in *CHEST* in 2013. In particular, Tables 1 and 2 describe extensively the common causes and medications that are associated with rhabdomyolysis. They accurately describe the common treatment recommendations and lack of Level 1 data to guide practitioners. Zimmerman JL, Shen MC, Rhabdomyolysis. *CHEST* 2013; **144**(3): 1058–1065.

IVF resuscitation

- Cho *et al.* randomized 28 patients to LR vs NS resuscitation for doxylamine succinate induced rhabdomyolysis. This anticholinergic drug is used for insomnia and is seen in 25% of drug overdose patients in Korea. There was no difference in time to normalization of CK levels; however, patients resuscitated with NS did develop a metabolic acidosis and required more sodium bicarbonate to achieve urine alkalinization. Patients treated with LR did not develop significant hyperkalemia. Cho YC, Lim H, Kim SH, Comparison of lactated Ringer's solution and 0.9% saline in the treatment of rhabdomyolysis induced by doxylamine intoxication. *Emerg Med J* 2007; **24**(4): 276–280.

Role of diuretics

- Brown *et al.* looked at 2083 trauma admissions who had CK levels >5000 U/L. There was no difference in rates of renal failure, need for dialysis or mortality in patients who received bicarbonate and mannitol prophylactically and those who did not. Brow CV, Rhee P, Chan L, Evans K, Demetriades D, Velmahos GC, Preventing renal failure in patients with rhabdomyolysis: do bicarbonate and mannitol make a difference? *J Trauma* 2004; **56**(6): 1191–1196.

8. Gastrointestinal

Chapter **8-(i)**

Nutrition in the Critically Ill

Michael A. Maccini, MD* and Ernest E. Moore, MD[†]

*Surgical Resident, University of Colorado School of Medicine
*†Professor of Surgery and Vice-Chair of Surgical Research, University of Colorado
School of Medicine*

Take Home Points

- Nutritional assessment, support, and monitoring are essential in the care of the critically ill. Ongoing monitoring of the patient's nutritional status and appropriate adjustments to the nutritional regimen are essential.
- The physiologic stress of critical illness results in a complex hypercatabolic state and metabolic derangements which must be taken into account when estimating patients' nutritional requirements.
- The goal of nutritional support is to maintain positive nitrogen balance to attenuate loss of protein in the form of muscle mass.
- Generic nutrition goals should be 25 non-protein calories/kg per day and 2 g/kg protein per day, based on the patient's adjusted feeding weight. Further protein needs may result from additional external losses; e.g., open wound, hemodialysis, ascitic or lymphatic leak.

Contact information: (Michael A. Maccini) 777 Bannock St, MC 0206, Denver, CO 80204; (Ernest E. Moore) 655 Broadway, Ste. 365, Denver, CO 80203; Tel.: 303-602-1820, email: Ernest.moore@dhha.org; Michael.Maccini@dhha.org

- Enteral feeding should not be held for surgical procedures in mechanically ventilated patients (airway is already secure).
- Enteral nutrition is superior to total parenteral nutrition and should be initiated early in hospitalization.
- Total parenteral nutrition may be necessary if enteral nutrition is contraindicated, but is associated with an increased risk of complications. Patients on TPN require close monitoring for evidence of complications.
- Hyperglycemia should be minimized by ongoing monitoring and corrected in critically ill patients.

Background

- Patients with prolonged ICU stays are vulnerable to substantial protein deficits. Measurable loss of muscle mass has been documented in ICU patients within a few days. Weakness due to these deficits is associated with prolonged mechanical ventilation, and immunosuppression which increases the risk of infection.
- Critically ill patients have increased energy expenditures due to the hypermetabolic state resulting from underlying acute illness or injuries.
  - o Levels of stress hormones (cortisol, epinephrine, norepinephrine, glucagon, etc.) are elevated and increase systemic metabolic activity, including gluconeogenesis.
  - o In addition, increased levels of tissue necrosis factor (TNF), and other cytokines such as IL-1 and IL-6 increase systemic inflammation and, thus increases metabolic demands.
  - o Growth hormone and insulin-like growth factor 1 (IGF-1) are anabolic hormones whose levels are suppressed following injury, shifting the overall metabolic balance to catabolism and increasing the body's use of amino acids for gluconeogenesis.
  - o Finally, the central nervous system responds to afferent signals alerting it to injury by stimulating sympathetic "fight or flight" responses, resulting in further release of pro-inflammatory mediators and catecholamines via activation of the hypothalamic-pituitary-adrenal axis.
- Malnutrition in the critically ill is due to abnormal processing of nutrients. The objective of nutritional support in the ICU is to maintain muscle/protein mass by minimizing catabolism, with the goal of preserving as much functionality as possible. Without addressing the underlying injury and other

sources of inflammation, even adequate nutritional supplementation cannot preserve lean body mass.

Main Body

- Nutritional Assessment
  - o Accurate assessment of a patient's nutritional status and needs requires a history, physical exam, and interpretation of laboratory data.
    - *History of present illness* should include a list of the patient's current injuries with level of severity, which allows for estimation of the patient's level of physiologic stress. *Medical and surgical histories* provide a picture of the patient's baseline level of function, pre-existing conditions — including weight loss and other signs of malnutrition — and potential anatomic alterations that may affect nutrition administration. *Social history* provides information regarding a patient's drug and alcohol use, as well as a support network to aid in discharge planning once inpatient care is no longer required.
    - *Physical exam* should include an estimation of the patient's muscle mass, caloric reserves, and fluid status. Body Mass Index (BMI) is an important measure, as underweight and obesity are both forms of malnutrition affecting nutritional needs and interventions.
    - Pertinent *laboratory data* may include albumin, prealbumin, transferrin, LFTs, electrolyte levels, CBC, and ABGs.
      - ⇨ Albumin, prealbumin and transferrin are constitutive proteins produced by the liver, and levels of production tend to drop in the acute post-surgical period or after injury as synthesis switches to production of acute phase proteins. Adequate nutritional support in conjunction with treatment of acute illness facilitates stress response resolution and inflammation reduction, and should ultimately result in normal serum protein levels. Acute phase protein monitoing, however, has limited clinical utility until systemic inflammation has resolved. Interpretation of serum protein levels may be less reliable in patients with underlying liver dysfunction and resulting baseline serum protein level derangements.

- Determination of nutritional requirements
  - o Indirect calorimetry is the gold standard for determination of metabolic energy expenditure. It is most useful in stable patients with an inspired FiO$_2$ of 50% or less and requires specialized equipment and personnel not universally available. It is very resource-intensive, however, and rarely used except for research. Thus, equations have been developed for estimating patients' caloric needs and are widely used (Harris-Benedict, etc.). Reasonable estimates of daily caloric requirements in surgical patients are as follows:
    - Normal and underweight patients: 25 kcal/kg
    - Obese patients: 20–25 kcal/kg
      - ⇨ For obese patients, use adjusted feeding weight (AW): AW = Ideal weight + [(actual weight – ideal weight) x 0.25]
        — Ideal weight (male) ≈ 50 kg + (2.3 x height in inches – 60)
        — Ideal weight (female) ≈ 45.5 kg + (2.3 x height in inches – 60)
  - o *Protein requirements* vary with the degree of catabolism in hypermetabolic critically ill patients. The goal is to provide enough protein to match protein catabolism.
    - Estimates of protein needs are as follows:
      - ⇨ Normal adult: 0.8 g/kg
      - ⇨ Mild stress: 1.2–1.4 g/kg
      - ⇨ Moderate stress: 1.5–1.7 g/kg
      - ⇨ Severe stress: 1.8–2.5 g/kg
    - Most surgical ICU patients require at least 2 g/kg of protein daily.
    - A more accurate determination of protein requirements can be obtained by calculating the patient's nitrogen balance, but is rarely helpful:
      - ⇨ NB = (Protein (g/24h)/6.25) – (24h urine urea nitrogen (g/24h) + 4)
      - ⇨ Goal is to maintain a 4–6 g positive nitrogen balance
    - In patients with *hepatic encephalopathy*, protein intake should be limited to 0.6–0.8 g/kg. Other causes of encephalopathy should be ruled out first, however, because patients with liver dysfunction who are not encephalopathic can tolerate more normal protein intake and needlessly withholding protein may be detrimental.
    - Patients with *renal failure* (especially those on dialysis) require increased protein intake (typically 2–2.5 g/kg daily) to maintain a

positive nitrogen balance, due to loss of serum proteins in urine and in dialysis.

o   Non-protein calories (NPC) should be provided to prevent protein catabolism. If inadequate overall calories are provided, a portion of the protein in the diet will be consumed for energy, leading to a negative nitrogen balance.

o   It is also important to avoid overfeeding, as this has been associated with hypercapnea and resulting prolonged weaning from mechanical ventilator support, hyperglycemia, hyperlipidemia, liver dysfunction, and increased risk of infections.

- Enteral Nutrition

  o   Enteral nutrition should be initiated as soon as possible once it has been determined that the patient will not be able to meet their caloric needs by mouth. We generally aim to initiate enteral nutrition within 24 hours of hospitalization.

    ▪   Contraindications for enteral feeding include prolonged shock, major GI bleed, ileus, mechanical bowel obstruction, or bowel in discontinuity. Recent GI tract surgery with an anastomosis is not a contraindication.

    ▪   Absence of bowel sounds and absence of flatus or bowel movements are not contraindications to starting enteral nutrition.

    ▪   Enteral nutrition is superior to total parenteral nutrition, reducing infectious complications and reducing costs of care.

  o   Options for *enteral access* include nasogastric or nasoduodenal tubes, or percutaneous gastrostomy or jejunostomy tubes which can be placed at bedside, in the operating room, or in interventional radiology.

    ▪   Prokinetic agents (erythromycin and metoclopramide) improve feeding tolerance rates in patients with elevated gastric residual volumes but have not demonstrated associated decreases in pneumonia, duration of ICU stay, or mortality [Chapter 8-(ii)].

    ▪   Post-pyloric feeding may also be better tolerated and allow administration of more calories than gastric feeding in the acute post-surgical or post-injury setting when there is delayed gastric emptying.

  o   Choice of enteral formula is determined by the patient's medical history and clinical status. The general classes of formulas include polymeric, (e.g. Jevity, Osmolite) which are standard formulas appropriate for the majority of patients; concentrated (e.g. Two-Cal), which deliver higher caloric density per unit volume for patients on fluid restrictions; and elemental (e.g. Vivonex), which are composed of partially digested proteins and simple carbohydrates and are appropriate for patients with short gut or other malabsorptive conditions.

- Reduced carbohydrate formulas are not necessary in patients with a history of diabetes unless unable to maintain good glycemic control.

o Calculation of goal tube feed rates should start with estimation of non-protein calorie requirements (see above). Using the total NPC requirement in conjunction with NPC per unit volume of the selected enteral formula allows determination of the total daily volume of formula needed, which can then be divided over the time period of feeding administration (typically 24 hours in ICU patients). Protein supplementation may be required depending on the patient's daily protein requirements.

- Example: 75 kg male with goal 25 NPCs/kg and goal 2 g/kg protein

$$75kg \times 25\frac{NPC}{kg} = 1875\ NPC$$

$$\frac{1875\ \dfrac{NPC}{day}}{0.98\ \dfrac{NPC}{mL}} = 1913\ \frac{mL}{day} \approx 80\ mL/hr$$

Protein content of tube feed regimen:

$$\frac{1.913\ L \times 55.5\ g_{protein}}{L} = 106\ g_{protein}$$

$$2\frac{g}{kg} \times 75\ kg = 150\ g - 106\ g \approx 44\ g_{protein}$$

Thus, the patient would have a goal rate of 80 mL/hr with 44 g of supplemental protein added to meet his nutritional needs.

o *Gastric residual volumes* should be monitored while providing NG or PEG tube feeds. If residual volumes are greater than 200 mL, consider starting prokinetic medications; if volumes are greater than 500 mL, hold feeds for at least 4 hours and then re-assess and restart at a lower infusion rate. In patients with repeated high residual volumes, consider obtaining small bowel enteral access.

- o In mechanically ventilated patients receiving enteral nutrition, there is no need to discontinue enteral feeding perioperatively unless bowel surgery is planned.

- Parenteral nutrition
  - o If a patient is unable to tolerate enteral nutrition due to GI dysfunction (i.e. ileus, obstruction, short gut, shock), they require nutritional support via parenteral route. Parenteral nutrition should be initiated on hospital day seven if the patient cannot receive enteral nutrition, or earlier if the patient has preadmission malnutrition.
  - o Parenteral nutrition solutions require central access due to their high osmolarity. Ideally, a dedicated lumen should be used and sterile technique observed when administering TPN.
  - o Although approximately 30% of calories are provided by fats in enteral nutrition, parenteral lipid emulsions carry increased risk of infection and are prone to oxidation, which can result in oxidative cell injury and exacerbate the already pro-inflammatory post-surgical/post-injury state. Thus, the minimum of 3–4% of daily calories from lipids required to prevent essential fatty acid deficiency should generally be sufficient and lipid emulsions should actually be avoided in the initial/acute setting. The role of omega-3 versus omega-6 remains controversial.
  - o Monitoring of patients on TPN should include daily basic metabolic profile with particular attention to calcium, magnesium, and phosphorus levels, and glucose. The TPN formula should be adjusted based on these electrolyte levels and normoglycemia maintained with supplemental insulin.
  - o *Complications* associated with TPN administration include risk of central line infection, electrolyte abnormalities, impaired glucose metabolism, liver dysfunction, hypercapnea (seen with overfeeding), and gut atrophy (due to absence of nutrients in the bowel lumen).

- Hyperglycemia
  - o Critically ill patients are at increased risk of developing hyperglycemia due to stress-induced abnormalities of glucose metabolism. Patients receiving total parenteral nutritional support are at further increased risk due to the inherent changes in glucose metabolism seen with TPN.
  - o Blood glucose should be monitored and a goal blood glucose of less than 180 maintained with intravenous insulin infusion if required, with transition to sliding scale insulin once insulin requirements have stabilized. More stringent control with lower blood glucose goals does not appear to be beneficial and may be harmful.

- Glutamine
  - o Glutamine is an important nutrient for bowel mucosa, and is included in many enteral formulas. However, glutamine is usually not provided in TPN because it must be delivered as a dipeptide. Production of glutamine decreases in the acute high physiologic stress state, however, so including supplemental glutamine in critically ill patients (enteral or parenteral) may help preserve the small bowel mucosa and reduce bacterial translocation.

Practical Algorithm(s)/Diagrams

Basic Nutrition Algorithm

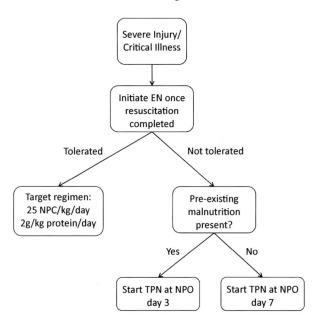

Fig. 1. Basic algorithm for nutritional support in the critically ill, with caloric and protein goals and timing of TPN initiation.

Review of Current Literature with References

History

- *Benefit of Early Enteral Feeding*: A prospective, randomized trial in 1986 demonstrated that patients receiving immediate enteral nutrition following emergent exploratory laparotomy for abdominal trauma had a lower incidence of sepsis [Moore E, Jones T. "Benefits of immediate jejunostomy feeding after major abdominal trauma — a prospective, randomized trial" *J Trauma* **26**: 10 (1986): 874–881].

- *Enteral vs Parenteral Nutrition*: A 1989 prospective, randomized trial demonstrated that patients receiving enteral nutrition had a lower rate of infections and lower rate of septic morbidity. Multiple subsequent randomized trials have duplicated this result. [Moore F *et al*. "TEN vs TPN following major abdominal trauma — reduced septic morbidity" *J Trauma* **29**: 7 (1989): 916–922].
- *Early Parenteral Nutrition*: Early initiation of parenteral nutrition does not improve mortality rates or hospital length of stay [Doig *et al*. "Early parenteral nutrition in critically ill patients with short-term relative contraindications to early enteral nutrition" *JAMA* **309**: 20 (2013): 2130–2138].

Controversial issues

- *Glutamine supplementation in TPN*: A 2010 meta-analysis demonstrated that adding glutamine to parenteral nutrition regimens shortened hospital length-of-stay and reduced morbidity from infection [Wang Y *et al*. "The impact of glutamine dipeptide-supplemented parenteral nutrition on outcomes of surgical patients: a meta-analysis of randomized clinical trials" *J Parenteral and Enteral Nutrition* **34**: 5 (2010): 521–529].
- *Gastric Residual Volume:* A 2013 randomized controlled trial demonstrated that not monitoring gastric residual volumes in mechanically ventilated patients and only holding tube feeds in the presence of regurgitation/vomiting did not result in an increase in ventilator-associated pneumonia. The intervention group had a higher proportion of patients receiving 100% caloric goal [Reignier J *et al*. "Effect of not monitoring residual gastric volume on risk of ventilator-associated pneumonia in adults receiving mechanical ventilation and early enteral feeding: a randomized controlled trial" *JAMA* **309**: 3 (2013): 249–256].
- *Anti-Inflammatory Enteral Formulas*: A randomized, double-blind, placebo-controlled trial demonstrated no improvement in ventilator-free days or other outcomes in ventilated patients who received omega-3 fatty acid, γ-linoleic acid, and antioxidant supplementation. This is in contrast to three prior studies demonstrating reduction in ventilator days, organ dysfunction, and mortality. The intervention group did suffer more diarrhea [Rice *et al*. "Enteral omega-3 fatty acid, γ-linoleic acid, and antioxidant supplementation in acute lung injury" *JAMA* **306**: 14 (2011): 1574–1581].

Chapter 8-(ii)

Tube Feed Intolerance

Anna Kristina Melvin, PA-C Janis Sandlin,
PA-C† and Walter L. Biffl, MD‡*

* Physician Assistant, Boulder Community Hospital

† Physician Assistant, Boulder Community Hospital

*‡ Professor of Surgery, University of Colorado School of Medicine,
Associate Director of Surgery, Denver Health Medical Center*

Take Home Points

- Diarrhea, emesis, or high gastric residual volumes (GRV) (>200 mL/4 hours) are examples of tube feed intolerance.
- Once tube feed intolerance has been recognized, it is important to consider organic causes such as intraabdominal infectious processes, or inadequate tube placement.
- Tube feeds that have been stopped may be resumed after symptoms improve or when GRVs are <200 mL/4 hours.
- Erythromycin and metoclopramide are first-line prokinetic agents.
- If gastric ileus is recalcitrant to prokinetic agents, consider post-pyloric tube placement or gastrostomy.

Contact information: (Anna Kristina Melvin and Janis Sandlin) Boulder Community Hospital, 1100 Balsam Ave, Boulder, CO 80304; (Walter L. Biff) Department of Surgery, Denver Health Medical Center, 777 Bannock St., MC 0206, Denver, CO 80204; Tel.: 303-602-1861, email: walter.biffl@dhha.org; Anna.Kristina@bch.org; Janis.Sandlin@bch.org

Background

- Feeding intolerance in critically ill patients in the ICU can lead to prolonged hospital stays, increased hospital costs, and a higher rate of morbidity. Early recognition is imperative.
- Etiologies of tube feed intolerance can include opioid use, recent abdominal surgery, increased age, preexisting comorbidities, prolonged ventilation, fluid/electrolyte imbalance, or poor underlying nutritional status.
- Diagnosis is subjective and can include the presence of:
  - High GRVs (>200 mL/4 hour)
    - Although the importance of measuring GRVs has been questioned recently, we still feel this is a safe approach particularly in high-risk patients.
  - Abdominal pain
  - Abdominal distension
  - Diarrhea
  - Emesis

Main Body

Nutritional support is an essential component of critical care. The most critically ill, who need support the most, are often unable to take nutrition by mouth (i.e., eat). Consequently, the critical care provider must provide support. Enteral nutrition is preferred over parenteral; various routes include:

- Eating
- Nasogastric tube
- Nasojejunal tube
- Gastrostomy tube

An awake, verbal patient can communicate lack of appetite, or nausea; however, critically ill patients are also often unable to tell the provider that they are not tolerating nutritional support. Thus, we must rely on signs and symptoms of intolerance. These may reflect either hyper- or hypomotility and include:

  - High GRVs (>200 mL/4 hour)
    - Although the importance of measuring GRVs has been questioned recently, we still feel this is a safe approach particularly in high-risk patients.

o Abdominal pain
o Abdominal distension
o Diarrhea
o Emesis

If signs or symptoms of feeding intolerance are observed, it is important to stop feeding due to the high risk of patient aspiration. It is important to exclude mechanical obstruction as well as to consider organic causes such as intraabdominal infectious processes or suboptimal tube placement prior to initiating promotility agents. Tube feeds that have been stopped may be resumed after symptoms improve or when GRV's are <200 mL/4 hours.

Hypermotility may be treated by altering the dietary formula or rate of administration. Prokinetic agents such as metoclopramide and erythromycin should be initiated in patients who have high GR volumes and who are not actively having diarrhea or emesis.

The two most common prokinetic agents used in the U.S. are metoclopramide and erythromycin. Metoclopramide is a dopamine D2 receptor antagonist which enhances gastric antral contractions and decreasing postprandial fundus relaxation. It carries potential side effects including anxiety, restlessness, and QT interval prolongation, and extrapyramidal side effects (dystonia and tardive dyskinesia) which have led to a FDA black box warning. Erythromycin is a macrolide antibiotic and motilin agonist which induces high amplitude gastric propulsive contractions and stimulates contractility of the fundus. Side effects of erythromycin include emergence of resistant bacteria, as well as ototoxicity, QT prolongation, and sudden death. In critically ill patients, erythromycin may be more efficacious, but both agents lose effectiveness over time and are sometimes used in combination.

If patient has recalcitrant gastric ileus, consider post-pyloric tube placement. This may be an effective way to introduce nutrients to the GI tract and potentially avoid some of the symptoms associated with gastric feeding tubes as mentioned above. In the authors' ICU, endoscopic positioning of postpyloric (nasojejunal) tubes allows the added benefit of ruling out proximal obstruction and diagnosing gastric pathology (e.g., gastritis, ulcers). Percutaneous endoscopic gastrostomy is employed for long-term care, allowing feeding as well as decompression.

Practical Algorithm(s)/Diagrams

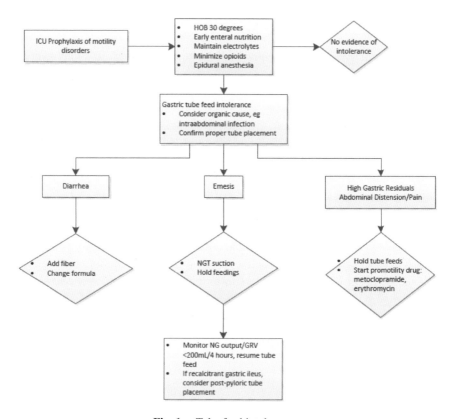

Fig. 1. Tube feed intolerance.

Review of Current Literature with References

- Rohm KD, Boldt J, Piper SN. Motility disorders in the ICU: recent therapeutic options and clinical practice. *Curr Opin Clin Nutr Metab Care* 2009; **12**: 161–167.

  o This represents the therapeutic options for motility disorders.

- Nguyen NQ, Chapman MJ, Fraser RJ *et al*. Erythromycin is more effective than metoclopramide in the treatment of feed intolerance in critical illness. *Crit Care Med* 2007; **35**: 483–489.

  o Prospective randomized trial demonstrating an advantage for erythromycin.

- Kim H, Stotts N, Froelicher ES *et al.* Why patients in critical care do not receive adequate enteral nutrition? A review of the literature. *J. Crit Care* 2012; **27**: 702–713.

  o A pertinent review of existing literature in regards to the nutritional status of critically ill patients.

- Reignier J, Mercier E, Le Gouge A *et al.* Effect of not monitoring residual gastric volume on risk of ventilator-associated pneumonia in adults receiving mechanical ventilation and early enteral feeding. A randomized controlled trial. *JAMA* 2013; **309**: 249–256.

  o Evaluation of the utility of measuring gastric residual volumes in patients on mechanical ventilation and those receiving early enteral feeding.

Chapter 8-(iii)

Gastrointestinal Ischemia

Jennifer A. Salotto, MD*

*Fellow, Trauma and Acute Care Surgery, Denver Health Medical Center

Take Home Points

- Acute mesenteric ischemia (AMI) is a life-threatening condition which occurs when perfusion of the viscera fails to meet metabolic demand.
- This disease process exists on a spectrum, ranging from ischemia, necrosis, and intestinal perforation to sepsis and death.
- Successful outcomes depend on a high index of clinical suspicion, early diagnosis and prompt treatment.
- Overall mortality remains high despite broadening options for therapy.
- The four underlying causes of AMI include arterial embolism, arterial thrombosis, mesenteric venous thrombosis, and non-occlusive mesenteric ischemia. It is important to distinguish between these causes because the treatments vary.
- Arterial embolism, specifically to the superior mesenteric artery (SMA), is the most common cause of AMI and may present with the sudden onset of

Contact information: Denver Health Medical Center, University of Colorado Health Sciences Center, 777 Bannock Street, MC 0206, Denver, CO 80204; Tel.: 857-928-4766, email: jennifer.salotto@ucdenver.edu

abdominal pain or classically, pain out of proportion to exam. Often the patient can give a history of prior embolic events or arrhythmia. It is treated with surgical embolectomy.

- SMA thrombosis is seen in patients with risk factors for atherosclerosis. Treatment is an arterial bypass around the obstruction.
- In those centers with interventional capabilities, endovascular therapy for AMI is no longer reserved for those at high risk. Patients who do not demonstrate peritonitis or clinical features of bowel ischemia may be candidates for definitive endovascular therapies including angioplasty, stenting, or thrombolysis. Laparotomy or laparoscopy may be used to assess bowel viability after an endovascular intervention.
- Non-occlusive mesenteric ischemia is inadequate visceral perfusion in the absence of an obstructing lesion. It is most commonly seen in ICU patients with severely depressed cardiac output or those receiving high-dose vasoconstrictors such as epinephrine or vasopressin. The mainstay of therapy is catheter-directed intra-arterial infusion of vasodilators such as papaverine.
- Mesenteric venous thrombosis (MVT) accounts for a small percentage of all mesenteric ischemic events and is usually limited to the SMV. MVT is noted in those with a hypercoagulable state, post-trauma, or post-splenectomy. It can present in an acute or a chronic form, depending on the etiology. Treatment is systemic anticoagulation.
- Bowel ischemia may occur after an open or endovascular abdominal aortic aneurysm repair due to disruption of the mesenteric arterial supply or from dislodgement of thrombus to the mesenteric vessels. Patients will present with acidosis, abdominal pain and bloody diarrhea in the acute post-operative period after an abdominal aneurysm repair. Diagnosis is made with a bedside flexible sigmoidoscopy and the treatment is bowel resection.
- Methods for assessing intestinal viability include visual inspection of bowel color and bleeding from divided tissue edges, assessing Doppler signals within the mesentery, and a fluorescein uptake evaluation. These tests are not completely reliable: bowel ischemia may progress and the serosa may appear healthy despite an ischemic mucosa. The decision to return to the operating room 24–48 hours after first operation for a second look exploration is left to the discretion of the surgeon. This second look allows time for demarcation of bowel ischemia and an opportunity to reassess bowel viability.

Background

- The arterial and venous anatomy of the GI tract

  o The arterial supply to the gastrointestinal tract stems from the abdominal aorta's three major branches, the celiac trunk, the superior mesenteric artery, and the inferior mesenteric artery.

  o The celiac artery provides blood flow to the foregut, including the stomach and the duodenum just proximal to the ligament of Treitz.

  o The superior mesenteric artery provides blood flow to the midgut, including the jejunum, the ileum, the appendix, the ascending colon, and the transverse colon. Major named branches include the ileocolic artery, the appendicular artery, the right colic artery and the middle colic artery.

  o The inferior mesenteric artery supplies blood flow to the hindgut, which includes the descending colon, the sigmoid colon, and the upper rectum. Major branches include the left colic artery, the sigmoidal arteries and the superior rectal artery.

  o The internal iliac artery gives rise to the middle and inferior rectal arteries.

  o There exists a fair amount of redundancy and collatoralization among the artierial branches of the GI tract. The SMA and the IMA usually anastomose via the marginal artery of the colon in the area of the splenic flexure, commonly known as the artery of Drummond. The marginal artery is absent in approximately 5% of the population. There are macrovascular collaterals between the left and middle colic artery within the colonic mesentery and microvascular collaterals within the bowel wall.

  o The venae rectae form a venous arcade that drains the small bowel and the proximal colon through the ileocolic, middle colic and the right colic veins into the superior mesenteric vein. Distally, the left colic, sigmoid, and rectosigmoid veins drain into the inferior mesenteric vein. The superior mesenteric vein, inferior mesenteric vein, and splenic vein all converge to become the portal vein.

- Gastrointestinal physiology

  o The layers of the bowel wall include the serosa, a longitudinal muscle layer, a circular muscle layer, the submucosa, and the mucosa.

  o The blood vessels of the gastrointestinal system are part of a vascular system known as the splanchnic circulation, which supplies the gut, the liver, the pancreas, and the spleen.

o The splanchnic circulation receives approximately 25% of the resting cardiac output and 35% of the postprandial cardiac output.
o Normal oxygen supply to the gut can be maintained at only 20% of maximal blood flow.
o Decreased oxygen concentration in the gut wall can increase local blood flow by 50–100%.
o Mesenteric blood flow is auto-regulated by the autonomic nervous system as well as by endogenous hormones in the bloodstream such as epinephrine, norepinephrine, vasopressin, and acetylcholine.
o The mucosa of the intestinal tract itself releases vasodilatory peptide hormones including cholecystokinin, vasoactive intestinal peptide, gastrin, and secretin. Gastrointestinal glands also release kallidin and bradykinin which are also powerful vasodilators.

- Pathophysiology of acute mesenteric ischemia

o The musocal and submucosal layers are most vulnerable to ischemia. Mucosal edema and hemorrhage may progress to sloughing and ulceration of the mucosa.
o As ischemia progresses, these ulcers go on to full thickness necrosis and eventually to perforation.

Main Body

- Etiology and presentation of acute mesenteric ischemia

o Mesenteric ischemia occurs when perfusion of the gastrointestinal tract fails to meet metabolic needs.
o Mesenteric arteries are subject to atherosclerosis in the same manner as both systemic and coronarey arteries. The same risk factors apply and should be solicited in the evaluation of the patient with suspected AMI.
o There are four etiologies for acute mesenteric ischemia: embolus, arterial thrombosis, non-occlusive ischemia, and venous thrombosis. An additional specific etiology of AMI occurs in patients who have had an abdominal aortic aneurysm repair in which the inferior mesenteric artery has been sacrificed, resulting in ischemic colitis. It is important to distinguish between each of these entities as the treatments vary.
o In an acute embolic occlusion, the SMA is the most common destination for mesenteric emboli due to the acute angle from which it comes off the aorta. These emboli tend to lodge a few centimeters distal to the origin of the SMA, usually after the takeoff of both the first jejunal branches

and the middle colic artery. Consequently, with an embolic event, both the proximal jejunum and transverse colon are spared. This is in contradistinction to the pattern of injury observed in the case of an acute thrombosis (discussed below).

o Superior mesenteric artery thrombosis occurs in the most proximal SMA, (usually within 2.5 centimeters of the ostia of the SMA off of the aorta) due to turbulent flow at the bifurcation (as seen in both carotid and femoral arterial disease). Given the more proximal nature of these occlusions, larger lengths of bowel are generally affected, including the proximal jejunum and transverse colon. For this reason, thrombotic occlusions, as compared to emboli, are associated with a higher mortality.

o Mesenteric venous thrombosis is generally limited to the superior mesenteric vein, and can be classified as either primary or secondary. Primary MVT is idiopathic, while secondary can be attributed to a prothrombotic state, an intra-abdominal inflammatory state such as pancreatitis, postoperative states (especially post-splenectomy), and in conditions of venous stasis including cirrhosis and portal hypertension. Oral contraceptives are also responsible for episodes of MVT in younger women.

o Clinical manifestations of MVT will depend on the size and location of the thrombus and the extent of the bowel involved. Acute venous thrombosis carries a risk of bowel necrosis, whereas chronic thrombosis allows time for collaterals to develop and therefore has a more subtle onset and a benign course.

o Non-occlusive mesenteric ischemia is malperfusion of the gastrointestinal tract in the absence of an obstruction. This form of AMI is most often noted in elderly patients with cardiogenic shock requiring agents such as vasopressin which constrict splanchnic blood flow.

o Both open and endovascular repair of abdominal aortic aneurysm can be complicated by AMI. During an aortic abdominal aneurysm repair, the inferior mesenteric artery (IMA) may be sacrificed. If little or no collateralization to the colon exists preoperatively, the loss of the IMA blood supply may result in colonic infarction. GI ischemia may also result from disruption and embolization of thrombus within the aneurysm. Finally, low-flow states associated with aortic clamping and/or hypotension secondary to aortic rupture may predispose the colon to ischemia. Patients who have undergone emergent repair of a ruptured AAA have a much greater likelihood of developing colonic ischemia when compared with those undergoing elective repair.

- History and physical exam
  - o Signs and symptoms of AMI exist on a spectrum dependent upon the severity of the ischemia: signs and symptoms of early ischemia are usually relatively non-specific, whereas the presentation of a patient with bowel necrosis and perforation is rarely subtle, including tachycardia, hypotension, peritonitis, leukocytosis, and the accumulation of the byproducts of anaerobic metabolism.
  - o It is necessary to have a high clinical suspicion for AMI when evaluating an ICU patient with abdominal pain. The history, physical, and labs may be non-specific. Exam may be confounded by sedation, paralytics, or delirium.
  - o The hallmark of AMI is pain out of proportion to physical exam.
  - o Both weight loss and food fear suggest chronic stenosis of mesenteric vessels due to atherosclerosis.
  - o Additional clinical findings include diffuse abdominal pain, nausea, vomiting, anorexia, diarrhea, melena or hematochezia.
  - o Pain may become localized and patient may develop tenderness, rebound and guarding with bowel ischemia or perforation.
  - o Onset of abdominal pain may be sudden in onset (embolic/thrombotic) or insidious (SMV thrombosis).
  - o Certain aspects of the history may aid in differentiation between the different types of AMI.
    - ▪ Embolic: atrial fibrillation, prior embolic events, recent peripheral or coronary catheterization, valvular heart disease, myocardial ischemia or infarction.
    - ▪ Thrombotic: older age, hypertension, smoking, diabetes, CAD/PVD, food fear, weight loss.
    - ▪ SMV Thrombosis: trauma, hypercoagulable state, post-splenectomy, pancreatitis, family history of deep vein thrombosis or pulmonary embolus.
    - ▪ NOMI: cardiogenic shock, hypovolemia, heart failure, vasoconstrictors, cocaine, digoxin, dialysis.
- Early interventions
  - o Initiate intravenous fluid resuscitation with close attention to endpoints of resuscitation [see Chapter 5-(iv)]. Maintain NPO status.
  - o Labs should include a complete blood count, basic metabolic panel, amylase and lipase, lactate and an arterial blood gas. Labs may indicate

an anion-gap metabolic acidosis. Correct electrolyte abnormalities and acid-base abnormalities.

- Laboratory derrangements occur relatively late in the course of ischemia.
- Do not wait for lab abnormalities before pursuing further diagnostic or interventional modalities.

o Obtain an EKG to evaluate cardiac rhythm.

o Obtain blood cultures and initiate broad-spectrum antibiotics with coverage against intestinal pathogens (typically gram negative rods and anaerobs).

o If suspicion is high and bleeding risk is low, initiate systemic anticoagulation empirically.

o Obtain an upright CXR to assess for intra-peritoneal air (suggesting intestinal perforation).

o Abdominal films may show semi-opaque indentations of the bowel lumen ("thumb-printing") which is indicative of mucosal edema.

o For patients requiring vasopressors in the face of suspected mesenteric ischemia, use dopamine or epinephrine.

- Diagnosis

o Patients with shock and/or diffuse peritonitis (i.e. "acute abdomen") do not require any additional diagnostic maneurvers and should undergo exploratory laparotomy promptly.

o In the remainder of cases, diagnositic imaging studies include CTA, angiography, duplex ultrasonography, endoscopy, and laparoscopy.

o A mesenteric duplex is rarely helpful in the evaluation of acute mesenteric ischemia due to the presence of bowel gas.

o Although contrast angiography has traditionally been considered the gold standard for diagnosis of mesenteric ischemia, it is costly, invasive, potentially nephrotoxic, and may not be readily available. In the absence of a hybrid operating room, it may also delay operative intervention.

o Thin-slice computed tomography angiography (CT-A) has replaced traditional angiography as a fast and highly sensitive means of diagnosing arterial and venous occlusions of the mesenteric vasculature. It easily rules out other sources of abdominal pain.

o CT-A may be considered in cases where the patient is hemodynamically stable and does not show any evidence of peritonitis, warranting a prompt surgical intervention.

- o In cases of acute mesenteric ischemia, a CT scan may demonstrate arterial or venous occlusion, thickened bowel loops, or free fluid. Pneumatosis intestinale, portal venous air, and free air are late findings.
- o A CT scan is highly sensitive for cases of mesenteric ischemia secondary to embolus, thrombosis of the arterial inflow or thrombosis of the venous outflow.
- o In most cases, angiography is limited to the minority of cases in which:
  - findings from less invasive means of imaging are equivocal.
    - ⇨ This line of therapy has been selected over operation (e.g., poor operative risk). Non-occlusive mesenteric ischemia is highly likely. In this case, a formal angiogram followed by catheter-based intervention is the most efficient means of diagnosis and treatment. The hallmark on angiogram of NOMI is diffuse mesenteric vasospasm with the absence of a complete occlusion.
- o In those patients with crampy abdominal pain, unexplained acidosis, or bloody stool after an abdominal aortic aneurysm repair, the diagnostic test of choice is bedside flexible sigmoidoscopy to evaluate the mucosa for signs of ischemia.
  - Findings on endoscopy may include: mild colitis with hemorrhagic mucosa, a moderate colitis with patchy ischemia limited to the mucosa, or a continuous area of full thickness ischemia.
- o Diagnostic laparoscopy may be considered in the relatively rare instance in which the diagnosis of AMI is still in question despite imaging with either CTA or angiography. It is important to remember that the bowel serosal layer (the only layer of the bowel that is visible via laparoscopy) is the least susceptible to ischemia. Therefore, normal appearing bowel serosa does not rule out AMI.
- Treatment
  - o Thrombotic vs. embolic
    - Heparinization.
    - In the OR: resect dead bowel, restore blood flow to bowel.
      - ⇨ bypass for thrombosis.
      - ⇨ embolectomy with Fogarty catheters for embolic event.
    - May anastomose or leave blind ends.

- A second look procedure should generally be performed in 24–48 hours, although the decision is ultimately left to the discretion of the operating surgeon.
- In certain cases where interventional resources and capabilities are available, therapies including endovascular thrombolysis, mechanical thrombectomy, angioplasty and stenting may be considered.

o Mesenteric venous occlusion

  - Heparinization.

    ⇨ bolus with 5000 U of heparin then begin a continuous infusion with a goal activated partial-thromboplastin time more than twice the normal level.

  - IVF for fluid shifts.
  - NGT and bowel rest.
  - Surgical exploration if clinically warranted.
  - In cases where the clinical picture continues to decline despite full anticoagulation, there is a role for endovascular clot lysis and mechanical aspiration if interventional radiology is available.

o Non-occlusive mesenteric ischemia

  - The treatment mainstay is intra-arterial instillation of papaverine performed in the interventional radiology suite.

    ⇨ bolus of 60 mg directly into the SMA, then infuse 30–60 mg/hr until resolution of symptoms.

  - After vasodilatory therapy, it is necessary to perform a follow-up angiogram to document resolution.
  - Adjuncts to intra-arterial therapies include maximizing oxygen delivery to tissues, improving cardiac output, and minimizing vasoconstrictors.

- Colonic ischemia after repair of an abdominal aortic aneurysm

  o Once this diagnosis of colonic ischemia after an abdominal aneurysm repair is considered, a bedside flexible sigmoidoscopy is the gold standard for diagnosis. Findings of mucosal edema, hemorrhage, ulceration, or necrosis would support the diagnosis.

  o For those patients with mild or moderate findings (hemorrhagic mucosa, patchy mucosal ischemia), it is appropriate to hydrate and clinically observe in the absence of sepsis or peritonitis, following up with a repeat sigmoidoscopy at 12-hour intervals. Caution should be taken with these patients, as delay in resection of a truly ischemic segment may result in full thickness necrosis and perforation. Any attempt to manage these patients conservatively should be aborted if the clinical picture worsens.

o   For those patients with severe findings on sigmoidoscopy, the treatment is returning to the operating room for a colectomy, resecting the necrotic portions of the bowel and creating a temporary end colostomy.

- Outcomes

o   Morbidity and mortality of acute mesenteric ischemia remain high despite advancing surgical and endovascular techniques.

o   After AMI, survival often depends on the age of a patient, comorbidities, timing of intervention, and the degree and extent of bowel ischemia.

o   Postoperative complications include sepsis, ongoing ischemia requiring repeat resections, wound infection, and short-gut syndrome in those requiring extensive small bowel resections.

o   Non-occlusive mesenteric ischemia carries a mortality near 50% due to underlying cardiac disease.

o   The mortality rate of mesenteric venous thrombosis was quoted by Kumar *et al.* to range from 20–50%. Recurrences are most common 30 days after presentation. These patients require at least six months to a year of systemic anticoagulation.

o   In a large observational study looking at over 87,000 patients with abdominal aortic aneurysm (AAA) repairs, the mortality of colonic ischemia post-AAA repair was noted to be around 37%. Those patients undergoing ruptured, open, or endovascular AAA repair without colonic ischemia were found to have an overall mortality of 6.7%.

Practical Algorithm(s)/Diagrams

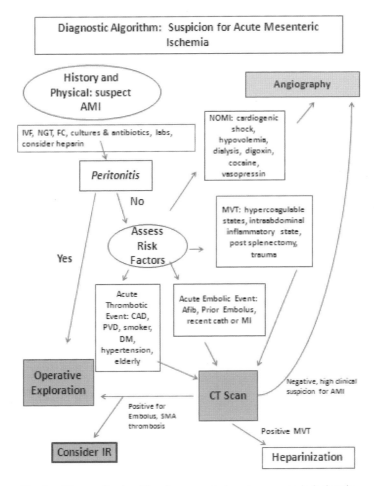

Fig. 1. Diagnostic algorithm for suspected acute mesenteric ischemia.

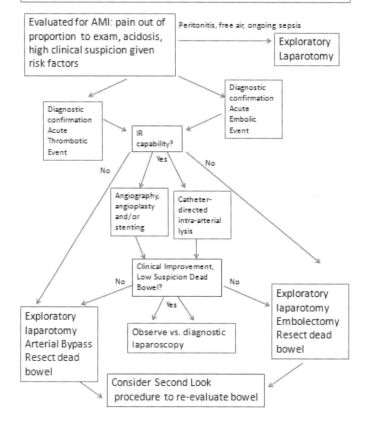

Fig. 2.   Treatment algorithm, thrombotic and embolic AMI.

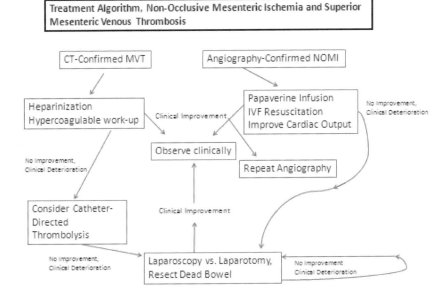

Fig. 3. Treatment algorithm, NOMI and SMV thrombosis.

Review of Current Literature with References

- In 2002, a retrospective study out of the Mayo Clinic described their ten-year experience with the clinical presentation of 58 patients with acute mesenteric ischemia. 95% presented with abdominal pain, 44% with nausea, 35% with diarrhea and vomiting, 16% had blood per rectum. The mean white blood cell count was elevated at 20.3 x 10⁹/mL and was abnormal in 98% of the patients. Base deficit was elevated in 52% and lactate was elevated in 91%, with a mean value of 4.7 mmol/L. In this patient population they noted a 32% 30-day mortality rate (Park WM, Gloviczki P, Cherry Jr KJ *et al.* Contemporary management of acute mesenteric ischemia: factors associated with survival. *J Vasc Surg* 2002; **35**: 445–452).

- An observational study by Perry *et al.* looked at the records of over 89,000 patients undergoing abdominal aortic aneurysm repair from the 2003–2004, utilizing the Nationwide Inpatient Sample database. They found the overall incidence of colonic ischemia to be 2.2%. The incidence after ruptured AAA repair was 8.9%, after open repair incidence was 1.9%, and after endovascular repair incidence was 0.5%. They reported mortality rates increased from two- to four-fold, quoting mortality from colonic ischemia post-AAA around 37% (Perry RJ, Martin MJ, Eckert MJ, Sohn Vr, Steele SR. Colonic ischemia complicating open versus endovascular abdominal aortic aneurysm repair. *J Vasc Surg* 2008; **48**: 272–277).

- A systematic review and meta-analysis published in 2010 evaluated the utility of multi-detector computerized tomography in the evaluation of acute mesenteric ischemia. They included three prospective and three retrospective studies for a total of 619 cases. They found an overall pooled sensitivity of 93.3% and a pooled specificity of 95.9% and concluded that this modality can be safely used as a first-line agent in evaluating AMI (Menke J. Diagnostic accuracy of multidetector CT in acute mesenteric ischemia: systematic review and meta-analysis. *Radiology* 2010; **256**: 93–101).

- A single-institution retrospective cohort review from the Cleveland Clinic described 56 of 70 patients with arterial embolic or thrombotic etiologies of AMI who underwent initial endovascular therapies. Successful endovascular treatment was achieved in 87%, defined as return of bowel perfusion without laparotomy, or with laparotomy but without open embolectomy or bypass. They demonstrated a statistically significant difference between in-hospital mortality with endovascular treatment (36%) as compared with traditional open therapy (50%). Factors associated with increased risk of death included advanced age, history of coronary artery disease, peripheral arterial disease, and an initial lactate >2.2 mmol/L (Arthurs ZM, Titus J, Bannazadeh M, Eagleton MJ, Srivastava S, Sarac TP, Clair DG. A comparison of endovascular revascularization with traditional therapy for the treatment of acute mesenteric ischemia. *J Vasc Surg* 2011; **53**: 698–705).

Hepatopancreaticobiliary

Carlton C. Barnett, MD* Brandon C. Chapman, MD[†]
and Edward L. Jones, MD[†]

* Professor of Surgery, University of Colorado School of Medicine
[†] Surgical Resident, University of Colorado School of Medicine

Take Home Points

- Acute liver failure can be a primary indication for ICU care as well as a significant co-morbidity and its management is driven by the etiology. Unfortunately, acute liver failure is resolved in only 40% of cases, leaving a significant number of patient in need of liver transplantation (Chapter 26).
- Chronic liver failure (cirrhosis) is a common co-morbidity that complicates ICU patient care.
- Cirrhosis is divided into two stages: compensated and decompensated. The median survival of patients with decompensated cirrhosis and a Child-Pugh score ≥ 12 or a model of end stage liver disease (MELD) score ≥ 21 is ≤ 6 months compared to a median survival of patients with compensated cirrhosis of >12 years. Decompensated cirrhosis often requires liver transplant for survival.

Contact information: Denver Health Medical Center, University of Colorado Health Sciences Center, 777 Bannock Street, MC 0206, Denver, CO 80204; Tel.: 303-436-5402, email: Carlton.barnett@dhha.org; edward.jones@ucdenver.edu; Brandon.Chapman@ucdenver.edu

- The differential diagnosis of patients with acute jaundice associated with critical illness can be broadly divided into three groups: extrahepatic bile duct obstruction, increased bilirubin production (or re-absorption), and impaired excretion due to hepatocellular dysfunction, hepatitis, or intrahepatic cholestasis.
- Biliary disease can be difficult to diagnose and often takes the form of acalculous cholecystitis [Chapter 10-(vi)].
- The management of biliary obstruction can be treated via endoscopic or percutaneous approaches and surgery is rarely indicated except in cases of life-threatening hemorrhage from biliary-arterial fistula.
- Acute pancreatitis is an inflammatory condition of the pancreas that ranges from mild edema to life-threatening necrosis. The mortality rate for severe acute pancreatitis has been reported as high as 15–30%. Early aggressive resuscitation is required to minimize morbidity and mortality.
- Contrast enhanced computed tomography (CT) should not be routinely performed in patients with acute pancreatitis and is indicated only in patients who show clinical signs of sepsis, fail to improve on supportive therapy, or regress after an initial period of improvement.
- Antibiotic prophylaxis has not been shown to reduce mortality, protect against infected necrosis, or reduce the need for surgical intervention and is not routinely indicated in patients with severe acute pancreatitis, including those with sterile pancreatic necrosis.
- Enteral nutrition has been shown to lower the incidence of infections, reduced surgical interventions to control pancreatitis, and a reduced length of hospital stay. It is the preferred route of nutritional support in patients with severe acute pancreatitis and can be given via nasogastric or nasojejunal routes.
- Early surgical debridement of necrotic pancreatic tissue is only indicated for FNA-proven infected necrosis or patients with surgical complications such as massive bleeding or bowel perforation.
- Measurements of intra-abdominal pressure should be done liberally as abdominal compartment syndrome (ACS) has been reported in up to 55% of patients with severe pancreatitis [Chapter 8-(vi)].

Background

- Acute liver failure is defined as either encephalopathy or hepatic synthetic dysfunction (INR > 1.49) in a patient without a history of pre-existing liver disease and lasting < 26 weeks in duration.

- The most common cause of acute liver failure is acetaminophen overdose followed by idiosyncratic drug reaction.
- Cirrhosis develops as a result of progressive hepatic fibrosis that is characterized by distortion of the hepatic architecture and formation of regenerative nodules. Although early treatment of the cause of liver disease may improve or reverse cirrhosis, advanced cirrhosis is irreversible.
- Patients with cirrhosis who have not developed major complications are classified as compensated cirrhosis
- Decompensated cirrhosis is a life-threatening condition that is characterized by one of the following complications: variceal hemorrhage, ascites, spontaneous bacterial peritonitis, hepatic encephalopathy, hepatocellular carcinoma, hepatorenal and hepatopulmonary syndrome.
- Patients with bleeding, infection, alcohol intake, medications, dehydration, and constipation are at increased risk of developing decompensated cirrhosis.
- The MELD score is based on three biochemical variables: serum bilirubin, serum creatinine, and either international normalized ratio (INR) or prothrombin time. It has been shown to accurately predict 3-month mortality from liver disease and should be used for allocation of liver donors.
- Eighty percent of daily bilirubin production is derived from hemoglobin. Heme from senescent red blood cells is converted to bilverdin via the rate limiting enzyme heme oxygenase. Bilverdin is subsequently converted to unconjugated bilirubin via bilverdin reductase and is carried to the liver via binding to albumin. Unconjugated bilirubin is taken up in the hepatocytes via facilitated diffusion and is conjugated by uridine diphosphoglucuronosyltransferase (UGT), which is secreted across the canalicular membrane of the hepatocyte via canalicular multi-drug resistant protein 2 (MRP2). Bacterial enzymes in the intestine reduce bilirubin into urobilinogen and stercobilinogen.
- Although not routinely indicated, contrast enhanced CT of the abdomen is the gold standard for diagnosing acute pancreatitis and its associated complications. Necrosis is characterized by focal or diffuse areas of diminished pancreatic parenchymal enhancement (<50 Hounsfield Units).
- Pancreatic necrosis is associated with pancreatic infection in up to 30–70% of cases, which is the most important risk factor for death.
- Several prognostic scoring systems including Ranson's Criteria, Glascow (Imrie) score, and APACHE II have been developed to predict clinical outcomes of acute pancreatitis, but frequent clinical assessment is mandatory.
- The Balthazar score is used in CT severity index (CTSI) for grading of acute pancreatitis and includes grading of pancreatitis (A-E) and the extent of pancreatic necrosis.

o Mild pancreatitis (interstitial): Balthazar B (enlargement of pancreas), Balthazar C (inflammatory changes in pancreas and peripancreatic fat), without pancreatic or extrapancreatic necrosis.

o Intermediate (exudative): Balthaazar D (ill defined single fluid collection), Balthazar E (two or more poorly defined fluid collections), without pancreatic necrosis; peripancreatic collections are due to extrapancretic necrosis.

o Severe (necrotizing): pancreatic necrosis.

Main Body

• *Acute Liver Failure*

o An acute injury (<26 weeks) to the liver demonstrated by encephalopathy and impaired synthetic function (INR >1.49) in a patient without pre-existing liver disease.

o Determination of the etiology begins with a careful history, hepatic function tests (bilirubin, aminotransferases, alkaline phosphatase), prothrombin time, viral hepatitis serology, autoimmune panel and specific medication levels as indicated by history.

o Common patterns of presentation in liver function tests are available in Table 1.

o The most common cause is acetaminophen toxicity followed by idio-syncratic drug reaction and viral hepatitis.

o Common etiologies can be remembered using the "ABCs" pneumonic:

A — Hepatitis A, Autoimmune, *Amanita phalloides* (mushroom poisoning).
B — Hepatitis B, Budd-Chiari.
C — Hepatitis C, cytomegalovirus infection.
D — Hepatitis D, Drugs (acetaminophen, isoniazid, halothane, pheny-toin, labetalol and many others).
E — Epstein-Barr virus.
F — Fatty liver of pregnancy, Reye's syndrome.
G — Genetic (Wilson's disease).
H — Hypoperfusion (sepsis), HELLP syndrome, HSV, hepatectomy.

o The appropriate management is directed towards rectifying the underlying cause. In addition, aggressive treatment of the common electrolyte abnormalities (hypokalemia, hyponatremia, hypophosphatemia and hypo-glycemia) as well as closely monitoring for cerebral edema (intra-cranial pressure monitors or transcranial Doppler ultrasound) and treatment when indicated.

o Seizures, acute renal failure and pulmonary infections and edema are other common complications. Treatment is supportive.

o Prognosis is most consistently associated with the grade of hepatic encephalopathy. Spontaneous recovery by gade. Grade I–II (mild to moderate confusion, minimal asterixis): 70% (mild-moderate confusion, minimal asterixis). Grade III (incoherent, arousable but sleeping): 50% Grade IV (comatose): <20%.

o Acetaminophen toxicity, hepatitis A, ischemia/shock or pregnancy-related acute liver failure as well as age 11–39 have higher likelihood of spontaneous recovery in contrast to hepatitis B, autoimmune hepatitis, Wilson disease, Budd-Chiari or malignancy.

o Prognostic models include the King's College Criteria as well as the MELD but must be used with caution as the sensitivity and specificity of these models have varied widely in the literature.

o If consideration is given for liver transplantation, then patients should be rapidly triaged and transferred to transplant centers.

- *Decompensated Cirrhosis*

  o Variceal hemorrhage:

    ▪ Prevention: non-selective beta blocker.
    ▪ Signs and symptoms: hematemesis and/or melena.
    ▪ Treatment: Endoscopic variceal band ligation.

  o Ascites

    ▪ Presentation: circulatory, vascular, functional, and biochemical abnormalities.
    ▪ Treatment: diuretics and sodium restriction, therapeutic pericentesis, and/or TIPS placement.

  o Spontaneous bacterial peritonitis

    ▪ Prevention: diuretics, aggressive treatment of localized infections, avoidance of proton pump inhibitors, prophylactic antibiotics.
    ▪ Presentation: fever, abdominal pain, abdominal tenderness, altered mental status, positive ascitic fluid bacterial culture and/or an elevated ascitic fluid absolute polynmorphonuclear leukocyte count (≥ 250 cells/mm^3).
    ▪ Treatment: Antibiotics.

  o Hepatic encephalopathy

    ▪ Prevention: avoidance of variceal bleeding, infection, sedatives, hypokalemia, and hyponatremia.

- Presentation: disturbance in diurnal sleep pattern, asterixis, hyperactive deep tendon reflexes, and transient decerebrate posturing.
- Treatment: treatment of predisposing conditions, synthetic disaccharides (lactulose), and non-absorbable antibiotics (rifaximin).

o Hepatocellular carcinoma

- Prevention: surveillance ultrasound every six months.
- Presentation: pain, early satiety, obstructive jaundice, a palpable mass, or marked elevations of serum alpha-fetoprotein (AFP).
- Treatment: hepatic resection, radiofrequency ablation, chemoembolization, or liver transplant determined by the size and number of lesions as well as patient performance.

o Hepatorenal syndrome

- Prevention: avoid nephrotoxic agents and excessive diuresis.
- Presentation: very low rate of sodium excretion, progressive rise in the plasma creatinine concentration.
- Treatment: prognosis is poor without liver transplant.

o Hepatopulmonary syndrome

- Presentation: triad of liver disease, increased alveolar-arterial gradient while breathing room air, and intrapulmonary vascular dilatations.
- Treatment: no effective medical treatments thus requiring liver transplant.

- *Acute Jaundice in the Critically Ill Patient*
  o History and physical examination
  o Laboratory evaluation

  - Normal alkaline phosphatase and aminotransferases — unlikely to be due to hepatic injury or biliary tract disease. Hemolysis characterized by an increased reticulocyte count, peripheral blood smear, positive Coombs test, increased lactate dehydrogenase, and decreased haptoglobin or inherited disorders of bilirubin metabolism should be considered.
  - Predominant alkaline phosphatase elevation — suggest biliary obstruction or intrahepatic cholestasis. Abdominal ultrasound to evaluate for intra- or extra-hepatic bile duct dilation should be obtained. Computed tomography or MRI can be used in patients in whom sonographic findings are equivocal if other intra-abdominal pathology needs to be excluded, or if ductal dilatation is seen on US without a clearly defined etiology.

- Predominant aminotransferase elevation — suggests intrinsic hepatocellular disease. Serologic testing to evaluate for viral hepatitis, alcoholic liver disease, and metabolic liver disease should be obtained. A liver biopsy may also be diagnostic.
  - o Differential Diagnosis (See Table 2).
- *Acute Pancreatitis (AP)*
  - o Etiology: Gallstones (45%), alcohol (35%), other rare causes include drug reactions, pancreatic/ampullary tumors, hypertriglyceridemia, hypercalcemia, hypothermia, congenital abnormalities, trauma, ERCP, and infectious/parasitic organisms.
  - o The diagnosis should be suspected in patients presenting with acute upper abdominal pain and tenderness, nausea, vomiting, elevated lipase and amylase.
  - o Ultrasound should be considered as initial test in all patients with pancreatitis to rule out a biliary etiology.
  - o Pancreatic necrosis on contrast-enhanced CT scan is characterized by focal or diffuse areas of diminished pancreatic parenchymal enhancement (less than 50 Hounsfield units).
  - o Due to the risk of contaminating sterile necrosis, fine needle aspiration (FNA) should only be performed in patients who show clinical signs of sepsis, fail to improve on supportive therapy, or regress after an initial period of improvement.
  - o CRP levels greater than 150 have been associated necrosis and an elevated serum procalcitonin may predict later organ dysfunction.
  - o Initial management focuses on aggressive intravascular resuscitation as sequestration of fluid into extravascular extracellular compartment (third-spacing) can lead to significant plasma volume.
  - o Frequent evaluation of abdominal compartment syndrome should be utilized due to the large amount of fluid required.
  - o Antibiotic prophylaxis has not been shown to reduce mortality, protect against infected necrosis, or reduce the need for surgical intervention and is not routinely indicated in patients with severe acute pancreatitis.
  - o Patients with mild AP should begin oral supplementation within a few days of presentation.
  - o Enteral nutrition has been shown to lower the incidence of infections, reduced surgical interventions to control pancreatitis, and a reduced length of hospital stay. It is the preferred route of nutritional support in patients with severe acute pancreatitis and can be given via nasogastric or nasojejunal.

o   Historically, early surgery was thought to improve outcome by removing necrotic tissue and decrease the stimulus for systemic inflammation; however, this has been disapproved by more recent clinical trials.

o   Open necrosectomy has been associated with a high morbidity (34–95%) and mortality (11–39%); thus, early surgical debridement of necrotic pancreatic tissue is only indicated for FNA proven infected necrosis or patients with surgical complications such as massive bleeding or bowel perforation.

o   A recent randomized control trial comparing a "step-up approach," characterized by initial percutaneous drainage followed by minimally invasive retroperitoneal necrosectomy if needed, to open necrosectomy demonstrated a lower complication rate, less organ failure, lower rates of incisional hernias, lower incidence of diabetes mellitus, and 35% of patients were successfully treated with percutaneous drainage alone.

o   Complications of acute pancreatitis include abdominal compartment syndrome, acute respiratory distress syndrome (ARDS), pancreatic and peri-pancreatic fluid collections, pancreatic necrosis, pancreatic pseudocyst, and pancreatic abscess.

Practical Algorithm(s) / Diagrams

Table 1. Common laboratory derangements in liver failure.

Test	Toxic or ischemic	Viral	Alcohol	Chronic biliary obstruction	Acute biliary obstruction	Infiltrating cancer
Aminotransferases (IU/L)	1000–10,000	100–1000	50–150	35–150	35–1000	35–100
Alkaline phosphatase (IU/L)	150–450	150–450	150–1000	300–3000	50–150	150–3000
Total Bilirubin (mg/dL)	2–10	2–60	2–60	2–60	0.5–2.5	0.5–10
PT	Prolonged	Prolonged	Prolonged	May be Prolonged	Normal	Normal
Responsive to Vit K	No	No	No	Yes	Yes	Yes
Examples:	Acetaminophen overdose, Shock or Sepsis	Hepatitis A, B or D	Alcohol	Pancreatic or Ampullary Carcinoma	Choledocholithiasis, Hepaticolithiasis	Cholangiocarcinoma, Mycobacterium avium-intracellulare infection

Table 2.   Differential diagnosis and management of acute jaundice.

Classification for acute jaundice associated with critical illness

Primary etiology	Examples	Treatment
Extrahepatic bile duct obstruction	Choledocholithiasis Common Bile Duct Stricture Traumatic or iatrogenic common bile duct injury Acute pancreatitis Malignancy (ampullary carcinoma)	Decompression, stone retrieval, stricture dilation, stent placement via ERCP or PTC
Increased bilirubin production	Massive transfusion Resorption of blood collections (hematomas, hemoperitoneum) Acute hemolysis (DIC, Immune mediated)	Treat underlying condition
Impaired excretion due to hepatocellular dysfunction, hepatitis, or intrahepatic cholestasis	Drug or alcohol-induced hepatitis Drug-induced intrahepatic cholestasis Drug-induced hepatocellular necrosis	Discontinue offending agent
	Gilbert's syndrome	No intervention needed
	Sepsis and other causes of inflammation Viral hepatitis	Treat underlying cause
	Total parenteral nutrition	Consider Enteral nutrition
	Ischemic Hepatitis	Treat underlying cause and maximize cardiac output to improve tissue oxygenation

Adapted from Vincent, Jean-Louis; Abraham, Edward; Kochanek, Patrick; Moore, Frederick A.; Fink, Mitchell P. (2011-05-12). Textbook of Critical Care: Expert Consult Premium (Kindle Locations 8657–8658). Elsevier Health Sciences. Kindle Edition.

Review of Current Literature with References

- Ostapowicz *et al.* published a prospective cohort study in 17 tertiary care centers as part of the U.S. Acute Liver Failure Study Group. Over a 41-month period, they analyzed 308 consecutive patients and reported that acetaminophen overdose was the most common cause of acute liver failure (39%) followed by idiosyncratic drug reactions (13%) and hepatitis A/B (12%). Survival at three weeks was just 67% and 29% underwent transplantation. Transplant-free survival ranged from 68% in acetaminophen toxicity to 25% for drug reactions and 17% of indeterminate cause. *Ann Intern Med.* 2002; **137**(12): 947.

- Wiesner *et al.* prospectively applied the MELD score to estimate the 3-month mortality to 3,437 adult liver transplant candidates with chronic liver disease who were added to the OPTN waiting list at 2A or 2B status between November 1999 and December 2001. Twelve percent of the patients died during the 3-month follow-up period and the waiting list mortality increased directly in proportion to the listing MELD score. Patients with a MELD score <9 had a mortality of 1.9% versus patients with a score ≥ 40 having a mortality of 71.3%. Thus, the MELD score can accurately predict 3-month mortality and should be used for allocation of donor livers. *Gastroenterology.* 2003; **124**: 91–96.

- A meta-analysis of 263 patients from six randomized controlled comparing enteral nutrition with parenteral nutrition in patients with acute pancreatitis demonstrated the enteral nutrition was associated with a significantly lower incidence of infections (RR 0.45; 95% CI 0.26–0.78, $p=0.004$), reduced surgical interventions to control pancreatitis (0.48, 0.22–1.0, $p=0.05$), and a reduced length of hospital stay (mean reduction of 2.9 days, 1.6 to 4.3 days, $p<0.001$). There were no significant differences in mortality (RR 0.66, 0.32–1.37, $p=0.03$) or non-infectious complications (0.61, 0.31–1.22, $p=0.16$) between the two groups. Based on these findings, enteral nutrition is the preferred route of nutritional support. *BMJ*, doi:10.1136/bmj. 38118.593900.55 (published 2 June 2004)

- A meta-analysis of 502 patients from eight studies comparing the clinical outcomes of patients with severe acute pancreatitis treated with prophylactic antibiotics compared with that of patients not treated with antibiotics demonstrated no protective effect of antibiotic treatment on mortality (RR 0.76; 95% CI 0.49–1.16), protection against infected necrosis (0.79: 0.56–1.11), or surgical intervention (0.88; 0.65–1.20). However, there was a benefit to non-pancreatic infections (0.60; 0.44–0.82). Based on these findings, antibiotic prophylaxis is not routinely indicated in patients with severe acute pancreatitis. *Am J Surg*. 2009; **197**: 806–813.

- In a multicenter study, 88 patients with necrotizing pancreatitis and suspected or confirmed necrotic tissue were randomly assigned to undergo primary open necrosectomy or a step-up approach consisting of percutaneous drainage followed, if necessary, by minimally invasive retroperitoneal necrosectomy. The primary end-point was a composite of major complications (new onset multiple organ failure or multiple systemic complications, perforation of a visceral organ or enterocutaneous fistula, or bleeding) or death and occurred in 31 of 45 patients (69%) assigned to open necrosectomy and in 17 of 43 patients (43%) assigned to the step-up approach. However, the rate of death did not differ significantly between the groups. The step-up approach should be considered in patients with infected necrotic tissue. *N Engl J Med*. 2010; **362**(16): 1491–1502.

Chapter $8\text{-}\left(v\right)$

Colorectal

Robert T. Stovall, MD*

*Assistant Professor of Surgery, University of Colorado School of Medicine

Take Home Points

- Acute colonic pseudo obstruction (ACPO) is a result of an ongoing process. This process should be identified and corrected.
- To diagnose acute colonic pseudo obstruction, mechanical obstruction and toxic mega-colon must be excluded as the cause.
- Toxic mega colon (TMC) is a potentially lethal final common pathway of severe colon inflammation that can be caused by a variety of initial processes.
- The diagnosis of TMC is clinical — a dilated, non-obstructed colon in the setting of and causing severe systemic toxicity.

Background

- Acute colonic psuedo obstruction (ACPO) (Ogilvie's syndrome) can complicate the course of many medical and surgical patients, but the exact incidence is unknown.
- It is believed to be more likely in elderly patients.

Contact information: Denver Health Medical Center, 777 Bannock Street, MC 0206, Denver, CO 80204. Tel.: 303-436-4029, email: robert.stovall@dhha.org

- Multiple conditions are associated with the development of ACPO.
- TMC is the final common pathway of many inflammatory colon disease processes.
  - o Commonly described as a result of inflammatory bowel disease but other inflammatory processes also can lead to TMC.
  - o Perhaps fulminant Clostridium dificile is one of the more common infectious etiologies that can cause TMC in the ICU setting.

Main Body

- Clinical Presentation of ACPO
  - o Nausea, vomiting and/or pain in the awake patient.
  - o Distended abdomen.
  - o No stool output or possibly diarrhea.
  - o Signs or symptoms of systemic toxicity should raise the suspicion of another diagnosis.
  - o The presence of peritonitis should raise of the suspicion of other diagnosis or ACPO complicated by perforation.
- Diagnosis of ACPO
  - o Need to maintain a high level of clinical suspicion.
  - o To be ACPO must rule out mechanical obstruction and toxic mega colon.
  - o History and physical exam.
    - ▪ Usually ongoing illness or recent surgery.
    - ▪ "Non-toxic."
    - ▪ Abdominal distention without signs of peritonitis.
  - o Labs
    - ▪ No diagnostic labs.
    - ▪ Assessment of electrolytes and acid base status can be helpful in both diagnosis and additional supportive measures.
  - o Abdominal plain films
    - ▪ Distended colon, specifically the cecum and transverse.
    - ▪ Possibly less distended left colon.
    - ▪ May show free air with perforation.
  - o Contrast Enema evaluation
    - ▪ Less used with current generation CT scanners.

- Can rule out distal obstruction.
- In certain cases may have therapeutic benefit.
   o CT Scan of the Abdomen and pelvis
      - Will show distention of colon without evidence of distal obstruction.
      - Useful to rule out additional diagnoses such as abscess or perforation.
- Differential Diagnosis of ACPO
   o Large bowel obstruction (e.g. tumor, volvulus, stricture).
   o Toxic mega-colon (e.g. from Inflammatory bowel disease, infectious etiology).
   o Both of these must be ruled out as ACPO is usually considered a diagnosis of exclusion.
- Treatment of ACPO
   o Evidence of perforation, ischemia, and/or peritonitis necessitate urgent surgical intervention.
   o Identify and correct likely underlying precipitating factors.
   o Nothing by mouth (NPO), nasogastric tube decompression, fluid resuscitation.
   o Consider possible rectal tube or fecal management system.
   o Close monitoring with serial exams, radiographs and laboratory assessments.
   o Correct electrolyte abnormalities.
   o Discontinue narcotic usage as possible and other sedatives or anitcholinergics.
   o Minimize all poly-pharmacy as possible.
   o Prone positioning and alternation of positioning may have benefits in the more mobile patient.
   o Pharmacologic options (after assuring no distal obstruction or toxic megacolon).
      - First-line therapy often considered to be neostigmine.
      - Neostigmine — 2 mg IV given over 3–5 minutes with possible repeat dose.
         ⇨ Cardiovascular monitoring should be used during and following administration. Atropine should be at the bedside.
         ⇨ Usual response if fairly rapid after administration of drug.
         ⇨ Timing of repeat dose a matter of debate.
         ⇨ Relapse rate of around 15–40%.
      - Other possible pharmacological options or if neostigmine fails.

⇨ Repeat neostigmine or neostigmine drip.

⇨ Polyethylene glycol has some support in preventing recurrence after neostigmine has initially been successful.

⇨ Pyridostigmine may have promise.

⇨ 10 to 30 mg pyridostigmine two times a day.

⇨ Increasing interest in peripheral opioid receptor antagonist but unclear benefit at this time.

⇨ Erythromycin, metoclopramide or cisapride have fallen out of favor for the treatment of ACPO.

o Endoscopic Therapies

- Colonoscopic decompression with or without the placement of a decompression tube.

    ⇨ Used when there is a failure of pharmacologic intervention.

    ⇨ Usual pre-colonoscopy bowel preparation is not used in ACPO.

    ⇨ Complication rates and mortality rates after colonoscopy for ACPO are higher than after colonoscopy for other indications.

    ⇨ Initial success rate fairly high, but recurrence requiring repeat decompression occurs in up to 40% of patients.

    ⇨ Passing scope all the way to cecum not felt to be indicated, only to hepatic flexure.

    ⇨ Can leave a decompression tube in the transverse colon but not clear that this improves outcome.

    ⇨ No hard indications for when to attempt colonoscopic decompression.

        — Likely no definite size criteria as indication for colonoscopy but more related to rate of increase in size and duration of dilation.

        — Usually after 9–12 cm consideration for colonoscopic decompression should be entertained.

- Colonoscopic decompression with the placement of a cecostomy tube has been described.

o Surgical Options

- Always indicated for evidence of perforation or ischemia.
- May be indicated if diagnosis is not clear.
- Outside of these indications, used in extreme circumstances.
- Pharmacologic and endoscopic decompression should be entertained prior to operative intervention.

- Options include
    - ⇨ Cecostomy to the skin.
    - ⇨ Cecostomy tube.
    - ⇨ Colectomy.
        - — If performed, usually recommended that end ostomy and mucous fistula are created and anastomosis avoided.
    - ⇨ Laparoscopic or open approaches are described. Depending on the size of the colon, laparoscopic is made more difficult.
- Clinical Presentation of TMC
    - o Affects all ages and sexes.
    - o History of IBD common, but can be first presentation.
    - o Antecedent diarrhea usually bloody, abdominal pain, cramping, distention.
    - o Ongoing resistant colitis may have been present leading up to the development of TMC.
    - o Patient will appear 'toxic'
        - Altered mental status.
        - Fever, tachycardia, possibly lower blood pressure.
        - Peritonitis may or may not be present.
        - Consider ongoing treatments and how they may affect presentation.
- Diagnosis of TMC
    - o High index of suspicion.
    - o Diagnosis is clinical in the setting of dilated, non-obstructed colon and a toxic patient.
    - o History
        - May include IBD, chronic diarrhea, acute diarrhea, known infections, recent travel.
        - Current and recent therapies should be evaluated — recent antibiotics, steroids or other immunosuppressant drugs or diseases.
    - o Physical Exam
        - May or may not have peritonitis.
        - Will have distention, and possible tenderness, abdominal pain.
        - Fever, tachycardia, hypotension, altered mental status.
    - o Labs
        - Should be drawn as parts of the work-up of the toxic patient, but no diagnostic lab test, all support the overall picture.

- Labs will be consistent with an inflammatory picture.
- Stool cultures should be sent to work-up the diarrhea for infectious etiologies (including *C. difficile*).
- Other cultures such as blood and urine should likely also be drawn in the workup.

o Radiology

- Plain radiographs of the abdomen are crucial early to evaluate colonic source of abdominal distention.
  - ⇨ Colon dilated (dilation >6 cm).
  - ⇨ Usual haustra may be present but are often disturbed.
  - ⇨ Small bowel dilation and possible large and small bowel fluid levels.
- Computed Tomography
  - ⇨ Can be helpful in assessing the colon and may help rule out mechanical causes of colonic dilation.
  - ⇨ Colon will be thickened, may have "accordion or target signs."
  - ⇨ Pericolonic fat stranding.
  - ⇨ May help evaluate other intra-abdominal processes and complications of mega colon.
- Literature is developing on the use of ultrasound to help diagnosis TMC.

o Endoscopy

- May have a limited role in the diagnosis of TMC if diagnosis is unclear.
- Usually felt that full colonoscopy in this setting is high-risk and thus limited exams only may be indicated.

• Treatment of TMC

o Multi-disciplinary approach is critical from an early stage.

o Medical treatment

- Depends on the underlying cause (e.g. IBD or *C. diff.* or CMV).
- Includes fluid resuscitation, bowel rest, correction of lab abnormalities and treatment of underlying cause.
- Minimize any drugs that may decrease colonic activity.
- Goals to reduce inflammatory source and prevent complications of severe colitis and to prevent death.
- Early surgical consultation is critical for a multi-disciplinary approach.

- Some have advocated patient positioning changes in the more mobile patient.
  - o Surgical treatment
    - Subtotal colectomy with end ileostomy is preferred when surgery indicated.
      - ⇨ Some lavage and diversion procedures for *C. difficile* have been advocated and are situation dependent (See section on treatment of *C. difficile*).
    - Earlier surgery (especially prior to perforation) has been shown to decrease mortality.
    - The decision for when to proceed to surgery is very challenging and the overall status of the patient must be considered as must the underlying diagnosis and underlying comorbidities of the patient.

Practical Algorithm(s)/Diagrams

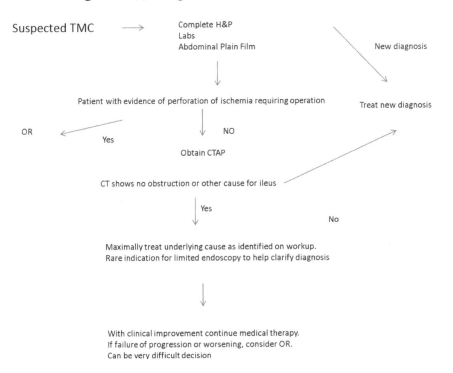

Fig.1. Suspected TMC.

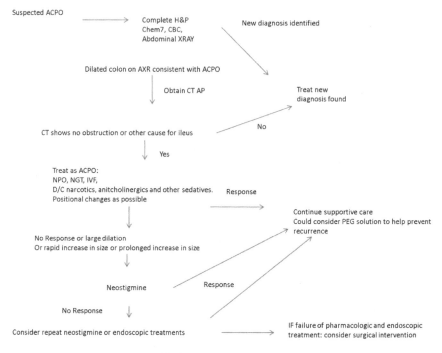

Fig.2.   Suspected ACPO.

Review of Current Literature with References

- Jain A, MD, Vargas, D. Advances and challenges in the management of acute colonic pseudo-obstruction (ogilvie syndrome). *Clin Colon Rectal Surg* 2012; **25**: 37–45.

  o Overview of Ogilvie's syndrome, pathophysiology, diagnosis and treatment.

- Autenrieth DM, Baumgart DC. Toxic mega colon. *Inflamm Bowel Dis* 2012; **18**: 584–591.

  o Recent review of TMC.

Chapter 8-(vi)

Abdominal Compartment Syndrome

Clay Cothren Burlew, MD*

*Director of Surgical Intensive Care Unit, Denver Health Medical Center,
Professor of Surgery, University of Colorado School of Medicine

Take Home Points

- Abdominal compartment syndrome (ACS) is defined as the combination of intraabdominal hypertension (IAH) with end organ dysfunction.
- Clinical indices of end-organ derangement such as decreased urine output, increased pulmonary pressures, decreased preload, cardiac dysfunction, and elevated intracranial pressure are fundamental to the identification of ACS.
- ACS is typified by IAH due to either intraabdominal injury (primary) or following massive resuscitation (secondary).
- Increasing abdominal pressure may develop before, during or after surgery, typically within the first 24–48 hours after injury.
- Physical examination cannot definitively diagnose IAH or its severity; a diagnosis of IAH can be obtained by measuring the patient's bladder pressure.

Contact information: Department of Surgery, Denver Health Medical Center, 777 Bannock Street, MC 0206, Denver, CO 80204; Tel.: 303-436-6558, Fax: 303-436-6572, email: clay.cothren@dhha.org

- With the recognition that ACS is a late event in the evolution of IAH, monitoring at-risk patients is advocated; this permits intervention in patients with IAH in an attempt to prevent the sequelae of ACS.
- Trauma patients that develop the "bloody vicious cycle" of hypothermia, acidosis, and coagulopathy are particularly susceptible to ACS and damage control operative technique should be considered.
- Once a patient is diagnosed with ACS, emergent decompression is indicated; this is typically accomplished via a midline laparotomy incision with evisceration of the bowel and egress of the accumulated peritoneal fluid or blood.
- Patients with marked intraperitoneal fluid as the primary component of their ACS may be effectively decompressed via a percutaneous drain placed using bedside ultrasound.

Background

- In the late 1800's, physicians identified the entity of increased abdominal pressure, and recognized that this increase in abdominal pressure could have systemic effects.
- The impact of intraabdominal pressure was largely ignored until the 1940s when Dr. Gross and his colleagues recognized that early forced closure of omphalocele defects, with reduction of the abdominal contents under extreme pressure, would lead to an infant's cardiovascular collapse.
- Despite this recognition, 35 additional years lapsed before the concept of intraabdominal hypertension (IAH) and its associated end-organ sequelae were discussed in the literature again with regularity.
- Kron et al. made the significant clinical contribution, that abdominal pressure, itself, could be used to determine need for abdominal decompression, and that this intervention could be lifesaving.
- Although Kron et al. are often credited with coining the term abdominal compartment syndrome (ACS), the first report of this term in the literature was not until five years later.
- The original description of ACS was in four patients who had undergone ruptured abdominal aortic aneurysm repair; postoperatively, when the patients' abdominal distension, increased airway pressures, increased central venous pressure, and oliguria, the surgeons reopened the patients' abdomen with resolution of the end-organ derangements.

Main Body

- Etiology and physiology

  o The etiology of ACS is multifactorial, typified by IAH due to either intraabdominal injury (primary) or following massive resuscitation (secondary).

  o The most common scenario for ACS is the multiply injured trauma patient who requires a large volume resuscitation, including both crystalloid and blood products; IAH in these patients is due to resuscitation-associated bowel edema, retroperitoneal edema, and large quantities of ascitic fluid combined with any associated intraabdominal pathology.

  o Increased abdominal pressure affects the cardiovascular system (decreased venous return to the right heart, decreased preload, decreased cardiac output, increased systemic vascular resistance, diminished stroke volume, decreased hepatic and intestinal perfusion), the pulmonary system (cephalad displacement of the diaphragm, increased intrathoracic pressures, decreased thoracic compliance, elevated airway pressures, hypoxemia), the renal system (relative obstruction to renal venous drainage, increased renal vascular resistance, decreased urine output), and the central nervous system (increased intracranial pressures) (Fig. 1).

- Diagnosis

  o Evidence of end-organ derangement such as decreased urine output, increased pulmonary pressures, decreased preload, cardiac dysfunction, and elevated intracranial pressure should herald the development of ACS.

  o With a multitude of etiologies that could cause a patient to have low urine output and cardiopulmonary woes, screening at-risk patients for IAH is paramount.

  o Patients identified to be at risk for IAH include those who have received 10 units of packed red cells or 10 L of crystalloid.

  o Physical examination cannot definitively diagnose IAH or its severity, as the patient's exam maybe reliable only about 40% of the time.

  o A diagnosis of IAH is typically obtained by measuring the patient's bladder pressure.

    ▪ The bladder acts as a passive reservoir, hence transmitting intraabdominal pressure without imparting any additional pressure from its own musculature.

- The technique as described by Kron *et al.* involves the installation of 25 cc of saline into the bladder via the aspiration port of a 3-way Foley catheter with the drainage tube clamped; after waiting for 30–60 seconds to allow the detrusor musculature to relax, pressure measurement with a manometer at the pubic symphysis is performed.
- Although the manometer technique is a single measurement in time, continuous monitoring is also an option.
- There are several conditions in which the bladder pressure may not be reflective of the intraabdominal pressure: external compression on the bladder due to pelvic packs, bladder rupture, marked adhesive disease, or neurogenic bladder.

- A grading system based on bladder pressure measurements was developed to aid in the diagnosis and subsequent treatment of ACS (Fig. 2).
- Abdominal perfusion pressure, defined as the mean arterial pressure minus the intraabdominal pressure, has also been advocated to diagnose IAH and ACS; to date, this has not been widely adopted in clinical practice.

- Treatment

  - There is not a single IAH pressure that mandates intervention; organ failure can occur over a wide range of recorded bladder pressures.
  - If the patient has ACS, however, emergent decompression is indicated; mortality is directly affected by decompression.
  - Patients with significant intraabdominal fluid, determined by bedside ultrasound, as the primary component of their ACS may be candidates for decompression via a percutaneous drain.
  - Abdominal decompression is typically performed via a midline laparotomy incision which allows egress of peritoneal fluid or blood as well as evisceration of the edematous bowel (Fig. 3).
  - Following laparotomy, temporary coverage of the viscera is necessary; one option for temporary abdominal closure is the use of a steri-drape and occlusive Ioban (Fig. 4).

    - The bowel is covered with a fenestrated subfascial 1010 steri-drape (3M Health Care, St. Paul, MN).
    - Small holes are cut in the plastic drape with a scalpel to allow intraabdominal fluid to pass through the drape.
    - The steri-drape is placed over the bowel and tucked under the fascia.
    - Two Jackson-Pratt drains are placed along the fascial edges to control reperfusion-related ascitic fluid; the drain tubing should exit cephalad to permit better occlusion between the Ioban and skin.

- The open abdomen, steri-drape, and drains are then covered using a large ioban (3M Health Care, St. Paul, MN).

o Despite temporary closure of the abdomen, a patient may develop recurrent ACS; leaving "expansion space" for the bowel in the temporary covering is critical. Additionally, bladder pressures should be monitored in at-risk patients.

Practical Algorithm(s) / Diagrams

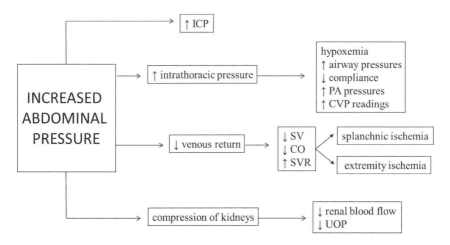

Fig. 1.   ACS affects multiple organ systems and physiologic parameters.

ICP = intracranial pressure; PA = pulmonary artery; CVP = central venous pressure; SV = stroke volume; CO = cardiac output; SVR = systemic vascular resistance; UOP = urine output.

ACS GRADE	Bladder Pressure	
	mm Hg	cm H$_2$O
I	10–15	13–20
II	16–25	21–35
III	26–35	36–47
IV	>35	≥48

Fig. 2. Grading system for intraabdominal pressure measurements in ACS.

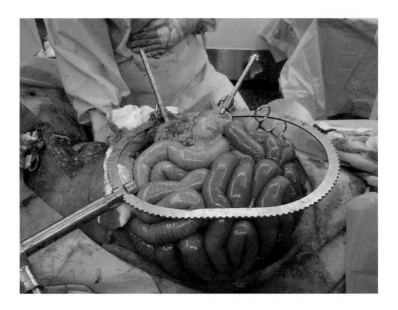

Fig. 3. Midline laparotomy permits decompression with egress of intraabdominal fluid/ blood and edematous bowel.

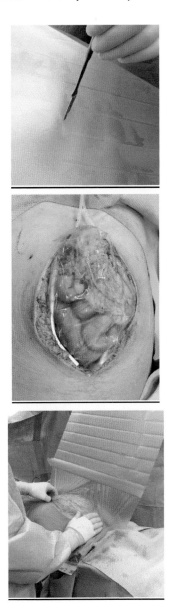

Fig. 4. Temporary abdominal closure using a fenestrated steri-drape, 2 JP drains, and an occlusive Ioban covering.

Review of Current Literature with References

- In 2013, Kirkpatrick *et al.* updated their 2006 consensus definitions of IAH and ACS and included practice guidelines. Their recommendations include intra-abdominal pressure measurement and protocolized monitoring, decompressive laparotomy for overt ACS, and negative pressure wound therapy to promote fascial closure. Other topics in the article include medical management of IAH, percutaneous drainage for ACS management, and red cell to plasma ratios (*Intensive Care Med* 2013; **39**: 1190–1206).

- In a meta-analysis of 14 studies with 2,500 patients, multiple risk factors for IAH and ACS were identified across a spectrum of patient populations; in trauma and surgical patients, large volume resuscitation was the most common risk factor for ACS (*Crit Care* 2013; **17**: R249). Madigan *et al.* had previously identified early, large volume crystalloid administration as the greatest predictor of secondary ACS (*J Trauma* 2008; **64**: 280–285).

- Balogh *et al.* noted in their single institution study that not only can ACS be predicted early but the rates of multiple organ failure in this population are markedly higher, >50% versus 12% in a non-ACS comparative group (*J Trauma* 2003; **54**: 848–859). Cotton *et al.* suggest that the rates of both multiple organ failure and the incidence of open abdomen management may be mitigated by the use of a massive transfusion protocol early in the patient's hospital course (*J Trauma* 2009; **66**: 41–48).

- In this single institution study, Cheatham *et al.* demonstate that percutaneous catheter decompression is effective in decreasing intraabdominal pressure; in their evaluation, a significant proportion of patients avoided decompressive laparotomy, particularly those with >1000 mL of drain output in 4 hours (*Chest* 2011; **140**: 1428–1435).

9. Hematology

Intensive Care Unit Anemia and Packed Red Blood Cell Transfusion

Fredric M. Pieracci, MD, MPH *

* *Acute Care Surgeon, Denver Health Medical Center*

Take Home Points

- Intensive care unit (ICU) anemia is nearly universal; 95% of patients who spend at least three days in the surgical ICU become anemic.
- The etiology of ICU anemia is multi-factorial; the most common contributing factors in critically ill surgical patients are hemorrhage, serial phlebotomy, hemodilution, impaired erythropoiesis, decreased erythrocyte lifespan, and deranged iron metabolism.
- Inflammation results in anemia via alterations in erythropoietin synthesis and sensitivity, decreased erythrocyte longevity, and hepcidin-mediated induction of a functional iron deficiency, in which iron is shunted from the bone marrow into storage as ferritin. This constellation of effects is termed the anemia of inflammation, and occurs within hours of ICU admission.

Contact information: Denver Health Medical Center, 777 Bannock Street, MC 0206, A388, Denver, CO 80206. Email: Fredric.Pieracci@dhha.org

- Although ICU anemia is associated with adverse outcomes, correction of anemia via allogeneic packed red blood cell (pRBCs) transfusion does not improve oxygen consumption, morbidity, or mortality, except in cases of either severe (hemoglobin < 7.0 g/dL) anemia or hemorrhagic shock.
- Despite these observations, pRBCs transfusion for stable ICU anemia remains a common practice in surgical ICUs; transfusions for stable ICU anemia outnumber those for hemorrhagic shock approximately five-fold at most academic trauma centers.
- Blood product transfusions are toxic: they induce an acute inflammatory response, are pro-thrombotic, and cause immunosuppression.
- Patients in hemorrhagic shock should receive pRBCs transfusions until the bleeding has stopped. Clinical markers of resuscitation should take precedence over an arbitrary hemoglobin transfusion trigger.
- For all other ICU patients, level I evidence exists to support a hemoglobin transfusion trigger of 7.0 g/dL, including patients in non-hemorrhagic shock, those with cardiac comorbidities, those with tachycardia, and those with traumatic brain injury.
- One exception may be patients with acute coronary syndromes [Chapter 5-(vii)], for which level II evidence exists supporting a hemoglobin transfusion trigger of 8.0 g/dL.
- Current data do not support routine supplementation of anemic ICU patients with recombinant erythropoietin, although important limitations to the literature should be recognized.
- Current data do not support routine iron supplementation (either enteral or parenteral) of anemic, critically ill surgical patients.

Background

- ICU anemia is exceedingly common: nearly all critically ill surgical patients become anemic within 72 hours of ICU admission.
- The etiology of ICU anemia is multi-factorial, including hemorrhage from trauma or surgical procedures, hemodilution with resuscitative fluids, serial phlebotomy, and the effects of inflammatory cytokines on erythropoiesis.
- Daily serial phlebotomy may exceed 250 mL of blood in some surgical ICU patients.
- Transfusion of pRBCs is also a common occurrence in the surgical ICU. Approximately one half of critically ill surgical patients receive at least one pRBCs transfusion during their ICU stay. Approximately 85% of all pRBCs transfusions in surgical ICUs are for ICU anemia (the other 15% are for acute hemorrhage).

- Although ICU anemia is correlated with adverse outcomes, a causal relationship has been difficult to demonstrate. Many confounders, such as severity of injury, comorbidities, and number of procedures, exist. In general, mild to moderate anemia (Hgb 7 – 12 g/dL) is well-tolerated, and may even be beneficial rheologically. Furthermore, there are no convincing data that correction of mild to moderate anemia with pRBCs transfusion improves outcomes.
- The inflammatory response associated with critical illness has a profound effect upon both erythropoiesis and erythrocyte longevity; these changes persist for months after ICU discharge.
- Inflammatory cytokines decrease erythropoietin synthesis and the sensitivity of the bone marrow to erythropoietin. Furthermore, these same cytokines decrease erythrocyte longevity. This results in inhibition of bone marrow erythropoiesis, and accelerated hemolysis.
- Inflammation also causes cytokine-mediated alterations in iron metabolism; specifically, iron is shunted from bone marrow sites of erythropoiesis into storage as ferritin within the reticuloendothelial system.
- This shunting is believed to be secondary to upregulation of the hepatic acute phase reactant hepcidin, which in turn down-regulates ferroportin, trapping iron within both duodenal enterocytes and macrophages.
- These changes result in a functional iron deficiency, in which little iron is available for incorporation into erythrocytes, although total body iron in storage is markedly elevated.
- The characteristic pattern of iron markers seen in inflammatory-mediated, functional iron deficiency is: (1) hypoferremia (serum iron concentration <50 ug/dL); (2) decreased transferrin saturation (<20%); (3) hyperferritinemia (serum ferritin concentration > 400 ng/mL, and often markedly elevated to >1000 ng/mL); and (4) increased byproducts of iron-deficient erythropoiesis, including erythrocyte zinc protoporphyrin and hypochromic erythrocytes.
- This pattern is also frequently observed in patients with chronic inflammatory conditions, such as systemic lupus erythematous, and was formally termed "anemia of chronic disease." However, because it is now appreciated that these changes occurs within hours of the inflammatory insult, the term "anemia of inflammation" has been adopted, and is more representative of the pathophysiology.
- Laboratory derangements seen in functional iron deficiency are nearly identical to those seen in absolute iron deficiency anemia, with the exception of the serum ferritin concentration (low in IDA and normal or high in functional iron deficiency), and the serum transferrin receptor concentration (low in IDA and normal in functional iron deficiency). The clinical scenario will also help differentiate between IDA and functional iron deficiency secondary to inflammation.

Main Body

- The best treatment for ICU anemia is prevention. Each tube of blood adds up, so think critically about the utility of every test that is ordered.
- In most cases, surgical ICU patients demonstrate a predictable, slow, regular decline in hemoglobin of 0.2 g/dL – 0.5 g/dL per day. This pattern is due to the aforementioned factors, is expected, and should not prompt an expensive workup as to the etiology of worsening anemia.
- In the minority of cases in which anemia is either unexplained or refractory to pRBCs transfusion, several laboratory tests may aid in the diagnosis. These tests will help categorize the anemia into one of three broad etiologies: (1) impaired erythropoiesis; (2) accelerated erythrocyte loss; or (3) both. These laboratory tests include:
  - Complete blood count, including both mean corpuscular volume (MCV) and mean corpuscular hemoglobin concentration. An elevated MCV (macrocytic anemia) suggests either vitamin B12 or folate deficiency. A depressed MCV (microcytic anemia) suggests iron deficiency (either absolute or functional).
  - Markers of hemolysis, including bilirubin (both direct and indirect), and haptoglobin.
  - Reticulocyte count/reticulocyte index: a low reticulocyte index suggests impaired erythropoiesis as opposed to accelerated erythrocyte loss.
  - Iron markers (discussed in *Background* section).
- The most common therapy for ICU anemia is pRBCs transfusion. Over the last three decades, the use of pRBCs transfusion in the treatment of ICU anemia has decreased dramatically. This decrease is due to the recognition that: (1) mild to moderate anemia is relatively well-tolerated by critically ill patients; (2) pRBCs transfusion does not impact significantly oxygen consumption in stable cases of mild to moderate anemia; and (3) blood product transfusion causes both inflammation and immunosuppression.

Theoretical basis for pRBCs transfusion

- Aerobic cellular metabolism may be characterized as a balance between oxygen delivery and oxygen consumption [Chapter 5-(i)].
- Normally, oxygen delivery far exceeds oxygen consumption. In this case, incremental increases in oxygen delivery are of no benefit. Conversely, when oxygen needs exceed delivery, shock and eventual cell death ensue. In this case, a prompt increase in oxygen delivery is necessary to preserve life.
- Oxygen delivery is the product of cardiac output and arterial oxygen content.

- The great majority of arterial oxygen content is achieved through binding of oxygen to hemoglobin within erythrocytes.
- The hemoglobin concentration is thus directly related to oxygen delivery.
- Accordingly, if one were to rely simply on mathematics, any increase in the hemoglobin concentration via pRBCs transfusion should result in an increase in oxygen delivery and ultimately oxygen consumption. However, this reasoning is flawed for several reasons:

  o It assumes that the patient's oxygen consumption is dependent upon oxygen delivery. This assumption is not true if either (1) the patient is not in shock or (2) the etiology of the patient's shock is not impaired oxygen delivery (e.g., septic shock).
  o Increasing hemoglobin improves oxygen content at the price of an increase in blood viscosity, which in turn decreases cardiac output. The net effect on oxygen delivery is unpredictable.
  o Transfused pRBCs do not behave as endogenous pRBCs *in vivo*. Rather, due to morphologic changes, as well as the accumulation of byproducts of storage, these transfused cells are clumsy, sticky, and stingy with respect to oxygen offloading. These changes are exacerbated by storage time.
  o pRBCs are thrombogenic. They increase blood viscosity, platelet adhesion and margination, and thrombin generation. These properties may be particularly deleterious to patients with acute coronary syndromes (ACS) secondary to atherosclerotic plaque disruption.

- Therefore, although the numeric calculation of oxygen delivery may increase following pRBCs transfusion, the actual delivery at the capillary level, and subsequent consumption by cells, is marginal.
- This hypothesis has been corroborated by several prospective studies, which have reported no change in either oxygen delivery or consumption after pRBCs transfusion.
- What, then, is a reasonable approach to pRBCs transfusion of critically ill patients with ICU anemia? Currently, the most commonly applied approach utilizes an absolute hemoglobin transfusion trigger of 7 g/dL (see *Review of Current Literature* section for discussion of this literature).
- This transfusion trigger has been challenged in several specific clinical circumstances, the two most common of which will be discussed herein:

  o *Acute coronary syndromes* are defined as unstable angina, ST-elevation myocardial infarction (MI), or non-ST-elevation MI.
  o These conditions share in common a reduction in myocardial oxygen delivery due to an unstable atherosclerotic plaque within the coronary arteries.

o It is argued that the hemoglobin transfusion trigger should be raised in patients with ACS (anywhere from 8 g/dL to 12 g/dL) because: (1) increased oxygen delivery is more important in this situation; and (2) although oxygen delivery may not change with pRBCs transfusion, increasing the arterial oxygen content will result in a decrease in cardiac output to maintain the same level of oxygen delivery, thereby placing less stress on the myocardium.

o These theoretical concerns have not been borne out in clinical investigation. There are many reasons for this disrecpancy, not the least of which is the thrombogenic properties of pRBCs transfusion, which are particularly dangerous in patients with ACS.

o Currently, and based on two prospective studies, a reasonable hemoglobin transfusion trigger for patients with ACS is 8 g/dL. There are no data to support transfusing to a higher hemoglobin.

o *Traumatic brain injured* patients are particularly vulnerable to secondary brain injury, caused by hypotension, hypothermia, and hypoxia. Accordingly, it has been argued that TBI patients should be transfused to a higher hemoglobin concentration than 7 g/dL.

o Approximately 50% of TBI patients receive at least one pRBCs transfusion.

o Studies of the effect of pRBCs transfusion on cerebral oxygen delivery and consumption have reported a variable, unpredictable, transient relationship.

o A subgroup analysis of the TRICC trial (discussed in *Review of Current Literature* section) limited to patients with moderate to severe TBI showed equivalent outcomes between the liberal (transfuse for Hgb < 10 g/dL) and restrictive (transfuse for Hgb < 7.0 g/dL) groups.

o See Chapter 32 for discussion of hemoglobin transfusion trigger following micro-vascular procedures.

• Treatment of ICU anemia with recombinant human erythropoietin has been studied extensively, most notably in three large, multi-center, randomized clinical trials by Corwin *et al.*

• In summary, these three trials showed a modest hemoglobin increase for the erythropoietin group as compared to placebo group, on the order of 0.5 g/dL. This increase in hemoglobin did not translate into a decrease in transfusion requirement.

• Mortality between groups was unchanged, with the exception of a subgroup analysis of trauma patients in the latest trial, in which erythropoietin therapy was associated with a significantly decreased mortality. This benefit is likely non-hematologic and requires further investigation.

- One limitation of the erythropoietin trials involves inadequate documentation of bone marrow iron delivery. Insufficient iron substrate may have hindered the ability of erythropoietin to improve anemia.

- Standard dosing of iron supplements (either enteral or parenteral) are not sufficient to overcome the functional iron deficiency associated with critical illness.

- The optimal therapy for functional iron deficiency may involve a combination of higher, goal-directed dosing, and hepcidin antagonism. Studies are ongoing.

- Standard dosing of iron supplements do not increase the risk of infection during critical illness.

- Blood product transfusion (including pRBCs transfusion) is independently associated with an increased likelihood of infection, organ failure, and death.

- Many of the deleterious effect of blood product transfusion stem from immunomodulation.

  o Passenger immune cells and cytokines attack recipient organ systems. In the case of the lungs, this results in transfusion-associated lung injury (TRALI). In the case of the immune system, this results in immunosuppression and infection.

  o By contrast, recipient immune cells and cytokines attack transfused pRBCs, resulting in the elaboration of further immune response, inflammation, and organ damage.

- Currently, no synthetic, hemoglobin-based oxygen carrier is FDA-approved for use in the U.S.

Practical Algorithm(s)/Diagrams

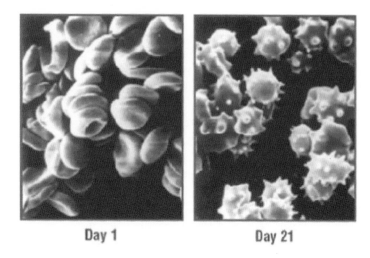

Day 1   Day 21

Fig. 1.   The packed red blood cell storage lesion.

Review of Current Literature with References

- The CRIT study reported that, among 4,892 critically ill patients, 44% received at least one pRBCs transfusion while in the ICU. The number of pRBCs transfusions was an independent predictor of worse outcome (Corwin *et al. Crit Care Med* 2004;**32**:39–52).
- The transfusion requirements in critical care (TRICC) trial compared restrictive (hemoglobin <7.0 g/dL) and liberal (hemoglobin <9.0 g/dL) transfusion triggers among 838 critically ill patients. Although inclusion criteria did not specify ongoing resuscitation, 37% of patients were in shock at the time of enrollment as evidenced by the need for vasoactive drugs. No difference in 30-day mortality was observed between groups. However, in-hospital mortality, as well as mortality among less severely ill patients (Acute Physiology and Chronic Health Evaluation II Score <20) and younger patients (age <55 years) was significantly lower in the restrictive transfusion group. It thus appears that a hemoglobin concentration of >7g/dL is at least as well-tolerated, and perhaps better tolerated, than a hemoglobin concentration of >9g/dL among critically ill patients (Herbert *et al. New Engl J Med* 1999;**340**:409–417).
- The CRIT Randomized Pilot Study randomized 45 patients with acute myocardial infarction to liberal (transfuse when hematocrit <30%) or conservative

(transfuse when hematocrit <24%) transfusion strategies. More patients in the liberal than the conservative arm were transfused (100% vs. 54%, respectively, $p<0.01$). The primary clinical safety measurement of in-hospital death, recurrent myocardial infarction, or new or worsening congestive heart failure occurred more commonly in the liberal arm as compared to the conservative arm (38% vs. 13%, respectively, $p=0.05$) (Cooper *et al. Am J Cardiol* 2011; **108**:1108–1111).

- The third, large randomized clinical trial of recombinant erythropoietin involved 1,460 critical ill patients. Comparing the erythropoietin and placebo groups, there was no difference in either the transfusion requirement or the number of patients transfused. Erythropoietin marginally increased the hemoglobin at day 29 as compared to placebo (1.6 g/dL vs. 1.2 g/dL, respectively, $p<0.01$) (Corwin *et al. New Engl J Med* 2007;**357**:965–976).

- We randomized 150 anemic, critically ill trauma patients to iron sucrose 100 mg IV thrice weekly or placebo for up to two weeks. Although ferritin increased significantly for the iron as compared to the placebo group, there was not discernable effect on iron-deficient erythropoiesis, anemia, pRBCs transfusion requirement, or mortality (Pieracci *et al. Crit Care Med* 2014;**42**: 2048–2057).

Chapter 9-(ii)

Diagnosis and Management of Coagulopathy

Eduardo Gonzalez, MD* and Ernest E. Moore, MD[†]

*Surgical Resident, University of Colorado School of Medicine

[†]Professor of Surgery and Vice-Chair of Surgical Research, University of Colorado School of Medicine

Take Home Points

- Appreciation of the underlying biologic mechanisms of hemostasis is central to the diagnosis and management of patients with coagulopathic bleeding.

- An endogenous coagulopathy, present upon ED arrival, has been identified in 25% of trauma patients; hypothermia, acidosis, and on-going shock worsen this already deranged hemostatic system.

- Hyper-fibrinolysis results in a 52–92% mortality rate, and should be identified promptly. Thrombelastography (TEG) is currently the best assay to diagnose hyper-fibrinolysis.

- Optimal management of coagulopathy starts with its prompt identification, or of those patients at risk of coagulopathy. Time is the main catalyst of coagulopathy, as the bloody vicious cycle perpetuates itself with every minute untreated.

Contact information: (Eduardo Gonzalez) 777 Bannock St. MC 0206, Denver, CO 80204; (Ernest E. Moore) 655 Broadway, Ste. 365, Denver, CO 80203; Tel.: 303-602-182; Emails: ernest.moore@dhha.org; Eduardo.Gonzalez@dhha.org

- All bleeding patients should be initially approached with the universal A-B-C (airway, breathing, circulation) assessment and management strategy, regardless of their coagulation status, as efforts to achieve hemostasis will be futile if these principles are not addressed.
- Viscoelastic hemostasis assays such as TEG provide prompt information on coagulation parameters that reflect all phases of clot formation; from the time it takes to form the first strands of fibrin, to clot breakdown by fibrinolysis.
- Patients with coagulopathic hemorrhage should be resuscitated with blood products when available, until bleeding has been controlled or coagulation parameters corrected. In these patients, crystalloid and colloid can worsen coagulopathy.
- Transfusion of blood products should be performed according to a massive transfusion protocol, ideally goal directed.
- Factor replacement (e.g., factor VIIa, prothrombin complex concentrate) and hemostatic medications should be used only as adjunct therapy to blood products and not as a substitute of them. They currently only have a role as salvage therapy in those patients with bleeding secondary to excessive anticoagulation, particularly those with intracranial hemorrhage.
- Tranexamic acid is an anti-fibrinolytic medication that when used adequately, can reduce mortality in trauma patients with documented hyper-fibrinolysis (TEG-LY30 >3.0%).

Background

- Severe bleeding is a frequently encountered challenge in the surgical intensive care unit. Although the etiology is diverse, the management based on the recent trauma experience is applicable to most bleeding scenarios.
- As much as 40% of injury-related mortality is attributable to hemorrhage.
  - ○ In both the civilian and military settings, uncontrolled bleeding is the most preventable cause of death.
  - ○ In trauma patients, there is compelling evidence that 25% of seriously injured patients have an endogenous coagulopathy, evidenced by deranged coagulation assays upon emergency department (ED) arrival; now generally referred to as trauma induced coagulopathy (TIC).
- Hemostasis is the physiologic cessation of bleeding achieved by the fluid and cellular components of the clotting system.
- The physiological mechanisms of hemostasis are complex. Our attempts to manage coagulopathy have so far parted from our basic comprehension of clot formation under homeostatic conditions; however unique mechanisms of

protein function and cell signaling exist under physiologic extremis, and remain poorly understood.

- Cell-based model of hemostasis (Fig. 1).
  - The traditional division of the clotting cascade into the intrinsic, extrinsic, and common pathways is medieval and has little *in vivo* validity.
  - Hoffman and Monroe advanced our conceptualization of *in vivo* hemostasis with the cell-based model of hemostasis, emphasizing the key interactions of the extravascular tissues, endothelium, platelets, and other blood cells, with plasma coagulation proteins. This allows cells to regulate hemostasis through receptors and signaling, and interact with other systems such as inflammation.
  - The cell-based model of hemostasis is conceptualized into three phases (initiation, amplification, and propagation), with most enzymatic reactions occurring on the phospholipid surfaces of cells.
  - Initiation
    - Exposed sub-endothelial collagen localizes circulating platelets by binding to the platelet's GP-VI receptor and $\alpha_2\beta_1$ integrin, adhering platelets to the site of injury (also referred to as primary hemostasis).
      - ⇨ At high shear rates (arterial circulation), circulating von-Willebrand (vW) factor binds to exposed sub-endothelial collagen and platelet adhesion is further re-enforced by binding of this collagen/ vonWillbrand factor complex to the platelet receptor GP Ib-IX-V.
    - With endothelial disruption, extra-vascular tissue factor (TF) binds circulating factor VII. The TF/VIIa complex activates factor X, which generates thrombin (factor IIa) from prothrombin.
      - ⇨ This initial amount of thrombin is insufficient to cleave fibrinogen and form a clot, but capable of activating factors V and VIII, and further activating adhered platelets via the protease activated receptors 1 and 4 (PAR-1 and PAR-4).
    - Amplification
      - ⇨ Factors Va and Xa which were activated during the initiation phase then form the pro-thrombinase complex (Va/Xa), and activated factors VIIIa and IXa form the tenase complex (VIIIa/IXa). The purpose of the tenase complex is to feed more Xa into the pro-thrombinase complex in order to yield a substantial amount of thrombin during the propagation phase.
        - — Factor IXa can originate from activation either through the TF/ VIIa complex or through factor XIa. This represents an overlap

between the classic description of mutually exclusive extrinsic (TF, VII) and intrinsic (XII, XI, IX) pathways.

- Propagation
  - ⇨ As tenase and pro-thrombinase potentiate each other, the so-called thrombin burst occurs. This amount of thrombin can now cleave fibrinogen into fibrin (fibrin then integrates activated platelets into the clot by binding to the GP-IIb-IIIa receptor), activates factor XIII (which polymerizes fibrin), and generates more Va and VIIIa (which further potentiates thrombin generation). This amount of thrombin also further activates platelets, generating a stable and growing clot.
- A sub-fraction of red blood cells are also capable of generating thrombin through the meizothrombin pathway.
○ Endogenous anti-coagulant system
  - Endogenous anti-coagulant proteins ensure microvascular integrity during hemostasis; protein-C, protein-S, tissue factor pathway inhibitor (TFPI), thrombomodulin (TM), and anti-thrombin (AT) have been well-characterized.
  - Heparan sulfate, heparin co-factor II, alpha-2-macroglobuliln, alpha-1-antitrypsin also enhance endogenous anti-coagulation.
  - AT directly inhibits thrombin, and most coagulation protein factors.
  - TFPI inhibits factor Xa and the VIIa/TF complex.
  - TM, an endothelial trans-membrane protein, binds and inactivates thrombin.
    - ⇨ The thrombin/TM complex activates protein-C that is attached to the endothelial protein-C receptor (EPCR).
    - ⇨ Activated protein-C cleaves Va and VIIIa, preventing their assembly into the pro-thrombinase and tenase complexes, thus hindering thrombin generation (Fig. 2).
    - ⇨ Through TM, thrombin is diverted from its pro-coagulant role to an anti-coagulant one, the so-called thrombin switch.
○ Fibrinolysis
  - Fibrinolysis is clot breakdown executed by plasmin-mediated cleavage of fibrin.
  - Plasmin is generated from tissue plasminogen activator (tPA) or urokinase plasminogen activator (uPA) cleavage of plasminogen.
  - Anti-plasmin (plasmin inhibitor), plasminogen activator inhibitor (PAI-1)(tPA inhibitor), and thrombin-activated fibrinolysis inhibitor

(TAFI)(down-regulates fibrinolysis), are endogenous anti-fibrinolytics that keep fibrinolysis in check (Fig. 3).

o Platelet function

  ▪ Platelet function is conceptualized into adhesion, activation, and aggregation for its study and understanding.

    ⇨ Adhesion: attachment to sub-endothelial collagen via the platelet receptors GP-VI, GP-1b-IX-V, and the integrin $\alpha_2\beta_1$.

    ⇨ Activation (secretion): platelet adhesion and thrombin (via PAR-1 and PAR-4) cause platelet activation.

      — Thrombin is the most potent platelet activator.

      — Activated platelets undergo a cytoskeletal change becoming more spherical with extended pseudopods, thus spreading over the exposed sub-endothelium.

      — The eicosanoid pathway is activated (via thromboxane-A2) and the content of platelet granules is released (alpha-granules: vW factor, factor V, fibrinogen, vitronectin, platelet factor-4, PAI-1)(dense bodies: ADP, serotonin, calcium).

      — Negatively-charged phospholipid micro-particles are transported to the outer surface (via a calcium dependent mechanism), which favors enzymatic assembly of coagulation proteins leading to thrombin generation.

    ⇨ Aggregation: activated platelets attach to fibrin via the GP-IIb-IIIa receptor, which tethers them to other platelets, leading to formation of a stable platelet and fibrin rich clot.

Main Body

• Inherited coagulopathies

  o The most common inherited bleeding disorder is Von Willebrand disease (vWD)(1–2% general population)(autosomal dominant).

    ▪ vW factor is a carrier of circulating factor VIII, and binds platelets to exposed blood vessel collagen via the GP-1b-IX-V receptor.

    ▪ Type 1: partial quantitative deficiency, type 2: qualitative deficiency, type 3: total quantitative deficiency.

    ▪ Bleeding manifestations are bruising and hemorrhage from mucous membranes such as menorrhagia, gastrointestinal (GI) bleeding, epistaxis, and severe post-partum bleeding.

- Diagnosis is by vWF quantification (vWF antigen) and function (ristocetin co-factor activity).
- Treatment should be managed through a hematology consultation. Urgent empiric treatment during severe hemorrhage in a patient with known vWD irrespective of type: 50 units/kg of VIII/vWF concentrate or cryoprecipitate at 1–2 bags/10 kg of body weight. Desmopressin (DDAVP) should not be used for an acute hemorrhagic event.

o Hemophilia A and B [deficiency of factor VIII and IX(Christmas factor), respectively](X-linked recessive)(A and B are indistinguishable clinically, hemophilia A is more common).

- Hemarthrosis during childhood is the most common clinical manifestation.
- Males with history of severe, unexplained bleeding after surgical or dental procedures, history of hemarthrosis, spontaneous retroperitoneal hematoma, or with a family history of hemophilia warrant a diagnostic workup.
- Diagnosis is by plasma factor VIII and IX quantitative assays.
- Mild hemophilia (residual factor level >5%, diagnosed as young adult after major surgery or trauma, spontaneous bleeding rare), moderate hemophilia (residual factor level 1–5%, diagnosed in childhood after minor trauma or surgery, hemarthrosis common), severe hemophilia (residual factor level <1%, diagnosed as neonate, severe spontaneous bleeding).
- Treatment should be managed through a hematology consultation. Emergent treatment during severe hemorrhage in a patient with a known diagnosis of hemophilia A or B is with 50 units/kg of body weight of factor VIII or IX respectively (elevates factor concentrations to >80%). Cryoprecipitate at 1–2 bags/10 kg may be used for hemophilia A but not hemophilia B (does not contain factor IX). Prothrombin complex concentrate (factors II, VII, IX, and X) can be used for hemophilia B, if factor IX is not available.
- Factor concentrations of 30–50% are required for surgical hemostasis; however higher levels may be desired for major trauma, intracranial hemorrhage, major surgery, and neurosurgical procedures.

o Factor XII (Hageman factor), prekallikrein, and kininogen deficiencies significantly prolong the partial thromboplastin time (PTT); however they are not associated with bleeding, even after surgery or trauma.

- ○ Prolonged prothrombin time (PT) with normal PTT: factor VII deficiency (rare). Normal PT with prolonged PTT: hemophilia A and B. Prolonged PT and PTT: factor V deficiency (rare), factor X deficiency (rare), and dys- or hypo-fibrinogenemia.
- ○ Hereditary disorders of platelet function (rare; 1:1,000,000).
  - Bernard-Soulier syndrome: GP 1b-IX-V receptor deficiency, autosomal recessive, low platelet counts since childhood, family history of low platelet counts, platelet size is large on smear, high mean platelet volume (MPV) on CBC.
  - Glanzmann thrombasthenia: GP IIb-IIIa receptor deficiency, autosomal recessive, normal platelet count and morphology.
  - Bleeding manifestations are bruising and hemorrhage from mucous membranes such as menorrhagia, GI bleeding, epistaxis, and severe post-partum bleeding.
  - Treatment of bleeding complications is with platelet transfusion; however, patients with multiple previous transfusions develop antibodies against the deficient receptor, limiting their effectiveness. In this scenario, factor VIIa, DDAVP, or PCC can be used as salvage therapy.

- Pathophysiology
  - ○ Trauma induced coagulopathy (TIC)
    - The "bloody vicious cycle" described in 1981 by the Denver General group (later referred as "lethal triad" by others) was characterized as clinical and experimental research data indicated that hypothermia and acidosis were conspicuous factors associated with early mortality in coagulopathic trauma patients. This notion has been integrated into the contemporary understanding of coagulopathy described in Fig. 4.
      - ⇨ A pH <7.25 significantly decreases enzymatic coagulation factor assembly and decreases the yield of thrombin generation.
      - ⇨ A core temperature <34°C compromises coagulation factor enzymatic activity and platelet function. PT/INR and PTT assays are done with samples warmed to 37°C, and do not detect these effects.
      - ⇨ Acidosis mostly affects enzymatic coagulation, while hypothermia mostly affects platelet function.
    - Although decreased concentration of coagulation factors has been reported after trauma/hemorrhagic shock and with fluid and blood

administration, recent data demonstrates that clotting is not compromised, as measured by viscoelastic parameters, until resuscitation
with crystalloid fluids achieves 50% hemodilution *in vivo*.

- 25% to 35% of trauma patients have been reported to have deranged
  coagulation assays upon ED arrival, and prior to fluid and blood
  product administration.

- Hypothermia, acidosis, hemodilution, and factor consumption are not
  primary drivers of coagulopathy but they rather exacerbate an already
  endogenously deranged hemostatic system.

- Protein-C activity: Brohi, Cohen *et al.* demonstrated increased
  protein-C activity in trauma patients with prolonged PT and PTT upon
  ED arrival. It has been proposed that increased protein-C activation
  results from tissue hypoperfusion, since patients with no base deficit
  had normal PT and PTT without increase in protein-C activation.

  ⇨ In a mouse model of trauma and hemorrhagic shock, prolongation
     of PTT was prevented by antibody-mediated inhibition of protein-C,
     and synergism of tissue injury and shock were required for prolon-
     gation of PTT when protein-C was not inhibited.

- The endothelium: elevated circulating syndecan-1, an endothelial
  glycocalyx protein that serves as a marker of endothelial injury, has been
  associated with a prolonged PTT, increased protein-C activity, increased
  circulating catecholamines, and is an independent predictor of mortality.

  ⇨ Syndecan-1 serves as a peptide backbone where heparan sulfate chains
     are attached. Circulating heparan sulfate has the potential of causing
     heparin-like endogenous anti-coagulant effects by potentiating AT.

- Platelet dysfunction is evident upon ED arrival in 45% of trauma patients
  by multi-plate impedance aggregometry. Early platelet dysfunction is
  characteristic of patients with traumatic brain injury (TBI).

  ⇨ Thrombelastography (TEG) platelet mapping has demonstrated
     86% inhibition of adenosine diphosphate (ADP) mediated platelet
     aggregation and 44% arachidonic acid (AA) inhibition in trauma
     patients. In TBI patients, ADP inhibition correlates strongly with
     severity of TBI, and distinguishes between survivors and non-survi-
     vors of TBI.

  ⇨ Platelet dysfunction has been attributed to early excessive platelet
     activation with subsequent exhaustion, as evidenced by elevated
     circulating CD40L (a soluble platelet ligand) early after injury
     and/or shock.

⇨ It remains unclear whether platelet dysfunction after injury and hemorrhagic shock is independent of enzymatic coagulation dysfunction.

- Fibrinolysis is a conspicuous factor in patients with TIC with the highest hemorrhage-related mortality.

  ⇨ Fibrinolysis can be physiologic (protecting the microvasculature and preventing systemic clot propagation), pathologic (premature clot breakdown from hyper-fibrinolysis), or shut-down (impaired fibrinolytic system that favors un-regulated clotting).

  — This is evidenced by recent clinical evidence that in trauma patients, there is a u-shaped distribution of mortality based on fibrinolysis quantified upon ED arrival; those with hyper-fibrinolysis and fibrinolysis shutdown have increased mortality compared to those with fibrinolysis within a physiologic range.

  ✓ Early mortality is seen in those with hyper-fibrinolysis and late mortality is seen in those with fibrinolysis shutdown.

  ⇨ Hyper-fibrinolysis is associated with a 52–92% mortality rate.

  ⇨ It has been proposed that excessive tPA derived from endothelial ischemia may bind all available PAI-1; this tPA/PAI-1 complex is subsequently cleared by the liver, favoring un-inhibited tPA leading to hyper-fibrinolysis.

  ⇨ Hyper-fibrinolysis has not yet been fully integrated into the currently proposed mechanisms of TIC, as a mechanistic link is lacking.

○ Disseminated intravascular coagulation (DIC) is a clinico-pathological syndrome characterized by generalized generation of fibrin leading to organ failure due to microvascular occlusion, and in more severe forms, concomitant consumption of coagulation factors and platelets, and occasionally hyperfibrinolysis, leading to coagulopathic bleeding.

- The initiating event for DIC is excessive tissue factor exposure leading to thrombin generation that overwhelms endogenous anticoagulants. Conditions with increased activation or expression of tissue factor: sepsis (TF expressed by cytokine-activated monocytes), meningococcemia, TBI, tumor emboli, myeloproliferative disorders, fat emboli, certain snake venoms, placental abruption, fetal demise, and amniotic fluid emboli.

- During sepsis, endothelial cells have a dysfunctional anti-coagulant surface glycocalyx, as well as dysfunctional endothelial cell-surface proteins such as TM which impairs protein-C activation. This favors widespread un-regulated thrombin generation throughout the microvasculature.

- Most cases of DIC do not manifest hyper-fibrinolysis, however it has been reported in the most severe cases. The mechanism under which DIC leads to fibrinolysis remains to be elucidated.

- Coagulation assessment
  - Optimal management of coagulopathy starts with prompt diagnosis. Time is the main catalyst of coagulopathy, as the bloody vicious cycle perpetuates itself with every minute untreated.
  - Patients with coagulopathic bleeding (or with high clinical suspicion of) should be initially evaluated with a CBC (Hgb/Hct and platelet count) and a viscoelastic assay such as TEG (or PT/INR, PTT, fibrinogen, and D-dimer when not available).
  - Conventional coagulation assays
    - PT/INR and PTT: initially developed to screen for heritable coagulopathies and later used to monitor anticoagulation therapy.
      - ⇨ They are performed on platelet-poor plasma and the end point for these tests is the time (in seconds) until the earliest formation of fibrin is detected. They do not assess the evolution of the clot beyond the formation of the first strands of fibrin.
      - ⇨ PT/INR and PTT have shown to correlate poorly with bleeding risk in elective general and vascular surgeries.
      - ⇨ PT/INR and PTT value thresholds used to define coagulopathy: PT>18 seconds, INR>1.5, PTT>38 seconds, or any of these values at a threshold of 1.5 times their reference value.
      - ⇨ In trauma patients, the prevalence of a prolonged PT is higher, but prolongation of the PTT is more specific. Adjusted odds ratio for mortality: 1.35 for PT and 4.26 for PTT prolongation.
    - Fibrinogen: concentrations >1.5g/L should be maintained in actively bleeding patients. In patients with TIC, fibrinogen concentrations decrease much earlier than other coagulation proteins.
    - Coagulopathic bleeding may exist in patients with normal values of PT/INR, PTT, fibrinogen, or platelet count.
      - ⇨ A study of markers of coagulopathy in 80 trauma patients identified that increasing injury severity correlated with elevated markers of endothelial glycocalyx damage, protein C activation, and clotting factor consumption even when INR and PTT values were in the normal range.

⇨ Nevertheless, in an actively bleeding patient, if any of these parameters are deranged they certainly contribute to hemorrhage and should be corrected.

o Viscoelastic hemostatic assays (VHA) (Fig. 5; Table 1)

- TEG provides data on the viscoelastic changes of whole blood as it clots in a 360 microliter plastic cup in which a rotational pin is suspended; increasing resistance generated by the clot is detected by the rotating pin and generates a characteristic tracing (Fig. 5).

    ⇨ The amplitude of the tracing (y-axis) represents the mechanical strength of the forming clot plotted over time (x-axis).
    ⇨ The clot is evaluated in a dynamic way; from the earliest mechanical resistance provided by the first strands of fibrin, to loss of strength secondary to fibrinolysis.

- Blood coagulation in TEG is initiated by contact of whole blood to the foreign surface of the TEG cup. Addition of coagulation activators such as kaolin (kaolin-TEG) or tissue factor (rapid-TEG) will expedite generation of results. Most TEG parameters can be obtained within ten minutes when using rapid-TEG (Table 1).

- The temperature at which VHA are performed can be adjusted to match that of the patient's.

- Clot formation via TEG is dependent on thrombin, mostly because clotting initiation is via contact of whole blood with the foreign surface of the cup and because of addition of activators such as kaolin and TF. Given that thrombin is the most potent platelet activator, inhibited platelets (e.g., with acetyl-salicylic acid or clopidogrel), may still generate enough clot strength to yield normal parameters due to the presence of thrombin. The TEG-platelet mapping assay (see below) has been developed to increase the sensitivity of TEG to platelet inhibition.

- Rotational thromboelastometry (ROTEM) is another viscoelastic assay that is based on the same principle as TEG, however it is mostly used in Europe. Its graphical output appears similar to that obtained with TEG; however, values of parameters are not interchangeable and separate treatment algorithms must be used.

- Limitations of VHA: (1) these assays do not reflect interactions between the fluid phase of coagulation and the endothelial cell surface; this dynamic is clearly present in the coagulopathic patient, however it remains to be fully understood; (2) pharmacologic platelet inhibition may not be evident with the standard assays, unless thrombin is inhibited and platelet agonists are utilized in the TEG-platelet mapping assay; (3) results can be operator dependent and subject to sampling and/or processing errors, as well as inter-sampling variability.

○ Platelet assays

- Incidence of thrombocytopenia (<150,000/mcl) in ICU patients ranges from 35% to 70%; it is due to increased consumption, destruction, sequestration, and suppressed bone marrow production.
- Platelet counts correlate with shock, trauma, and sepsis severity, mostly decreasing during the first four days of critical illness.
- Thrombocytopenia is an independent predictor of ICU mortality in multivariate analyses (relative risk: 1.9–4.2); particularly in those patients who fail to increase platelet counts after the first four days of illness (stronger predictor of mortality than the APACHE-2 score).

  ⇨ This may not be directly related to coagulopathy as the cause of mortality.

  ⇨ Platelet counts are not reflective of platelet function, and bleeding from dysfunctional platelets may occur regardless of platelet count, particularly in settings of acute physiologic extremis such as hemorrhagic shock.

  ⇨ 30% of the total platelet volume is pooled in the spleen of normal individuals. >50% of platelets can be sequestered in patients with splenomegaly.

- Platelet aggregometry (evaluates platelet aggregation by collagen, ADP, and epinephrine under high shear rates through microscopic aperture) is the gold standard for assessment of platelet function; however its results are not immediately available, and it has not been validated clinically during resuscitation.
- VHA such as TEG have been modified to evaluate platelet function (TEG-platelet mapping).

  ⇨ In this assay, heparin is used to eliminate the thrombin contribution to clot formation and platelet aggregation is then stimulated with AA or ADP. A separate assay from the same sample is done using reptilase and factor XIIIa to generate a pure fibrin clot. The maximum amplitude (MA) from the fibrin clot is then subtracted from the AA or ADP-generated MA, isolating the platelets' contribution to clot formation.

⇨ Effects of endogenous or pharmacological (aspirin, clopidogrel) platelet inhibition can be evaluated with TEG-platelet mapping. However, it has not been validated clinically during resuscitation.

o Disseminate intravascular coagulation (DIC)

   ▪ The diagnosis of DIC is one of exclusion and consequently scoring systems have been developed.
   ▪ Laboratory parameters in conjunction with clinical suspicion are employed to establish the diagnosis of DIC (score >5 compatible with DIC, <5 suggestive of DIC).
      ⇨ Platelet count (>100,000/mcl=0, <100,000/mcl=1, <50,000/mcl=2).
      ⇨ D-dimer (no increase=0, moderate increase=2, strong increase=3).
      ⇨ PT (elevation from normal range)(<3 sec=0 , 3–6 sec=1, >6 sec=2).
   ▪ Fibrinogen (>1.0g/L=0, <1.0g/L=1).
   ▪ 35% of ICU patients will meet the criteria for DIC.
   ▪ The cornerstone for management of DIC is correction of the underlying cause (e.g., sepsis).

• Management: all bleeding patients should be initially approached with the universal A-B-C (airway, breathing, circulation) assessment and management strategy, regardless of their coagulation status, as efforts to achieve hemostasis will be futile if these principles are not addressed. Particular attention to treatment of hypothermia while resuscitation is ongoing is imperative.

o Crystalloid and colloid administration to coagulopathic patients worsens their coagulopathy.

   ▪ *In vitro* studies have demonstrated increased fibrinolysis with crystalloid and colloids.
   ▪ In particular, hydroxyethyl starch can precipitate coagulopathy, and has been associated with increased mortality when used in patients at risk for coagulopathy.
   ▪ Patients with coagulopathic hemorrhage should be resuscitated with blood products when available, until bleeding has been controlled or coagulation parameters corrected.

o Blood products (Table 2)

   ▪ Blood transfusion risks in the U.S.: HIV (1:1,800,000), hepatitis C (1:1,600,000), hepatitis B (1:220,000), bacterial contamination (platelets, 1:75,000), hemolytic reaction (1:25,000), mis-transfusion (1:19,000), transfusion-related acute lung injury (TRALI) (1:5,000), fever/allergic reaction (1:100).

- Red blood cells
  - ⇨ As a general consensus, it is recommended that a hemoglobin level above 10 g/dl (Hct >30%) be maintained in patients with active hemorrhage.
- Hemostatic blood products (plasma, cryoprecipitate, and platelets) should be transfused as indicated by a massive transfusion protocol (MTP) or by a VHA, and in their absence based on the individual parameters described below.
- Plasma
  - ⇨ Hemostasis can be achieved when the coagulation factor activity is at least 30% of normal; this can be achieved with administration of a 15 mL/kg dose of plasma. Repeated or higher doses may be needed in patients with ongoing hemorrhage.
  - ⇨ By traditional tests and practice, and in the absence of VHA, in a patient with active hemorrhage, plasma is transfused to maintain an INR<1.5 and PTT<45 seconds.
  - ⇨ Plasma transfusion is more effective in correcting significant INR elevations (>2.0) and less effective with moderate elevation; the INR of donor plasma ranges between 1.0 and 1.3.
  - ⇨ Available data do not support the efficacy of FFP as prophylaxis for invasive procedures or surgery in patients with an INR<1.9.
- Intracranial, spinal, and ophthalmologic surgery or procedures are exceptions in which correction of coagulation parameters to a normal level may be warranted.
  - ⇨ Plasma transfusions in patients with severe liver failure are only effective for several hours because of the short half-life of factor VII (4–6h).
  - ⇨ Half-life (hours) of coagulation factors in plasma after transfusion: Fibrinogen (96h), II (60h), V (24h), VII (4-6h), VIII (10h), IX (22h), X (35h), XI (60h), XIII (144h), vWF (10h). All factors are stable *in vitro* except V and VIII, which are labile.
- Cryoprecipitate
  - ⇨ A fibrinogen level >150 mg/dL (>1.5g/L) should be maintained during active hemorrhage.
- Platelets (transfusion thresholds)
  - ⇨ <100,000/mcl: active hemorrhage, severe or multi-system trauma, TBI, intracranial hemorrhage, major surgery, or neurosurgical procedures.

⇨ <50,000/mcl: minor surgery or interventional procedures.

⇨ <10,000/mcl: non-bleeding patients (spontaneous bleeding rarely occurs with platelets >10,000/mcl).

○ Massive transfusion protocols (MTP) (Fig. 6)

- MTP allow for immediate processing of blood products by the blood bank and their systematic delivery to the patient's bedside. They create uniform treatment strategies to be easily followed by all medical providers across all disciplines.

- MTP's are either based on fixed plasma:RBC, cryoprecipitate:RBC, and/or PLT:RBC ratios agreed upon an institution, or goal directed by traditional coagulation assays or VHA.

- MTP activation criteria, their method of coagulation assessment (traditional coagulation tests vs. VHA), and their blood product ratio vary widely between institutions.

- Studies have demonstrated a survival benefit with a RBC:FFP ratio between 1:1 and 1:2. However, it remains unclear at which specific ratio within this range does administration of higher plasma ratios become no longer beneficial.

  ⇨ These studies have been criticized, particularly for methodological flaws that include survival bias (e.g., patients who did not survive were not transfused with plasma, and hence survivors had a higher plasma to RBC ratio) and heterogeneity between studies.

- While the optimal ratio remains a matter of debate, and randomized clinical trials are in progress, the majority of the data supports a 1:2 ratio.

  ⇨ Achieving this ratio requires early transfusion of plasma.

  ⇨ It appears that the benefit from a 1:2 or 1:1 ratio is not necessarily the ratio of blood products given *per-se*, but the fact that plasma is being transfused earlier.

- This increased use of plasma is not risk-free, since the incidence of transfusion-related acute lung injury is increased, as may be the risk of the acute respiratory distress syndrome and transfusion related circulatory overload (TACO).

- Liberal criteria for activation of MTP, or lack of re-assessment of these patients' hemodynamic and hemostatic status, may lead to indiscriminate administration of blood products.

- For trauma patients, the Denver Health Medical Center MTP (Fig. 6) is initiated based on field and ED vital sign criteria established by the

Research Outcomes Consortium (ROC), with the addition of high-risk injury patterns such as penetrating torso wounds, unstable pelvic fracture, or abdominal ultrasound with evidence of bleeding in more than one region. It is a goal-directed, TEG-guided protocol.

- Pediatric patients <40kg of actual body weight meeting criteria for MTP activation, are managed according to the pediatric MTP algorithm in Fig. 7.

○ Factor component replacement and hemostatic medications

- Current evidence supports the use of factor replacement and hemostatic medications only as adjunct therapy to blood products (with very specific indications), and not as a substitute of them.
- Factor VIIa

⇨ Its use is mostly limited to promptly reverse coagulopathy of therapeutically anti-coagulated patients with severe hemorrhage or intracranial hemorrhage, or as salvage therapy when blood products are being delivered and hemostasis needs to be achieved more rapidly.

⇨ When used, it is important to correct acidosis, hypothermia, thrombocytopenia, and hypofibrinogenemia, in order for it to be effective.

⇨ Dose: 60–90 mcg/kg i.v., can be repeated in two hours if needed.

- Prothrombin concentrate complex (PCC)

⇨ Concentrate of factors II, VII, IX, and X.

⇨ Its use is mostly limited to promptly reverse coagulopathy of therapeutically anti-coagulated patients with severe hemorrhage or intracranial hemorrhage, or as salvage therapy when blood products are being delivered and hemostasis needs to be achieved more rapidly.

⇨ Preparations vary worldwide; with the U.S. receiving FDA approval for "3-factor" PCC (II, IX, X) whereas many clinical studies conducted outside the U.S. used "4-factor" PCC, which includes activated factor VII.

⇨ When using a 3-factor PCC, supplementation with a plasma transfusion or factor VIIa (20 mcg/kg) has been recommended.

⇨ Median time for correction of INR to normal levels is 30 min.

⇨ Dose: INR 2.0–3.9 = 25 units/kg i.v. (max. dose: 2500 units), INR 4.0–5.9 = 35 units/kg i.v. (max. dose: 3500 units), INR >6.0 = 50 units/kg i.v. (max. dose: 5000 units).

- Factor VIIa and PCC administration should be administered with extreme caution and at the clinician's discretion, given their cost and possibility of associated thromboembolic complications.
- DDAVP
  - ⇨ Causes release of endothelial Weibel-Palade bodies, which contain vW factor, thus improving platelet adhesion.
  - ⇨ Used in the treatment of type 1 von Willebrand disease, and uremic bleeding in renal failure patients.
  - ⇨ In the absence of these conditions, there is no data to support its use; however it has been used as salvage therapy during coagulopathic hemorrhage.
  - ⇨ Preliminary animal studies show that desmopressin improves hypothermia and acidosis-induced platelet dysfunction, but clinical validation is lacking.
  - ⇨ Dose: 0.3 mcg/kg i.v., can be repeated in four hours.
- o Anti-fibrinolytics
  - Tranexamic acid (TXA) is a lysine analogue that prevents fibrinolysis by binding to plasminogen, preventing its interaction with fibrin, and activation by tPA into plasmin.
  - TXA should only be used in patients with coagulopathic hemorrhage and documented hyper-fibrinolysis (TEG-LY30 >3.0%).
    - ⇨ Empiric use of TXA when a TEG is not available or has not been resulted should be restricted to two conditions: patients at high risk of hyper-fibrinolysis (severe injury with SBP <75 mmHg), and patients in hemorrhagic shock not achieving adequate hemostasis despite appropriate blood product resuscitation.
  - Administration of TXA >3h from injury is harmful as it results in increased mortality.
  - TXA should be administered with extreme caution given the possibility of associated thromboembolic complications and other potential non-thrombotic complications.
  - Dose: 1000 mg i.v. If fibrinolysis persists despite initial dose (rare), a continuous infusion of 1000 mg i.v. over eight hours can be used.
- o Hemorrhage in anticoagulated patients [Table 3 in Chapter 9-(iii) describes pharmacokinetics of anticoagulation agents].
  - Major spontaneous bleeding is most commonly gastrointestinal, genitourinary or intracranial, otherwise bleeding in anticoagulated patients occurs after trauma or surgery.

- Identification of anticoagulation should be performed with a specific assay according to the pharmacologic agent used or suspected:
  - ⇨ Unfractionated heparin: PTT, LMWH: anti-Xa activity levels, fondaparinux: anti-Xa activity levels, rivaroxaban and apixaban: anti-Xa activity levels, dabigatran: ecarin clotting time or thrombin time (a normal PTT may exclude anticoagulation with dabigatran), bivalirudin and argatroban: PTT, warfarin: INR.
  - ⇨ TEG-ACT (rapid-TEG) or TEG R-time (kaolin-TEG) can be used to identify anticoagulation with most anticoagulant agents.
  - ⇨ Platelet inhibition with aspirin, clopidogrel, ticlopidine, prasugrel, ticagrelor, abciximab, eptifabatide, or tirofiban can be quantified with TEG-platelet mapping or platelet aggregometry (not available in most clinical settings).
- Hemorrhage with unfractionated heparin anticoagulation
  - ⇨ Life-threatening or intracranial hemorrhage: protamine dose estimated based on UFH half-life (50 mg max-dose).

Time elapsed	Protamine to neutralize 100 units of heparin
Immediate	1.0 mg
30–60 min	0.5 mg
>2 h	0.25 mg

  - ⇨ When heparin is given as a continuous i.v. infusion, only heparin given in the preceding several hours should be considered (e.g., a patient receiving heparin at 1250 units/hour will require ~20 mg of protamine for reversal of heparin given in the last 2–2.5h).
  - ⇨ Rapid infusion of protamine may result in hypotension and a systemic inflammatory state.
- Hemorrhage with LMWH anticoagulation
  - ⇨ Life-threatening or intracranial hemorrhage: enoxaparin administered in ≤8 hours: 1 mg of protamine neutralizes 1 mg of enoxaparin (e.g., dose of protamine should equal the last dose of enoxaparin administered). Administered in > 8 hours: 0.5 mg of protamine for every 1 mg of enoxaparin.
  - ⇨ Protamine completely reverses factor II inhibition by LMWH, however only 75% of Xa inhibition is reversed by protamine.

- Hemorrhage with warfarin anticoagulation

  ⇨ Life-threatening or intracranial hemorrhage: 10 mg vitamin K (phytonadione) i.v. and PCC or factor VIIa (if no PCC or factor VIIa available transfuse a 20 mL/kg dose of plasma).

  ✓ Not administering vitamin K may result in a rebound coagulopathy.

  ⇨ For mild or moderate bleeding oral vitamin K administration along with local bleeding control and supportive measures is adequate.

  ⇨ Treatment with high doses of vitamin K may make it difficult to resume effective anticoagulation with warfarin for days to weeks after the bleeding episode has been controlled.

- Hemorrhage with direct thrombin inhibitor (argatroban, dabigatran, bivalirudin) anticoagulation

  ⇨ There is no reversal agent for direct thrombin inhibitors.

  ⇨ Life-threatening or intracranial hemorrhage: PCC and factor VIIa have been proposed as salvage therapy.

  ⇨ Argatroban and bivalirudin have short half-lives (<1h); however can be increased to 4h with liver failure (argatroban) and renal failure (bivalirudin).

  ⇨ Dabigatran has a 16h half-life and clearance can be prolonged with renal dysfunction. This drug can be cleared by emergent hemodialysis in cases associated with hemorrhage.

- Hemorrhage with fondaparinux anticoagulation

  ⇨ There is no reversal agent for fondaparinux.

  ⇨ Life-threatening or intracranial hemorrhage: PCC and factor VIIa have been proposed as salvage therapy.

- Hemorrhage with rivaroxaban and apixaban anticoagulation

  ⇨ There is no reversal agent for apixaban or rivaroxaban.

  ⇨ Life-threatening or intracranial hemorrhage: PCC and factor VIIa have been proposed as salvage therapy.

- Hemorrhage with pharmacologic platelet inhibition (aspirin, clopidogrel, ticlopidine, prasugrel, ticagrelor, abciximab, eptifabatide, tirofiban).

  ⇨ There is no reversal agent for platelet inhibitors.

  ⇨ It is important to remember that the platelet inhibitory half-life of aspirin and clopidogrel exceeds their pharmacokinetic half-life.

⇨ Life-threatening or intracranial hemorrhage: platelet transfusion. DDAVP and vW factor administration have been proposed as salvage therapy.

- Immune thrombocytopenic purpura (ITP)

  ○ Abrupt onset of thrombocytopenia, no explained by medications, illness, or other causes.
  ○ Petechiae, bruising, mucosal bleeding.
  ○ Most commonly chronic and relapsing in adults, acute in children.
  ○ Autoimmune etiology; antibodies against platelet membrane glycoproteins.
  ○ Clinical diagnosis by exclusion.
  ○ Acute treatment is with corticosteroids: prednisone (1 mg/kg per day orally) or dexamethasone (40 mg/day orally for four days, repeated every 14 to 28 days as needed).
  ○ Patients with life-threatening hemorrhage and ITP-induced thrombocytopenia require platelet transfusion.
  ○ Splenectomy should be only considered for those patients who do not respond to corticosteroid treatment. Rituximab (thrombopoiesis-stimulating agent) can be used in patients who are not candidates for splenectomy.

- Thrombotic thrombocytopenic purpura (TTP) with hemolytic uremic syndrome (HUS)

  ○ Suspect in patients with microangiopathic hemolytic anemia and thrombocytopenia without an apparent alternative etiology.
  ○ Pentad of signs (only present in 25% of patients): thrombocytopenia, microangiopatic hemolytic anemia, fever, neurologic signs or symptoms, and renal dysfunction.
  ○ Caused by deficiency of the vW factor cleaving enzyme (ADAMTS-13), resulting in persistence of large multimeric vWF leading to increased platelet adhesion and consumption.
  ○ Can be congenital from decreased ADAMTS-13 synthesis or acquired from autoantibodies against ADAMTS-13.
  ○ Platelet thrombi in the microvasculature lead to organ dysfunction (e.g., stroke, renal dysfunction) and intravascular hemolysis.
  ○ Diagnosis is clinical and supported by laboratory findings of schistocytes on peripheral blood smear, elevated LDH, and indirect hyperbilirubinemia.
  ○ Diagnosis may be confirmed by ADAMTS-13 level, however not necessary to initiate treatment.
  ○ >90% mortality rate without treatment.

- o Managed with emergent plasma exchange upon diagnosis, replacement fluid must be plasma, continue daily until LDH and platelet count have normalized for two days.
- o Transfuse plasma (4–6 units in adults) if plasmapheresis is delayed.

Practical Algorithm(s)/Diagrams

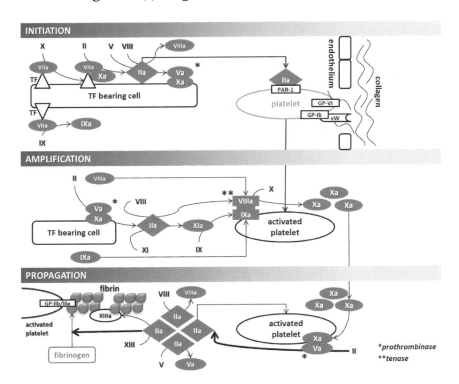

Fig. 1. Cell-based model of hemostasis.

TF: tissue factor, PAR-1: protease activated receptor 1.

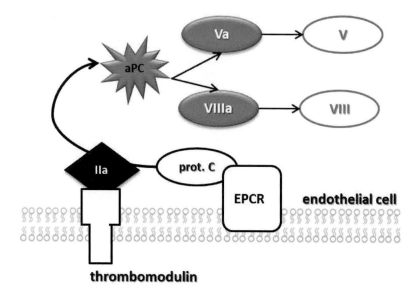

Fig. 2. Protein-C activation system.

EPCR: endothelial protein-C receptor, IIa: thrombin, aPC: activated protein-C.

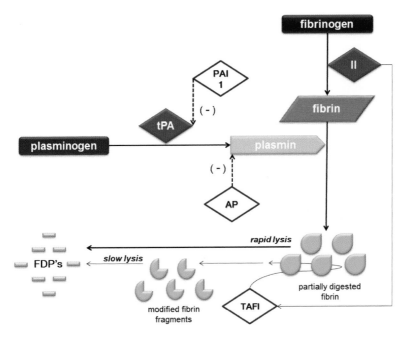

Fig. 3. Fibrinolysis system.

PAI-1: plasminogen activator inhibitor, tPA: tissue plasminogen activator, AP: anti-plasmin, II: thrombin, TAFI: thrombin activated fibrinolysis inhibitor, FDP's: fibrin degradation products.

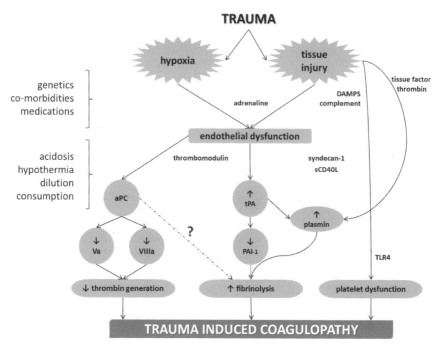

Fig. 4. Current understanding of the pathophysiology of trauma induced coagulopathy. APC: activated protein-C, PAI-1: plasminogen activator inhibitor, tPA: tissue plasminogen activator, DAMPs: damage-associated molecular pattern molecules TLR-4: toll-like receptor 4.

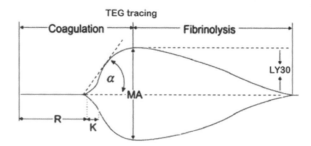

Fig. 5. Thrombelastography (TEG) tracing (see Table 1 for description of variables).

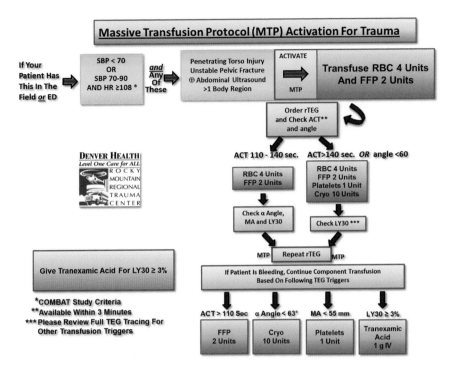

Fig. 6.   Denver Health Medical Center massive transfusion protocol (MTP).

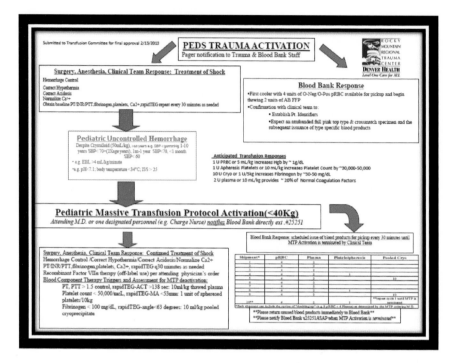

Fig. 7. Pediatric massive transfusion protocol (MTP).

Table 1.   Thrombelastography (TEG) parameters.

TEG Parameter	Significance	Unit of Measure	Normal Range
R-time	Time elapsed from the initiation of the test until the point where the onset of clotting provides enough resistance to produce a 2-mm amplitude reading on the TEG tracing.	minutes	kaolin-TEG: 3.8–9.8
ACT	Used as a surrogate of R-time in the rapid-TEG assay which uses tissue factor to obtain a quicker reading.	seconds	rapid-TEG: 78–110
K-time	Time interval from the R time to the point where fibrin cross-linking provides enough clot resistance to produce a 20-mm amplitude reading. Reflects potentiation of enzymatic factors yielding clot strengthening mostly derived from fibrin.	minutes	rapid-TEG: 0.5–2.0 kaolin-TEG: 0.5–3.5
alpha-angle	Angle of a tangent line between the initial split point of the tracing and the growing curve. Reflects potentiation phase of enzymatic factors yielding clot strengthening mostly derived from fibrin.	degrees	rapid-TEG: 66–82 kaolin-TEG: 47–77
MA	Point at which clot strength reaches its maximum measure in millimeters on the TEG tracing. Reflects the end result of maximal platelet-fibrin interactions.	millimeters	rapid-TEG and kaolin-TEG: 50–72
G	Overall total clot strength resulting from all coagulation interactions, calculated from MA; G=(5000*MA)/(100-MA).	dynes/cm2	rapid-TEG and kaolin-TEG: 5.3–12.4
LY-30	Percentage of clot strength loss 30 minutes after reaching maximal amplitude. Reflects amount of fibrinolysis.	percent	rapid-TEG and kaolin-TEG: <3.0%

R-time: reaction time; K-time: coagulation time; MA: maximum amplitude; G: total clot strength; LY-30: lysis at 30 minutes.

Table 2. Blood products.

Product	Volume Per Unit	Content**	Details
RBC	200–350 mL	1 unit RBC: Hct of 60%	Transfused RBC have a half-life of 30 days in the absence of bleeding or hemolysis. 1 unit increases Hgb by 1g/dL and Hct by 3%, in the absence of ongoing bleeding or hemolysis. In neonates and children transfusion dose is 10–15 mL/kg with an expected 2–3 g/dLHgb rise.
Plasma	200–350 mL	1 unit plasma: 600 mg of fibrinogen, 1 IU/mL of all coagulation factors and coagulation inhibitors.	FFP*: frozen within 8h of collection (contains functional quantities of all coagulation factors). F24*: frozen within 24h of collection (may contain variably reduced levels of factor VIII, 40–80% of normal)
Cryoprecipitate	15 mL	1 unit of cryoprecipitate: 200 mg of fibrinogen, 100 IU of factor VIII, 100 IU of vWF, and 75 IU of factor XIII.	Each unit or "bag" of cryo is obtained from precipitation of one unit of plasma. In most centers it is delivered as pre-pooled "10-packs"* (10 units or "bags," 150 mL), "5-packs," or as individual units*. A "10-pack" will increase the recipient's fibrinogen by 70–100 mg/dL. Neonates and children dose: 1–2 "bags" or units/10 kg.
Platelets	300 mL (SDP) 60 mL (RDP)	1 unit SDP: 3.5 × 10^{11} platelets 1 unit RDP: 5.5 × 10^{10} platelets	SDP* are obtained by apheresis of a single donor (also called "apheresis platelets"). RDP* are obtained by centrifugation, 4–6 units from different donors are then pooled. 1 unit of SDP is equivalent to 6 RDP units. 1 SDP unit (or 6 RDP units) increases the recipient's platelet count by 50,000/mcl.[†]

RBC: red blood cells, IU: international units, vWF: von-Willebrand factor, SDP: single-donor platelets, RDP: random-donor platelets.

* depends on local blood banking practices; DHMC products: plasma F24, cryoprecipitate "10-packs," SDP apheresis platelets.

** the average of the accepted range value is used.

[†] at 1h post-transfusion, accounts for estimated 30% splenic secuestration, and assumes no platelet destruction or ongoing bleeding.

Table 3. Anticogulants.

Drug	Mechanism of action	Indications (FDA Approved)	Dose	Route	Half-life	Metabolism	Excretion	Detection of anti-coagula-tion	Drug interactions[†]	Unique Issues
Warfarin	Vitamin K epoxide reductase inhibition	— Post-VTE risk reduction (acute management of DVT or PE should be done with an agent of fast therapeutic onset).	2–10 mg/d. See table # for dosing adjustments.	oral	36 h (very variable, range 20–60 h) (peak plasma levels reached 72–96 h)	hepatic (CYP–2C9)	biliary	INR	CYP450: 1A2, 2C9, 3A4 inhibitors and inducers	— 2C9 and VKORC1 genetic variations influence dose response and impact bleeding risk. — 99% bound to plasma albumin. — No hepatic dose adjustment needed (however, marked dose response in liver desease). — No renal dose adjustment needed.

(*Continued*)

Table 3 (*Continued*)

Drug	Mechanism of action	Indications (FDA approved)	Dose	Route	Half-life	Metabolism	Excretion	Detection of anti-coagulation	Drug interactions[†]	Unique issues
Heparin (unfractionated)	Thrombin and factor Xa inhibition (anti Xa/ thrombin ratio: 1.0)	— VTE prophylaxis. — DVT and PE tx (only for acute management, transition to warfarin for post-VTE risk reduction). — NSTEMI or unstable angina. — STEMI.	— VTE prophylaxis: 5,000 units q 8–12h subq (recommended dose is 5000 units q8h; 5000 units q12h can be used to minimize bleeding risk, but efficacy is comparable to placebo in high VTE risk patients). — DVT and PE tx (only for acute management, transition to warfarin for post-VTE risk reduction): 80 units/kg bolus i.v., then 18 units/kg/h continuous i.v. infusion. — NSTEMI or unstable angina: 60 units/kg bolus i.v., then 12 units/kg/h continuous i.v. infusion. — STEMI: adjunct to fibrinolysis; 60 units/ kg bolus i.v., then 12 units/kg/h continuous i.v. infusion.	parenteral (intravenous and sub-cutaneous)	— i.v. infusion:1.5h (increased with renal impairment). — i.v. bolus (dose dependent): 25 units/kg = 30min, 100 units/kg = 60 min.— subq: 1.5–3.0 h.	hepatic	mostly renal	PTT	No significant interactions	— No hepatic dose adjustment needed. — No renal dose adjustment needed. — VTE prophylaxis for BMI ≥40: 7500 units subcutaneous q8h. — Anti-Xa prophylactic goal (measured 4 h after dose): 0.1–0.4. — Anti-Xa therapeutic goal (measured 4 h after dose): 0.3–0.7. — Relationship between anti-Xa and PTT is variable by institution, however usually the therapeutic PTT is 2.0–2.5 times the control PTT.

| Enoxaparin (LMWH) | Thrombin and factor Xa inhibition (anti Xa/thrombin ratio: 3.3) | — VTE prophylaxis. — DVT and PE tx (only for acute management, transition to warfarin for post-VTE risk reduction). — NSTEMI or unstable angina. — STEMI. | parenteral (subcutaneous) | — VTE prophylaxis: 40 mg/d (for ICU-trauma, post-op hip and knee replacement, hip and pelvic fracture patients: 30 mg q12h). — DVT and PE tx (only for acute management, transition to warfarin for post-VTE risk reduction): 1mg/kg q12h or 1.5 mg q24h. — NSTEMI or unstable angina: 1 mg/kg q12h with concurrent aspirin tx. — STEMI: 30 mg bolus (i.v.), then 1mg/kg q12h (subq) (>75 y.o.: no bolus and 0.75 mg/kg q12h) | 3.5h (up to 8h in renal impairment) | hepatic | mostly renal | anti-Xa | No significant interactions | — VTE prophylaxis for BMI 40–49: 40 mg q12h, BMI ≥50: 60 mg q12h. — No hepatic dose adjustment needed. — Avoid if Cr clearance <30mL/min. — LMWH efficacy reduced by vasopressor use. — Anti-Xa prophylactic goal (measured 4h after dose): 0.2–0.6 (q12h or q24h dosing). — Anti-Xa therapeutic goal (measured 4h after dose): 0.6–1.0 (q12h dosing), 1.0–2.0 (q24h dosing). |

(Continued)

Table 3 (*Continued*)

Drug	Mechanism of action	Indications (FDA approved)	Dose	Route	Half-life	Metabolism	Excretion	Detection of anti-coagulation	Drug interactions[†]	Unique issues
Dalteparin (LMWH)	Thrombin and factor Xa inhibition (anti Xa/ thrombin ratio: 2.0)	— VTE prophylaxis. — DVT and PE tx (only for acute management, transition to warfarin for post-VTE risk reduction(except cancer patients)). — Post-VTE risk reduction (cancer patients only). — MI (non-Q wave) or unstable angina.	— VTE prophylaxis: 5000 units/d — DVT and PE tx: 200 units/kg daily (transition to warfarin for post-VTE risk reduction in non-cancer patients). — Post-VTE risk reduction (cancer patients only): 200 units/kg daily for 1 month, then 150 units/ kg daily for months 2–6. — MI (non-Q wave) or unstable angina: 120 units/kg Q12h (max. dose: 10,000 units q12h) with concurrent aspirin tx.	parenteral (subcutaneous)	4 h (up to 8 h in renal impairment)	hepatic	mostly renal	anti-Xa	No significant interactions	— VTE prophylaxis for BMI ≥40: 6500 units/d. — No hepatic dose adjustment needed. — Avoid if Cr clearance <30mL/min. — LMWH efficacy reduced by vasopressor use. — Anti-Xa prophylactic goal (measured 4 h after dose): 0.2–0.5. — Anti-Xa therapeutic goal (measured 4 h after dose): 0.5–1.5.

| Bivalirudin | Thrombin inhibition | — HIT tx.
— PCI for ACS in HITT or HITT-risk patients.
— Cardiopulmonary bypass in HIT patients. | — HIT tx: 0.1–0.2 mg/kg continuous i.v. infusion (goal PTT 2.0–2.5 times control) (start warfarin once therapeutic goal reached and PLT count $\geq 150 \times 10^9$, and continue bivalirudin until INR within desired range; stop bivalirudin and check INR in 4h, if INR is below desired range then resume bivalirudin and repeat until desired INR is reached on warfarin alone).
— PCI for ACS in HIT: 0.75 mg/kg bolus i.v.,1.75 mg/kg/hour for the duration of procedure and up to 4h post-procedure. | 25 min (up to 3h with renal insufficiency) | parenteral (intravenous) | blood proteases | 20% renal, proteolysis | PTT | No significant interactions | — Transition to warfarin may be delayed based on bleeding risk and need for interventional procedures.
— Critically ill patients require lower doses.
— No hepatic dose adjustment needed.
— Renal dose adjustment required: CrCL 30–60 mL/min = 0.08–0.1 mg/kg/hour; CrCL <30 mL/min = 0.04–0.05 mg/kg/hour.
— Hemodialysis removes 25%. |

(*Continued*)

Table 3 (*Continued*)

Drug	Mechanism of action	Indications (FDA approved)	Dose	Route	Half-life	Metabolism	Excretion	Detection of anti-coagula-tion	Drug interactions†	Unique issues
Argatroban	Thrombin inhibition	— HIT tx. — PCI for ACS in HIT or HIT-risk patients.	— HIT tx and prophy-laxis: 0.5–2.0 mcg/kg/min continuous i.v. infusion (goal PTT 2.0–2.5 times control) (start warfarin once therapeutic goal reached and PLT count ≥150 × 10⁹ and continue argatroban until INR is ≥4; stop argatroban and check INR in 4 h, if INR is below desired range then resume argatroban and repeat until desired INR is reached on warfarin alone). — PCI for ACS: 350 mcg/kg bolus i.v., 25 mcg/kg/min continuous i.v. infusion.	parenteral (intravenous)	45 min (up to 2 h in hepatic impairment)	hepatic	22% renal, 65% fecal	PTT	No significant interactions	— Transition to warfarin may be delayed based on bleeding risk and need for interventional procedures. — Will also significantly increase INR. — No renal dose adjustment needed. — Avoid with impaired liver function. — Can be used (off-label) for pre-filter administration during CRRT in HIT patients.

| Dabigatran | Thrombin inhibition | — Stroke and systemic embolism prevention in non-valvular AF. | 150 mg q12h | oral | 16h | hepatic | 80% renal, 20% fecal | Ecarin cloting time (ECT) or thrombin time (TT) | P-glycoprotein inhibitors, PPI** | — Avoid if Cr clearance <30mL/min or with impaired liver function.
— Dialyzable. |
| Fondaparinux | Factor Xa inhibition (indirect) | — VTE prophylaxis.
— DVT and PE tx (only for acute management, transition to warfarin for post-VTE risk reduction).
— HIT tx. | — VTE prophylaxis: 2.5 mg/d.
— DVT or PE tx: 7.5 mg/d (weight 50–100 kg), 10 mg/d (weight >100 kg).
— HIT tx: 7.5 mg/d (weight 50–100 kg), 10 mg/d (weight >100 kg) (start warfarin once PLT count ≥150 x 10^9 and continue fondaparinux for at least 5 days, and until INR is ≥2 for at least 24h). | parenteral (subcutaneous) | 20h | unknown (non-hepatic) | 77% renal | anti-Xa | No significant interactions | — Contraindicated if body weight <50 kg.
— Long-term use (>14 days) has not been studied.
— Avoid if CrCL<30mL/min.
— Dialyzable.
— Anti-Xa prophylactic goal (measured 3h after dose): 0.3–0.5.
— Anti-Xa therapeutic goal (measured 3h after dose): 1.2–1.3. |

(Continued)

Table 3   (Continued)

Drug	Mechanism of action	Indications (FDA approved)	Dose	Route	Half-life	Metabolism	Excretion	Detection of anti-coagulation	Drug interactions[†]	Unique issues
Rivaroxaban	Factor Xa inhibition (direct)	— VTE prophylaxis — DVT or PE tx. — Stroke and systemic embolism prevention in non-valvular AF.	— VTE prophylaxis:10 mg/d (14 d for knee, 35d for hip) — DVT or PE tx: 15 mg Q12h for 3 weeks then 20 mg/d (duration of tx per ACCP 9th Ed.). — Stroke and systemic embolism prevention in non-valvular AF: 20 mg/d.	oral	8h (12h in elderly)	hepatic	66% renal, 33% fecal	anti-Xa	P-glycoprotein inhibitors, CYP-3A4 inhibitors	— Avoid if CrCL<30mL/min or with impaired liver function. — Not dialyzable
Apixaban	Factor Xa inhibition (direct)	— Stroke and systemic embolism prevention in non-valvular AF.	5 mg Q12h (2.5mg if 2 of the following present: ≥80 y.o, weight ≤60 kg, or Cr≥1.5 mg/dL)	oral	12h	hepatic	25% renal, 75% fecal	anti-Xa	CYP-3A4 inhibitors	— Avoid if CrCL<30mL/min or with impaired liver function. — Not dialyzable

P-glycoprotein inhibitors*: rifampin, amiodarone, verapamil. CYP-3A4 inhibitors*: ketoconazole, itraconazole, voriconazole, fluconazole (mostly 2C9 inhibitor, weak 3A4), ciprofloxacin, metronidazole, erythromycin, ritonavir, amiodarone.

CYP-1A2 inhibitors*: ciprofloxacin, ethanol. CYP-2C9 inhibitors*: amiodarone, TMP/SMX, metronidazole, fluconazole, fluvastatin, isoniazid, lovastatin, setraline, gemfibrozil. CYP-2C9 inducers**: rifampin, carbamazepine, phenytoin, phenobarbital.

U.S. brand names: enoxaparin (Lovenox), dalteparin (Fragmin), bivalirudin (Angiomax), dabigratan (Pradaxa), fondaparinux (Arixtra), apixaban (Eliquis), rivaroxaban (Xarelto).

*May increase anti-coagulant concentration and/or effect.

**May decrease anti-coagulant concentration and/or effect.

[†]Combination of any two medications that affect hemostasis is considered a significant interaction as they increase bleeding risk.

tx: treatment, DVT: deep vein thrombosis, PE: pulmonary embolism, VTE: venous thrombo embolism, MI: myocardial infarction, STEMI: ST-segment elevation myocardial infarction, NSTEMI: non-ST-segment elevation myocardial infarction, PTT: partial thromboplastin time, LMWH: low molecular weight heparin, PCI: percutaneous coronary intervention, ACS: acute coronary syndrome,

Review of Current Literature with References

- In a prospective cohort study of major trauma patients studied upon ED arrival, Brohi, Cohen, *et al*. (*Ann Surg* 2007; **245**: 812–818) identified that patients without tissue hypoperfusion were not coagulopathic, irrespective of the amount of thrombin generated. Prolongation of PT and PTT was only observed with an increased base deficit (BD). An increasing BD was associated with high soluble thrombomodulin and increased protein-C activity. High thrombomodulin and increased protein-C activity were significantly associated with increased mortality, blood transfusion requirements, acute renal injury, and reduced ventilator-free days.

- The Ben-Taub group studied outcomes before and after implementation of a TEG-guided MTP (Tapia, Mattox *et al.*, *J Trauma Acute Care Surg* 2013; **74**: 378–385). These investigators compared outcomes of a fixed 1:1:1 (RBC:FFP:PLT) ratio MTP to a goal-directed TEG-guided MTP. A significant survival benefit was identified in penetrating trauma patients receiving >10 units of RBC in the TEG-guided MTP group compared to the fixed-ratio MTP group. Blunt trauma patients who received >10 units of RBC received less FFP when a TEG-guided MTP protocol was used compared to a fixed-ratio MTP, with no difference in mortality. There was no difference in volume of blood products or mortality in patients receiving <10 units of blood.

- In two studies that used a statistical analysis technique of pattern-finding and data reduction, known as principal components analysis (Kutcher, Cohen *et al.*, *J Trauma Acute Care Surg* 2013 **74**: 1223–1230)(Chin, Moore *et al. Surgery* 2014;**156**(3): 570–577), patterns of TIC based on coagulation factors, endogenous anticoagulants, and VHA parameters were identified. Two distinct patterns of TIC were described: (1) global coagulation factor depletion, which was associated with penetrating injury as well as injury severity, and predicted coagulopathy and mortality; (2) hyperfibrinolysis, which was associated with hemorrhagic shock, and predicted mortality. These data suggests distinct and possibly overlapping patterns of TIC; however their biological mechanisms remain to be understood, particularly regarding fibrinolysis.

- In the clinical randomization of an anti-fibrinolytic in significant hemorrhage (CRASH-2) trial (*Lancet* 2010; **376**: 23–32), an absolute mortality reduction of 1.5% was identified in trauma patients receiving empiric tranexamic acid (TXA) compared with placebo. Enrollment criteria included adult trauma patients within eight hours of injury with a SBP<90 mmHg or HR>110, or those who were considered to be at risk of significant hemorrhage. Early TXA (<1h from injury) administration was associated with the greatest reduction in hemorrhage-related mortality. TXA given 3h after injury was associated with an increased risk of death (4.4% vs. 3.1%; RR, 1.44; 95% CI, 1.1–1.8). No coagulation assays were used to describe the degree of coagulopathy and/or fibrinolysis of the patients enrolled, or to characterize the effect of the studied drug. The characteristics of the population studied are the primary criticism of this trial; only 50% of patients met inclusion criteria and only half of those received a blood transfusion. Furthermore, there was no significant reduction in transfusion requirements in the treatment arm of the study.

- In a comprehensive analysis of the data of all clinical studies using TXA as an anti-fibrinolytic in trauma patients performed by Napolitano, Moore *et al.* (*J Trauma Acute Care Surg* 2013; **74**: 1575–1586), only a modest effect on the overall population treated was observed; all-cause mortality was reduced from 16.0% to 14.5%(number-needed-to-treat, 67), and the risk of death caused by bleeding overall was reduced from 5.7% to 4.9%(number-needed-to-treat, 121). TXA's greatest impact on mortality was in those in the severe shock group (SBP<75 mmHg). Furthermore, the mechanism by which TXA reduced mortality in the CRASH-2 trial (*Lancet* 2010; **376**: 23–32) remains unclear given that fibrinolysis and coagulation assessments were not part of the study design. This calls for caution of indiscriminate use of anti-fibrinolytic drugs and raises the question of whether coagulation assessments should be performed prior to their administration.

Prevention and Management of Venous Thromboembolism

Eduardo Gonzalez, MD* and Ernest E. Moore, MD†

*Surgical Resident, University of Colorado School of Medicine
†Professor of Surgery and Vice-Chair of Surgical Research, University of Colorado School of Medicine

Take Home Points

- Surgical intensive care unit patients by definition are at the highest risk for venous thromboembolic events (VTE) and should be managed with pharmacologic and mechanical prophylaxis if no contraindications exist.

- High-risk conditions independently associated with VTE: increasing age, trauma (spinal fracture or cord injury, pelvic fracture, vascular injury), cancer, total knee arthroplasty, total hip arthroplasty, and presence of an indwelling central venous catheter. History of a VTE is the strongest predisposing risk factor.

- The choice of prophylactic anticoagulant agent should be made based on the evidence available for each high-risk group (e.g., trauma, orthopedic surgery, surgical oncology patients).

Contact information: (Eduardo Gonzalez) 777 Bannock St. MC 0206, Denver, CO 80204; (Ernest E. Moore), 655 Broadway, Ste. 365, Denver, CO 80203; Tel.: 303-602-1820, Fax: 303-602-1817, email: ernest.moore@dhha.org; Eduardo.Gonzalez@dhha.org

- The timing at which pharmacologic VTE prophylaxis benefits patients with traumatic brain injury over an increased risk of intracranial hemorrhage progression has not been adequately studied. The decision of when to start prophylaxis should be made on a case-by-case basis.
- Duplex ultrasound is the diagnostic test of choice when there are clinical findings of deep vein thrombosis.
- Computed tomography (CT) angiography is the diagnostic test of choice when there are clinical findings of a pulmonary embolism (PE) in a normotensive patient, while other diagnostic strategies are available for patients with contraindications for CT, or those who are hypotensive.
- The presence of hypotension associated with a PE has been defined as a threshold for thrombolysis. A careful consideration of contraindications due to bleeding risk should be had.
- If there is a high index of suspicion for PE, anticoagulation should be started while proceeding with diagnostic testing.
- Intravenous unfractionated heparin is the anticoagulant agent of choice for treatment of a DVT or PE in surgical ICU patients.
- Post-VTE risk reduction therapy should be continued with warfarin for at least three months in most cases.
- Heparin induced thrombocytopenia typically causes a >50% decrease in platelet count, that usually occurs 5–10 days after heparin exposure. It is associated with a 50% incidence of thrombotic complications, and should be treated with anticoagulation using a non-heparin agent.

Background

- Despite implementation of guidelines for the prevention and treatment of venous thromboembolisms (VTE), pulmonary embolisms (PE) remain the most common preventable cause of hospital death (appx. 150,000–200,000 deaths/year in the United States).
- Virchow's triad, consisting of stasis, endothelial injury, and hypercoagulability (inherited or acquired), is the basic pathophysiological process driving VTE.
- Mechanisms of activation of the coagulation system following critical illness, surgery, or trauma are incompletely understood, but may include decreased venous blood flow in the lower extremities, immobilization, release or exposure of tissue factor, increased platelet activity, endothelial cell activation, depletion of endogenous anticoagulants such as antithrombin and protein C, and compromised fibrinolysis.
- The reported incidence of clinically diagnosed VTE in intensive care unit (ICU) patients ranges from 1.3 to 7.6% despite administering recommended

pharmacological and/or mechanical prophylaxis. However, the true incidence of all VTE's is substantially higher if routine screening with imaging
is performed:

- o   A 10% prevalence of VTE upon ICU admission has been reported.
- o   In trauma patients, screening with venography detected a DVT incidence
      of 58% in patients who were not receiving VTE prophylaxis.
- o   A single-center study that used computed tomography (CT) scanning to
      screen for asymptomatic PE in trauma patients (ISS ≥9) detected an inci-
      dence of 24% (54% of patients with a detected asymptomatic PE were
      receiving pharmacologic prophylaxis).

- Failure to significantly decrease the incidence of VTE despite adopting the
  recommended prophylactic strategies may be due to inadequate heparin dosing, failure to address platelet activation, and shutdown of fibrinolysis.

  - o   The lack of efficacy of thromboprophylaxis with heparin has been largely
        attributed to decreased bioavailability due to peripheral edema, vasocon-
        striction, decreased cardiac output, and obesity.
  - o   Studies have shown anti-Xa levels to be below recommended thresholds
        for prophylaxis despite using recommended doses.
  - o   ICU patients experience a substantial progressive increase both in the
        concentration as well as the function of fibrinogen, which independently
        enhances coagulation.
  - o   Fibrinogen binds heparin and reduces its bioactivity; there is an inverse
        correlation between fibrinogen levels and the efficacy of heparin.
  - o   Activated platelets also contribute to hypercoagulability, and heparin
        administration appears to paradoxically increase platelet activation.
  - o   Suppressed endogenous fibrinolytic activity, also referred to as fibrinoly-
        sis shutdown, has been documented in ICU patients, and may be
        implicated in driving VTE formation.

- Characterization of hypercoagulability has been achieved clinically with
  thrombelastography (TEG) in ICU trauma patients.

  - o   Both enzymatic (driven by fibrinogen and coagulation factors) and plate-
        let hypercoagulability are concomitantly present.
  - o   Citrated-kaolin TEG values of clot strength maximum amplitude (MA)
        >72 mm, and shear elastic modulus strength (G) >12.4 dynes/cm^2, have
        been established as markers of post-injury hypercoagulability associated
        with increased risk of VTE.
  - o   This hypercoagulable threshold is reached by 48 h from ICU admission in
        most trauma patients.

Main Body

- VTE risk assessment
  - ○ Risk assessment should be performed upon every patient's admission to the ICU. When contraindications for VTE prophylaxis exist, a daily re-assessment of bleeding and thrombosis risk should be performed.
  - ○ Omission of prophylaxis at 24 h from ICU admission has been associated with a 3-fold increase in VTE incidence, and with an estimated attributable mortality effect of 3.9 to 15.4%.
  - ○ DVT event rates in the absence of prophylaxis based on systematic screening studies with imaging: acute spinal cord injury 90%, trauma 58%, elective hip surgery 50%, major general surgery 25%, neurosurgical patients 22%.
  - ○ The Caprini Risk Assessment Model, described in Table 1, is the most commonly utilized VTE risk assessment tool in surgical patients and has been modified for its use in the 2012 American College of Chest Physician's VTE prophylaxis guidelines.
    - ▪ Although this tool is useful to identify those patients who will benefit from VTE prophylaxis, surgical ICU patients by definition are high risk (mostly due to a major surgical procedure, central venous catheter [CVC], immobility, and/or trauma) and should be managed as such.
    - ▪ Of note, this model was not developed using rigorous statistical methods, and includes some variables that were later found not to be associated with VTE risk. Furthermore, it does not include specific criteria for trauma patients.
  - ○ In trauma patients, the Greenfield risk assessment profile (RAP) score has been developed to identify those patients at high risk for VTE ($\geq$5 points) who will benefit from VTE prophylaxis. Table 2 describes the RAP score.
  - ○ Hereditary hypercoagulable disorders: activated protein-C resistance from factor V Leiden (most common, 5% general population), prothrombin gene mutation 20210A, protein C and S deficiency, elevated homocysteine, antithrombin deficiency, and elevated coagulation factors VIII, IX, and XI.
    - ▪ The total incidence of one of these inherited thrombophilias in subjects with a VTE range from 24% to 37% compared with approximately 10% in controls.
  - ○ The Asian population has a lower incidence of VTE compared to other ethnicities.
  - ○ Acquired hypercoagulable disorders: anti-phospholipid antibody syndrome, polycythemia vera, essential thrombocytosis, paroxysmal nocturnal hemoglobinuria, Cushing syndrome.

o Polycythemia vera patients have a high incidence of portal and mesenteric vein thrombosis, mostly due to hypercoagulability resulting from increased blood viscosity. Hence, adequate hydration perioperatively is crucial in preventing thrombosis in these patients.

o Malignancy is the most common acquired condition predisposing to VTE.

o Major risk factors that have been independently associated with increased VTE incidence: increasing age, spine fracture, spinal cord injury, pelvic fracture, severe femur or tibial fracture, vascular injury (risk highest with venous repair or ligation), sepsis, >72 hours of mechanical ventilation, prolonged neuromuscular blockade (repeated dosing or continuous infusion), indwelling central venous catheters (CVC), prolonged vasopressor requirements, obesity, congestive heart failure, and end-stage renal disease. History of a previous VTE is the strongest risk factor.

o Medications associated with a hypercoagulable state: oral and transdermal contraceptives, estrogen (+/− progestin) replacement therapy, tamoxifen, raloxifene, L-asparaginase, chemotherapeutic agents, bevacizumab (Avastin; VEGF monoclonal antibody used in colon cancer).

o In ICU patients with CVC, there is a 33% prevalence of catheter-related DVT reported by studies using ultrasound (US) screening.

■ Incidence of CVC-related DVT by catheter location: femoral vein > internal jugular vein > subclavian vein.

■ Peripherally inserted central venous catheters (PICC) are associated with an increased risk of catheter related DVT's compared to that of CVC's (OR 2.55) (80% of PICC-related DVT's occurred within 14 days from insertion).

■ Prevalence of a CVC-related DVT is elevated when a central line associated blood stream infection (CLABSI) is present, and conversely there is a 2.6-fold higher risk of sepsis when CVC related DVT is present.

■ Misplaced CVC (catheter tip in the innominate vein or junction of the innominate vein with the superior vena cava) are associated with a higher risk of CVC related DVT than properly positioned catheters (catheter tip in distal superior vena cava or junction with right atrium).

• VTE prophylaxis

o Anticoagulant medications and dosing are described in Table 3.

o Very-low, low, and moderate VTE risk patients should be managed according to Table 1.

o High-risk patients, in addition to pharmacologic prophylaxis, should receive lower extremity intermittent pneumatic compression (IPC) if no contraindications exist (skin breakdown, wounds, grafts, fractures, external fixators, or casts).

- IPC use prevents venous stasis, and also decreases circulating plasminogen activator inhibitor-1 (PAI-1) levels which favors endogenous tissue plasminogen activator (tPA) activity.
- In high VTE risk patients, use of IPC in addition to pharmacologic prophylaxis reduces VTE risk more than either treatment alone.

o Pharmacologic prophylaxis is recommended with low-dose unfractionated heparin (UFH) or low molecular weight heparin (LMWH) for high-risk patients.

o Selection of low-dose UFH vs. LMWH should be made based on evidence for each specific patient population:

- General and abdominal/pelvic surgery (excluding surgery for cancer).
  - ⇨ Meta-analyses have shown equal efficacy of low-dose UFH (5000 units q8h) vs. LMWH in prevention of VTE's, with no significant differences in bleeding complications.

- Trauma
  - ⇨ Studies have demonstrated no benefit of low-dose UFH (5000 units q12h) when compared to no prophylaxis at all in trauma patients (injury severity score, ISS ≥9).
  - ⇨ Use of LMWH (enoxaparin 30 mg q12h) in trauma patients (ISS ≥9), is associated with a decreased incidence of DVT (detected by screening venography) compared to low-dose UFH (5000 units q12h) (33% vs. 41%, $p = 0.01$). No differences in PE or mortality.
  - ⇨ It has been suggested that addition of low-dose aspirin (81–160 mg), as well as extended heparin prophylaxis (2–5 weeks) in patients at highest VTE risk (spinal fracture or cord injury, pelvic fracture, and vascular injury requiring repair or ligation) could be beneficial.

- Neurosurgery and spine surgery:
  - ⇨ Patients at highest risk for VTE include: craniotomy or spinal surgery for malignant disease, combined anterior-posterior spinal approach, paresis, spinal fracture or cord injury, and traumatic brain injury (TBI) associated with poly-trauma.
  - ⇨ It is unclear to what degree bleeding risk may exceed the benefit of VTE pharmacologic prophylaxis in the first 48 hours after intracranial hemorrhage (ICH), severe TBI, craniotomy, or spine surgery.

— The most benefit of pharmacologic VTE prophylaxis is seen when started within 72 hours. Given the lack of data, timing of pharmacologic prophylaxis should be based on a patient-specific daily bleeding vs. thrombosis risk assessment.

— These patients still benefit from VTE prophylaxis with IPC until bleeding risk allows initiation of pharmacologic prophylaxis.

⇨ Although most studies investigating the effectiveness and safety of pharmacologic VTE prophylaxis in neurosurgery and spine surgery (non-traumatic) have been done with LMWH, there are no studies to support LMWH over low-dose UFH regarding efficacy and bleeding risk.

- Orthopedic surgery:

⇨ Patients at highest risk for VTE include: total hip arthroplasty, total knee arthroplasty, and hip or pelvic fracture surgery.

⇨ There is more data to support the efficacy of LMWH over other agents, with no difference in bleeding events.

⇨ Most benefit from pharmacologic prophylaxis is seen when started 12h post-operatively, if hemostasis is adequate.

⇨ Median time to VTE is 3.5 weeks.

⇨ Extended pharmacologic prophylaxis recommended for 2–5 weeks post-operatively for highest risk patients (total knee arthroplasty, total hip arthroplasty, and hip or pelvic fracture surgery).

— LMWH is the preferred agent for extended prophylaxis, but rivaroxaban, adjusted-dose warfarin (INR goal 2.0–2.5), or aspirin are acceptable alternatives when lack of patient compliance with injections or cost is an issue.

- Surgical oncology:

⇨ 33% of VTE occur after hospital discharge in surgical oncology patients.

⇨ Extended pharmacologic prophylaxis for four weeks post-operatively is recommended after abdominal or pelvic cancer surgery.

— Studies supporting this extended duration recommendation have only been done with LMWH.

⇨ No difference was observed in DVT, PE, bleeding complications, and survival in a meta-analysis comparing peri-operative LMWH vs. low-dose UFH (5000 q8 hours) for VTE prophylaxis in surgical oncology patients (prophylaxis limited to hospital stay).

⇨ The risk of thrombosis may be further increased in patients with malignancy and a CVC or PICC, in which the incidence of a symptomatic VTE is as high as 12%.

⇨ Particular attention to bleeding risk must be placed on patients with liver resections (proportional to the number of segments resected), pancreatic or bile leak, more than one enteric anastomosis, and with a sentinel bleed.

- Obese and bariatric surgery patients:

  ⇨ The volume of distribution of heparin in obese patients differs from non-obese patients since adipose tissue has a lower blood volume than lean tissue; as a result, heparin dosing requirements do not increase linearly with body weight.

  ⇨ Table 3 reviews the dose adjustments needed for a BMI ≥40. Routine prophylactic doses can be used for BMI <40.

  ⇨ There is no preferred agent, however limited studies have shown that LMWH is more efficacious in preventing post-operative VTE than low-dose UFH after bariatric surgery, with no differences in bleeding risk.

  ⇨ Extended pharmacologic prophylaxis for 1–2 weeks post-operatively after bariatric surgery rather than prophylaxis limited to hospital stay is recommended.

- In hospitalized high-VTE risk patients, routine discontinuation of prophylactic anti-coagulation before an interventional or surgical procedure (except for neurosurgery, spine, or ocular surgery) is not recommended.

○ Bleeding risk

- Definition of a major bleeding event according to the International Surgical Thrombosis Forum: fatal bleeding, symptomatic bleeding in critical organ, new or increased intracranial hemorrhage, retroperitoneal bleeding, bleeding causing hemodynamic instability, bleeding causing decrease in hemoglobin ≥2 g/dL, bleeding requiring ≥2 units of blood transfusion, bleeding requiring and interventional or surgical procedure.

- Incidence of bleeding complications from pharmacologic VTE prophylaxis: injection site bruising (6.9%), wound hematoma (5.7%), drain site bleeding (2.0%), hematuria (1.6%), gastrointestinal tract bleeding (0.2%), retroperitoneal bleeding (0.1%), need for subsequent operation (0.9%).

- Non-surgical/non-trauma risk factors associated with bleeding complications from VTE prophylaxis: active gastro duodenal ulcer (OR 4.1), bleeding event within last 3 months (OR 3.6), history of esophageal variceal bleeding (OR 3.5), admission platelet count <50,000 (OR 3.3), age >85 years (OR 2.9), liver failure (OR 2.1), renal failure (OR 2.0).
  - If LMWH and LDUH are contraindicated due to allergy or history of HIT, fondaparinux or aspirin (325 mg) can be used for prophylaxis along with IPC in high VTE risk patients.
  - Routine prophylactic use of IVC filters is not recommended in high VTE risk patients.
  - In selected high VTE risk patients (e.g., spinal cord injury, pelvic fracture), in whom pharmacologic VTE prophylaxis is contraindicated or will be delayed for a significant period of time, an IVC filter can be considered.
- VTE diagnosis
  - Figure 1 describes a DVT diagnostic and therapeutic algorithm.
  - Clinical findings associated with a high probability of a DVT are: unilateral extremity pain (associated with at least one physical exam finding), unilateral pitting edema, neck or facial swelling, extremity circumference greater than contralateral extremity (>3 cm difference for lower extremity, >2 cm for upper), tenderness upon muscle compression, and prominent superficial veins.
  - Surgical ICU patients with clinical findings of a DVT should be evaluated with Duplex ultrasound.
    - Ultrasound findings diagnostic of a DVT are: decreased vein compressibility (most sensitive and specific finding), abnormal Doppler color flow, presence of an echogenic band, and abnormal change in diameter during Valsalva maneuver.
  - D-dimer levels (a degradation product of cross-linked fibrin) have a 95% diagnostic sensitivity for VTE. Levels are frequently increased in non-thrombotic conditions (e.g., malignancy, increasing age, sepsis, pregnancy, following surgery or trauma, atrial fibrillation, and stroke), making it a non-specific assay, and should not be used as a standalone test to rule out or diagnose a VTE in critically ill and surgical patients.
  - Distal DVT's (distal to the popliteal vein trifurcation or to the axillary vein) are associated with a low risk of pulmonary embolization. However, there is a 15–23% probability of extension to more proximal veins (popliteal, femoral, iliac, axillary, brachiocephalic). This probability of proximal extension may be even higher in patients with non-modifiable VTE risk factors.

- Risk factors for proximal extension of a distal DVT: thrombus >5 cm in length, thrombus >7 mm in diameter or involving multiple veins, history of previous VTE, active cancer or receiving cancer treatment, expected prolonged immobility, and critically ill patients.
- Patients with any risk factor of proximal extension should receive therapeutic anticoagulation for distal DVT.
- If there are no risk factors for extension (provided symptoms are not severe), patients can undergo weekly ultrasound surveillance (two negative follow-up ultrasounds are needed to rule-out proximal extension).
- If risk factors of extension are present, but bleeding risk contraindicates anticoagulation, patients can undergo weekly ultrasound surveillance or placement of an IVC filter.

o Patients with isolated calf muscle vein thrombosis (soleal or gastrocnemius vein) have a lower risk of proximal extension compared to distal DVT, and provided symptoms are not severe, can be managed with weekly ultrasound surveillance to rule-out proximal extension.

o At 12 months after a proximal DVT has been diagnosed, 50% of patients have residual non-compressibility of the involved vein on ultrasound. When recurrence is suspected, diagnosis is challenging when there is no previous ultrasound study available for comparison. Recurrence can be excluded by a low d-dimer, however if elevated, venography should be performed.

o If an iliac, pelvic, IVC, or brachiocephalic DVT is suspected despite a negative ultrasound, CT-venography is recommended, given the technical limitations of ultrasound in these proximal anatomical regions.

o Unprovoked upper extremity DVT (UEDVT) is much less common compared to lower extremity DVT. Most UEDVT are associated with a CVC, transvenous pacemaker or defibrillator leads, upper extremity trauma, thoracic outlet syndrome, Paget-Von Schroetter-effort thrombosis, or malignancy. If none of these risk factors are present, they warrant a hypercoagulable workup.

o Routine ultrasound screening for DVT (in patients with no clinical findings) is not advised.

o Figure 2 describes a PE diagnostic and therapeutic algorithm.

o Clinical findings associated with a PE are: dyspnea, tachypnea, pleuritic chest pain, hemoptysis, tachycardia, hypoxemia, and syncope; albeit these findings have low specificity. A loud P2 heart sound and new-onset jugular vein distension are the only two clinical findings with high specificity, and indicate right ventricle (RV) dysfunction.

o Inverted T-waves on anterior leads is the most common EKG finding in patients with a PE (present in 68%).

o A high-index of suspicion based on clinical findings of a PE should prompt immediate initiation of anticoagulation therapy (if no contraindications exist) followed by evaluation with pulmonary imaging.

  ▪ Clinical prediction models of VTE for risk stratification of patients based on pre-test probability have not been validated in ICU patients.

o CT angiography is the preferred diagnostic modality for surgical ICU patients in whom a PE is suspected; it is performed in a brief period of time, results are readily available, and other non-thrombotic pathologies can be excluded. However, the patient transportation required maybe unsafe for the hemodynamically unstable.

o Ventilation/perfusion lung scintigraphy (V/Q scan) allows visualization of pulmonary perfusion by injection of albumin labeled with technetium-99, and paired with ventilation scintigraphy, can identify mismatch defects (perfusion defect with normal ventilation), which usually represent a PE.

  ▪ The interpretation of V/Q scan findings is classified into three categories: normal (no PE), high probability (PE), and non-diagnostic.

  ▪ Any pulmonary pathology that narrows the airways or fills them with fluid will cause reactive vasoconstriction, resulting in a non-thrombotic perfusion defect, limiting the positive predictive value of this test.

  ▪ The limited availability in urgent situations, as well as the limited specificity in surgical and critically ill patients given the frequent prevalence of pulmonary abnormalities (e.g., atelectasis, pneumonia, bronchospasm, respiratory failure), limits the use of V/Q scans in these patient populations.

o Although echocardiography has only a sensitivity of 60% for diagnosing a PE, it can serve as a useful tool in hypotensive patients suspected to have a PE who cannot safely undergo pulmonary imaging; lack of RV dysfunction accurately rules-out a PE as the source of hypotension.

  ▪ Findings on echocardiography suggestive of a PE are: RV dilation (without hypertrophy), RV hypokinesis, paradoxical septal systolic motion, Doppler evidence of pulmonary hypertension, and RV thrombus.

  ▪ It has prognostic implications in normotensive patients with PE when RV dysfunction is identified.

o   In patients in which radiation or contrast exposure should be avoided (pregnant patients, renal insufficiency, contrast allergy) but have clinical findings of a PE, and are normotensive, finding a DVT by ultrasound is sufficient evidence to warrant therapeutic anticoagulation without further pulmonary imaging.

  ▪   31% of patients with a PE have a DVT at the time of diagnosis.
  ▪   No evidence of a DVT on ultrasound (US) does not rule-out a PE and pulmonary imaging (CT or V/Q scan) must be performed.

o   The origin of a PE is from proximal lower extremity DVT in 90% of cases. However, it has been recently demonstrated that a number of PE that were thought to be embolic in origin are in fact in-situ pulmonary thrombi.

o   The clinical severity of a PE depends on two factors: the size of the thrombus and the patient's underlying cardiopulmonary function.

  ▪   Similar hemodynamic and clinical outcomes will manifest from an anatomically large PE in a patient with normal cardiopulmonary function and from an anatomically small one in a patient with impaired cardiopulmonary function.

o   The term "massive" has been used interchangeably to describe anatomically large PE's (a finding only loosely correlated to clinical outcome), or to describe PE's associated with hypotension (regardless of the thrombus size). Because of the ambiguity of this terminology, a new classification related to clinical outcomes and management options has been proposed (Task Force for the Diagnosis and Management of Acute Pulmonary Embolism):

  ▪   High-risk PE (previously massive): provoking hypotension (5% of cases, 15–30% mortality, 70% if presenting with cardiac arrest).
  ▪   Intermediate-risk PE (previously sub-massive): normotensive, however, provoking RV strain (RV dilation, RV hypokinesis, paradoxical septal systolic motion) (30% of cases, 5% mortality).
  ▪   Low-risk PE (previously non-massive): normal blood pressure, normal RV function (65% of cases, <1% mortality).

•   VTE management

o   Figure 1 describes a DVT diagnostic and therapeutic algorithm.
o   The aims of VTE treatment are three-fold: (1) to prevent death from a PE, (2) to prevent VTE recurrence, and (3) to prevent post-thrombotic complications.
o   Untreated proximal DVT are associated with a 17% incidence of symptomatic PE, and 50% incidence of an asymptomatic PE in studies using screening pulmonary imaging.

o If diagnostic testing or results for a suspected DVT are going to be delayed >4 h, then therapeutic anticoagulation should be started while awaiting study or results.

o Intravenous UFH is the agent of choice for treatment of DVT and PE in surgical ICU patients (Table 3 describes other anticoagulant agents and dosing).

- An initial bolus of 80 units/kg should be given, followed by continuous infusion at 18 units/kg/hr.

- Bolus can be withheld or reduced if significant bleeding risk exists.

- The recommended goal therapeutic range is 0.3–0.7 units/mL of anti-Xa activity at 4 h from initiation, or a PTT range adjusted to these anti-XA values (the relationship between anti-Xa and PTT values is variable by institution, however usually the therapeutic PTT is 2.0–2.5 times the control PTT).

- Intravenous UFH is preferred in surgical patients given its short half-life, allowing for windows of decreased anticoagulation if risk of bleeding needs to be decreased temporarily.

- In non-surgical patients, LMWH at therapeutic doses can be used.

o Sub-therapeutic dosing at 24 h from VTE diagnosis results in a significantly greater frequency of recurrence when compared to those patients who reach a therapeutic target within 24 h, with no difference in bleeding complications when titration protocols are followed.

o Requirement of unusually large doses of heparin in order to achieve therapeutic anticoagulation (>35,000 units of heparin per 24 hours, excluding initial bolus doses), should prompt testing for antithrombin deficiency; if confirmed, anticoagulation should be performed with a direct thrombin inhibitor such as bivalirudin or argatroban.

o Patients with worsening DVT symptoms despite therapeutic anticoagulation, those with phlegmasia cerulea dolens (described below), ilio-femoral DVT, and in some cases recurrence of DVT in the same site, should be considered for DVT thrombolysis or thrombectomy (surgical or percutaneous).

- Removal of the clot by thrombolysis or thrombectomy, almost immediately restores venous outflow and reduces the incidence of post-thrombotic syndrome by early reestablishment of venous patency and preservation of valves.

o Acute DVT treatment should be transitioned to post-VTE risk reduction therapy with warfarin as soon as possible.

- It is recommended for warfarin to be started simultaneously with initiation of parenteral anticoagulation, however this can be delayed based on bleeding risk and need for surgical or interventional procedures.
  - ⇨ Delaying initiation of post-VTE risk reduction therapy with warfarin significantly prolongs patients' hospital stay.
- Once warfarin is started, parenteral anticoagulation should be continued for a minimum of 5 days and until an INR ≥2.0 is achieved for at least 24 h.
  - ⇨ Once warfarin has achieved therapeutic levels, INR initially increases mostly due to inhibition of synthesis of factor VII (4 h half-life); however thrombosis risk may still exist despite elevated INR if factors II and X (72 h and 36 h half-life, respectively) are not inhibited by continuing heparin anticoagulation.
- Warfarin should be adjusted to a target INR of 2.5 (range 2.0–3.0). Table 4 describes dosing titration of warfarin.
- In patients with cancer, post-VTE risk reduction therapy can be performed with LMWH rather than warfarin given improved efficacy with no differences in bleeding events reported by studies in this patient population.

○ Table 5 describes duration of VTE therapy.
○ Figure 2 describes a PE diagnostic and therapeutic algorithm.
○ Cardiogenic shock resulting from a PE should be initially approached with the universal A-B-C (airway, breathing, circulation) assessment and management strategy.

- Resuscitation with volume should be judicious, as this can further worsen RV function.
- There is no reported optimal vasopressor for PE-induced hypotension; however, norepinephrine has the benefit of producing less tachycardia than other inotropic agents.

○ When a PE is suspected in a surgical ICU patient, anticoagulation should be started immediately (if no contraindications exist) before proceeding with a diagnostic approach.
○ The presence of hypotension (systolic blood pressure, SBP<90) associated with a PE has been defined as a threshold for thrombolysis.

- Successful thrombolysis allows for faster normalization of hemodynamic parameters compared to anticoagulation alone, at the cost of increased incidence of major bleeding events (6.2% vs. 1%).

⇨ With risk of major bleeding events being the main drawback of thrombolysis, a careful consideration of potential contraindications should be had when considered, limiting its use in patients with recent surgery or trauma.

- Thrombolysis is also indicated if a patient deteriorates hemodynamically from a PE while being treated with anticoagulation.
- If thrombolysis is used, treatment via peripheral vein is suggested over pulmonary artery catheter, and short infusion times (2 h) are preferred over longer infusion times (24 h).
- If thrombolysis fails to improve hemodynamic instability, if contraindicated because of bleeding risk, or if it is thought that shock will result in death before thrombolysis is effective, embolectomy (surgical or endovascular, depending on available resources and expertise) is indicated.

o 30% of normotensive patients with acute PE have echocardiographic findings of RV dysfunction at presentation (intermediate-risk PE). These patients have a 10% rate of subsequent PE-related hypotension despite being treated with anticoagulation and a 5% mortality rate, in contrast to a benign prognosis seen in patients with no findings of RV dysfunction (low-risk PE).

- Studies have suggested that these normotensive patients with PE and RV dysfunction could benefit from initial thrombolytic therapy rather than receiving anticoagulation alone, based on findings of quicker resolution of RV dysfunction with thrombolysis. However, there were no differences in mortality in these studies.
- It remains unclear whether normotensive patients presenting with a PE should be screened with echocardiography, as some might benefit from thrombolysis if RV dysfunction is diagnosed.

o If an asymptomatic DVT or PE is diagnosed, treatment should be the same to that of a symptomatic DVT or PE.
o If distal DVT is treated, treatment should be the same to that of a proximal DVT.
o Treatment of UEDVT is similar to that of lower extremity DVT.
o In patients with a proximal DVT of the leg in whom anticoagulation is contraindicated, placement of an IVC filter is recommended.

- A conventional course of therapeutic anticoagulation for DVT should be started once risk of bleeding allows, even while IVC filter is still in place.

o In patients with a PE in whom anticoagulation is contraindicated, placement of an IVC filter is recommended.

- A conventional course of therapeutic anticoagulation for PE should be started once risk of bleeding allows, even while IVC filter is still in place.
  - o In addition, IVC filter placement may be considered in patients with a PE when their underlying hemodynamic or respiratory compromise is severe enough that another PE may be lethal, regardless of the initial mode of treatment.
- Catheter related VTE
  - o In patients with a CVC related DVT, routine catheter removal is not recommended, provided it is needed, remains functional, and well-positioned.
  - o A CVC-related DVT involving the axillary or more proximal veins should be treated with anticoagulation.
  - o When removing a catheter responsible for a CVC-related DVT, it has been suggested that at least a brief period of therapeutic anticoagulation should precede removal, in order to minimize risk of embolization. There is no data to validate this concept.
  - o Patients who have had prior UEDVT should be screened for patency of the central veins prior to placement of a subsequent catheter.
  - o Table 5 describes duration of CVC-related DVT therapy.
- Complications of VTE
  - o Phlegmasia cerulea dolens
    - Venous gangrene resulting usually from an extensive proximal (e.g., ilio-femoral) DVT (can also occur in upper extremity).
    - Clinical diagnosis based on severe pain, tenderness, swelling, and cyanosis.
    - Unilateral limb discoloration or cyanosis in a patient with a known or suspected DVT is the hallmark sign.
    - Thrombolysis or thrombectomy along with anticoagulation should be the first-line of therapy.
    - Delay in treatment may result in secondary arterial compromise, development of compartment syndrome, or limb loss.
  - o Post-thrombotic syndrome (PTS)
    - PTS is a frequently unrecognized chronic sequela of DVT developing in 20–50% of patients, even when treated appropriately with anticoagulation.
    - Symptoms range from persistent swelling to severe pain, ulceration, and venous claudication.
    - The underlying pathophysiology of PTS is lack of venous patency and venous valve incompetency resulting in venous hypertension.

- Patients at highest risk are those with ilio-femoral DVT (90% incidence) and those with recurrence of DVT in the same location, justifying consideration of thrombolysis or thrombectomy rather than anticoagulation alone as the initial treatment in these patients.
- PTS can be prevented by decreasing DVT recurrence with adequate anticoagulation regimens, and with use of a graduated elastic compression stocking or sleeve on the affected limb beginning at the time of diagnosis.

o DVT can lead to paradoxical arterial embolizations in patients with a PFO (27% of population), and has been reported as a cause of non-hemorrhagic cryptogenic stroke in critically ill patients.

o Chronic thromboembolic pulmonary hypertension (CTPH)

- Characterized by persistence of thrombi and vascular remodeling in the pulmonary circulation secondary to pulmonary embolism; diagnosed by V/Q scan and confirmed by right heart catheterization (mean pulmonary artery pressure >25 mm Hg in the absence of an elevated wedge pressure [<15 mm Hg]).
- Three months after an acute PE, 19% of patients treated with anticoagulation have some residual perfusion obstruction.
- Patients at increased risk for CTPH are those with PE recurrence, >50% amputation of pulmonary artery or main branch at time, and unprovoked or idiopathic PE.
- Patients present with chronic dyspnea and subsequently develop heart failure.
- Treated with surgical pulmonary endarterectomy.

- Special populations

o Renal disease

- Patients with renal disease experience both bleeding and thrombotic complications, conditions that often overlap.
- Renal disease leads to increased levels of fibrinogen, factor VIII, von-Willebrand factor (vWF), and homocysteine, with decreased levels of protein C and antithrombin, all of which favor thrombosis.
- Risk of thrombosis is highest in those patients with end-stage renal disease requiring hemodialysis.
- Bleeding complications secondary to anticoagulation often result from inadequate dosing or choice of medication based on renal function.
- General guidelines for VTE prophylaxis should be followed with particular attention to dosing and choice of anticoagulant based on renal function. UFH can be used in patients with renal disease.

- LMWH, fondaparinux, dabigatran, rivaroxaban, and apixaban should be avoided in patients with renal disease.
- End stage renal disease patients who require hemodialysis are at high risk of HIT, given the repeated exposure to heparin during dialysis and vascular access procedures.
- Patients with renal disease and HIT can receive treatment with either argatroban (if liver function is normal) or bivalirudin (adjusted to renal function).
- In patients with HIT requiring hemodialysis, argatroban should be used as an alternative to heparin in the filter and extracorporeal circuit. Catheters should not be locked with heparin, alternatively citrate can be used.

○ Liver disease

- The coagulopathy and thrombocytopenia seen in liver disease do not necessarily protect these patients from thrombosis.
- Because both pro-coagulant and anti-coagulant proteins are diminished in unpredictable ratios during liver disease, the predilection for either bleeding or thrombosis is difficult to assess.
- Hepatic dysfunction leads not only to decreased synthesis of fibrinogen and coagulation factors (II, VII, IX, and X), but also to decreased levels of the anticoagulant proteins C, S, and antithrombin, as well as plasminogen.
- In cirrhosis, elevated levels of PAI-1, factor VIII, and vWF, are also seen, potentially representing an endothelial response to inflammation.
- Patients with cirrhosis are at increased risk of portal thrombosis; this risk is highest when these patients experience sepsis, severe trauma, and major surgery.
- Patients with esophageal varices secondary to portal hypertension are at the highest risk of bleeding secondary to anticoagulation.
- Guidelines on indications for VTE prophylaxis of cirrhotic patients are lacking based on the paucity of data.
- Pharmacologic VTE prophylaxis should be started based on a patient-specific bleeding vs. thrombosis risk assessment. Low-dose UFH and LMWH can be used in patients with liver disease.
- The effectiveness of anticoagulation in cirrhotic patients may be affected by lower levels of antithrombin and a larger volume of drug distribution.
- Dose adjustment to anti-Xa target levels is recommended whenever prophylactic or therapeutic anticoagulation is indicated in critically ill cirrhotic patients or those with acute liver failure. Anti-Xa traget ranges are described in Table 3.

- Argatroban, dabigatran, rivaroxaban, and apixaban should be avoided in patients with liver disease.
- Patients with liver disease and HIT can receive treatment with either fondaparinux (if renal function is normal) or bivalirudin.

o Pediatric patients

- The strongest acquired risk factors for a first-time VTE in children are: CVC, malignancy, and trauma.
    ⇨ Two-thirds of all pediatric VTE's are associated with the use of a CVC.
- Two serious DVT complications are seen more often in children than in adults:
    ⇨ Intra-cardiac extension into the right atrium of a CVC-related DVT.
    ⇨ Paradoxical embolization of a venous clot into the arterial circulation given the prevalence of a patent foramen ovale and septal defects.
- Given extensive venous collateralization, extremity swelling resulting from a DVT is less common than in adults.
- Often, marked dilation or visibility of superficial veins is the only sign of a DVT.
- For pediatric trauma patients, we recommend VTE prophylaxis with LMWH for ≥14 y.o., given the lower VTE incidence in younger patients.
    ⇨ For patients <50 kg, prophylactic doses should be adjusted to an anti-Xa levels described in Table 3.
    ⇨ For patients ≥50 kg, adult prophylactic doses can be used and do not require routine anti-Xa dose adjustments.
- Initial treatment for acute VTE is recommended with intravenous UFH.
    ⇨ An initial bolus of 75 units/kg should be given, followed by continuous infusion at 18–20 units/kg/hr.
    ⇨ Bolus can be withheld or reduced if significant bleeding risk exists.
    ⇨ Transition to dose-adjusted warfarin for post-VTE risk reduction therapy should be similar to adult patients.
- LMWH can also be used in pediatric patients.
- When indicated, therapeutic doses of aspirin in children should be used in the dose range of 1.0–2.0 mg/kg/day.

○ Pregnancy

- Pregnancy is associated with an increased risk of thrombosis that may be due in part to obstruction of venous return by the enlarged uterus, as well as a hypercoagulable state associated with pregnancy. Estimates of the age-adjusted incidence of VTE range from 5 to 50 times higher in pregnant versus non-pregnant women.
- Hypercoagulability seen during pregnancy occurs in part because of activated protein C resistance, and increased levels of fibrinogen, factors V, VII, VIII, IX, X, and PAI-1.
- LMWH is the preferred agent, over UFH, for prophylaxis and VTE treatment when indicated (mostly due significant variability in dose-response to UFH given increase in heparin-binding proteins and plasma volume changes seen in pregnancy, as well as higher incidence of osteoporosis with long-term use of UFH).
- 85% of pregnancy-related DVT occur during pregnancy (incidence highest in the third trimester), while 85% of PE occur in the post-partum period (incidence highest in those undergoing cesarean delivery).
- 90% of pregnancy-related DVT occur in the left lower extremity, and the majority involve a proximal vein.
- Post-VTE risk reduction therapy should be performed with LMWH and can be transitioned to dose-adjusted warfarin post-partum, with a minimum total anti-coagulation period of three months, and at least six weeks of post-partum anti-coagulation.
- Anticoagulation should be held 24 hours prior to induction of labor or cesarean section, and re-started at 12 h post-operatively if hemostasis is adequate.
- All patients with a history of a prior VTE, those with factor V Leiden, prothrombin 20210A mutation, or a first-degree relative with a VTE, should undergo post-partum prophylaxis with LMWH for six weeks.
- Low-dose UFH and LMWH do not cross placenta.
- Warfarin crosses placenta and has the potential to cause fetal wastage, bleeding in the fetus, and teratogenicity.
- Oral direct thrombin and Xa inhibitors should be avoided during pregnancy. Fondaparinux is restricted for pregnant patients with HIT or severe allergic reactions to heparin. Experience with argatroban and bivalirudin during pregnancy is limited.
- Use of thrombolytics to manage PE is associated with a 15% incidence of fetal loss and 30% of pre-term labor. This should not preclude the use of thrombolytics, when indicated, for a life-threatening PE.

o Neuraxial anesthesia.

- Neuraxial anesthesia can be used with pharmacologic prophylaxis with cautious patient selection as follows: avoiding patients with known clotting disorders, avoiding patients receiving thienopyridine platelet inhibitors (clopidogrel and ticlodipine) within two weeks of placement, waiting until trough blood levels for those already receiving pharmacologic prophylaxis, delaying prophylaxis (at least 24 h) if a hemorrhagic aspirate is performed, and monitoring for symptoms of spinal hematoma when using spinal anesthesia and pharmacologic prophylaxis.

- Spinal catheter placement or removal should be delayed from last administered dose: 2 h for i.v. UFH (normal PTT should be documented), 4 h for low-dose UFH, 12 h for LMWH.

- After spinal catheter placement or removal, the next dose should be given at least 2 h after for intravenous or subcutaneous UFH, and 6 h for LMWH.

- Given increased risk of bleeding, patients on therapeutic dose LMWH, q12 h prophylactic dose LMWH, and fondaparinux, should not receive neuraxial anesthesia, or should transition to UFH or daily LMWH dosing prior to placement.

- Patients receiving more than one medication affecting hemostasis (including NSAID's) should generally not receive neuraxial anesthesia.

- Patients receiving aspirin can have spinal catheters placed or removed without delaying dosing, as long as they are not receiving, or expected to receive, another medication affecting hemostasis while the spinal catheter is in place.

- Heparin induced thrombocytopenia (HIT)

  o Generation of IgG antibodies directed against circulating complexes of platelet factor-4 (PF4) bound to heparin resulting in thrombocytopenia and in some patients, thrombosis.

  - PF4 is a cytokine released by alpha-granules when platelets are activated that inhibits endogenous heparinoids on the endothelial surface, and consequently has a high affinity for exogenous heparin.

  - Antibodies against the heparin/PF4 complex appear in serum at a median of 4 days from a first-time heparin exposure.

  - A pro-thrombotic state occurs when platelets are activated by the Fc region of the antibody bound to the heparin/PF4 complex, this also causes the platelets to release pro-coagulant microparticles that promote thrombin generation.

- Platelets with these antibody complexes attached are then cleared by macrophages and the reticuloendothelial system.
○ HIT occurs in 5% of patients exposed to heparin, regardless of the dose, schedule, or route of administration.
○ The frequency of HIT is variable and influenced by the type of patient population: cardiac surgery>vascular surgery>trauma>medical>obstetrical, sex: female>male, type of heparin used: bovine unfractionated>porcine unfractionated>LMWH>fondaparinux, duration of exposure: the risk decreases if it has not occurred at 10–14 days of continuous exposure, timing of exposure in relation to surgery post-operative>pre-operative, and BMI: high BMI>low BMI.
  - The highest incidence of HIT is seen in patients on extracorporeal circulatory support and with ventricular assist devices receiving heparin (10%).
○ Thrombocytopenia is the most common finding of HIT, and typically occurs between 5–10 days from beginning of heparin exposure.
  - In patients who have been exposed to heparin within the last 3 months, thrombocytopenia can occur in <24 h with heparin re-exposure.
  - A platelet count drop of >50% of baseline is typical, the mean nadir is a count of 60×10^9, and counts rarely decrease <20×10^9.
○ The pro-thrombotic state induced by HIT leads to a 50% incidence of thrombotic complications in serologically confirmed HIT:
  - DVT (50%), PE (25%), aorto-iliac thrombosis (10%), thrombotic stroke (7%), adrenal hemorrhagic infarction from adrenal vein thrombosis (3%), cerebral sinus thrombosis (3%), mesenteric thrombosis (3%).
○ Skin necrosis (typically seen at subcutaneous injection sites) is common in patients with HIT, and should prompt an evaluation for HIT when noted in high-risk patients.
○ Acute systemic reactions to heparin (most commonly seen with a heparin bolus) are common in patients with HIT, and range from mild allergic reactions to anaphylaxis with cardiopulmonary collapse. Acute systemic reactions to heparin should prompt an evaluation for HIT when noted in high-risk patients.
○ Clinical suspicion of HIT should be followed by serologic testing if there is an intermediate or high pretest probability. Table 6 describes the 4T pre-test probability model.

o   A low pretest probability represents a minimal possibility of HIT, and does not require serologic testing, however monitoring of platelet counts and for clinical findings of thrombosis should continue.

o   Serologic testing for PF4/heparin antibodies (PF4-ELISA) (reported in optical density, OD) has a strong negative predictive value, however it has low specificity.

   ▪   An OD value ≤0.4 has a ≤0.5% risk of HIT and can exclude this diagnosis.

   ▪   An OD value ≥2.0 has a ≥90% risk of HIT and does not require further testing.

   ▪   0.5–1.9 OD values are considered indeterminate and require a platelet activation assay (serotonin-release assay, SRA) to confirm diagnosis.

   ▪   There is a high degree of false positivity post-cardiopulmonary bypass or aortic balloon pump.

o   A presumptive diagnosis of HIT based on clinical findings (moderate or high 4T score) should be treated for HIT while awaiting serologic confirmation. Presumptive treatment includes the following:

   ▪   All forms of heparin should be discontinued (including LMWH, heparin flushes, and heparin-bonded catheters).

   ▪   Because of the high risk of thrombosis associated with HIT, therapeutic anticoagulation with a non-heparin anticoagulant should be initiated (unless contraindicated by bleeding risk), even if the original indication for anticoagulation no longer exists.

      ⇨   Patients with normal renal and hepatic function can receive fondaparinux (subcutaneous), argatroban (intravenous), or bivalirudin (intravenous).

      ⇨   Patients with renal dysfunction can be treated with argatroban.

      ⇨   Patients with hepatic dysfunction can be treated with fondaparinux or bivalirudin.

      ⇨   Patients with renal and hepatic dysfunction can be treated with bivalirudin (dose adjusted to renal function).

      ⇨   Specific dosing for each agent is described in Table 3.

   ▪   Warfarin should not be started until therapeutic anticoagulation has been achieved, and the platelet count is ≥150 × 10^9 in order to avoid the transient increase in hypercoagulability initially induced by warfarin (due to the rapid inhibition of protein C).

   ▪   Warfarin should be dose-adjusted to a target INR of 2.5 (range 2.0–3.0).

- Optimal duration of anticoagulation with warfarin for HIT patients has not been studied. It has been recommended that:
  - ⇨ Patients with serologically confirmed HIT, with no thrombotic complications, should receive 1–3 months of anticoagulation.
  - ⇨ Patients with serologically confirmed HIT, who developed thrombotic complications, should receive 3–6 months of anticoagulation.
- Thrombocytopenia resolves in a median of 7 days from nadir (range 4–14 days).
- ○ If the diagnosis of HIT is excluded by serology, heparin can be resumed (if the original indication for anticoagulation persists).

Practical Algorithm(s)/Diagrams

Table 1.   Caprini venous thromboembolism risk assessment.

1 point	2 points	3 points	5 points
○ Age 41-60 y ○ Minor surgery ○ BMI >25 kg/m2 ○ Swollen legs or varicose veins ○ Pregnancy or postpartum ○ History of unexplained or recurrent spontaneous abortion ○ Oral contraceptives or hormone replacement ○ Sepsis (<1mo) ○ Serious lung disease, including pneumonia (<1mo) ○ Abnormal pulmonary function ○ Acute myocardial infarction ○ Congestive heart failure (<1mo) ○ History of inflammatory bowel disease ○ Medical patient at bed rest	○ Age 61-74y ○ Arthroscopic surgery ○ Major open surgery (>45min) ○ Laparoscopic surgery (>45min) ○ Malignancy ○ Confined to bed (>72h) ○ Immobilizing plaster cast ○ Indwelling central venous catheter	○ Age >75y ○ History of VTE ○ Family history of VTE ○ Factor V Leiden ○ Prothrombin gene mutation 20210A ○ Lupus anticoagulant ○ Anticardiolipin antibodies ○ Elevated serum homocysteine ○ Heparin-induced thrombocytopenia ○ Other congenital or acquired thrombophilia	○ Stroke (<1mo) ○ Elective arthroplasty ○ Hip, pelvis, or leg fracture ○ Acute spinal cord injury (<1mo)

score	risk group	risk of symptomatic VTE if no prophylaxis used*	recommended prophylaxis modality (ACCP 9th ed. 2012)
0	VERY LOW	<0.5%	*early and frequent ambulation*
1-2	LOW	1.5%	*IPC and ambulation*
3-4	MODERATE	3.0%	*IPC OR* *pharmacologic prophylaxis***
≥5	HIGH	≥6.0%	*pharmacologic prophylaxis* *AND IPC*

* risk calculated from post-operative incidence of VTE's in general surgery patients
** Pharmacologic prophylaxis is preferred over intermittent pneumatic compression (IPC) only by Denver Health consensus guidelines in the absence of significant bleeding risk

Table 2. Trauma venous thromboembolism risk assessment profile (RAP).

	Points
Underlying condition	
obesity	2
malignancy	2
coagulation disorder	2
previous VTE	3
Iatrogenic factors	
femoral venous line	2
transfusion >4 units	2
operation >2h	3
major venous repair	3
Injury-related factors	
chest AIS >2	2
abdomen AIS >2	2
head AIS >2	2
spinal fractures	3
GCS <8	3
severe lower extremity frac-ture	4
pelvic fracture	4
spinal cord injury	4
Age	
40–59	2
60–74	3
>75	4

AIS: Abbreviated injury score, GCS: Glasgow coma scale
Adapted from Greenfield *et al.*, J Trauma 1997;42:100–3.

Table 3. Anticoagulants.

Drug	Mechanism of action	Indications (FDA approved)	Dose	Route	Half-life	Metabolism	Excretion	Detection of anti-coagula-tion	Drug interactions[†]	Unique issues
Warfarin	Vitamin K epoxide reductase inhibition	— Post-VTE risk reduction (acute management of DVT or PE should be done with an agent of fast therapeutic onset).	2–10 mg/d. See table # for dosing adjustments.	oral	36h (very variable, range 20–60 h) (peak plasma levels reached 72–96 h)	hepatic (CYP-2C9)	biliary	INR	CYP450: 1A2, 2C9, 3A4 inhibitors and inducers	— 2C9 and VKORC1 genetic variations influence dose response and impact bleeding risk. — 99% bound to plasma albumin. — No hepatic dose adjustment needed (however, marked dose response in liver desease). — No renal dose adjustment needed.

Heparin (unfractionated)	Thrombin and factor Xa inhibition (anti Xa/ thrombin ratio: 1.0)	— VTE prophylaxis. — DVT and PE tx (only for acute management, transition to warfarin for post VTE risk reduction). — NSTEMI or unstable angina. — STEMI.	— VTE prophylaxis: 5,000 units q 8–12 h subq (recommended dose is 5000 units q8h; 5000 units q12 h can be used to minimize bleeding risk, but efficacy is comparable to placebo in high VTE risk patients). — DVT and PE tx (only for acute management, transition to warfarin for post-VTE risk reduction): 80 units/kg bolus i.v., then 18 units/kg/h continuous i.v. infusion. — NSTEMI or unstable angina: 60 units/kg bolus i.v., then 12 units/kg/h continuous i.v. infusion. — STEMI: adjunct to fibrinolysis; 60 units/kg bolus i.v., then 12 units/kg/h continuous i.v. infusion.	parenteral (intravenous and subcutaneous)	— i.v. infusion:1.5 h (increased with renal impairment). — i.v. bolus (dose dependent): 25 units/kg = 30 min, 100 units/kg = 60 min. — subq: 1.5–3.0 h.	hepatic	mostly renal	PTT	No significant interactions	— No hepatic dose adjustment needed. — No renal dose adjustment needed. — VTE prophylaxis for BMI ≥40: 7500 units subcutaneous q8 h. — Anti-Xa prophylactic goal (measured 4 h after dose): 0.1–0.4. — Anti-Xa therapeutic goal (measured 4 h after dose): 0.3–0.7. — Relationship between anti-Xa and PTT is variable by institution, however usually the therapeutic PTT is 2.0–2.5 times the control PTT.

(Continued)

Table 3. (*Continued*)

Drug	Mechanism of action	Indications (FDA approved)	Dose	Route	Half-life	Metabolism	Excretion	Detection of anti-coagulation	Drug interactions[†]	Unique issues
Enoxaparin (LMWH)	Thrombin and factor Xa inhibition (anti Xa/ thrombin ratio: 3.3)	— VTE prophylaxis. — DVT and PE tx — NSTEMI or unstable angina. — STEMI.	— VTE prophylaxis: 40 mg/d (for ICU-trauma, post-op hip and knee replacement, hip and pelvic fracture patients: 30 mg q12h). — DVT and PE tx (only for acute management, transition to warfarin for post-VTE risk reduction): 1 mg/kg q12h or 1.5 mg q24h. — NSTEMI or unstable angina: 1 mg/kg q12h with concurrent aspirin tx. — STEMI: 30 mg bolus (i.v.), then 1 mg/kg q12h (subq) (>75 y.o.: no bolus and 0.75 mg/kg q12h)	parenteral (sub-cutane-ous)	3.5 h (up to 8 h in renal impairment)	hepatic	mostly renal	anti-Xa	No significant interactions	— VTE prophylaxis for BMI 40–49: 40 mg q12h, BMI ≥50: 60 mg q12h. — No hepatic dose adjustment needed. — Avoid if Cr clearance <30 mL/min. — LMWH efficacy reduced by vasopressor use. — Anti-Xa prophylactic goal (measured 4 h after dose): 0.2–0.6 (q12h or q24h dosing). — Anti-Xa therapeutic goal (measured 4 h after dose): 0.6–1.0 (q12h dosing), 1.0–2.0 (q24h dosing).

| Dalteparin (LMWH) | Thrombin and factor Xa inhibition (anti Xa/thrombin ratio: 2.0) | — VTE prophylaxis. — DVT and PE tx (only for acute management, transition to warfarin for post-VTE risk reduction(except cancer patients)). — Post-VTE risk reduction (cancer patients only). — MI (non-Q wave) or unstable angina. | — VTE prophylaxis: 5000 units/d — DVT and PE tx: 200 units/kg daily (transition to warfarin for post-VTE risk reduction in non-cancer patients). — Post-VTE risk reduction (cancer patients only): 200 units/kg daily for 1 month, then 150 units/kg daily for months 2–6. — MI (non-Q wave) or unstable angina: 120 units/kg Q12h (max. dose: 10,000 units q12h) with concurrent aspirin tx. | parenteral (subcutaneous) | 4 h (up to 8 h in renal impairment) | hepatic | mostly renal | anti-Xa | No significant interactions | — VTE prophylaxis for BMI ≥40: 6500 units/d. — No hepatic dose adjustment needed. — Avoid if Cr clearance <30mL/min. — LMWH efficacy reduced by vasopressor use. — Anti-Xa prophylactic goal (measured 4 h after dose): 0.2–0.5. — Anti-Xa therapeutic goal (measured 4 h after dose): 0.5–1.5. |

(Continued)

Table 3. (Continued)

Drug	Mechanism of action	Indications (FDA approved)	Dose	Route	Half-life	Metabolism	Excretion	Detection of anti-coagulation	Drug interactions†	Unique issues
Bivalirudin	Thrombin inhibition	— HIT tx. — PCI for ACS in HITT or HITTI-risk patients. — Cardiopulmonary bypass in HIT patients.	— HIT tx: 0.1–0.2 mg/kg/hr continuous i.v. infusion (goal PTT 2.0–2.5 times control) (start warfarin once therapeutic goal reached and PLT count $\geq 150 \times 10^9$, and continue bivalirudin until INR within desired range; stop bivalirudin and check INR in 4 h, if INR is below desired range then resume bivalirudin and repeat until desired INR is reached on warfarin alone). — PCI for ACS in HIT: 0.75 mg/kg bolus i.v.,1.75 mg/kg/hour for the duration of procedure and up to 4 h post-procedure.	parenteral (intravenous)	25 min (up to 3 h with renal insufficiency)	blood proteases	20% renal, proteolysis	PTT	No significant interactions	— Transition to warfarin may be delayed based on bleeding risk and need for interventional procedures. — Critically ill patients require lower doses. — No hepatic dose adjustment needed. — Renal dose adjustment required: CrCL 30–60 mL/min = 0.08–0.1 mg/kg/hour; CrCL <30 mL/min = 0.04–0.05 mg/kg/hour. — Hemodialysis removes 25%.

Argatroban	Thrombin inhibition	— HIT tx. — PCI for ACS in HIT or HIT-risk patients.	— HIT tx and prophylaxis: 0.5–2.0 mcg/kg/min continuous i.v. infusion (goal PTT 2.0–2.5 times control) (start warfarin once therapeutic goal reached and PLT count ≥150 × 10^9 and continue argatroban until INR is ≥4; stop argatroban and check INR in 4h, if INR is below desired range then resume argatroban and repeat until desired INR is reached on warfarin alone). — PCI for ACS: 350 mcg/kg bolus i.v., 25 mcg/kg/min continuous i.v. infusion.	parenteral (intravenous)	45 min (up to 2h in hepatic impairment)	hepatic	22% renal, 65% fecal	PTT	No significant interactions	— Transition to warfarin may be delayed based on bleeding risk and need for interventional procedures. — Will also significantly increase INR. — No renal dose adjustment needed. — Avoid with impaired liver function. — Can be used (off-label) for pre-filter administration during CRRT in HIT patients.
Dabigatran	Thrombin inhibition	— Stroke and systemic embolism prevention in non-valvular AF.	150 mg q12h	oral	16 h	hepatic	80% renal, 20% fecal	Ecarin clotting time (ECT) or thrombin time (TT)	P-glycoprotein inhibitors, PPI**	— Avoid if Cr clearance <30mL/min or with impaired liver function. — Dialyzable.

(Continued)

Table 3. (*Continued*)

Drug	Mechanism of action	Indications (FDA approved)	Dose	Route	Half-life	Metabolism	Excretion	Detection of anti-coagulation	Drug interactions†	Unique issues
Fondaparinux	Factor Xa inhibition (indirect)	— VTE prophylaxis. — DVT and PE tx (only for acute management, transition to warfarin for post-VTE risk reduction). — HIT tx.	— VTE prophylaxis: 2.5 mg/d. — DVT or PE tx: 7.5 mg/d (weight 50–100 kg), 10 mg/d (weight >100 kg). — HIT tx: 7.5 mg/d (weight 50–100 kg), 10 mg/d (weight >100 kg) (start warfarin once PLT count $\geq 150 \times 10^9$ and continue fondaparinux for at least 5 days, and until INR is ≥ 2 for at least 24h).	parenteral (subcutaneous)	20 h	unknown (non-hepatic)	77% renal	anti-Xa	No significant interactions	— Contraindicated if body weight <50 kg. — Long-term use (>14 days) has not been studied. — Avoid if CrCL <30 mL/min. — Dialyzable. — Anti-Xa prophylactic goal (measured 3 h after dose): 0.3–0.5. — Anti-Xa therapeutic goal (measured 3 h after dose): 1.2–1.3.
Rivaroxaban	Factor Xa inhibition (direct)	— VTE prophylaxis (only for post-op knee and hip replacement). — DVT or PE tx. — Stroke and systemic embolism prevention in non-valvular AF.	— VTE prophylaxis: 10 mg/d (14d for knee, 35d for hip). — DVT or PE tx: 15 mg Q12h for 3 weeks then 20 mg/d (duration of tx per ACCP 9th Ed.). — Stroke and systemic embolism prevention in non-valvular AF: 20 mg/d.	oral	8 h (12 h in elderly)	hepatic	66% renal, 33% fecal	anti-Xa	P-glycoprotein inhibitors, CYP-3A4 inhibitors	— Avoid if CrCL <30 mL/min or with impaired liver function. — Not dialyzable

| Apixaban | Factor Xa inhibition (direct) | — Stroke and systemic embolism prevention in non-valvular AF. | 5 mg Q12h (2.5 mg if 2 of the following present: ≥80 y.o., weight ≤60 kg, or Cr≥1.5 mg/dL). | oral | 12h | hepatic | 25% renal, 75% fecal | anti-Xa | CYP-3A4 inhibitors | — Avoid if CrCL <30mL/min or with impaired liver function. — Not dialyzable |

P-glycoprotein inhibitors*: rifampin, amiodarone, verapamil. CYP-3A4 inhibitors*: ketoconazole, itraconazole, voriconazole, fluconazole (mostly 2C9 inhibitor, weak 3A4), ciprofloxacin, metronidazole, erythromycin, ritonavir, amiodarone.

CYP-1A2 inhibitors*: ciprofloxacin, ethanol. CYP-2C9 inhibitors*: amiodarone, TMP/SMX, metronidazole, fluconazole, fluvastatin, isoniazid, lovastatin, setraline, gemfibrozil. CYP-2C9 inducers**: rifampin, carba-mazepine, phenytoin, phenobarbital.

U.S. brand names: enoxaparin (Lovenox), dalteparin (Fragmin), bivalirudin (Angiomax), dabigatran (Pradaxa), fondaparinux (Arixtra), apixaban (Eliquis), rivaroxaban (Xarelto).

* May increase anti-coagulant concentration and/or effect.

** May decrease anti-coagulant concentration and/or effect.

†Combination of any two medications that affect hemostasis is considered a significant interaction as they increase bleeding risk.

tx: treatment, DVT: deep vein thrombosis, PE: pulmonary embolism, VTE: venous thrombo embolism, MI: myocardial infarction, STEMI: ST-segment elevation myocardial infarction, NSTEMI: non-ST-segment eleva-tion myocardial infarction, PTT: partial thromboplastin time, LMWH: low molecular weight heparin, PCI: percutaneous coronary intervention, ACS: acute coronary syndrome,

Table 4. Warfarin dosing.

	INR	Warfarin daily dose
day 1		5 mg[*]
day 2	<1.5	5 mg
	1.5–1.9	2.5 mg
	2.0–2.5	1.0–2.5 mg
	>2.5	no warfarin[**]
day 3	<1.5	5–10 mg
	1.5–1.9	2.5–5.0 mg
	2.0–3.0	0–2.5 mg
	>3.0	no warfarin[**]
day 4	<1.5	10 mg
	1.5–1.9	5.0–7.5 mg
	2.0–3.0	0–5.0 mg
	>3.0	no warfarin[**]
day 5	<1.5	10 mg
	1.5–1.9	7.5–10 mg
	2.0–3.0	0–5.0 mg
	>3.0	no warfarin[**]
day 6	<1.5	7.5–12.5 mg
	1.5–1.9	5.0–10 mg
	2.0–3.0	0–7.5 mg
	>3.0	no warfarin[**]

[*] Consider a first dose of 2.5 mg for patients <50 kg, liver disease, or of asian ethnicity.
[**] Omit doses until INR <2.5.

Table 5. Duration of post-VTE risk reduction therapy.

Venous thromboembolic event	Duration of therapy
Provoked DVT (e.g., associated with surgery, trauma)	3 months
Provoked PE (e.g., associated with surgery, trauma)	3 months
CVC-related DVT	3 months (and as long as CVC is in place)
Idiopathic DVT*	3 months minimum, consider indefinite
Idiopathic PE*	3 months minimum, consider indefinite
VTE associated with cancer	Indefinite or as long as cancer is active or requiring therapy
Recurrent VTE	Indefinite therapy
HIT** without thrombosis	1–3 months
HIT** with thrombosis	3–6 months

*After 3 months of treatment perform hypercoagulable workup and evaluate for risk-benefit ratio of extended prophylaxis.

**diagnosis confirmed serologically.

DVT: deep vein thrombosis, PE: pulmonary embolism, CVC: central venous catheter, HIT: heparin induced thrombocytopenia.

Table 6.   Heparin induced thrombocytopenia 4T pre-test probability.

	2	1	0
Thrombocytopenia	>50% fall and nadir $\geq 20 \times 10^9$	30–50% fall or nadir 10–19×10^9	<30% fall or nadir $<10 \times 10^9$
Timing of platelet count decrease (1st day of heparin exposure = day 0)	days 5–10 (or $\leq$ day 1 if prior heparin exposure within last 30 days)	> day 10, or timing unclear (or > day 1 if prior heparin exposure within 30–100 days)	< day 5 (no prior heparin exposure within last 100 days)
Thrombosis	new thrombosis (arterial or venous), adrenal hemorrhage, skin necrosis, or acute systemic reaction after heparin bolus	suspected thrombosis, or recurrence of previous thrombosis	none
Other causes of Thrombocytopenia	none evident	possible	definite (e.g., hemodilution, other medications, sepsis)

Pre-test probability of HIT: $\geq$6 points = HIGH, 4–5 points = INTERMEDIATE, $\leq$3 points = LOW.

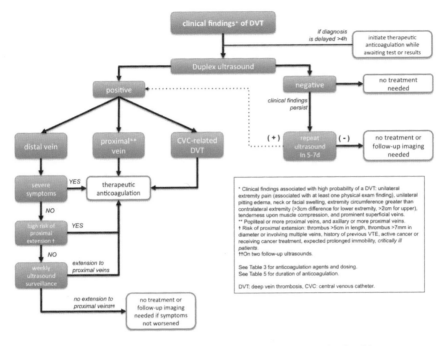

Fig. 1.   Deep vein thrombosis diagnostic and therapeutic algorithm.

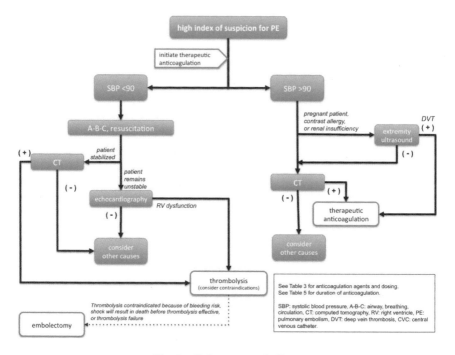

Fig. 2. Pulmonary embolism.

Review of Current Literature with References

- American College of Chest Physicians Evidence-Based Clinical Practice Guidelines 2012 9th Ed. Guidelines. Antithrombotic therapy and prevention of thrombosis. *Chest* 2012; **141**:e227S–e277S.

- In a Cochrane review, data from two trials involving 331 major trauma patients demonstrated that LMWH (enoxaparin 30 mg q12h) appeared to reduce the risk of DVT compared to low-dose UFH (5000 units bid) (RR 0.68; 95%CI 0.50–0.94). Routine DVT screening was performed on all studied patients. There was no statistically significant difference in risk of incidence of PE, bleeding complications, and in mortality when comparing LMWH vs. UFH. People who received both mechanical and pharmacological prophylaxis had the lowest risk of DVT (RR 0.34; 95% CI 0.19 to 0.60). *Cochrane Database Syst Rev.* 2013; **28**:CD008303.

- A multicenter, randomized, blinded, placebo-controlled trial compared an additional three weeks of pharmacologic VTE with a LMWH (bemiparin) to no additional prophylaxis in 626 patients who underwent abdominal or pelvic surgery for cancer, all of whom initially received 1 week of prophylaxis with once-daily LMWH. Surveillance venography was performed after three weeks, and patients were followed clinically for three months. The primary outcome was a composite of any DVT (including asymptomatic and distal DVT), PE, and death from any cause. Although the risk of the composite outcome was 24% lower and the risk of proximal DVT was 88% lower in the extended prophylaxis group, there were no differences in symptomatic or fatal VTE events. *J Thromb Hemostasis*. 2010;1223–1229.

- Jamjoon *et al.* performed a systematic review of the literature reporting on the timing of pharmacologic prophylaxis in TBI patients. The authors dichotomized the timing of prophylaxis to early and late at 72 h post-injury. A total of five retrospective cohort studies were included in the review with a total of 1,624 patients, of which 713 received early prophylaxis and 911 received late prophylaxis. There was a VTE risk reduction of 0.52 (95%CI 0.37–0.73) for those receiving early prophylaxis. Assessing safety, the relative risk of ICH progression in the early vs. the late group was 0.64 (95%CI 0.35–1.14). Based on the available literature, the authors conclude that prophylaxis by 72 hours reduces the risk of VTE without affecting progression of ICH. The retrospective nature of the studies included in this review and the variability in the measurement of ICH progression (some studies described it as progression on head CT obtained for clinical suspicion or need for craniotomy, another study described it as progression on head CT routinely obtained after prophylaxis initiation) limit the interpretation of the data. Other studies have reported progression of ICH when prophylaxis is started before 48 hours. No randomized controlled studies on timing of prophylaxis exist to date. *J Neurotrauma*. 2013; **30**: 503–511.

- Consensus guidelines for VTE prophylaxis in pediatric trauma patients are lacking. Overall, the incidence of post-injury VTE in pediatric patients is lower than that of adults. However, the age cut-off at which this difference is no longer significant has not been studied. In an evidence-based review of the literature Streck *et al.* identified that the mean age of patients with a VTE was 16.6 years vs. 12.1 years ($p < 0.01$) in those who did not develop VTE, independent of other risk factors. By multivariate logistic regression those <14 years of age had a decreased risk of VTE (OR 0.2, 95%CI 0.1–0.9). With the limitations of the data available, this is the first study that identifies an age cut-off (≥ 14 y.o.) at which VTE prophylaxis in pediatric trauma patients could be beneficial. *J Pediatr Surg* 2013;1413–1421.

10. Infectious Disease

Chapter **10-(i)**

Evaluation of Fever

Robert T. Stovall, MD*

*Assistant Professor of Surgery, University of Colorado School of Medicine

Take Home Points

- Fever is a sign of inflammation, not necessarily infection.
- A thorough history and physical exam will usually identify the likely source of infection.
- Routine "knee jerk" batteries of tests to workup a fever are often not warranted.
- Imaging, labs or cultures should be obtained based on risk factors identified in the history and physical exam.

Background

- Fever is common after a surgical procedure, occurring in 50% of patients.
- Up to 90% of critically ill patients with severe sepsis will experience fever during their stay in the intensive care unit.
- Significant cost can be accrued in the workup of the febrile ICU patient.
- Fever is a natural response to inflammation and may not itself be pathological depending on the setting.

Contact information: Denver Health Medical Center, 777 Bannock Street, MC 0206, Denver, CO 80204. Email: robert.stovall@dhha.org

Main Body

- Source of fever

  o Inflammation (both infectious and non-infectious).
  o Medications (common culprits).

- Definition of a fever

  o Normal temperature varies based on age, time of day, and method of measurement.
  o Temperature can be affected by various environmental factors and drugs in the ICU.
  o Fever is defined differently by different groups and is somewhat arbitrary and depends on patient characteristics and setting (e.g. immunosuppressed, post operatively).
  o A broadly defined generalization by the ACCM and IDSA suggests >38.3 deserves attention in an ICU setting.
  o If you want a more sensitive screen, use a lower workup threshold.
  o Our Surgical ICU uses 38.5 but this can vary based on clinical suspicion.

    ▪ Many post trauma/surgery patients have a large inflammatory burden which may cause fever of non-infectious origin.

- Non-infectious sources of fever

  o Up to 50% of fevers in the ICU are not related to infection.
  o Potential non-infectious fevers (any cause of inflammation)

    ▪ Pancreatitis, thromboembolism, drugs, alcohol withdrawal myocardial infarction, pneumonitis, pericarditis, cancer, surgery, autoimmune disease, adrenal insufficiency, ischemia, blood product transfusions, iatrogenic, transfusions, many others.

- Common ICU sources of infectious fever

  o All usual infections are present while the incidence of each type may vary based on ICU.
  o It is commonly reported that surgical site, respiratory, bloodstream, and urinary tract make up the vast majority of infectious sources of fever in the SICU.

    ▪ Surgical sites of any kind both superficial and deep.
    ▪ Respiratory — Pneumonia (ventilator associated and otherwise), empyema.
    ▪ Urinary tract infection (upper and lower), especially if instrumented.
    ▪ Bloodstream infections, especially with indwelling devices.

- Abdominal infections – abscesses, perforations, colitis, toxic mega-colon, *C. diff,* cholangitis, cholecysitis (calculus and acalculus), spontaneous bacterial peritonitis.
- Central nervous system (risk is higher with instrumentation or trauma).
- Sinusitis.

- Workup of the febrile ICU patient
  - Start with thorough history and physical examination.
    - Key points are past history as well as recent history/events.
    - Recent procedures/surgeries/trauma.
    - Any indwelling hardware or foreign bodies.
    - Recent infections.
    - Search for reasons for potential immunosuppression.
    - Physical examination emphasis on <u>surgical sites</u> and foreign bodies.
    - Evaluated front and back.
  - Use adjunctive studies (imaging, labs, and cultures) to help confirm or refute suspicious sources found on history and physical exam. Routine sets of labs, culture or imaging are less likely to be cost-effective in finding an infectious source of fever.
  - Cultures:
    - Respiratory cultures
      ⇨ Multiple methods of obtaining cultures are debated.
      ⇨ Broncho-alveolar lavage (BAL) or mini BAL felt to be appropriate.
      ⇨ Clinical scores exist to help stratify the risk/benefit of obtaining respiratory cultures in ventilated febrile ICU patients, but no clear consensus exists as to optimal method.
      ⇨ Clinic suspicion is increased for respiratory source of infection when there has been worsening of respiratory parameters [e.g. hypoxia (decreased p/f ratio), increasing vent settings, new findings on CXR, long duration of intubation, etc.].
    - Urinary Tract Cultures
      ⇨ Instrumentation of the urinary tract is believed to increase the risk of infection similar to other body systems.
      ⇨ Urinalysis (UA) has been proposed as a rapid screen of infection; however the utility of this test as a screen for infection is patient and setting dependent. Conflicting literature exists as to its use in the ICU.

⇨ We use the UA as a screen for infection in the catheterized trauma patient in our ICU as a negative UA in this population greatly reduces the chance of a positive urine culture in the workup of a fever. If additional suspicion exists however, a culture needs to be sent.

⇨ Urine cultures should be sent when the suspicion of a urinary tract source of infectious fever is present.

- Blood Cultures

  ⇨ Incidence of bacteremia in the ICU varies based on population.

  ⇨ CCM/IDSA guidelines recommend blood cultures for every fever, but the evidence for this is lacking.

  ⇨ Factors that suggest need for blood cultures include: long term indwelling intravascular devices, immunosuppression, possibly rigors.

- Additional Cultures

  ⇨ If the history and physical exam suggest alternative sources of fever, especially surgical sites or other instrumented sites, effort should be made to assess these sites and cultures should be sent.

- Imaging

  ⇨ Chest X-ray (CXR): Commonly ordered as respiratory infections are common. Evidence suggests this is not necessary in every post-operative patient without other risk factors. However, most would agree that a newly febrile intubated patient should have a CXR.

  ⇨ Computed Tomography: Very useful when dictated by history and physical but not a routine part of every fever workup.

- Septic Patient Caveat: When a patient is febrile and septic, the risk-benefit profile of additional testing shifts as finding the source of infection and assuring appropriate antibiotics have survival benefit.

- Treatment

  o The treatment of fever is usually to treat the underlying cause. Treatment of the fever itself is of unclear benefit and may have some detrimental effects (e.g. in sepsis).

  - However, in certain situations, such as increased intracranial pressures, a fever can have deleterious effects and the risk benefit likely favors attempts to bring the temperature down.

  - Also, at very high levels, arguments are made to bring down the temperature as life-threatening complications can ensue (e.g., rhabdomyolysis). This usually represents a different clinical scenario.

o The need to treat a fever for the fever's sake is variable and situation dependent.

- **Summary**

 o A systematic and measured approach to the workup of a fever in the ICU is the optimal management strategy. Routine batteries of test should not be instituted. A thorough history and physical is warranted with each fever and adjunctive studies should be ordered based on this assessment.
 o Fever plus risk factors should prompt adjunctive studies.
 o Treatment of a fever should be directed at treating the underlying cause. In certain clinical situations, attempts to lower patient temperature directly may be warranted.

Practical Algorithm(s)/Diagrams

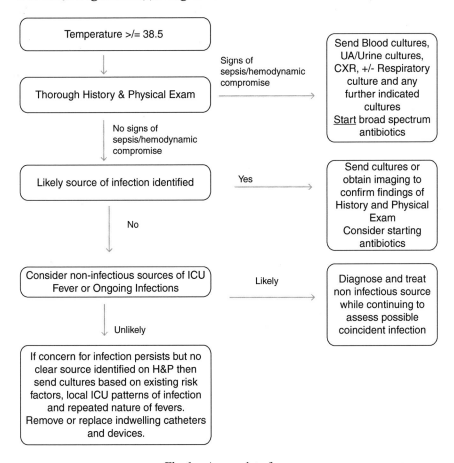

Fig. 1. Approach to fever.

Review of Current Literature with References

- O'Grady N, Barie PS, Bartlett JG *et al*. Guidelines for evaluation of new fever in critically ill adult patients: 2008 update from the American College of Critical Care Medicine and the Infectious Diseases Society of America. *Crit Care Med* 2008; **36**: 1330–1349.

    o Consensus guideline from large society. Defines fever as >38.3°C. Recommends blood culture and CXR on all febrile ICU patients. Reviews components of other potential ICU causes of fever

- Dimopoulos G, Falagas ME. Approach to the febrile patient in the ICU *Infect Dis Clin North Am* 2009; **23**: 471–484.

    o Review of fever assessment in ICU. Similar to CCM/IDSA guideline.

- Perlino, Carl A. Postoperative Fever. *Med Clin North Am* **85**: 1141.

    o Reviews general post-operative fever workup. Not specific to the ICU patient, but may apply to situations in the ICU.

Chapter 10-(ii)

Antimicrobial Stewardship

Michelle K. Haas, MD* and Timothy Jenkins, MD*

*Assistant Professor of Medicine, University of Colorado School of Medicine

Take Home Points

- Antimicrobial stewardship is defined as a systematic approach for optimizing antibiotic use in order to improve individual patient outcomes while minimizing adverse events associated with antibiotic use.
- Antibiotic use has dramatically increased over the past 10 years reaching a peak in 2010. This increase has been associated with: development of resistant organisms, *C. difficile* infection, adverse drug events, catheter-associated complications, and excess medical costs. Prevention of unnecessary antibiotic use can minimize all of these unintended consequences.
- Emergence of antibiotic resistance has been associated with: increased morbidity and mortality, increased length of hospitalization and increased hospital costs when compared with infections due to susceptible organisms.

Contact information: Denver Health Medical Center, University of Colorado Health Sciences Center, 777 Bannock Street, MC 0206, Denver, CO 80204; Tel.: 303-602-5052, email: Michelle.Haas@dhha.org; Timothy.Jenkins@dhha.org

- Unnecessary antibiotic use can be prevented by ensuring an appropriate indication for antibiotic therapy exists, selection of the appropriate antibiotic and dose, and use of the shortest effective duration of therapy.
- Providers can improve antibiotic use further by ensuring judicious use of broad-spectrum agents such as carbapenems as well as participating in the development and implementation of institutional guidelines to further streamline care.
- For critically ill patients who have an unknown source of infection, use of broad-spectrum empiric antimicrobial therapy is appropriate initially but should consider local resistance patterns.
- In critically ill patients who receive broad spectrum antibiotic therapy, de-escalate to the narrowest spectrum of activity as soon as possible as microbiological cultures and clinical status allow.
- Treat for the shortest appropriate duration, referring to local and national guidelines where appropriate.
- Maximize the ability to use diagnostic tests for decisions about antibiotic therapy by making all attempts to obtain appropriate microbiologic specimens for culture prior to starting empiric treatment.
- Take an "antibiotic time-out" on rounds each day to ask three key questions: Is this an appropriate indication for an antibiotic? Is this the optimal antibiotic choice/dose? What is the shortest effective duration of therapy?

Background

- While a lack of appropriate empiric antibiotics can be associated with increased mortality,[1] up to 50% of antibiotic use in healthcare settings may be inappropriate, which can be associated with substantial negative effects including the emergence of resistance, increased risk of *C.difficile* infection and adverse drug events.
- Antibiotic use creates a selective pressure leading to emergence of resistance in individual patients, intensive care units, hospitals and within communities. The proportion of pathogens causing hospital-onset infections that are resistant to target antimicrobial drugs continues to increase at an alarming rate. Cabapenem resistant gram negatives were uncommon in 2001 and now have been described in most states. *Pseudomonas* resistance has been associated with all-carbapenem use, including use of "*Pseudomonas*-sparing" carbapenems such as ertapenem. Over the 10-year period from 1995–2004, the proportion of enterococcal infections among ICU patients that were resistant to vancomycin doubled from less than 15% to 30%. Within the Denver Health

system, use of fluoroquinolones for urinary tract infections has been associated with emergence of fluoroquinolone resistance in *E.coli*. Infections with drug resistant organisms are associated with increased morbidity and mortality, increased length of hospitalization and increased costs compared to infections due to susceptible organisms.

- *Clostridium difficile* infection (CDI) has shown a 4-fold increase in incidence in elderly since mid-1990s with an associated increase in severe cases necessitating colectomy (1.2 to 3.4 per 1,000 cases). Mortality has increased due to CDI, at a rate of 35% between 1999–2004. The risk of CDI increases with increasing cumulative doses of antibiotics, days of antibiotic exposure and the number of antibiotics used. Not all antibiotics confer equal risk, with the highest risk seen with 2nd/3rd generation cephalosporins and beta-lactam+ inhibitor combinations.

- Antibiotics are a leading cause of adverse events such as renal failure, neutropenia, severe drug eruptions, fevers and in rare cases, death. Vancomycin use can be associated with the development of acute renal failure and neutropenia. B-lactam antibiotics can be associated with drug-induced cholestasis and hepatitis. Fluoroquinolones can cause QT prolongation and use has been associated with serious arrhythmia. Azithromycin use has been associated with an increased risk of sudden cardiac death.

- In 2007, the Infectious Disease Society of America (IDSA) recognized the importance of promoting the rational use of antibiotics through developing guidelines for implementing antimicrobial stewardship programs in the inpatient setting. Denver Health instituted an antimicrobial stewardship program in 2008.

- The primary goal of hospital antimicrobial stewardship programs is to facilitate optimizing antibiotic use to improve patient outcomes. Stewardship programs also aim to limit the emergence of resistant organisms associated with excessive use of antibiotics and to control healthcare costs. This is accomplished through strategies such as promoting judicious use of broad spectrum antimicrobials, reviewing provider antibiotic prescriptions and giving feedback to providers, education and the implementation of guidelines.

- Data regarding the impact of implementing the aforementioned strategies has met with success, decreasing broad spectrum antibiotic use while limiting the emergence of resistance. There are limited data regarding the impact on mortality. However, studies evaluating the impact of antimicrobial stewardship in the intensive care unit have been associated with improved prescribing practices and one study has shown reductions in length of stay, mechanical ventilation days and mortality.[2,3]

- Within the Denver Health system, our surgical intensive care unit has worked closely with the antimicrobial stewardship program to implement strategies promoting the judicious use of antibiotics. This effort has been associated with success in reducing total antibiotic use, use of antibiotics with broad spectrum activity and decreased costs (see Fig. 1).
- Providers can optimize antibiotic use in critically ill patients through daily review of the appropriateness of antibiotic therapy including indication for therapy, antibiotic choice, dose, and duration of therapy.

Main Body

- Choosing an empiric antimicrobial regimen
  - o The importance of early goal directed therapy and adequacy of resuscitation cannot be over-emphasized for critically ill patients with severe sepsis/shock. For an in-depth discussion, refer to Chapter 5-(iv). Initial empiric antibiotic therapy should be broad-spectrum to avoid failure to cover the infecting pathogen and resultant increased mortality.[1,4–6] The most common reasons for inadequate coverage are failure to cover MRSA and failure to cover resistant gram negatives, therefore knowing local resistance patterns is essential. However, while broad coverage is appropriate, use of two gram negative agents did not offer any additional benefit over one broad spectrum agent in one randomized controlled trial.[7] Narrower-spectrum therapy, which decreases selective pressure for the development of resistant organisms, decreases risk of *C. difficile*, and decreases costs, must be weighed against the risk of creating a gap in coverage in critically ill patients with severe sepsis/shock and an unknown source of infection.
  - o Optimizing dosing of empiric antibiotic regimens will avoid undertreatment of infections and excessive antibiotic use. For example, central nervous system infections may require higher dosing of certain agents. Many antibiotics need dose adjustments in the context of renal failure to avoid toxic adverse effects. Dose adjustments are rarely needed for patients with end stage liver disease.
  - o Institutional guidelines or clinical pathways should be followed when applicable, to standardize and streamline care, improve antimicrobial prescribing, and decrease medical costs.
- Maximizing the ability to safely de-escalate therapy
  - o In order to allow informed de-escalation of antibiotic therapy, it remains important to maximize the yield and accuracy of diagnostic tests. Cultures

should be obtained from blood for culture prior to antibiotic administration when possible and should avoid cultures from central lines given the increased risk of false positive cultures. Depending on the suspected source of infection, additional cultures such as bronchoalveolar lavage (BAL) may be appropriate and should ideally be obtained prior to administration of antibiotic therapy. Use of urinalysis alone may be sufficient in SICU patients to exclude the presence of infection.[8]

o Isolation of an organism from culture does not necessarily indicate that it is contributing to the patient's infectious process. Cultures from non-sterile sites such as wound swabs must be interpreted with great caution with consideration for the clinical context of the patient for they often do not reflect the causative organism. Similarly, bronchoalveolar lavage (BAL) specimens in patients who have been intubated for prolonged periods of time may reflect organisms colonizing the airway.

o Procalcitonin (PCT) is a biomarker that is significantly increased in the setting of a bacterial infection compared to viral or non-infectious inflammatory processes where the level of elevation correlates with disease severity. Use of PCT is a promising aid for clinical decision-making, particularly in the setting of acute lower respiratory tract infections and sepsis. Data on the utility of procalcitonin to guide antibiotic therapy are limited in immunocompromised individuals, pregnancy, parasitic infections and in gram negative infections such as *Pseudomonas* and *Acinetobacter*. Use in septic patients in surgical ICUs has been limited; however one randomized trial demonstrated a reduction in duration of therapy without a negative effect on clinical outcomes.[9] While more data are needed, there may still be a role in cautious use of PCT to guide discontinuation of antimicrobial therapy in SICU patients.

• Narrowing therapy when an organism is isolated

o Once susceptibilities are determined, antibiotic therapy should be narrowed to the most effective, narrow spectrum agent. Interpreting susceptibility reports should also consider the clinical context. Not all antibiotics have equal penetration into certain preserved sites, such as the central nervous system (CNS). Cefazolin, while appropriate for many cases of methicillin susceptible *S. aureus* (MSSA) bacteremia, does not penetrate well into the CNS and thus is not appropriate treatment for meningitis or a brain abscess.

o Other organism-specific examples of the importance of narrowing therapy include rapid de-escalation from vancomycin to a B-lactam when MSSA is isolated. Vancomycin is clearly inferior for MSSA and use is associated with relapse rates of 20% as well as excess mortality compared to B-lactam therapy. Therefore even in penicillin-allergic patients, every attempt should be taken to administer B-lactam therapy for serious *S. aureus* infections, including desensitization if needed.

o Conversely, some organisms may be associated with emergence of resistance to overly narrow spectrum therapy. *Enterobacter* has a propensity for developing resistance while on therapy with 3rd generation cephalosporins. Therefore, treatment with these agents should be avoided even if reported as susceptible. A broader spectrum agent such as a carbapenem may be indicated depending on the clinical context.

o Use of infectious diseases consultation has been associated with improved outcomes for *S. aureus* bacteremia, including reductions in mortality. Therefore where questions remain for de-escalating therapy, consultation with your antimicrobial stewardship team or infectious disease specialists is recommended.

o While considering narrowing therapy, certain antibiotics have excellent oral-bioavailability such as fluoroquinolones, azoles, macrolides and clindamycin. Whenever appropriate, IV therapy should be changed to oral therapy to limit adverse events associated with intravenous administration as well as to reduce costs.

• De-escalating therapy if cultures are negative

o At 48–72 hours, discontinue vancomycin in clinically stable patients when no resistant gram-positive pathogens have been identified. Despite recent trends in decreasing isolation of MRSA nationally, vancomycin is often unnecessarily continued in antibiotic regimens despite absence of cultured or suspected resistant gram-positive pathogens.

o Absence of growth of gram-negative organisms from all microbiological cultures should prompt consideration of de-escalation from dual gram-negative therapy to a single agent.

o Negative cultures and studies may be useful in patients with selected suspected infections. In patients in whom ventilator-associated pneumonia was suspected, negative cultures at 72 hours obtained off antibiotics suggests an alternative cause of the clinical syndrome. Current Infectious Diseases Society of America/American Thoracic Society guidelines for healthcare-associated pneumonia advocate for cessation of antibiotic therapy in stable patients with no other source of infection. Within our SICU, a clinical pulmonary infection score (CPIS) of 6 or greater would be an indication to initiate antibiotic therapy. Antibiotics are discontinued in patients with CPIS scores of less than 6 for three days with negative cultures and no other source of infection. SICU patients with suspected urinary tract infections, a negative urinalysis has a very high negative predictive value, essentially excluding the presence of infection.

- Be patient. Allow sufficient time for a clinical response prior to changing antibiotic regimens in clinically stable patients

  o Clinical improvement is not always immediately apparent, even with appropriate therapy. Patients with *S. aureus* bacteremia may take up to 7 days to clear despite appropriate therapy and source control. Patients with pyelonephritis may continue to have fevers for up to 72 hours after initiating appropriate therapy. Multiple changes to antibiotic regimens without adequate time to determine the effect of a regimen can confuse the clinical picture.

  o Conversely, slow clinical improvement could indicate an undrained focus of infection such as an intra-abdominal abscess and need for surgical intervention. Clinically stable patients who are thought to be responding slower than expected to therapy should have a careful evaluation for undrained focus of infection and non-infectious causes of fever prior to changing antibiotic therapy. Escalating antibiotic therapy should be reserved for patients with precipitous development of septic shock without obvious source.

- Treat for the shortest effective duration for a given infection

  o Shorter course of therapy are less likely to select for antibiotic resistant organisms, reduce the risk of *C.difficile* infection and limit the emergence of adverse drug events associated with cumulative doses.

  o Duration of therapy may vary depending on the organism involved and the site of infection as well as host factors. Current guidelines for the management of sepsis recommend 7–10 days with the caveat that longer courses may be needed in selected clinical scenarios such as *S. aureus* bacteremia, fungal infections and those with immunodeficiences. While exceptions remain for certain non-lactose fermenting gram negative infections and *S. aureus*, ventilator-associated pneumonia can be treated for 7–8 days in the majority of cases. Catheter-associated blood stream infections have established durations of therapy summarized in the Infectious Diseases Society of America guidelines which depend on several factors including the organism isolated. For infections requiring prolonged intravenous antibiotic therapy such as *S. aureus* bacteremia or intracranial abscess infectious disease consultation is recommended.

- o Counting the days of therapy, while a simple task can be challenging in the reality of frequent hand-offs and multiple changes in antibiotic regimens. The first day of effective therapy should be counted as day one, and the duration should include all current and prior effective therapy. Therapy prescribed at discharge or recommended upon transfer from the ICU should count these days of therapy, avoiding the tendency to reset the clock when patients change locations or providers. Every effort should be made to communicate both days of therapy and anticipated total duration of therapy, including involving the patient, ancillary care teams as well as documenting in the medical record. Failure to keep an accurate record of days of appropriate antibiotic therapy commonly leads to unnecessary prolongation of therapy. Prolongation of antibiotic therapy has been associated with the emergence of resistance and increases the risk of adverse events such as *C. difficile* colitis and drug toxicities.

- o Many experts advocate for an antibiotic time-out each day on rounds to ask three fundamental questions to ensure optimization of antibiotic therapy: (1) Is this an appropriate indication for an antibiotic? (2) Is this the optimal antibiotic choice/dose? (3) What is the shortest appropriate duration of therapy?

- Prevent infections

  - o Patients who do not develop infectious-related complications in the intensive care unit are less likely to be exposed to antibiotic therapy. Therefore every attempt should be made to reduce risk of infections in the following ways:

    - Hand hygiene before and after every patient contact will limit spread of resistant organisms between patients.

    - Remove vascular and urinary catheters as soon as possible as both are associated with increased infections over time.

    - Prevent hospital-acquired pneumonia through the use of incentive spirometry, ambulation if able, elevation of the head-of-bed and avoidance of unnecessary use of proton pump inhibitors.

Practical Algorithm(s)/Diagrams

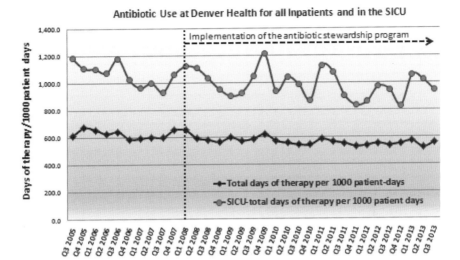

Antibiotic Use at Denver Health for all Inpatients and in the SICU

16% decrease in antibiotic use in the SICU since 2008
37% decrease in use of cefepime, piperacillin-tazobactam, levofloxacin and imipenem in the SICU since 2008

Fig. 1. Antibiotic use over time after implementation of an antibiotic stewardship program at a public safety net hospital. Monitoring antibiotic use in healthcare facilities coupled with antibiogram data can inform future interventions.

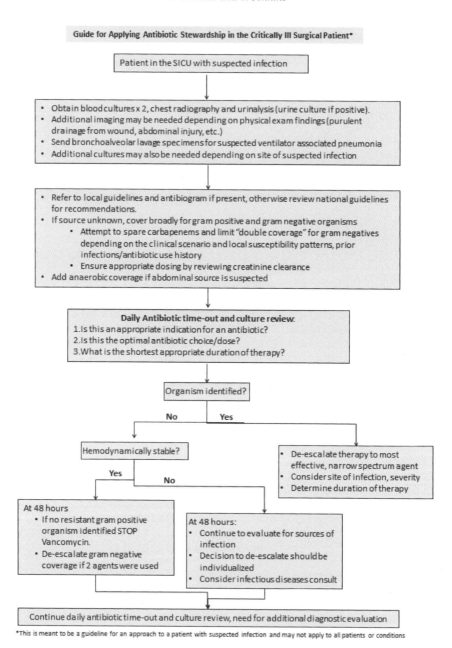

Guide for Applying Antibiotic Stewardship in the Critically Ill Surgical Patient*

Patient in the SICU with suspected infection

- Obtain blood cultures x 2, chest radiography and urinalysis (urine culture if positive).
- Additional imaging may be needed depending on physical exam findings (purulent drainage from wound, abdominal injury, etc.)
- Send bronchoalveolar lavage specimens for suspected ventilator associated pneumonia
- Additional cultures may also be needed depending on site of suspected infection

- Refer to local guidelines and antibiogram if present, otherwise review national guidelines for recommendations.
- If source unknown, cover broadly for gram positive and gram negative organisms
    - Attempt to spare carbapenems and limit "double coverage" for gram negatives depending on the clinical scenario and local susceptibility patterns, prior infections/antibiotic use history
    - Ensure appropriate dosing by reviewing creatinine clearance
- Add anaerobic coverage if abdominal source is suspected

Daily Antibiotic time-out and culture review.
1. Is this an appropriate indication for an antibiotic?
2. Is this the optimal antibiotic choice/dose?
3. What is the shortest appropriate duration of therapy?

Organism identified?

No   Yes

Hemodynamically stable?

Yes   No

- De-escalate therapy to most effective, narrow spectrum agent
- Consider site of infection, severity
- Determine duration of therapy

At 48 hours
- If no resistant gram positive organism identified STOP Vancomycin.
- De-escalate gram negative coverage if 2 agents were used

At 48 hours:
- Continue to evaluate for sources of infection
- Decision to de-escalate should be individualized
- Consider infectious diseases consult

Continue daily antibiotic time-out and culture review, need for additional diagnostic evaluation

*This is meant to be a guideline for an approach to a patient with suspected infection and may not apply to all patients or conditions

Fig. 2.   This represents one approach to applying antibiotic stewardship strategies in the critically ill surgical patient. As with all guidelines, this approach may not be appropriate for all patients and clinical judgment should determine its applicability.

Review of Current Literature with References

1. Kollef MH, Sherman G, Ward S, Fraser VJ. Inadequate antimicrobial treatment of infections: a risk factor for hospital mortality among critically ill patients. *Chest* 1999; **115**: 462–474.

   • This prospective study of 2,000 patients admitted to intensive care units evaluated the association between inadequate antimicrobial treatment of their infections and mortality. Hospital mortality rate of patients receiving inadequate treatment was 52.1% compared to 12.2% for those who received adequate treatment for their infection. Inadequate antimicrobial treatment was determined to be an independent factor associated with mortality after multivariate logistic regression analysis (OR 4.27, 95% CI 3.35–5.44, $p < 0.001$).

2. Katsios CM, Burry L, Nelson S *et al.* An antimicrobial stewardship program improves antimicrobial treatment by culture site and the quality of antimicrobial prescribing in critically ill patients. *Crit Care (London, England)* 2012; **16**: R216.

   • This retrospective study reviewed consecutive patients admitted to an intensive care unit over a two month period before and after the introduction of an antimicrobial stewardship program. The overall aim was to determine the impact of the stewardship program on documentation of antimicrobial use and decision to treat cultures from sterile sites compared to non-sterile sites. They found an increase in the treatment of sterile site cultures (64 vs. 83%, $p = 0.01$) and a reduction in the treatment of non-sterile site cultures (71 vs. 46%, $p = 0.002$.) There was no difference in the percentage of cultures form sterile vs. non-sterile sites in either period. There was an increase in the number of formally documented stop dates (53% compared to 71%, $p < 0.0001$) and regimen de-escalation (15% compared to 23%, $p = 0.026$).

3. Rimawi RH, Mazer MA, Siraj DS, Gooch M, Cook PP. Impact of regular collaboration between infectious diseases and critical care practitioners on antimicrobial utilization and patient outcome. *Crit Care Med* 2013; **41**: 2099–2107.

   • This retrospective study reviewed 246 patients admittted to a medical ICU who received antibiotics for suspected infection to evaluate the impact of of infectious disease fellow review of antibiotic prescribing. Patients were selected over a 3 month period before the intervention and then over the same 3 month period one year later. They evaluated antibiotic use, treatment duration and severity of illness, including mortality. While there were no differences in severity of illness between the two groups, significant differences were seen in broad spectrum antibiotic use including carbapenems and extended spectrum B-lactams. Additionally they demonstrated a significant reduction in mechanical ventilation days, length of stay and hospital mortality ($p = 0.0367$).

4. Kumar A, Ellis P, Arabi Y *et al*. Initiation of inappropriate antimicrobial therapy results in a fivefold reduction of survival in human septic shock. *Chest* 2009; **136**: 1237–1248.

   - In this retrospective study of 5,715 patients with septic shock in three countries, the aim was to determine the appropriateness of initial antimicrobial therapy. The site of infection and infecting pathogens were also reviewed and the major clinical endpoint reviewed was survival. The survival rate after appropriate therapy was 52% which fell to 10.3% in patients who received inappropriate therapy (OR, 9.45, 95% CI 7.74–11.54, $p<0.0001$). After adjustment for severity of illness, comorbid conditions and other risk factors, inappropriate therapy remained associated with the risk of death (OR 8.99, 95% CI 6.6–12.23)

5. Kumar A, Roberts D, Wood KE *et al*. Duration of hypotension before initiation of effective antimicrobial therapy is the critical determinant of survival in human septic shock. *Crit Care Med* 2006; **34**: 1589–1596.

6. Gaieski DF, Mikkelsen ME, Band RA *et al*. Impact of time to antibiotics on survival in patients with severe sepsis or septic shock in whom early goal-directed therapy was initiated in the emergency department. *Crit Care Med* 2010; **38**: 1045–1053.

7. Brunkhorst FM, Oppert M, Marx G *et al*. Effect of empirical treatment with moxifloxacin and meropenem vs meropenem on sepsis-related organ dysfunction in patients with severe sepsis: a randomized trial. JAMA 2012; **307**: 2390–2399.

   - In this randomized open label trial of 600 patients with severe sepsis or septic shock, the impact of use of meropenem alone compared to meropenem + moxifloxacin was evaluated on degree of organ failure. Secondary outcomes included 28 day and 90 day all cause mortality. There were 551 patients who were able to be evaluated at study closure and of these individuals there was no statistically significant differences in degree of organ failure, 28 day or 90 day mortality.

8. Stovall RT, Haenal JB, Jenkins TC *et al*. A negative urinalysis rules out catheter-associated urinary tract infection in trauma patients in the intensive care unit. *J Am College Surgeons* 2013; **217**: 162–166.

9. Schroeder S, Hochreiter M, Koehler T *et al*. Procalcitonin (PCT)-guided algorithm reduces length of antibiotic treatment in surgical intensive care patients with severe sepsis: results of a prospective randomized study. *Langenbeck's Archives of Surgery/Deutsche Gesellschaft fur Chirurgie* 2009; **394**: 221–226.

Sepsis

Heather Young, MD* and Connie Savor Price, MD†

*Assistant Professor of Medicine, University of Colorado School of Medicine
†Associate Professor of Medicine, University of Colorado School of Medicine

Take Home Points

- Surgical patients account for nearly one-third of sepsis cases in the United States and sepsis is the leading cause of death in non-cardiac intensive care units.
- Sepsis-related mortality remains prohibitively high (>40%).
- Early treatment is essential in the management of sepsis, and therapy should be started as soon as the syndrome is recognized.
- Adequate fluid resuscitation, antibiotic therapy, intubation and mechanical ventilation, and source control are key components of early sepsis therapy.
- Intravenous (IV) antibiotic therapy should be administered within 1 hour of identifying sepsis.
- The delivery of evidence-based care and rapid source control can improve patient outcomes.

Contact information: Denver Health Medical Center, University of Colorado School of Medicine, 777 Bannock Street, MC 4000, Denver, CO 80204; Tel.: (Connie Savor Price): 303-602-5016, email: Connie.Price@dhha.org; Heather.Young2@dhha.org

Background

- Surgical patients account for nearly one-third of sepsis cases in the United States. The mortality rate for septic shock in the perioperative period exceeds that of both myocardial infarction and pulmonary embolism.
- Risk factors for both the development of sepsis and death from sepsis included age older than 60 years, the need for emergency surgery, and the presence of comorbid conditions.
- Intraabdominal infection is the most common source of sepsis among surgical patients, accounting for approximately two-thirds of all cases.
- When septic shock follows sepsis, there is a 39% mortality rate among emergent surgical patients and a 30% mortality rate among elective surgical patients.
- The early identification of sepsis and implementation of early evidence-based therapies have been documented to improve outcomes and decrease sepsis-related mortality.
- The definition of sepsis is adapted from Levy MM, Fink MP, Marshall JC *et al.* 2001 SCCM/ESICM/ACCP/ATS/SIS International Sepsis Definitions Conference. *Crit Care Med* 2003; **31**: 1250–1256. Sepsis is defined as the presence (probable or documented) of infection together with systemic manifestations of infection, including:

  o General variables

     - Fever (>38.3°C)
     - Hypothermia (core temperature <36°C)
     - Heart rate >90/min–1 or more than two sd above the normal value for age
     - Tachypnea
     - Altered mental status
     - Significant edema or positive fluid balance (>20 mL/kg over 24 hr)
     - Hyperglycemia (Plasma glucose >140 mg/dL or 7.7 mmol/L) in the absence of diabetes

  o Inflammatory variables

     - Leukocytosis (WBC count >12,000 µL–1)
     - Leukopenia (WBC count <4000 µL–1)
     - Normal WBC count with greater than 10% immature forms
     - Plasma C-reactive protein more than two sd above the normal value
     - Plasma procalcitonin more than two sd above the normal value
     - Hemodynamic variables

- Arterial hypotension (SBP <90 mm Hg, MAP <70 mm Hg, or an SBP decrease >40 mm Hg in adults or less than two sd below normal for age)

  o Organ dysfunction variables

    - Arterial hypoxemia (PaO_2/FiO_2 <300)
    - Acute oliguria (urine output <0.5 mL/kg/hr for at least 2 hrs despite adequate fluid resuscitation)
    - Creatinine increase >0.5 mg/dL or 44.2 μmol/L
    - Coagulation abnormalities (INR >1.5 or aPTT >60 s)
    - Ileus (absent bowel sounds)
    - Thrombocytopenia (platelet count <100,000 μL–1)
    - Hyperbilirubinemia (plasma total bilirubin >4 mg/dL or 70 μmol/L)

  o Tissue perfusion variables

    - Hyperlactatemia (>1 mmol/L)
    - Decreased capillary refill or mottling

- Diagnostic criteria for sepsis in the pediatric population are signs and symptoms of inflammation plus infection with hyper- or hypothermia (rectal temperature >38.5°C or <35°C), tachycardia (may be absent in hypothermic patients), and at least one of the following indications of altered organ function:

  o Altered mental status
  o Hypoxemia
  o Increased serum lactate level
  o Bounding pulses

- Severe sepsis definition is defined from the same as sepsis-induced tissue hypoperfusion or organ dysfunction (any of the following thought to be due to the infection):

  o Sepsis-induced hypotension
  o Lactate above upper limits laboratory normal
  o Urine output <0.5 mL/kg/hr for more than 2 hrs despite adequate fluid resuscitation
  o Acute lung injury with PaO_2/FiO_2 <250 in the absence of pneumonia as infection source
  o Acute lung injury with PaO_2/FiO_2 <200 in the presence of pneumonia as infection source
  o Creatinine >2.0 mg/dL (176.8 μmol/L)

o Bilirubin >2 mg/dL (34.2 µmol/L)
o Platelet count <100,000 µL
o Coagulopathy (international normalized ratio >1.5)

Main Body

Modified from Dellinger RP, Levy MM, Rhodes A, et al. Surviving Sepsis Campaign: International Guidelines for Management of Severe Sepsis and Septic Shock: 2012. Crit Care Med 2013; 41: 580–637.

- Initial Resuscitation

  o This is discussed in more detail in Chapter 5-(iii), *Resuscitation.*

  o Resuscitation goals for patients with sepsis-induced tissue hypoperfusion during the first 6 hrs include:

    ▪ Central venous pressure (CVP), if available, 8–12 mm Hg in nonintubated patients. A higher target of 12 to 15 mm Hg should be the goal in mechanically ventilated patients or in circumstances of increased abdominal pressure.
    ▪ Mean arterial pressure (MAP) ≥65 mm Hg
    ▪ Urine output ≥0.5 mL/kg/hr
    ▪ Central venous (superior vena cava) or mixed venous oxygen saturation 70% or 65%, respectively.

  o In patients with elevated lactate, target resuscitation to normalize lactate

  o The above strategy (Fig. 1) is termed early goal-directed therapy, and is associated with reduced 28-day mortality

- Glucocorticoid therapy, nutritional support, and glucose control are additional issues that are important in the management of patients with severe sepsis or septic shock. Each is discussed separately [see Chapters 11-(ii), 8-(i) and 11-(iii), respectively].

- Screening for Sepsis

  o Early identification of septic patients is imperative if mortality rates are to be improved.

  o In the surgical patient, some of the early signs of sepsis are often attributed to other common problems seen in the postoperative period.

  o All potentially infected, seriously ill patients, should be routinely screened for severe sepsis to allow earlier implementation of therapy.

- Diagnosis
  - o Cultures as clinically appropriate before antimicrobial therapy if no significant delay (>45 mins) in the start of antimicrobial(s).
  - o Obtain at least two sets of blood cultures (both aerobic and anaerobic) before antimicrobial therapy, with at least one drawn percutaneously.
    - It is crucial to obtain the appropriate volume of blood for the culture system.
    - Obtaining blood cultures from all lumens of vascular access devices (VAD) in place for at least 48 hours may aid in diagnosis of a device associated bacteremia. If a VAD culture inoculated with the same amount of blood becomes positive at least 120 minutes before the peripheral cultures become positive, it is recommended that the device be removed because it is likely infected.
    - Cultures drawn from vascular access devices have a higher likelihood of becoming positive due to contamination and may prompt inappropriate antibiotic use [Chapter 10-(ii)]. Results should be interpreted in light of clinical scenario and peripheral culture results.
  - o Additional cultures from other sites (e.g., respiratory, urinary tract) and radiographic imaging are dictated by clinical suspicion.
  - o Although modern conventional culture techniques allow for enhanced growth of yeast, autopsy-based studies have not been reported, a diagnosis may take days. The β-D-glucan assay may be a useful adjunct to blood cultures and biopsy for patients with deep-seated candidiasis (e.g., intra-abdominal candidiasis) but false-positive reactions can occur with colonization alone.
  - o The potential role of biomarkers for diagnosis of infection in patients presenting with severe sepsis remains undefined. The utility of procalcitonin levels or other biomarkers (such as C-reactive protein) to discriminate the acute inflammatory pattern of sepsis from other causes of generalized inflammation (e.g., postoperative) has not been demonstrated.
  - o Imaging studies performed promptly to confirm a potential source of infection and potential sources of infection should be sampled as they are identified, in consideration of risk for patient transport and invasive procedures.
- Antimicrobial Therapy
  - o Administer effective intravenous (IV) antimicrobials within the first hour of recognition of septic shock and severe sepsis.

o   Inadequate initial antimicrobial coverage is associated with increased morbidity and mortality. Initial empiric anti-infective therapy of one or more drugs that have activity against all likely pathogens (usually bacterial and/or fungal) and that penetrate in adequate concentrations into tissues presumed to be the source of sepsis.

o   The selection of antimicrobial therapy should take into account the patient's history of drug allergies, recent antimicrobial exposure, suspected source of infection, and local antibiograms.

o   Antimicrobial regimen should be reassessed daily for potential deescalation [Chapter 10-(ii)].

o   Combination empirical therapy should be reserved for severe sepsis and/or for patients with suspected or confirmed difficult-to-treat, multidrug resistant bacterial pathogens such as *Acinetobacter* and *Pseudomonas* spp. A combination of beta-lactam and macrolide should be used for patients with septic shock from bacteremic *Streptococcus pneumoniae* infections (Table 1).

o   When indicated, empiric coverage for *Staphylococcus* spp typically should be active vs MRSA until either a staphylococcal etiology is ruled out or susceptibility is confirmed to be active vs β-lactam. We do not advocate use of vancomycin empirically against enterococcus due to our local antibiogram.

o   Empiric combination therapy should not be administered for more than 3–5 days. De-escalation to the most appropriate single therapy should be performed as soon as the susceptibility profile is known.

o   Duration of therapy should not exceed 7–10 days; longer courses may be appropriate in patients who have a slow clinical response, undrainable foci of infection, bacteremia with *S. aureus*; some fungal and viral infections, or infection in setting of immunologic deficiencies, including neutropenia.

o   Antimicrobial agents should not be used in patients with severe inflammatory states determined to be noninfectious.

•   Source Control

o   A specific anatomical diagnosis of infection requiring consideration for emergent source control should be pursued and excluded as rapidly as possible.

o   In surgical patients, the abdomen is the more frequent site of infection and often requires diagnostic imaging to identify the source and an operative procedure to attain control.

o   When source control in a severely septic patient is required, the effective intervention associated with the least physiologic insult should be used (e.g., percutaneous rather than surgical drainage of an abscess).

o If a diagnosis is made requiring source control, intervention should be taken within 12 hours.

o Patients presenting with septic shock requiring surgical intervention are suboptimal candidates for surgery due to hemodynamic instability. A "damage control laparotomy" (DCL) is a deliberate decision to address an identified source of infection in an abbreviated manner for sole purpose of controlling the infection, without a prolonged definitive operation, while undergoing continued resuscitation. Once the patient is stabilized, a definitive surgical procedure can be performed.

o When infected peripancreatic necrosis is identified as a potential source of infection, definitive intervention is best delayed until adequate demarcation of viable and nonviable tissues has occurred.

o If intravascular access devices are a possible source of severe sepsis or septic shock, they should be removed promptly after other vascular access has been established.

• Infection Prevention

o Implement careful infection control practices, including adherence to hand hygiene and standard (or appropriate transmission-based) precautions, during the care of septic patients.

o Prevention of device- and procedure-related infections used in the treatment of the septic patient is discussed in more detail in Chapter 10-(viii).

o Institute daily bathing of ICU patients with chlorhexidine gluconate (CHG) to reduce the rate of healthcare associated infections, including ventilator organisms, bloodstream infections, and ventilator-associated pneumonia.

o Routinely screen patients for multidrug resistant organisms of epidemiologic significance to your patient population. Screening can detect colonization states before clinical infection becomes apparent, allowing implementation of transmission-based precautions (e.g., contact isolation) before transmission can occur, and prevent the establishment of endemicity. Examples include admission and weekly peri-rectal swabs to detect carbepenem-resistant enterobacteriaceae (CRE) and anterior nares swabs for colonization with methicillin-resistant *Staphylococcus aureus* (MRSA).

o Consider decolonizing *S. aureus* nasal carriers using 2% mupirocin calcium ointment to bilateral nares for five days. *S. aureus* is a common cause of community and healthcare associated infections, difficult to treat, and when methicillin resistant, it has limited antibiotic options. Carriers of *S. aureus* have higher risk of infection from the organism with which they are colonized.

Practical Algorithm(s)/Diagrams

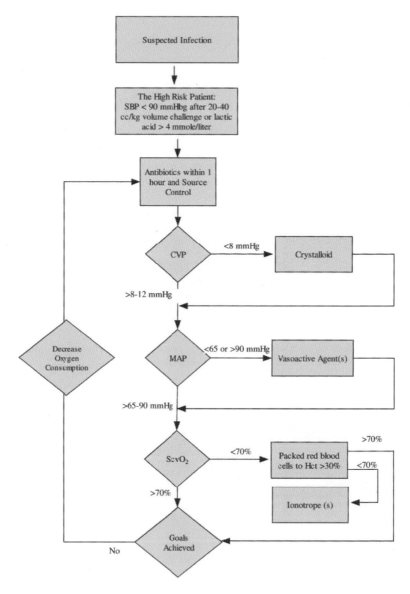

Fig. 1.   Early goal directed therapy.

Reproduced without permission from Otero RM, Nguyen HB, Huang DT. Chest 2006; **130**: 1579–1595

Table 1. Antibiotic agent selection for empiric treatment of the critically ill patient based on suspected site of infection, Denver Health, 2013.

Indication	Recommended empiric therapy	Alternative (use for mild-moderate β-lactam allergy)	Severe β-lactam allergy
Source unknown[1]			
Sepsis syndrome, unclear source and resuscitated (defined as SpO$_2$ >95% with respiratory support up to FiO$_2$ 40% and PEEP 5, off pressors) (*when source known or suspected, select empiric therapy for that source per recommendations below*)	Vancomycin weight-based IV dosing plus Cefepine 2gm IV Q12H[2] Add metronidazole if possible intra-abdominal source **Discontinue vancomycin if no MRSA identified at 48 hours**	No change	Vancomycin weight-based IV dosing plus Aztreonam 2gm IV Q8H Add metronidazole if possible intra-abdominal source **Discontinue vancomycin if no MRSA identified at 48 hours**
Septic shock and/or severe respiratory failure (refractory hypotension, PaO$_2$/FiO$_2$ ratio of <250) unclear source (*when source known or suspected, select empiric therapy for that source per recommendations below*)	Vancomycin weight-based IV dosing plus Cefepine 2gm IV Q12H[2] plus Amikacin 15mg/kg IV × 1 (up to 2 doses q 24 hours pending culture data. One dose only if renal failure is present or consider avoiding) Add metronidazole if possible intra-abdominal source **Discontinue vancomycin and 2nd gram-negative agent if no MRSA or resistant gram-negative organism, identified by 48 hours**	No change	Vancomycin weight-based IV dosing plus Aztreonam 2gm IV Q8H OR Levofloxacin 750mg IV Q24H plus Amikacin 15mg/kg IV × 1 (up to 2 doses q 24 hours pending culture data. One dose only if renal failure is present or consider avoiding) Add metronidazole if possible intra-abdominal source **Discontinue vancomycin and 2nd gram-negative agent if no MRSA or resistant gram-negative organism, respectively, identified by 48 hours**

(Continued)

Table 1. *(Continued)*

Indication	Recommended empiric therapy	Alternative (use for mild-moderate β-lactam allergy)	Severe β-lactam allergy
Pulmonary Infections			
Community-acquired pneumonia (NOTE: if septic shock present, refer to the recommendations for septic shock in the previous box)	Ceftriaxone 1gm IV Q24H plus Azithromycin 500mg PO/IV Q24H Consider addition of Vancomycin and ID consult if risk factors for MRSA pneumonia: necrosis/cavitation, post-influenza pneumonia or other clinical suspicion for *S. aureus* pneumonia	No change	Levofloxacin 750mg PO/IV Q24H[3] See recommendations regarding suspected MRSA in first box
Health care-associated/hospital-acquired pneumonia	Vancomycin weight-based IV dosing plus Cefepime 2gm Q8H[2] May consider addition of 2nd gram-negative agent (amikacin for patients in shock — see above recommendations) Obtain quantitative sputum culture and stop vancomycin if MRSA not identified within 48 hours	No change	Vancomycin weight-based IV dosing + Levofloxacin 750mg IV Q24H[3] May consider addition of 2nd gram-negative agent (amikacin for patients in shock — see above recommendations)
Confirmed MRSA pneumonia (blood or pleural fluid culture + sputum with >25 PMNs, culture + and no other organisms, BAL 10,000 cfu/mL in the presence of fever, leukocytosis and pulmonary infiltrates)	Vancomycin weight-based IV dosing; Indications for Linezolid 600 mg IV every 12 hours *where there is no clinical improvement with Vancomycin:* Vancomycin MIC >1, severe necrosis/cavitation. Consult Infectious Disease.	No change	No change

COPD exacerbation (without pneumonia)	Azithromycin 500 mg IV × 1, then 250 mg IV or PO Q24H OR Doxycycline 100 mg PO BID	No change	No change
Acute aspiration pneumonia	Ceftriaxone 1 gm IV Q24H	No change	Levofloxacin 750 mg IV Q24[3]
Lung abscess, aspiration pneumonia presenting from community	Unasyn 3 gm IV Q6H	Clindamycin 600 mg IV Q8H	No change
Skin and soft tissue infections			
Cellulitis WITHOUT cutaneous abscess, low clinical suspicion for necrotizing fasciitis[4]	Vancomycin weight-based IV dosing plus Cefepime 2gm IV Q12H[2]	Vancomycin weight-based IV dosing Plus Cefepime 2 gm IV Q12H	Vancomycin weight-based IV dosing plus Levofloxacin 750 mg IV Q24H
Cellulitis WITH cutaneous abscess, draining or to be drained	Vancomycin weight-based IV dosing	No change	No change
Necrotizing fasciitis, suspected or confirmed (consult General Surgery and ID)	Vancomycin weight-based IV dosing plus Piperacillin/tazobactam 4.5 gm IV Q6H plus Clindamycin 900 mg IV Q8H	Vancomycin weight-based IV dosing plus Cefepime 2 gm IV Q8H plus Clindamycin 900 mg IV Q8H	Vancomycin weight-based IV dosing plus Levofloxacin 750 mg IV Q24H plus Clindamycin 900 mg IV Q8H

(Continued)

Table 1. (*Continued*)

Indication	Recommended empiric therapy	Alternative (use for mild-moderate β-lactam allergy)	Severe β-lactam allergy
Diabetic foot ulcer infection	Vancomycin weight-based IV dosing plus Piperacillin/tazobactam 4.5 gm IV Q6H	Vancomycin weight-based IV dosing plus Cefepime 2 gm IV Q8H plus Metronidazole 500 mg IV Q8H	Vancomycin weight-based IV dosing plus Levofloxacin 750 mg IV Q24H plus Metronidazole 500 mg IV Q8H
Odontogenic space infection/ parapharyngeal abscess	Unasyn 3 gm IV Q6H	Clindamycin 600 mg IV Q8H	No change
Urinary tract infections			
Urinary tract infection from community-minimal risk for multi-drug resistant organism	Ceftriaxone 1gm IV Q24H Note: Agent of choice for pan-susceptible E. coli is cefazolin 1 gm IV Q8H	No change Note: Agent of choice for pan-susceptible E. coli is cefazolin 1 gm IV Q8H	Aztreonam 2 g IV every 8 hours +
Urinary tract infection from community-moderate to high risk of multi-drug resistant organism or from long-term care facility	Cefepime 2 gm IV Q8H[2]	No change	Aztreonam 2 g IV every 8 hours
Urinary tract infection, hospital-acquired	Cefepime 2 gm IV Q8H[2]	No change	Aztreonam 2 g IV every 8 hours

Intra-abdominal infections

Spontaneous bacterial peritonitis	Ceftriaxone 2 gm IV Q24H	No change	Levofloxacin 750 mg IV/PO daily
Upper GI bleed prophylaxis (only indicated in patients with cirrhosis)	Ceftriaxone 1 gm IV Q24H	No change	Levofloxacin 750 mg IV/PO daily
Uncomplicated intra-abdominal infection Examples: Appendicitis without perforation Acute biliary tract infection (cholecystitis, cholangitis)	Ceftriaxone 1 gm IV Q24H plus Metronidazole 500 mg PO Q8H	No change	Levofloxacin 750 mg IV/PO daily plus Metronidazole 500 mg PO Q8H
Complicated or healthcare associated intra-abdominal infection	Piperacillin/tazobactam 4.5 g IV q 6 hours + Vancomycin 30 mg/kg (max dose 2 g) IV × 1	Vancomycin weight based dosing plus cefepime 2 g IV q 12 hours plus metronidazole 500mg IV/PO q 8 hours	Vancomycin weight based dosing PLUS Levofloxacin 750 mg IV/PO daily plus metronidazole 500 mg I/v/PO q 8 hours

Central nervous system

Acute bacterial meningitis	Ceftriaxone 2 gm IV Q12H plus Vancomycin weight-based IV dosing plus Ampicillin 2 gm IV Q4H (if risk for Listeria)	Ceftriaxone 2 gm IV Q12H plus Vancomycin weight-based IV dosing plus TMP-SMX 20 mg/kg/day IV divided Q6H (if risk for Listeria)	Aztreonam 2 g IV ever 6 hours Plus Vancomycin weight-based IV dosing plus TMP-SMX 20 mg/kg/day IV divided Q6H (if risk for Listeria)

(Continued)

Table 1. (*Continued*)

Indication	Recommended empiric therapy	Alternative (use for mild-moderate β-lactam allergy)	Severe β-lactam allergy
Other clinical scenarios			
Febrile neutropenia	Cefepime 2 gm IV Q8H[2] Add vancomycin if risk factors for MRSA infection present	No change	Aztreonam 2g IV every 8 hours Add vancomycin if risk factors for MRSA infection present
Necrotizing pancreatitis	**Prophylaxis with a carbapenem is not recommended.** See recommendations for sepsis and septic shock depending on clinical condition.		

Notes: The antibiotic regimens shown are general guidelines and should not replace clinical judgment. Antibiotic doses shown are for normal renal function — adjust for renal insufficiency as appropriate.

1. Add micafungin 100 mg IV daily and consider ID consult if persistent fever and hemodynamic instability despite broad-spectrum antibacterial therapy and one or more of the following:
   • Candida colonization of multiple sites (urine + BAL for example)
   • Total parenteral nutrition (TPN)
   • Solid organ or hematopoietic cell transplantation
   • Prior surgery, especially abdominal
   • Underlying hematologic malignancy
   • Currently undergoing chemotherapy
   • Central venous catheter

2. May be associated with increased risk of non-convulsive status in patients over the age of 50 with significant CNS pathology, renal failure. Consult with ICU pharmacist for optimal dosing in these patients.

3. Fluoroquinolones have activity against Mycobacterium tuberculosis. If TB risk factors, call ID.

4. Cellulitis that is not the primary reason for ICU admission or is mild should be treated with Vancomycin alone, no additional gram negative coverage is necessary.

Review of Current Literature with References

- Kumar *et al.* conducted a retrospective cohort study between July 1989 and June 2004. Medical records of 2,731 adult patients with septic shock from fourteen intensive care units (four medical, four surgical, six mixed medical/surgical) and ten hospitals (four academic, six community) in Canada and the United States were reviewed. Effective antimicrobial administration within the first hour of documented hypotension was associated with increased survival to hospital discharge in adult patients with septic shock. The authors found that each hour in delay of antimicrobials was associated with an average decrease in survival of 7.6% (*Crit Care Med* 2006; **34**: 1589–1596).

- Rivers and colleagues randomly assigned 263 patients who arrived at an urban emergency department with severe sepsis or septic shock to receive either six hours of early goal-directed therapy or standard therapy (as a control) before admission to the intensive care unit. Clinicians who subsequently assumed the care of the patients were blinded to the treatment assignment. In-hospital mortality (the primary efficacy outcome), end points with respect to resuscitation, and acute physiology and chronic health evaluation (APACHE II) scores were obtained serially for 72 hours and compared between the study groups. In-hospital mortality was 30.5% in the group assigned to early goal-directed therapy, as compared with 46.5% in the group assigned to standard therapy ($p = 0.009$). The general application of this mortality benefit shown in a single center is unknown. Large randomized trials (e.g., Protocolized care for early septic shock [PROCESS] and Australasian resuscitation in sepsis evaluation [ARISE]) are ongoing and are designed to answer this question (*N Engl J Med* 2001; **345**: 1368–1377).

- A consensus conference of 55 international experts gathered to outline evidenced-based recommendations for the acute management of sepsis and septic shock in 2004, which were updated again in 2008. With a modified Delphi method, the experts used the grades of recommendation, assessment, development and evaluation (GRADE) system to guide assessment of quality of evidence from high (A) to very low (D) and to determine the strength of recommendations. There was strong agreement among a large cohort of international experts regarding many level 1 recommendations for the best current care of patients with severe sepsis (*Crit Care Med* 2008; **36**: 296–327).

Chapter 10-(iv)

Ventilator-associated Pneumonia

Fredric M. Pieracci MD, MPH*

*Acute Care Surgeon, Denver Health Medical Center

Take Home Points

- Ventilator-associated pneumonia (VAP) is the most common infection in mechanically ventilated, critically ill surgical patients.
- Despite this, culture of the lower respiratory tract is performed much less frequently than both blood and urine cultures during the course of a "fever workup" of an intensive care unit (ICU) patient. In many cases, this practice results in a delay in the diagnosis of VAP.
- Many strategies have been shown to effectively prevent VAP and should be incorporated into a "VAP bundle," which is then implemented in every ventilated ICU patient. These include head of bed elevation, maintenance of adequate endotracheal tube cuff pressure, oral decontamination, avoidance of routine stress ulcer prophylaxis, and daily interruption of sedation.
- Establishing the diagnosis of VAP is more complicated than for many other ICU infections, mostly because infection must be differentiated from respiratory colonization, which occurs universally in intubated patients.

Contact information: Denver Health Medical Center, 777 Bannock Street, MC 0206, A388, Denver, CO 80206. Email: Fredric.pieracci@dhha.org

- Screening criteria for VAP vary widely among ICUs; most protocols incorporate one or more variables from the clinical pulmonary infection score (CPIS): temperature, WBC count, oxygenation, respiratory secretions, and CXR findings.
- The current standard of care for diagnosing VAP involves derangement of one or more of the aforementioned clinical variables in addition to growth of one or more pathogens from a lower respiratory tract culture in densities of 10^4 cfu/mL–10^5 cfu/mL.
- Both sputum cultures and tracheal aspirates are not sufficiently specific to diagnose VAP and should not be used. Rather, culture of the lower respiratory tract via either blind ("mini") or bronchoscopic bronchoalveolar lavage, or protected brush specimen, should be used.
- Semi-quantitative cultures (i.e., light, medium, or heavy growth) are not sufficiently specific to diagnosis VAP; rather, quantitative cultures should be used, with the aforementioned thresholds.
- Both delays in the initiation of appropriate antimicrobial therapy and over-treatment for VAP are associated with adverse outcomes.
- Because of this, VAP protocols should strive for an initial period of high sensitivity (over-treat while waiting for the results of lower respiratory tract cultures), followed by a period of high specificity (de-escalate or discontinue antimicrobial therapy based upon final culture results).
- Choice of empiric antimicrobial therapy for VAP depends upon both risk factors for infection with multi-drug resistant (MDR) organisms and local ICU antibiograms.
- Most cases of VAP can be treated effectively with 8 days of antibiotics, with the exception of infection with a non-lactose fermenting gram negative rod; these cases should be treated for 14 days. Shorter (<8 days) courses of therapy are currently under investigation.

Background

- Pneumonia is defined as inflammation of the lung parenchyma caused by infection.
- Pneumonia is dichotomized into community acquired pneumonia (CAP) and healthcare-associated pneumonia (HCAP). This distinction is important with respect to likelihood of infection with MDR pathogens, duration of antimicrobial therapy, and overall prognosis. Healthcare-associated has replaced the prior term "nosocomial," in recognition of the fact that certain risk factors beyond inpatient hospitalization increase the likelihood of infection

with a MDR pathogen. These include recent hospitalization, residence in a long-term care facility, outpatient dialysis, outpatient chemotherapy, and homelessness.

- VAP represents a subset of HCAP, defined as pneumonia that occurs >48 hours after intubation. Pneumonia that occurs <48 hours after intubation is believed to be a consequence of factors separate from those of the endotracheal tube itself, and behaves clinically and microbiologically more like CAP.

- VAP is further subdivided into early (2–5 days from intubation) and late (>5 days from intubation). Again, this distinction is useful in terms of likelihood of infection with MDR pathogen and thus choice of empiric antimicrobial agents.

- The incidence of VAP is on the rise; it is currently the most common infection in mechanically ventilated, surgical ICU patients.

- VAP is believed to result from interruption of multiple host defense mechanisms by critical illness, and specifically an artificial communication between the oropharynx and the lower respiratory tract, which is normally sterile. These host defenses include the epiglottis, vocal cords, cough reflex, ciliated epithelium and mucus of the upper airways. Malnutrition, sedation, and neuromuscular paralysis further diminish the body's ability to ward off respiratory infection.

- The most effective way to prevent VAP is to avoid intubation. When intubation is necessary, prompt extubation is the next most effective step. During periods of prolonged intubation, the following strategies have been shown to decrease the risk of VAP: (1) head of bed elevation; (2) avoidance of routine stress ulcer prophylaxis; (3) oropharyngeal decontamination; (4) maintenance of tracheal tube cuff pressure > 20 cm H_2O; and (5) daily interruption of sedation. ICUs that incorporate these strategies into a routine "VAP bundle" have successfully reduced the incidence of VAP.

Main Body

Diagnosis

- There is no universally accepted screening algorithm for VAP.
- Suspicion for VAP usually begins with derangement of one or more of the following variables, which are grouped into a scoring system called the CPIS: (1) temperature; (2) WBC count; (3) oxygenation; (4) respiratory secretions; and (5) CXR findings (Table 1).
- The original description of the CPIS also included a microbiologic variable. Each of the six variables ranged from 0–2, for a total possible score of 12.

For screening purposes, the microbiologic variable is not useful as this information is not available at the time that the decision to screen is made.

- Consequently, a variation of the CPIS score that omits the microbiologic variable, termed $CPIS_{clinical}$, is what is most commonly used for screening. This score ranges from 0–10.
- The traditional threshold for $CPIS_{clinical}$ for screening, which is both reported in the literature and used in clinical trials of VAP, is 6. However, multiple studies have found that this threshold and the CPIS in general, lacks sensitivity for diagnosing VAP.
- Our group initiates screening for VAP in the presence of at least fever and leukocytosis. This increases sensitivity at the price of specificity.
- Once the decision to screen for VAP has been made, a lower respiratory tract culture is obtained and sent for quantitative microbiology.
- Lower respiratory tract cultures may be obtained via blind broncho-alveolar lavage, bronchoscopic broncho-alveolar lavage, or protected brush specimen. Each approach has both advantages and disadvantages, no one approach has been clearly shown superior to the others, and choice of method is dependent upon institutional resources.
- In contrast to lower respiratory tract cultures, upper respiratory tract cultures, such as sputum culture and tracheal aspirate, are likely to be contaminated with normal respiratory flora, and thus lack specificity. They should not be used in the diagnosis of VAP.
- Semi-quantitative cultures (i.e., light, medium, and heavy growth), also lack specificity and should not be used in the diagnosis of VAP.
- Whenever possible, lower respiratory tract cultures should be obtained prior to the initiation of antimicrobial therapy.
- The most commonly employed threshold for VAP is $>10^5$ clu/mL. A threshold of 10^4 cfu/mL may also be used, at the expense of specificity. Current data suggest that, in surgical patients, using a threshold off 10^5 cfu/mL is both safe and more specific than 10^4 cfu/mL.
- The threshold for diagnosing VAP should be lowered 10-fold if the culture was obtained while the patient was receiving antibiotics to which the pathogen is sensitive.
- Recently, the CDC put forth the "ventilator associated events" paradigm, which is intended for epidemiologic, rather than clinical purposes. Early reports indicate that VAP as defined by these new criteria is poorly correlated with VAP as diagnosed by the aforementioned clinical and microbiologic data.

Treatment

- Initiation of empiric antimicrobial therapy should follow immediately the acquisition of the lower respiratory tract culture.
- One possible exception to this rule involves the absence of organisms on gram stain in the early VAP window: 95% of these patients will not go on to have VAP.
- Choice of empiric antimicrobial therapy is based on both risk factors for infection with a MDR organisms and local antibiograms.
- In general, patients suspected of having early VAP (days intubated 2–5), and without risk factors for HCAP, should receive narrow-spectrum therapy. We use ceftriaxone 1 gm IV q8 hrs.
- Patients suspected of having late VAP, or those with risk factors for HCAP, should receive broad spectrum therapy with activity against both MRSA and resistant gram negative bacteria. We use vancomycin and cefepime.
- Empiric antimicrobial therapy continues for 1–3 days until final culture results become available.
- At this point, one of four possibilities may occur: (1) either no growth or insufficient growth to diagnosis VAP → discontinue antibiotics; (2) sufficient growth of one or more organisms that is only sensitive to the empiric therapy → complete definitive therapy with the empiric agent(s); (3) sufficient growth of one or more organisms that is sensitive to a more narrow-spectrum agent → de-escalate and complete definitive therapy with the narrowest spectrum agent; (4) sufficient growth of one or more organisms that are not sensitive to the choice of empiric therapy → change agent to which the organism is sensitive to complete definitive therapy. This last scenario should be minimized as it represents inappropriate initial choice of antimicrobial therapy.
- Most cases of VAP should be treated with 8 days of total therapy (empiric plus definitive). One exception is infection due to a non-lactose fermenting gram negative rod (e.g., *pseudomonas aeruginosa, acinitobacgter baumanii,* or *stenotrophomonas spp.*), which should be treated for 14 days.
- There are no convincing data that any pathogen should be "double covered," that is, definitive treatment with ≥1 antibiotic.
- If patients continue to demonstrate signs of infection despite negative, final lower respiratory tract cultures, empiric antibiotics for VAP should be stopped, a repeat lower respiratory tract culture should be obtained, and non-pulmonary sources of infection should be sought.

Practical Algorithm(s)/Diagrams

Table 1. Variables used to calculate $CPIS_{clinical}$ (range 0–10) and CPIS (range 0–12).

Parameter	Points
Temperature (°C)	
36.5 – 38.4	0
38.5 – 38.9	1
≥39.0 or <36.5	2
Blood Leukocytes, mm³	
4,000 – 11,000	0
<4,000 or >11,000	1
Bands ≥ 50%	2
Tracheal Secretions	
Scant	0
Non-purulent	1
Purulent	2
PaO_2:FiO_2	
>200	0
<200	2
Chest X-Ray	
No infiltrate	0
Diffuse or patchy infiltrate	1
Localized Infiltrate	2
Gram Stain*	
No organisms	0
≥1 organism	2

* Used only to calculate CPIS.

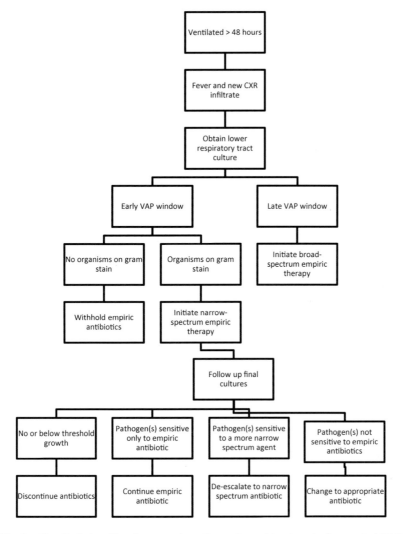

Fig. 1. Practical algorithm for screening, diagnosis, and treatment of suspected VAP.

Review of Current Literature with References

- In an analysis of 1,013 lower respiratory tract cultures, we showed that the CPIS score had poor discriminative ability for VAP (ROC area under the curve = 0.56). Furthermore, at the traditional cutoff of 6, sensitivity was approximately 20%. Screening based on fever, new CXR findings, and organisms on gram stain provided acceptable sensitivity (Pieracci *et al. Surg Infect* 2014; in press).

- Fagon *et al.* randomized 413 patients with suspected VAP to evaluation with bronchoscopic lower respiratory tract cultures, analyzed quantitatively (invasive group), or tracheal aspirates, analyzed semi-quantitatively (clinical group). Compared with the clinical strategy, patients in the invasive group demonstrated decreased 14-day mortality (16% vs. 25%, $p=0.02$), less antibiotic use, decreased sepsis-related organ failure, and decreased 28 day mortality. The clinical strategy also resulted in more and broader-spectrum antibiotic therapy, and increased emergence of fungi (Fagon *et al. Ann Int Med* 2000; **132**: 621–630).

- A randomized, multicenter trial of 401 patients with VAP assigned subjects to receive eight or 14 days of antibiotic therapy. Patients treated for eight days had equivalent mortality, ICU length of stay, duration of mechanical ventilation, and recurrence of infection despite significantly more antibiotic-free days. Recurrent infections were less likely to be caused by MDR pathogens in the eight day group. However, patients with VAP caused by non-lactose fermentive gram negative rods were more likely to develop recurrent VAP if treated with 8 days (*JAMA* 2002; **290**: 2588–2598).

- Croce *et al.* examined the diagnostic threshold for VAP among 1,372 lower respiratory tract cultures from trauma patients. VAP was defined as >105 cfu/mL, and a false negative culture was defined as any patient who had <105 cfu/mL and developed VAP with the same organism up to seven days after the previous culture. The false negative rate was 5%, and commonly involved non-lactose fermenting gram negative rods (*J Trauma* 2004; **56**: 931–936).

Urinary Tract Infection

Nicole Nadlonek, MD* and Robert T. Stovall, MD[†]

*Surgical Resident, University of Colorado School of Medicine
[†]Assistant Professor of Surgery, University of Colorado School of Medicine

Take Home Points

- Urinary tract infections (UTI) occur commonly in ICU patients at an approximate rate of 6%
- The presence of an indwelling bladder catheter or other urinary tract manipulation is a major risk factor for nosocomial UTI. Other risk factors include long duration of catheterization, diabetes mellitus, female gender, and inadequate catheter care.
- Prevention is of paramount importance with UTI. Use sterile technique to insert indwelling bladder catheters, use proper hygiene and avoid contamination of the collecting system, and remove catheters as soon as possible.

Contact information: (Nicole Nadlonek) 12631 E. 17th Ave, MC C302, Aurora, CO 80045; (Robert T. Stovall) Denver Health Medical Center, University of Colorado Health Sciences Center, 777 Bannock Street, MC 0206, Denver, CO 80204; Tel.: 303-436-1029, email: Nicole.nadlonek@ucdenver.edu; Robert.stovall@dhha.org

Background

- Urinary tract infections (UTIs) are reportedly the most commonly acquired nosocomial infections and common infection present in ICU patients.
- In the setting of trauma critical care, most patients have a urinary catheter or have recently had urinary catheterization which are believed to increase the risk of UTI.
- The Centers for Medicare and Medicaid stopped reimbursing for catheter associated UTI in 2008, as they deemed it to be a preventable complication.

Main Body

- Definitions
  - Asymptomatic bacteriuria occurs in a patient with or without an indwelling catheter who has $>10^5$ cfu/ml of uropathogenic bacteria in the absence of symptoms.
    - Symptoms with a catheter are commonly defined as a fever $>38°C$, suprapubic tenderness or costovertebral angle pain or tenderness.
  - CDC definition of Catheter associated UTI: Patient had an indwelling urinary catheter in place for >2 calendar days, with day of device placement being Day 1, and catheter was in place on the date of event and
    - at least one of the following signs or symptoms: fever ($>38°C$); suprapubic tenderness*; costovertebral angle pain or tenderness* with no other recognized cause and
    - a positive urine culture of $\geq10^5$ colony-forming units (CFU)/ml and with no more than two species of microorganisms.
  - Definitions of UTI are more difficult in the ICU setting as it is more common to have more than one simultaneous infection and symptoms in obtunded ICU patients are more difficult to identify. Index of suspicion plays a more important role in the ICU setting.
- Prevention
  - Avoid unnecessary catheterization and remove indwelling urinary catheters as soon as possible.
  - Use sterile insertion technique.
  - Prophylactic antibiotics during catheterization do not reduce the risk of infection.
  - Good catheter care and hygiene will help to keep from introducing bacteria into the collecting system.

- Diagnosis
  - o Because ICU patients with catheter associated bacteriuria may be otherwise asymptomatic, evaluation for UTI is appropriate when patients develop a fever or otherwise unexplained systemic manifestations suggesting infection, including altered mental status and hypotension.
  - o Ideally, urinalysis and culture should be obtained prior to starting antibiotics. If possible, the culture should be obtained by removing the indwelling catheter and obtaining a midstream specimen or changing the catheter and drawing the specimen from the port in the drainage system of the new catheter.
  - o It is possible that in certain patient populations, a UA can be an initial screening evaluation for UTI in febrile ICU patients as was shown in trauma patients. However, each patient population may be different and a urine culture is the ultimate answer if ongoing suspicion exists.

- Antibiotic therapy
  - o Should be based on culture results when available. If treatment is required prior to culture data, empiric antibiotics should be chosen based on urine gram stain, previous culture results, or the sensitivity patterns of organisms in the institution.
  - o Tailor antibiotic treatment once culture and susceptibility results are available. Duration of treatment has not been well studied. A seven-day regimen is currently suggested for patients presenting with symptoms consistent with lower tract infection, and a longer course of 10 to 14 days is recommended for patients with more severe presentations. For catheter associated infections treatment duration are usually recommended to be 10–14 days. However, in our institution we have had success with shorter durations of therapy. With catheter associated UTIs, when the catheter is changed, it is possible that 7 days is adequate. Clinical course would have to dictate and risk benefit of selecting resistance in the critically ill patient must be weighed against ongoing risk of UTI.

- Candiduria
  - o Its incidence is related directly to duration of catheter treatment. It is generally asymptomatic. If identified, the catheter should be changed.
  - o Most common organism is *Candida albicans*, which is generally susceptible to fluconazole. The second most common organism is *Candida glabrata* has significant resistance to fluconazole and thus should be treated with another agent. Obviously, local susceptibility patterns should be consulted.

o Patients who need treatment of candiduria are infants with low birth weights, patients undergoing genitourinary procedures, neutropenic patients, renal transplant patients, and symptomatic patients.
o Treatment should be with fluconazole for *C. albicans* and amphotericin is an alternative in fluconazole resistant species. The newer azoles and echinocandins are poorly filtered in the kidneys, and often have sub-therapeutic levels. The treatment course is usually recommended to be 7–14 days.
o Also, it is common that if yeast appears in multiple locations or sites in an ICU patient to treat as an infection.

Practical Algorithm(s)/Diagrams

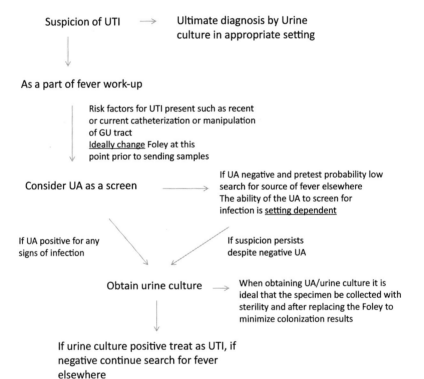

Review of Current Literature with References

- Laupland *et al.* performed a prospective trial of adult multidisciplinary ICUs examining the rate of ICU acquired UTI, defined as $>10^5$ cfu/ml or 1–2 organisms >48 hours after ICU admission. They found 9% of patients in their ICUs developed UTIs, with increased risk associated with female gender and extended ICU length of stay. Though nosocomial UTI was a marker of morbidity, they did not find an associated increase in mortality (*J Crit Care* 2002; **17**: 50–57).

- In a prospective trial of 405 patients admitted to a surgical intensive care unit that was designed to determine the incidence of nosocomial infections, the rate of urinary catheter associated UTI was 4.2% in symptomatic patients and 14% in asymptomatic patients. 25% of the patients had an infection, and 75% of those nosocomial infections were considered ICU acquired. UTI accounted for 28% of the nosocomial infections. Therefore, surveillance for UTI is an important part of care in the surgical intensive care unit (Wagenlehner *et al. Int J Antimicrob Agents* 2006; **28**: S86eS90).

- A retrospective review of 232 UAs from 112 trauma patients in the ICU showed that a negative urinalysis has a sensitivity of 100%, specificity of 65%, and a negative predictive value of 100% in the diagnosis of UTI. The sensitivity and specificity and NPV for any culture positivity were 90%, 66% and 98.5% respectively. Urinalysis appears useful to rule out UTI as a source of fever in a trauma patient in the ICU (Stovall *et al. J Am Coll Surg* 2013; **217**: 162–166).

- A retrospective review of trauma registry data from a Level I trauma center from 2003 to 2008 included 5,736 patients. It showed that 11.9% of these patients met criteria for UTI and that 71.6% were associated with indwelling urinary catheters. Furthermore, UTI predicted in-hospital mortality after proportional hazard regression modeling. This suggests that UTI is associated with an increased mortality in trauma patients (Monaghan *et al. J Trauma* 2011; **71**: 1569–74).

Intra-abdominal Infections

Edward L. Jones, MD* and Carlton C. Barnett, MD†

*Surgical Resident, University of Colorado School of Medicine
†Professor of Surgery, University of Colorado School of Medicine

Take Home Points

- Infections are common in intensive care unit patients and an intra-abdominal source must be ruled out no matter the initial reason for hospitalization.
- Rapid diagnosis is key and must be provoked by a high suspicion for an intra-abdominal source based upon persistent fever, abnormal laboratory tests (white blood cell count, elevated platelets, bicarbonate, total bilirubin/alkaline phosphatase, lactate etc.) and physical exam findings (e.g. tenderness, jaundice, peritonitis).
- Once the etiology is identified, the severity of disease must be defined in order to determine the appropriate course of treatment (antibiotics, surgery or radiographically-guided drainage).

Contact information: Denver Health Medical Center, University of Colorado Health Sciences Center, 777 Bannock Street, MC 0206, Denver, CO 80204; Tel.: 303-436-5402, email: Carlton.barnett@dhha.org; edward.jones@ucdenver.edu

- Delays in treatment of intra-abdominal infections are associated with poor outcome.
- Trends in common laboratory markers are more useful than individual, absolute measurements.
- While following the logic of Ockham's razor as stated by Ptolemy: "we consider it good principle to explain the phenomena by the simplest hypothesis possible," a missed infective source may result in the patient's rapid demise and so, a thorough search and rapid treatment of all infections is essential.

Background

- Acalculous cholecystitis is more common in critically ill patients and must be aggressively diagnosed, due to the high mortality (up to 45%), with ultrasound or a hepatobiliary (HIDA) scan.
- Management of cholecystitis includes broad spectrum antibiotics (blood cultures are positive in up to 90% of cases) and cholecystectomy or cholecystostomy (radiographically-guided drainage) if the patient is too unstable for surgery.
- Necrotizing pancreatitis should only be surgically debrided with evidence of infection (positive cultures or in the case of patient demise with confirmatory imaging).
- Suppression of gastric acid increases the risk of nosocomial pneumonia and clostridia infections that is not seen with binding agents (sucralfate).
- Increasing rates of *Clostridium difficile* infection (CDI) is closely related to increased use of broad spectrum antibiotics and should be suspected after antibiotic exposure with >5 watery stools/day.
- Initial treatment for non-severe CDI is oral metronidazole for 10–14 days. Recurrent or severe disease should be treated with oral vancomycin and/or intravenous metronidazole in patients with ileus.
- Severe CDI unresponsive to medical therapy for 48 hours or associated with multi-organ failure or peritonitis should undergo early surgical intervention, which includes subtotal colectomy or diverting loop ileostomy and colonic lavage based upon surgeon preference.
- Intra-abdominal abscesses are managed with immediate drainage, either in the operating room or via radiographically-guided catheters and broad spectrum antibiotics until the organism(s) is identified.

Main Body

Acute acalculous cholecystitis

- Acalculous cholecystitis accounts for just 5–15% of cases of acute cholecystitis but carries a high mortality (up to 45%).
- Prolonged bowel rest (~4 weeks), total parenteral nutrition and common medications (estrogens, anabolic steroids, chlorpromazine, erythromycin, penicillins and cholesterol-lowering statins) promote biliary stasis combined with gallbladder hypoperfusion, resulting in acalculous cholecystitis.
- Ultrasound is often the first diagnostic step as it can be performed at bedside and gallbladder distention and sludge are suggestive findings. Increasing gallbladder wall thickness and sloughed mucosa can be seen and are considered diagnostic.
- The "gold standard" hepatobiliary (HIDA) scan can be performed in borderline cases but requires transport to nuclear imaging suite.
- Once diagnosed (or in cases of high suspicion) prompt intervention is warranted.

  o Cholecystectomy should be performed in all patients if possible.
  o In unstable patients who would not tolerate cholecystectomy, percutaneous drainage (cholecystostomy) should be done with radiographic guidance.
  o Broad spectrum antibiotics should be started (piperacillin/tazobactam, imipenem or meropenem) and narrowed once gram stain, cultures or tissue reveal the organism and its sensitivity.

Necrotizing pancreatitis

- Pancreatic necrosis occurs in approximately 20% of patients secondary to inflammation and vascular compromise. Sterile necrosis does not necessarily lead to infection but can cause chronic fevers and PO intolerance.
- Secondary infection is usually heralded by worsening tachycardia, hypotension, fever and multi-organ failure and the bacterial or fungal infections are a result of translocation from the gastrointestinal tract or iatrogenic seeding from drainage/biopsy or invasive monitoring.
- Secondary infection can be minimized by early enteral feeding and protocolized removal of invasive monitors (central venous catheters, urinary catheters and mechanical ventilation). Diagnosis is more likely in the presence of air

bubbles in retroperitoneal necrosis on computed tomography and/or fine needle aspiration.

- The optimal time for surgical debridement is approximately four weeks after onset when delineation of live and dead tissue is easiest.
- Early necrosectomy may be required in unstable patients with infected pancreatitis but is associated with a morbidity rate of 72% and mortality ranging from 4–25% due to the maximal inflammatory response and hypervacularity. No matter the time of intervention, consideration should be given to cholecystectomy and/or cholangiography if a biliary source is suspected as well as placement of a jejunal feeding tube.
- Minimally invasive approaches continue to be investigated and include traditional laparosocpic retroperitoneal debridement by traveling transmesocolically. Also, video-assisted retroperitoneal debridement has been described whereby a previously placed percutaneous retroperitoneum drain is used as a guide/tract to follow a continuously irrigating cystoscope. This allows direct visualization of the retroperitoneum and debridement as well as placement of large bore drains. However, it does not allow simultaneous cholecystectomy or feeding jejunostomy placement.

Intrabdominal abscess

- The resident gastrointestinal flora are the cause of most intra-abdominal infections and as one progresses down the gastrointestinal tract, the number of micro-organisms increases from 10^3 organisms/gram in the stomach to 10^{11} in the colon.
- In the stomach and duodenum, most organisms are gram-positive cocci (streptococci, lactobacilli) and increasing numbers of enteric gram negatives (Escherichia, klebsiella and enterobacter) with a predominance of obligate anaerobes (bacteroides) in the colon.
- Most intra-abdominal infections result from perforations of gastrointestinal tract and, as a result, are polymicrobial in nature. *Escherichia coli* is the most common isolate followed by klebsiella, and gram positives (streptococcus).
- Initial antibiotic choice should be broad with antimicrobial action against aerobes, gram negatives, gram-positive cocci and obligate anaerobes. Common first-line agents are listed in Table 1.
- At the same time as antibiotic initiation, control of the source must be undertaken. For abscesses <2 cm in size, intravenous antibiotics may be adequate treatment. However, for large collections or patients with hemodynamic embarrassment, percutaneous or surgical drainage is warranted.

- Abscesses secondary to gastrointestinal perforation or anastomotic leak should be drained in addition to closing/repairing the perforation/leak. This may require proximal diversion in the case of distal anastomotic leak but remains at the clinician's discretion.
- The use of urokinase, alteplase or tissue plasminogen activator in percutaneous drains is safe and often decreases the number of drainage days, hospital stay and therefore, total cost.

Clostridium difficile infections

- The incidence of CDI continues to increase (30 per 100,000 in 1990 to 80+ per 100,000 in 2005) with 3 million cases annually and 14,000 deaths.
- *C. Difficile* is a spore-forming, gram-positive anaerobe bacillus that does not inhabit the intestines of healthy subjects but is able to proliferate when the normal microlfora has been altered.
- *C. Difficile* is transmitted by the fecal-oral route and is transmitted to the hospitalized patient via the hands of hospital personnel. This has prompted the strict adherence to so-called "contact precautions" including disposable gloves and gown use as well as 15-second hand-washing before and after patient contact. Of note: alcohol-based hand-sanitizers are ineffective against *C. Difficile* spores and as such are an ineffective substitute for hand washing.
- *C. Difficile* is not invasive but, once outnumbering the normal flora, produces cytotoxins that damage intestinal mucosa resulting in an intense inflammatory response creating plaque-like lesions known as "pseudomembranes" which is a marker of severe disease and inducing severe, watery diarrhea (often >10 bowel movements per day).
- The diagnosis is suspected in patients with multiple, watery bowel movements following recent antibiotic administration (often 1–2 weeks prior but single-dose, peri-operative antibiotics has resulted in CDI) and can be associated with a sudden, unexplained leukocytosis (often >16,000 white blood cells/mm^3).
- At our institution, the diagnosis is made by rapid enzyme immunoassay for *C. Difficile* antigen glutamate dehydrogenase (highly sensitive and results within 1 hour) and *C. Difficile* toxins A and B (sensitivity 75%, specificity 99%, results within a few hours). If the antigen alone is positive then a *C. Difficile* PCR is sent for confirmation (results within an hour but expensive). The gold standard for diagnosis is a cell culture cytotoxicity assay but it is labor and time intensive (at least two days until results return).

- Broad spectrum antibiotics and clindamycin are common inciting antibiotics and for mild disease, cessation or transition to other regimens may be all that is necessary for treatment.
- Patients with moderate disease the initial therapy is oral metronidazole (500 mg PO TID) for 10–14 days. Vancomycin (125 mg PO QID) is reserved for those intolerant to metronidazole (Table 2).
- Patients with severe or complicated CDI (diarrhea plus organ injury or failure), who can tolerate PO, should be given Vancomycin as first-line treatment due to faster symptom resolution and fewer treatment failures. Symptomatic improvement should be seen in 48–72 hours. Combination IV Metronidazole and PO +/- PR Vancomycin is given in refractory cases.
- For persistent/refractory cases without evidence of organ failure, sepsis or toxic megacolon fecal microbiota transplantation may be considered but is only available in select institutions. Success rates of 80% have been seen with multiple treatments but any evidence of hemodynamic instability should proceed to surgical intervention.
- With evidence of shock, perforation or toxic megacolon, a subtotal colectomy and diverting ileostomy should be performed. Due to extensive nature of surgery as well as the compromised patient status, the mortality remains high (up to 50%).
- Diverting loop ileostomy and colonic lavage has been described recently with reduced mortality, compared to historical control, but more trials are needed.

Practical Algorithm(s)/Diagrams

Table 1. Initial antibiotic choice for intra-abdominal abscesses.

Single agents	B-lactam/B-lactamase inhibitor	Carbapenems	Cephalosporins	Fluroquinolones	Glycycline
	ampicillin/sulbactam	doripenem	cefotetan	moxifloxacin	tigecycline
	piperacillin/tazobactam	ertapenem	cefoxitin		
	ticarcillin/clavulanate	Imipenem/cilastatin			
		meropenem			
Combination Agents					
Cephalosporin base	cefazolin/cefuroxime + metronidazole				
Fluroquinolone base	Cefotaxime/ceftriaxone/ ceftazidime/cefepime + metronidazole/clindamycin ciprofloxain/levofloxacin + metronidazole				
Aminoglycoside base	amikacin/gentamicin/ tobramycin + metronidazole/ clindamycin				

Table 2. Antibiotic treatment of clostridium difficile-assocaited disease in adults.

	1st Line	2nd Line	3rd Line
Initial(Mild) Disease	**Metronidazole 500 PO TID × 10–14 days**	**Vancomycin 125 mg PO QID × 10–14 days**	
1st Relapse	Metronidazole 500 PO TID × 10–14 days	Vancomycin 125 mg PO QID × 10–14 days	Fidaxomicin 200 mg PO BID × 10 days
2nd Relapse	Tapered Vancomycin Dosing (125 mg PO QID × 7d, BID × 7d, daily × 7d, every other day × 7d, every 3 days × 14d) +/- probiotics	Fidaxomicin 100 mg PO BID × 10 days	

Review of Current Literature with References

- Eatock *et al.* randomized 50 consecutive patients with severe acute pancreatitis based upon APACHE II and CRP measurements to either nasogastric (NG) or nasojejunal (NJ) feeding. Overall mortality was 24.5% with five deaths in the NG group and seven in the NJ. No statistically significant differences between the two groups were noted, therefore the cheaper and simpler method of NG feeding is recommended (*Am J Gastroenterol* 2005; **100**: 432).

- Yi *et al.* reviewed eight randomized controlled trials of total parenteral nutrition versus enteral nutrition in severe pancreatitis in this 2012 meta-analysis. Enteral nutrition was associated with decreased mortality, infectious complications, organ failure and need for surgical intervention (*Intern Med* 2012; **51**: 523–530).

- Cheng *et al.* performed a prospective, randomized controlled trial of alteplase vs. saline injection in percutaneous drains for loculated intra-abdominal abscesses. Twenty patients were included and abscess resolution was achieved in 80% of alteplase treated patients (2 mg or 4 mg twice daily for three days based upon abscess volume) vs. just 33% of saline-only treated patients (*J Vasc Interve Radiol* 2008; **19**: 906–911).

- Neal *et al.* reported a new minimally-invasive colon-preserving alternative to subtotal colectomy in patients with severe clostridium difficile-associated disease. Prospective review of 42 patients who underwent diverting loop ileostomy and colonic lavage (35 successfully) that resulted in reduced mortality compared to historical control (19% vs. 50%, OR 0.24, $p = 0.006$). The technique included laparoscopic diverting loop ileostomy, intra-operative colonic lavage with warm polyethylene glycol 3,350 via ileostomy and post-operative antegrade vancomycin flushes (*Ann Surg* 2011; **254**: 423–427).

Chapter 10-(vii)

Blood Stream/Central Venous Catheter-associated Infections

Marshall T. Bell, MD* and Robert T. Stovall, MD[†]

*Surgical Resident, University of Colorado School of Medicine
[†]Assistant Professor of Surgery, University of Colorado School of Medicine

Take Home Points

- Catheter related blood stream infections (CRBSI) are an important source of increased cost and morbidity in the intensive care unit.
- The risk of CRBSI is minimized by aseptic technique, appropriate catheter material, anatomic site and duration.
- Fevers in the setting of hemodynamic instability should prompt immediate catheter removal.
- Febrile patients with central venous catheters (CVC) should have blood cultures drawn from a peripheral line and the CVC.
- Upon diagnosis of CRSBI, antibiotics should be instituted and catheter should be removed.
- Patients with CRBSI who require continued central venous access should have new CVC placed for a fresh stick.

Contact information: University of Colorado Health Sciences Center, 12631 E. 17th Ave, C-305, Aurora, CO 80045; Tel.: (Marshall T. Bell) 303-990-1140, (Robert T. Stovall) 303-436-4029, email: Marshall.bell@ucdenver.edu; robert.stovall@dhha.org

505

Background

- Approximately 15 million CVC days occur in ICUs annually in the United States.
- All intravascular catheters are associated with risks of infection, phlebitis and bacteremia.
- Catheter related blood stream infections (occurring on average 5.3 times per 1,000 catheter days) are an important and preventable source increased cost and morbidity.
- The CDC defines CRBSI as "all blood stream infections occurring in patients with intravascular catheters when other sites of infections have been excluded."
- Of the intravascular devices used, non-tunneled, central venous catheters account for the overwhelming majority of blood stream infections in the ICU.
- These infections can occur from migration of skin flora, catheter or infusate contamination and hematogenous spread.

Main Body

- *Prevention*
  - Prevention of CTBSI relies on appropriate catheter selection, catheter location, aseptic technique and the duration of catheter usage.
  - **Catheter Material**
    - Microorganisms are able to adhere to catheters made of polyvinyl chloride or polyethylene more readily than those made of Teflon® or polyurethane. Thus, catheters made of polyvinyl chloride and polyethylene should be avoided.
    - Catheters coated with antimicrobial agents such as chlorhexidine/ silver sulfadiazine or minocycline/rifampin have been shown to reduce the risk of CRBSI.
  - **Catheter Location**
    - The concentration of skin flora at the insertion site is directly related to the development of CRBSI.
    - Infectious complications are least frequently observed for catheters placed in the subclavian vein and most frequently for femoral catheters. Catheters placed in the internal jugular vein have a slightly higher incidence infectious complications than subclavian catheters.

- The subclavian and internal jugular veins both represented viable options and when determining catheter placement the risk (i.e. arterial injury, and pneumothorax) and benefits of each location should be considered.
- Femoral catheters should be avoided if possible and those placed emergently should be removed as soon as clinically prudent.

o **Technique**

- "Insertion bundles" have been shown to reduce infectious complications of CVC. It is unclear which components of these bundles are most significant but likely, careful attention to detail and aseptic technique play a critical role.

- **Hand Hygiene**

  ⇨ Appropriate hand washing with antibacterial or alcohol-based solutions should be performed prior to insertion of all CVC.

- **Barrier Techniques**

  ⇨ Maximum barrier precautions including cap, mask, gown and sterile drape should be used.

- **Skin Antisepsis**

  ⇨ Of the commercially available agents, chlorhexidine, when compared to providine-iodine or 70% ETOH solutions, is associated with the lowest incidence of CRBSI.

- **Catheter Dressing**

  ⇨ All CVC should have a chlorhexidine-impregnated sponge (biopatch®) placed to reduce the risk of catheter colonization and CRBSI.

  ⇨ Following placement of CVC, the site should be dressed with sterile gauze or a transparent, semi-permeable dressing.

  ⇨ Change dressing at least once a week or if dressing becomes damp, loosened or soiled.

- **Team Considerations**

  ⇨ Educate of all bedside caregivers in appropriate care and surveillance of catheters and insertion sites.

  ⇨ Evaluate insertion sites daily.

o **Duration of Catheter Usage**

- All CVCs should be removed when no longer indicated.

- Catheters placed in emergent situations, where sterile technique was compromised, should be removed as soon as clinically reasonable.
- At Denver Health, line changes routinely performed at 10 days unless a contraindication exist. We also will change lines with unexplained fever.
- We do not practice the change of a line over a wire unless absolutely necessary.
- Studies have not demonstrated a decrease in CRBSI when catheters are routinely changed.

- *Diagnosis*
  - There is no minimum amount of time for a catheter to be in place for a CRBSI to develop.
  - A high-index of suspicion for a CRBSI should be maintained for all patient with CVC.
  - A variety of organism are associated with CRBSI. Among these gram positive cocci are the most common. Gram-negative bacteria (*E. coli, Pseduomonas, Enterobacter* and *Klebsiella)* as well as Candida species are also commonly associated with CRBSI.
  - **Special Consideration**
    - *Pseudomonal* species account for the majority of CRBSI in burn patients.
    - Gram-negative organisms are more common in patients with malignancies.
    - The majority of CRBSI in hemodialysis patients are caused by gram-positive organisms.

- *Treatment*
  - Febrile patients with hemodynamic instability should have all vascular catheters removed and replaced regardless of blood culture findings.
  - Treatment of CRBSI entails removal CVC and initiation of broad spectrum antibiotics, with coverage methicillin-resistant *S. aureus* prior to obtaining culture results but preferably started after cultures are obtained.
  - If central access is still indicated, exchange over a guide-wire should not be performed.
  - Surveillance cultures should be obtained 48 hours following diagnosis and at 48 hour interval until bacteremia has resolved. Appropriate antibiotic coverage should be maintained for 10–14 days.
    - Prolonged treatment may be indicated if surveillance cultures demonstrate persistent bacteremia.

o Patient who remain febrile with negative blood cultures and no other identified source of infection should have CVC removed.
o In general, antibiotic treatment is not indicated in the following situations:
  ▪ As prophylaxis for patients with CVC.
  ▪ Phlebitis without evidence of infection.
  ▪ Colonized catheter without clinical sign of infection (positive CVC culture with skin flora and negative peripheral cultures).
o **Special Consideration**
  ▪ Bacteremia from *S. aureus* is commonly complicated by infectious endocarditis. Transesophageal ultrasound should be performed in all patients with *S. aureus* bacteremia.
  ▪ Patients diagnosed with candidemia should have antifungal therapy for at least two week from last positive blood culture. Additionally, all patients should be evaluated by an ophthalmologist for endophthalmitis.

Practical Algorithm(s)/Diagrams

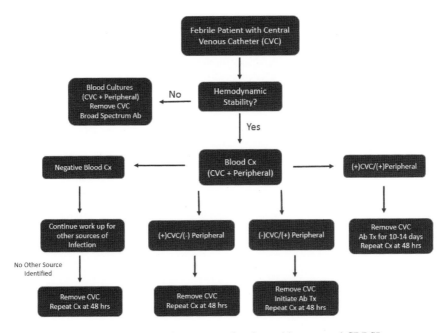

Fig. 1. Diagnosis and treatment of patient with suspected CRBSI.

Review of Current Literature with References

- Longitudinal cohort study assessing the impact of care provider education and implementation of prevention strategies for catheter related blood stream infections on ICU patients at a single institution. A comparison of infectious rates in 1,050 patients after implementation of preventions strategies to 2,104 in the control period. Provider education and implementation of insertion bundles was associated with a significant reduction of CRBSI (relative risk 0.33, 95% CI 0.20–0.56) (*Lancet* 2000, **355**: 1864–1868).

- Meta-analysis of 10 randomized controlled trials and cohort studies comparing infectious rates for central vein catheters placed in subclavian, internal jugular or femoral vein. Catheter associated blood stream infections per 1,000 catheter days were identified in the subclavian vein 1.3, jugular 2.6 and femoral 3.6. The analysis indicated the a significant reduction of CVC placed in the subclavian vein when compared to jugular ($p < 0.001$) and femoral site ($p < 0.001$) (*Crit Care Med* 2012, **40**: 1625–1633).

- Microbial patterns responsible for hospital acquired infections in 463 institutions. Of the 28,502 hospital acquired infections the CRBSI accounted for 35.5%. The 11,428 CRBSI's identified in this study are characterized by species and ICU prevalence (*Infect Control Hosp Epidemiol* 2009 **29**: 996–1011).

Chapter 10-(viii)

Necrotizing Soft Tissue Infection

Teresa Jones, MD* Edward Jones, MD* and Robert T. Stovall, MD†

*Surgical Resident, University of Colorado School of Medicine

†Assistant Professor of Surgery, University of Colorado School of Medicine

Take Home Points

- Necrotizing soft tissues infections (NSTI) are characterized by rapid and fulminant tissue destruction and high mortality.
- The rapid diagnosis is essential leading to early surgical intervention and broad-spectrum antibiotics.
- Increasing age, obesity, diabetes, immunosuppression, intravenous drug use, recent trauma or surgery increases the risk of a NSTI.
- The diagnosis of NSTI is a clinical one i.e., based upon the history and physical exam as no imaging or laboratory values have excellent sensitivity and specificity.
- The laboratory risk index for necrotizing fasciitis (LRINEC) score should be used to supplement the history and physical and borderline cases should undergo bedside fascial biopsy with frozen section looking for necrosis and performance of the "finger test."

Contact information: Denver Health Medical Center, 777 Bannock Street, MC 0206, Denver, CO 80204; Email: Teresa.jones@ucdenver.edu; edward.jones@ucdenver.edu; robert.stovall@dhha.org

- A high index of suspicion is needed as the "hard signs" of NSTI (bullae, skin necrosis, ecchymosis and crepitus) are often absent and imaging remains non-specific.
- The current treatment of a NSTI is emergent, radical surgical debridement of all involved tissue and broad spectrum intravenous antibiotics. Any delay is associated with a significant increase in mortality.
- Post-operatively patients should be re-examined every 2–4 hours and return to the operating room every 24 hours for repeat debridement until only healthy tissue remains.

Background

- Over 1,000 cases of necrotizing soft tissue infection (NSTI) are reported per year but it is likely under-reported after mandatory reporting was discontinued in 1991.
- Less than 15% of patients are admitted with the correct diagnosis.
- The progressive infection produces toxins that cause vascular occlusion, ischemia and tissue necrosis that may rapidly progress to systemic inflammation, sepsis and death.
- Mortality rates range from 12–35% and clostridial infections have been associated with increasing rates of limb loss (OR 3.9, 95% CI 1.1–12.8) and mortality (OR 4.1, 95% CI 1.3–12.3).
- A high index of suspicion is necessary for the early diagnosis and prompt surgical intervention of necrotizing soft tissue infections with associated septic shock as each hour delay in antimicrobial initiation and surgery is associated with a 7.6% increase in mortality.
- *Streptococcus spp.* remains the single most common causative organism; however, polymicrobial, gram-negative, and anaerobic bacteria are significant contributors with increasing methicillin-resistant *Staphylococcus aureus* (MRSA) being reported.
- Broad spectrum antibiotics should be initiated as soon as the diagnosis is suspected.
- Once diagnosed, the treatment is early surgical debridement to avoid mortality. Removal of all infection and necrosis to healthy tissue can be associated with significant morbidity including limb loss and need for skin grafting. In addition, these infections are associated with prolonged hospitalizations which increases the risk of concomitant nosocomial infections, respiratory failure, and/or acute renal failure.

Main Body

Presentation & diagnosis

- NSTI incidence increases with age, up to 12 per 100,000 patients once over the age of 80.
- The majority (85%) of NSTIs are community acquired; 10% hospital-acquired and 4% are encountered at long term care facilities.
- Most common sites of infection are the extremities.
- Risk factors:

  o Diabetes mellitus
  o Immune suppression
  o Cirrhosis
  o Chronic kidney disease
  o Malignancy
  o Intravenous drug use

- Most consistent clinical feature: pain out of proportion to exam findings.
- "Hard signs" (blistering, crepitus, obvious necrosis) are rare (10–40%) but should prompt immediate debridement and antibiotics.
- Evaluate history specifically for clues to causative organism although this is usually underwhelming:

  o Trauma including penetration lesions, insect bites, injection sites (*Clositridial* and polymicrobial infections)
  o Recent surgery (MRSA/polymicrobial infections)
  o Foreign travel including abnormal ingestions
  o Tonsillitis, impetigo (*Streptococcal* infections)

Lab values

- No specific laboratory values have been proven as diagnostic; however the laboratory risk indicator for necrotizing fasciitis (LRINEC) can be used for risk stratification.
- LRINEC (Fig. 1)
  o Originally derived from multiple cases of Virbo NF, not verified in RCT.
  o Max score: 13; C-reactive protein (CRP) elevation >149 mg/L accounting for 4 points.
  o >6 raises suspicion, PPV 92%, NPV 65%.
  o Subsequent studies failed to confirm the initial high predictive values.

Radiology: Do not let radiology delay surgery

- Plain radiographs demonstrate subcutaneous emphysema in 17–30%.
- Computed tomography often demonstrates non-specific inflammatory changes and remains non-diagnostic unless subcutaneous emphysema is present.
- Magnetic resonance imaging: demonstrates hyperintenses signal on T2 weight images but the delay associated with imaging can increase mortality.

Fascial biopsy and the finger test

- Should only be performed at bedside in borderline cases (LRINEC<5 and low clinical suspicion) in a hemodynamically stable patient. Otherwise, perform in operating room where you can progress directly to debridement.
- Make 2 cm incision in affected area and continue down to fascia sending a frozen section of a 1cm piece of fascia.
- Diagnosis confirmed grossly: obvious necrosis, no skin/subcutaneous bleeding (evidence of thrombosis due to bacterial toxin secretion), grayish/ "dishwater" fluid encountered.
- Finger test: sterile, gloved finger slides with minimal resistance along the deep fascial plane (place finger through the 1cm hole in the fascial that was sent for frozen section).

Pathology

- Histology: angiothrombosis of perforating vessels with necrosis, underlying thrombi, polymorphonuclear lymphocyte (PMN) infiltrate, vasculitis and/or bacteria.
- Gross: Thrombosed vessels with lack of bleeding or contracting muscle and easy separating of fascial planes with gentle finger pressure: "finger test."
- Several bacterial types of Necrotizing Soft Tissue Infections:
  - Type I (55–80%): Mixed infection, aerobic and anaerobic.
  - Type II infection (<20%): beta-hemolytic *streptococcus* or *staphylococcus aureus*.
    - Group A *streptococcus* progresses rapidly, often without an obvious focus.
    - 30–50% associated with toxic shock syndrome.

o Type III (depends upon geographic location)

   ▪ Gram-negative, monomicrobial.

   ▪ *Vibrio vulnificus* (near coasts/seawater), *Pasteurella spp.* (feline associated), *Haemophilus spp.*, *Klebsiella spp.*

- Type IV (after burns/trauma)

   ▪ Fungal, (*Mucor spp.* or *Rhizopus spp.*).

Treatment

- Rapid, early surgical debridement and broad spectrum antibiotics (see below).
- Airway, breathing and circulation per ATLS/ACLS protocols with aggressive fluid resuscitation.

Surgical debridement

- Surgical debridement is lifesaving if initiated early.
- Continue debridement until brisk bleeding of tissue is encountered. This includes removal of all necrotic skin, subcutaneous tissue, fascia and muscle if necessary. A wise surgeon once said "if you do not feel guilty after a wide debridement then you likely have not debrided enough to save their life."
- Amputation is required in up to 50% of cases (increased risk in lower extremity NSTIs).
- Any delay in early debridement is associated with up to a 9× increase in mortality.
- Repeat exploration and debridement of additional necrotic tissue should be every 24–48 hours until no infection remains.
- Reconstruction (muscle or skin flaps, skin grafting) should take place only in hemodynamically stable patients without evidence of infection (often at least 7–10 days after arrival).
- Consider Urologic/Gynecologic assistance and early, diverting colostomy in NSTIs of the perineum (Fournier's gangrene).

Antibiotics

- Empiric broad spectrum as soon as possible as each hour of delay in sepsis is associated with 7.6% increase in mortality.

- Coverage of gram-positive, gram-negative and anaerobic organisms with special consideration for group A *streptococcus* and *clostridum spp.*

  o Carbapenem or beta-lactam/beta-lactamase inhibitior (imipenem, meropenem, piperacillin/tazobactam or ticarcillin/clavulanate). Allergies: aminoglycoside/ fluroquinolone (gentamicin if renal function permits/levofloxacin) + metronidazole.
  o Clindamycin

    ▪ Efficacy not affected by the inculum size or stage of bacterial growth.
    ▪ Suppresses bacterial toxin synthesis and monocyte synthesis of tumor necrosis factor-alpha.

  o MRSA coverage (vancomycin, daptomycin or linezolid)

    ▪ Narrow antibiotics once gram stain, culuture and pathology returns with inciting orgranism(s) and sensitivities.
    ▪ Duration of treatment is undefined: recommend continuation until no further debridements are required and hemodynamic status is normalized.

Adjunctive measures: SHOULD NOT DELAY SURGERY

- Intravenous immune globulin (IVIG).

  o Antibodies thought to neutralize *streptococcal* superantigens and *Clostridal* toxins.
  o High dose (2 g/kg) for group A *Streptococcal* infections.
  o Supporting data is limited and mostly retrospective.

- Hyperbaric oxygen (HBO)

  o Thought to increase tissue oxygen tension with resultant increase in reactive oxygen species and improved polymorphonucelar lymphocyte bactericidal action.
  o Limits clostridial exotoxin and spore production as well as killing anaerobes.
  o HBO for clostridial infections improved survival in a dog model but studies in humans (retrospective reports with less than 50 patients) demonstrate mixed results.
  o DO NOT delay surgical debridement!

Practical Algorithm(s)/Diagrams

Laboratory Risk Indicator for Necrotizing Fasciitis (LRINEC) Scoring System

Variable	Score
C-reactive protein (mg/L)	
<150	0
>150	4
White blood cell count (/mm^3)	
<15	0
15-25	1
>25	2
Hemoglobin (g/dL)	
>13.5	0
11-13.5	1
<11	2
Sodium (mmol/L)	
≥135	0
<135	2
Creatinine (mg/dL)	
≤1.6	0
>1.6	2
Glucose	
≤180	0
>180	1

Fig. 1. A score of 6 is highly suspicious (PPV 92%, NPV 96%) for necrotizing soft tissue infections. Max score is 13. Interpret with caution in diabetics and patients with renal failure.

Review of Current Literature with References

- Ustin and Malangoni reviewed necrotizing soft tissue infections in a recent article that provides an excellent overview (*Crit Care Med* 2011;**39**:2156–2162).
- Wong *et al.* retrospectively identified 89 consecutive patients with severe cellulitis or abscess. Univariate and multivariate logistical regression were used to create the LRINEC score of independently predictive factors. Cutoff value for the LRINEC was 6 points with a positive predictive value of 92% and a negative predictive value of 96%. Model performance was very good with a Hosmer-Lemeshow statistic $p = 0.91$ but large subset of infections with *Vibrio spp.* warrants caution in use away from coastal areas (*Crit Care Med* 2004; **32**:1535–1541).

- Su *et al.* retrospectively reviewed 209 patients at a tertiatry care center and reported 15.8% mortality and 26.3% amputation rate for NSTIs over three years. LRINEC score 6 and greater was significantly associated with increasing mortality and amputation rates but sensitivity and specificity for mortality using a cutoff score of 6 was 66% and 58% respectively (*ANZ J Surg* 2008; **78**: 968–972).

11. Endocrine

Chapter 11-(i)

Endocrine Emergencies

Robert McIntyre, Jr., MD* Eric Peltz, DO[†]
and Maria Albuja Cruz, MD[†]

*Professor of Surgery, University of Colorado School of Medicine
[†]Assistant Professor of Surgery, University of Colorado School of Medicine

Take Home Points

- A common contributing issue in all endocrine emergencies is a precipitating factor which may be trauma, surgery, infection, and other medical illness.
- Endocrine emergencies may also be due to unrecognized or undertreated endocrine abnormality.
- The most common causes of thyrotoxicosis are Grave's disease, toxic nodular goiter or solitary toxic nodule, and thyroiditis. Less common causes are drug induced (amiodarone or iodinated contrast), exogenous hormone, and pituitary tumors.
- Treatment of thyroid storm is to stop hormone synthesis, inhibit hormone release, block peripheral hormone conversion, and blunt end organ effects.
- Goals of treatment of myxedema coma are to replace thyroid hormone, support vital functions, replace glucocorticoids, and treat precipitating factors.

Contact information: Department of Surgery, 12631 East 17th Ave, C313, Aurora, CO 80045. Email: Robert.mcintyre@ucdenver.edu; Erik.peltz@ucdenver.edu; Maria.albujacruz@ucdenver.edu

- Euthyroid sick syndrome is also referred to as non-thyoidal illness and refers to a group of changes in thyroid hormone and TSH levels that occur in critical illness and starvation.
- Treatment of euthyroid sick syndrome with T4 or T3 is controversial and there is no data that demonstrates a beneficial outcome.
- The etiologies of hypoglycemia can be divided into fasting and fed causes (reactive hypoglycemia).
- Manifestations of hypoglycemia can be divided into neuroglycopenic and adrenergic manifestations.
- Diabetic Ketoacidosis and Hyperosmolar Hyperglycemic Syndrome are at opposite ends of a spectrum.
- The triad of DKA is hyperglycemia, anion gap metabolic acidosis and ketonuria.
- The triad of HHS is hyperglycemia, hyperosmolarity and altered mental status.
- Diabetes insipidus (DI) comes in two varieties: central (decreased ADH) and nephrogenic (decreased responsiveness to ADH).
- The diagnosis of DI is simultaneous serum hypertonicity (>295 mOsm/kg) with hypernatremia (>145 mEq/L) and hypo-osmolar polyuria (<300 mOsm/kg).
- Syndrome of inappropriate antidiuresis (SAID) causes hyponatremia associated with a low plasma osmolarity (<280 mOsm/kg), high urine osmolarity (>100 mOsm/kg), and high urine Na (>40 mEq/L).
- Three rules apply to correction of water excess or deficit. Return the P_{Na} to normal at the relative speed that it became abnormal. If there are no symptoms of water or Na imbalance, there is no emergency. The degree of rapid P_{Na} correction should be towards normal until symptoms abate.
- Pheochromocytoma in the ICU usually involves a hypertensive crisis or postoperative care.
- Sepsis, respiratory insufficiency, hypertensive crises, or acute psychosis are the most frequent examples of presentation of Cushing's syndrome in the intensive care unit.

Main Body

Thyroid storm

- Thyroid storm is the extreme manifestation of thyrotoxicosis.
- The most common causes of thyrotoxicosis are Grave's disease, toxic nodular goiter or solitary toxic nodule, and thyroiditis. Less common causes are drug induced (amiodarone or iodinated contrast), exogenous hormone, and pituitary tumors.

- Thyroid storm usually occurs in a patient with unrecognized or inadequately treated thyrotoxicosis.
- A common contributing issue in all endocrine emergencies is a precipitating factor which may be trauma, surgery, infection, and other medical illness.
- Presenting symptoms include anxiety, confusion, psychosis, tremor, hyperreflexia, fatigue, weakness, tachycardia, chest pain, diaphoresis, heat intolerance, hyperthermia, dyspnea, weight loss, dry eyes, nausea, vomiting, diarrhea, jaundice, oligomenorrhea.
- Physical exam findings include fever, altered mental status, wide pulse pressure, atrial fibrillation, high output congestive heart failure, thyromegaly, and ophthalmopathy.
- Thyroid function testing reveals increased total T4 (TT4), free thyroxine index (FTI), and Free T4 (FT4) associated with a decreased thyroid stimulating hormone (TSH). The tri-iodothyronine (T3) may be normal or increased.
- Only a small percentage of thyroid hormone is free and unbound. Many conditions and drugs alter protein binding so free hormone levels are preferable in the diagnostic workup.
- Treatment of thyroid storm is to stop hormone synthesis, inhibit hormone release, block peripheral hormone conversion, and blunt end organ effects.

  o Interruption of thyroid hormone production utilizes anti-thyroid medications propylthiouracil (PTU) or methimazole. These drugs prevent organification of iodine to tyrosine and coupling of iodotyrosines. PTU also inhibits conversion of T4 to active T3, whereas methimazole does not. PTU is dosed 200 – 250 mg every 4–6 hours (orally, NGT, or rectal). Methimazole is 20–25 mg every 6 hours (orally, NGT, or rectal). Side effects include agranulocytosis, hepatotoxicity, rash, and vasculitis.

  o PTU has a black box warning because of hepatic toxicity; methimazole should be used initially in all patients except during the first trimester of pregnancy due to its association with birth defects.

  o There is stored hormone in the thyroid gland which can be released over months. Blocking release can be done using iodine (Lugol's solution, 8 drops every 8 hours; or potassium iodide, SSKI 5 drops every 8 hours), sodium iodide (1 gm iv over 24 hours) or corticosteroids (Dexamethasone 2 mg every 6 hours or Hydrocortisone 100 mg every 8 hours).

  o Conversion of T4 to active T3 is via the enzyme deiodinase in peripheral tissues. Deiodinase is inhibited by propranolol, steroids, and iopanoic acid.

  o End organ effects can be blocked using propranolol (nonselective β-blockade) which is the preferred agent or esmolol (selective β-blockade) which is very short-acting. Propranolol can be dosed 80–120 mg orally every 6 hours or 1–2 mg IV at 1 mg/min every 4–6 hours.

o In refractory cases plasmapheresis, charcoal hemoperfusion and plasma exchange rapidly reduce hormone levels.

- Supportive treatment includes ICU monitoring, treatment of the precipitating factor, control of dysrythmias, and cooling. You can use acetaminophen but should avoid salycilates, which increase free thyroid hormone levels.
- Mortality rates remain approximately 20%.

Myxedema

- Myxedema is the extreme manifestation of hypothyroidism and is usually due to autoimmune thyroid disease, iatrogenic, noncompliance, drug induced (amiodarone and lithium), and iodine deficiency.
- Myxedema coma is usually seen in a patient with unrecognized or inadequately treated hypothyroidism. Precipitating factors are common. A typical presentation is the elderly patient in the winter time.
- Manifestations include decreased mentation or coma, seizures, weakness, hypothermia, dry skin, coarse hair, coarse facial features, periorbital edema, goiter, bradycardia, decreased pulse pressure, CHF, hypoventilation, ileus, constipation or fecal impaction, renal insufficiency and urinary retention.
- Laboratory findings may include hypercarbia, hypoxia, hyponatremia, hypoglycemia and increased CPK. The TSH level will be elevated but does not correlate with severity. The TT4, FT4, and FTI will be decreased. T3 may be low or normal.
- Goals of treatment of myxedema coma are to replace thyroid hormone, support vital functions, replace glucocorticoids, and treat precipitating factors.

o Treatment may be with T4 IV, load with 200–300 mcg over 5 minutes followed by 50–100 mcg IV daily then convert to oral dosing when patient is able to take oral medications.

o T3 may be used alone or with T4. However, studies do not show much benefit of combination treatment over T4 alone. If used in combination T3 is 20–50 mcg IV over 5 minutes followed by 20–30 mcg per day, either IV or oral.

o Supportive measures may include ICU monitoring, respiratory support, fluid resuscitation, correction of electrolytes, vasopressors, and passive rewarming. Active rewarming should be avoided as it can cause hypotension. Cultures and empiric antibiotics should be initiated for suspected infection.

o Glucocorticoid replacement is done with hydrocortisone 100 mg IV every 8 hours.

- Mortality rates in recent studies vary from 0–45%.

Euthyroid sick syndrome

- Abnormal thyroid functions are common in critical illness. Euthyroid sick syndrome is also referred to as non-thyoidal illness and refers to a group of changes in thyroid hormone and TSH levels that occur in critical illness and starvation. These changes are due to alterations in thyroid hormone metabolism at the level of the hypothalamus, pituitary, thyroid, transport proteins and peripheral tissue.
- Thyroid hormone and TSH levels will vary according to severity of illness and the time course (Fig. 1). There is a decrease in T4 conversion to T3 primarily in the liver by decreased deiodinase type I activity, and T3 is converted to reverse T3 (rT3) which does not have hormone activity.
- Serum T3 is decreased more so than T4 and TSH, which are either normal or mildly decreased with an increase in rT3. In contrast primary hypothyroidism will manifest as a high TSH, and T4 is decreased more than T3.
- T3 resin uptake is usually increased from reduced binding of thyroid hormones to circulating proteins.
- During recovery, TSH levels will increase before normalization while FT4 decreases and T3 levels increase.
- Treatment with T4 or T3 is controversial and there is no data that demonstrates beneficial outcome. Euthyroid sick syndrome appears to be an adaptive response to decrease metabolism and preserve energy.
- Current evidence indicates that the severity of thyroid hormone changes can have prognostic value. Very low T3 levels are associated with higher mortality rates in critical illness.

Hypoglycemia

- The etiologies of hypoglycemia can be divided into fasting and fed causes (reactive hypoglycemia).

  o Fasting hypoglycemia can be due to insulin infusion, medications, ETOH, sepsis, hepatic failure, renal failure, malignancy, insulinoma, noninsulinoma pancreatogenous hypoglycemia syndrome, hormone deficiency and autoimmune antibodies.

    ○ Fed hypoglycemia can be due to insulin infusion, discontinuation of parenteral nutrition, β cell tumors, glucose intolerance, idiopathic reactive, dumping syndrome, fructose intolerance, and leucine.

- Manifestations of hypoglycemia can be divided into neuroglycopenic and adrenergic manifestations.

    ○ Neuroglycopenia symptoms include cognitive impairment, fatigue, visual changes, headache, slurred speech, nervousness, confusion, bizarre behavior, amnesia, seizures and coma.

    ○ Adrenergic manifestations are diaphoresis, tachycardia, palpitations, and tremor.

- Emergency treatment is IV injection of a bolus dextrose which may be followed by an infusion if the cause has not been corrected. If there is no IV access, an intramuscular injection of the counter-regulatory hormone glucagon (1 mg) can be given. Glucagon causes the glucose level to rise through its actions in the liver.

Diabetic ketoacidosis (DKA) and hyperosmolar hyperglycemic syndrome (HHS)

- DKA and HHS are at opposite ends of a spectrum. There may be some patients with features of both or you may consider that the syndromes have some overlap.
- The triad of DKA is hyperglycemia, anion gap metabolic acidosis and ketonuria.
- DKA patients are people that have no insulin and develop ketoacidosis. These patients are usually young adults with type I DM. Blood sugar is high (>250 mg/dl). Ketones are present in urine and serum, and they have an increased anion gap metabolic acidosis.
- The triad of HHS is hyperglycemia, hyperosmolarity and altered mental status.
- HHS patients have some insulin and therefore do not have ketoacidosis. These patients are generally older and have type II DM. The blood sugar may be extremely high (>600 mg/dl). They do not have ketones in urine or serum, and they do not have an acidosis. The serum osmolarity is often >320 mOsm/kg.
- Precipitating factors may be infection (pneumonia or urinary tract infection), noncompliance, new onset, and other medical illness such as gastrointestinal bleeding, myocardial infarction or stroke.

- Manifestations include polyuria, polydipsia, malaise, stupor, weakness, tachycardia, orthostatic hypotension, shock, anorexia, nausea, abdominal pain, seizures, and coma. Kussmaul breathing and an acetone breath occur only in DKA.
- Counter-regulatory hormones include catecholamines, glucagon, growth hormone, and cortisol. Levels are elevated in DKA which leads to gluconeogenesis and lipolysis. In HHS, the counter-regulatory hormones are generally not as high and there is less lipolysis and ketone production.
- In ketoacidosis, beta-hydroxybutyrate is metabolized to acetoacetate then to acetone. The first two are acids, the latter is not. Serum ketone measurement measures acetoacetate and acetone but not beta-hydroxybutyrate. Thus, ketone tests will be negative early in the course before significant acetoacetate generation. Further, ketone testing will remain positive even as the acidosis corrects.
- Average deficits in DKA are approximately 5 L of isotonic saline plus a free water deficit.
  - H_2O 6–7 L
  - Na   7–10 mmol/kg
  - K   3–5 mmol/kg
  - Cl   3–5 mmol/kg
  - PO_4 1–2 mmol/kg
  - Mg   1–2 mEq/kg
- Sodium adjusted to glucose correction is an estimate of the free water deficit.
  - Corrected Na = Current Na^+ [(1.6) × Glucose − 150/100]
- Management is to give intravenous fluids, replace electrolytes, IV insulin, and serial laboratory tests.
  - Insulin in DKA can be given 10 units IV push followed by an infusion of 0.1 u/kg/hr. Increase the insulin infusion to achieve ≥50 mg/dl/hr decrease in glucose. In older individuals, the infusion should be started at 0.5 u/kg/hr.
  - Anticipate a rapid drip in K. If patient is hypokalemic, give K before insulin is started.
  - Bicarbonate is not usually necessary and can lead to a paradoxical decrease in pH, sodium overload and hypokalemia. Consider it for pH <6.9 (50–100 mmol over 1.5–2 hours).
  - Replace phosphate with potassium phosphate.

- Monitoring DKA therapy includes hourly glucose and K with chemistries every 4–6 hours and urine ketones, anion gap and acid–base status. Venous blood gases can be used to avoid arterial puncture.
- When the glucose decreases to 250–300 mg/dl, a glucose infusion should be started.

  ○ Insulin therapy is continued to correct the ketoacidosis.
  ○ Half the insulin rate when the pH is >7.25–7.3.
  ○ Discontinue the insulin infusion once the anion gap is cleared, the ketones are negative or serum bicarbonate is ≥18 mEq/L.

- Cerebral edema can be a complication of DKA itself or due to rapid fluid expansion. Headache or sudden onset of confusion may be the presentation. Treatment is with mannitol 1 mg/kg.
- HHS patients require more fluid and less insulin than DKA.

Diabetes insipidus (DI)

- DI comes in two varieties: central (decreased ADH) and nephrogenic (decreased responsiveness to ADH).

  ○ Central DI is due to a lack of antidiuretic hormone (ADH) and occurs with head trauma, brain surgery, tumors, vascular diseases, brain hypoxia, and CNS infections.
  ○ Nephrogenic DI is a decrease in ADH action and can be from obstruction, polycyctic kidney, sickle cell disease, sarcoidosis, amyloidosis, and medications (lithium).

- DI leads to polyuria (hallmark), significant fluid loss, and hypernatremia.
- Polyuria is urine output > 3 L/day and may be due to psychogenic polydipsia, dipsogenicc DI (defect in thirst center), central DI, and nephrogenic DI. Polyuria may also occur from osmotic diuresis in diabetes mellitus (glucose), recovery from renal failure (urea), and IV infusions (saline, mannitol).
- Laboratory evaluation includes P_{Osm}, P_{Na}, P_{BUN}, $P_{glucose}$, U_{volume}, U_{Osm}, U_{Na}, and U_K.
- The diagnosis of DI is simultaneous serum hypertonicity (>295 mOsm/kg) with hypernatremia (>145 mEq/L) and hypo-osmolar polyuria (<300 mOsm/kg).
- In the presence of hypernatremia, urine osmolality <300 mOsm/kg is consistent with central DI. Urine osmolality is 300–800 mOsm/kg is partial central DI or nephrogenic DI. A hypernatremic patient with urine osmolality >800 mOsm/kg is hypovolemic.

- To differentiate central from nephrogenic DI, check urine osmolality then administer 1-desamino-8-D-arginine vasopressin (DDAVP) and recheck the urine osmolality a short time later.

  o If urine osmolality does not change, they have nephrogenic DI or do not have DI. If there is a 50% increase in urine osmolality, then they have central DI.

- Management requires careful monitoring of patient weight, electrolytes, and intake/output.
- Treatment is fluid replacement, correct electrolytes, treat the underlying cause, stop causative medications (lithium), thiazide diuretics and ADH replacement.
- DDAVP (Desmopressin) is given 1–2 mcg every 12–24 hours subcutaneous or iv, The nasal preparation is 5–10 mcg every 12–24 hours nasal spray.
- DDAVP is a V2 receptor agonist as opposed to V1 receptors which are found on arterioles and are activated by vasopressin. DDAVP does not have significant vasopressor effects.
- The risk of profound hyponatremia is significant if excess hypotonic fluids are given in the setting of DDAVP driven anti-diuresis. Thus, an increase in urine output should be allowed before a second dose of DDAVP is given.
- Three rules apply to correction of water excess or deficit:

  o Return the P_{Na} to normal at the relative speed that it became abnormal.
  o If there are no symptoms of water or Na imbalance, there is no emergency.
  o The degree of rapid P_{Na} correction should be towards normal until symptoms abate.

Syndrome of inappropriate antidiuresis (SAID)

- Syndrome of inappropriate antidiuresis (SAID) is characterized by euvolemic hyponatremia.
- Measure P_{Osm}, P_{Na}, U_{Osm}, U_{Na}, and U_K.
- The hyponatremia is real (vs pseudohyponatremia due to hyperglycemia or uremia) and associated with a low plasma osmolarity (<280 mOsm/kg), and high urine osmolarity (>100 mOsm/kg), and high urine Na (>40 mEq/L).
- SIADH is usually due to malignancy, a pulmonary or central nervous system disorder, or medications.
- Some medications may cause hyponatremia due to SIADH or SIADH-like mechanisms including ADH analogues (DDAVP, oxytocin), several antipsychotics and antidepressants, cyclophosphamide, nonsteroidal anti-inflammatory

drugs, haloperidol, selective serotonin reuptake inhibitors, proton pump inhibitors, and ecstasy.

- Hyponatremia may present with neurologic dysfunction due to increased intracranial pressure from brain edema. Symptoms may include seizures, respiratory arrest, hypoxia, noncardiogenic pulmonary edema.
- ADH results in increase brain water and edema. Initial adaption results in excretion of brain Na and K, which leads to decrease in brain water. Later ADH over 48–72 hours leads to more loss of brain Na and K as well as non-electrolyte osmolytes (such as amino acids) and idiogenic osmoles. These idiogenic osmoles take longer to get out of the brain but also take longer to get back in with treatment. This is the mechanism of neuronal shrinkage.
- Acute treatment of severe hyponatremia goals include two factors.

  o Cerebral edema is treated to relieve symptoms, prevent progression of neurologic dysfunction and prevent respiratory arrest.
  o Avoid excessive correction to prevent osmotic demyelination.

- Acute severe symptoms require emergency treatment.
- Treatment is according to symptoms and follows the three rules above under DI.

  o Asymptomatic: Fluid restriction and treat underlying cause
  o Mild symptoms: Saline and furosimide
  o Severe symptoms: Hypertonic saline

- Correct Na no more than 10–12 mEq/L per 24 hours and <18 mEq/L in 48 hours.

  o Rapid achievement of 2–4 mEq/L over 2–4 hours is safe.

- Osmotic demyelation syndrome rarely occurs if Na is >120 mmol/L.

  o Risk factors include alcohol abuse, malnutrition, hypokalemia, burn or liver transplant patients, elderly women especially those on thiazides.

- Calculate Na deficit = total body water × (target Na-current Na).

  o 100 ml bolus 3% NaCl can safely raise Na by ~2 mEq/L.
  o Monitor Na every 1–2 hours.

Pheochromocytoma

- Pheochromocytoma in the ICU usually involves a hypertensive crisis or post-operative care.

- Pheochromocytoma follows the rule of 10s: Malignant, familial, bilateral, multiple, and extra-adrenal.
- Most cases have episodic hypertension associated with headache, diaphoresis, palpitations, flushing, anxiety, or chest pain. Some patients have sustained hypertension and some patients may be normotensive.
- Approximately 20% of patients will present with crisis.

  o As with other endocrine emergencies, pheochromocytoma crisis may be due to elective surgery or other medical illness.
  o Crisis may be characterized by hypertension, hypotension, arrhythmias, myocardial ischemia or infarction, cardiomyopathy or cardiogenic shock, pulmonary edema, stroke, hypertensive encephalopathy, hypoglycemia, or multiorgan dysfunction.

- Drug treatment of the hypertensive crisis is done with the iv alpha antagonist phentolamine. Unopposed β blockade is to be avoided. Conversion to an oral agent utilizes the nonselective α_1- α_2 phenoxybenzamine or a selective α_1 blocker doxazosin or terazosin.

  o An alternative is calcium channel blockers.

- Crisis management may also include inotropes, intra-aortic ballon pump, and extracorporeal life support in rare cases.
- Catecholamine excess can be detected using 24 hour urine or plasma total and fractionated metanephrines (metanephrine and normetanephrine). Levels are typically three times above the upper limits of normal.

  o The ICU is generally not the place to make this diagnosis.

- Localization is done with CT or MRI. MIBG scintigraphy is helpful to localize extra-adrenal tumors.
- Emergency resection is not indicated.
- Most patients require 10–14 days of preoperative medical preparation. However, patients with mild normotensive presentation may undergo surgery without any preoperative preparation.
- Risk factors for hemodynamic instability during surgery include a high plasma norepinephrine level, larger tumor size, more profound postural blood pressure fall after α-blockade, and a mean arterial pressure above 100 mmHg.
- Following resection, ICU admission may be necessary for hypertension, hypotension, arrhythmia, or hypoglycemia.

Severe hypercortisolism

- Classic signs of Cushing's syndrome are central obesity, buffalo hump, easy bruising, abdominal striae, osteoporosis, proximal weakness, and glucose intolerance.
- Sepsis, respiratory insufficiency, hypertensive crises, or acute psychosis are the most frequent examples of presentation of Cushing's syndrome in the intensive care unit.
- Cushing's syndrome is most often due to exogenous steroids.
- The most frequent endogenous cause of Cushing's syndrome (70%) is an adrenocorticotropic hormone (ACTH) secreting adenoma of the pituitary gland, known as Cushing's disease. Cortisol-producing adenomas of the adrenal gland cause 15% of Cushing's syndrome. In approximately 15% of cases, Cushing's syndrome is attributable to an ectopic ACTH-producing tumor. The most common functioning adrenal cortical carcinoma produces cortisol.
- Testing may be done with serum cortisol and ACTH levels, nighttime salivary cortisol, overnight dexamethasone suppression testing, or 24 hour urine cortisol.
- Imaging for localization includes cerebral magnetic resonance imaging for evaluation of pituitary adenomas and abdominal computed tomography for imaging the adrenal glands. With suspicion of an ectopic ACTH-producing tumor, Chest CTS or PET scanning may be necessary to evaluate for malignancy.
- Enzyme inhibitors ketoconazole, metyrapone, and etomidate reduce cortisol.
  - o Etomidate blocks 11-beta-hydroxylation of deoxycortisol.
  - o Intravenous low-dose etomidate infusion rates for the treatment of hypercortisolaemia are 0.04–0.05 mg/kg/h, equating to 2.8–3.5 mg/h in a 70 kg patient with dose titration according to serum cortisol. Target cortisol level is 500–800 nmol/L in a stressed patient and 150–300 nmol/L in a nonstressed patient.
  - o Cortisol levels fall within 12–24 h. Frequent monitoring is necessary for serum cortisol levels to achieve either complete or partial blockade and to prevent hypoadrenalism.
  - o Sedation scoring is necessary every two hours.
  - o Intravenous hydrocortisone at 0.5–1 mg/h is required for complete blockade but then the patient will need steroid replacement with hydrocortisone. This may be more convenient than frequently altering the etomidate.
- Surgical treatment of the cause of Cushing's syndrome may include hypophysectomy, resection of malignancy, and adrenalectomy. Rescue bilateral adrenalectomy may be necessary in ACTH dependent severe disease.

Hypercalcemic crisis

- Hypercalcemic crisis is a life-threatening condition that describes the severely compromised patient with profound volume depletion, altered sensorium which may manifest as a coma, cardiac decompensation and abdominal pain that may mimic an acute abdomen, caused by deterioration of chronic or acute hypercalcemia.
- Overall, the most common causes of hypercalcemia in an inpatient are malignancy (70%) and primary hyperparathyroidism (20%).
- Simultaneous elevation of PTH levels and calcium (Ca) levels proves the parathyroid origin of the hypercalcemia. If PTH levels are low or suppressed, other causes of hypercalcemia should be investigated.
- Most patients with non-parathyroidal hypercalcemia have a malignancy. Approximately half of these patients will have elevated PTH-related protein (PTH-rp).
- Hypercalcemic crises are predominantly secondary to hyperparathyroidism (HPT); for this reason, HPT must be proven or ruled out. HPT requires parathyroidectomy.
- Malignancy related hypercalcemia is the most common cause of inpatient hypercalcemic crises (50%) and complicates 10–30% of malignancies. It is usually present in the context of advanced clinically obvious disease.
- Severe hypercalcemia is defined as a serum Ca level >14 mg/dl.
- Symptoms and signs of hypercalcemia relate both to the volume contraction that accompanies these findings and the neuromuscular dysfunction that occurs.

  - Polyuria, thirst, confusion, drowsiness, agitation, stupor, coma, myopathy, hypertension, bradyarrhythmias, heart block, constipation, nausea, anorexia, vomiting, and abdominal pain.

- There are four basics goals of therapy: (1) correct dehydration; (2) enhance renal excretion of calcium; (3) inhibit accelerated bone resorption; and (4) treat underlying disorder

  - The cornerstone of acute management of hypercalcemia is *fluid resuscitation*.

    - 0.9% NS IV 500–1000 ml over the first hour, and 2–6 L fluids over the first 24 hours to reverse the intravascular volume contraction and promote the renal excretion of calcium.
    - For those patients with renal failure or for those who cannot tolerate large-volume resuscitation, hemodialysis with a low-calcium dialysate is the treatment of choice.

○ Historical approaches advocated the use of **loop diuretics** to induce further renal calcium loses, more recent treatment strategies have avoided diuretics due to the risk of aggravating volume contraction. Loop diuretics have a role in those patients where vigorous resuscitation may provoke cardiogenic fluid overload.

○ Intravenous **biphosphonates** should be administered as soon as severe hypercalcemia is diagnosed because there is latency until peak effect of 2–5 days.

- The dose of pamidronate is based on the calcium level: 30 mg IV over 2h if Ca <12 mg/dl or significant renal impairment; 60 mg IV over 4h if Ca 12–14 mg/dl; and 90 mg IV over 6h if Ca>14.
- Zoledronic acid 4 mg IV as initial treatment, 8 mg on retreatment.
- Pamidronate and Zoledronate contraindicated if GFR <30 ml/min/1.73 m².
- Potential risk of IV biphosphonates use is osteonecrosis of the jaw (ONJ). ONJ is more likely in the setting of hypercalcemia associated with malignancy.
- Hypophosphatemia and hypomagnesemia are other potential complications.
- Biphosponates are not generally necessary in patients with PHPT as they often respond to rehydration. Biphosphonates should be particularly avoided if urgent parathyroidectomy is performed as their use can result in profound postoperative hypocalcemia.

• **Glucocorticoids** exert a calcium-lowering effect by inhibiting the effects of vitamin D, reducing calcium absorption, increase renal calcium excretion and inhibit osteoclast-activating factor. They are indicated for hypercalcemia caused by vitamin D (or its analogs) toxicity. They are ineffective in most cases of hypercalcemia associated with malignancy.

○ Hydrocortisone 100 to 300 mg/day IV for 3 to 5 days.

• **Calcitonin** acts quickly (within 24 to 48 hours) to lower serum calcium levels, though the absolute effect on serum calcium is small; however, it can be an early effective intervention since more definitive therapies (i.e. bisphosphonates) may take several days to become fully effective.

○ Calcitonin 4–8 IU/kg SC/IM every 6–12h.

○ Because preparations of calcitonin are extracted from salmon, patients with preformed antibodies or those with previous exposure to calcitonin can demonstrate an allergic reaction consisting of respiratory distress, flushing, nausea, vomiting, and tingling in the extremities.

- ***Phosphate infusion*** is only indicated in life-threatening cardiac arrhythmias or severe encephalopathy when dialysis is not immediately available.
- Contraindicated medications during hypercalcemia are digitalis and hydrochlorothiazides.
  - o Digitalis may cause cardiac arrest and potentiates arrhythmias.
  - o Thiazides reduce calciuria and thus, contribute to the severity of hypercalcemia.

Practical Algoritm(s)/ Diagrams

Serum hormone concentration in
Nonthyroidal illness

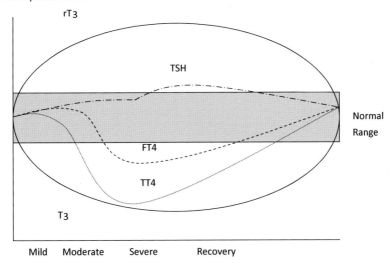

Fig. 1.

Review of Current Literature with References

Thyroid storm

- Landmark article published in 1993 by Burch and Wartofsky assigned a numerical score to each of the different signs and symptoms of thyroid storm and established diagnostic criteria based on the total score calculated. Because laboratory studies cannot distinguish thyroid storm from thyrotoxicosis, clinical features are the key to this diagnosis, and a scoring system helps clinicians determine when to make the diagnosis.

Burch HB, Wartofsky L. Life-threatening thyrotoxicosis. Thyroid storm. *Endocrinol Metab Clin North Am* 1993; **22**: 263–277.

- The Japan Thyroid Association surveyed the incidence of thyroid storm in Japan. Diagnostic criteria were based on combinations of CNS symptoms, fever, tachycardia, congestive heart failure, and gastrointestinal/hepatic disturbances. Tachycardia with a heart rate of higher than 130 was found in greater than 75% of the patients, and 84% of the patients had CNS symptoms, 69% of the patients had gastrointestinal manifestations, and 40% of the patients had heart failure. In all, 76% of the patients with thyroid storm had more than three major organ manifestations, consistent with multiple organ failure.

Akamizu T, Satoh T, Isozaki O *et al.* Diagnostic criteria, clinical features, and incidence of thyroid storm based on nationwide surveys. *Thyroid* 2012; **22**: 661–679.

Myxedema coma

- Twenty-three patients with myxedema coma from 1999–2006 were studied. Various predictors of mortality included hypotension and bradycardia, mechanical ventilation, hypothermia, sepsis, intake of sedative drugs, lower Glasgow Coma Scale, high acute physiology and chronic health evaluation II (APACHE II) score, and high sequential organ failure assessment (SOFA) score. Baseline and day 3 SOFA scores of more than 6 were highly predictive of poor outcome.

Dutta P, Bhansali A, Masoodi SR *et al.* Predictors of outcome in myxedema coma: a study from a tertiary care centre. *Crit Care* 2008; **12**: 1–8.

Euthyroid sick syndrome

- Four hundred and eighty consecutive patients without known thyroid diseases were followed. Baseline characteristics, including the acute physiology and chronic health evaluation II (APACHE II) score and thyroid hormone, N-terminal pro-brain natriuretic peptide (NT-proBNP) and C-reactive protein (CRP) levels were collected. Among the thyroid hormone levels, free T3 had the greatest power to predict ICU mortality better than NT-proBNP and CRP levels. Addition of FT3 to APACHE II improved the ability to predict mortality.

Wang F, Pan W, Wang H, Wang S, Pan S, Ge J. Relationship between thyroid function and ICU mortality: a prospective observation study. *Crit Care* 2012; **16**: R11.

Pheochromocytoma

- Seventy-three patients whom were operated on between 1995 and 2007 were studied. Parameters studied were catecholamine type and concentration, tumor diameter, mean arterial pressure (MAP) before and after pretreatment with α-antagonist, postural fall in blood pressure (BP) after pretreatment, type of α-blockade, type of operation, and presence of a familial syndrome. A correlation was found between hemodynamic instability and plasma norepinephrine levels, tumor diameter, postural BP fall, MAP at presentation and after α-blockade. Type of operation or α-blockade and presence of a familial polytumor syndrome were not related to HD instability.

  Bruynzeel H, Feelders RA, Groenland TH, van den Meiracker AH, van Eijck CH, Lange JF, de Herder WW, Kazemier G. Risk factors for hemodynamic instability during surgery for pheochromocytoma. *J Clin Endocrinol Metab.* 2010; **95**: 678–85.

- Twenty-five of 137 patients between 1993–2011 presented with crisis. Fifteen patients were stabilized and discharged, and 10 underwent urgent operation. Elective surgery patients had shorter length of stay, less complications, and less ICU admissions. There was no mortality.

  Scholten A, Cisco RM, Vriens MR, Cohen JK, Mitmaker EJ, Liu C, Tyrrell JB, Shen WT, Duh QY. Pheochromocytoma crisis is not a surgical emergency. *J Clin Endocrinol Metab.* 2013; **98**: 581–91.

Severe hypercortisolism

- This is an excellent review of the use of etomidate to manage severe hypercortisolism in cases with significant complications that include sepsis, severe hypertension, and psychosis.

  Preda VA, Sen J, Karavitaki N, Grossman AB. Etomidate in the management of hypercortisolaemia in Cushing's syndrome: a review. *Eur J Endocrinol* 2012; **167**: 137–143.

Hypercalcemia

- Eighty-eight out of 1,310 patients with PHPT between 1970–2009 presented with hypercalcemic crisis. Hypercalcemic crisis is appropriately treated by expeditious parathyroidectomy. Similar long-term outcomes on parathyroidectomy for patients with PHPT without hypercalcemic crisis were reported.

  Cannon J, Lew J.I, Solorzano CC. *Surgery* 2010; **148**: 807–813.

Chapter 11-(ii)

Adrenal Insufficiency

Daniel Lollar, MD*

* Fellow, Trauma and Acute Care Surgery, Denver Health Medical Center

Take Home Points

- The maximum production of cortisol from a healthy, stressed adrenal cortex is no more than 350 mg a day. This represents a significant increase from the normal daily release of 15–25 mg without stress. Replacement therapy should not surpass maximum physiologic output.
- There is no physiological difference between the hormone cortisol and the drug hydrocortisone; the difference is sematic and of historic interest only.
- The diagnosis of relative adrenal insufficiency (RAI) in the ICU is complicated. Laboratory evaluation of cortisol levels, while frequently performed and debated, do not accurately reflect the physiologic response of the hypothalamic-pituitary-adrenal (HPA) axis. A level of clinical suspicion, an accurate history and an appropriate clinical picture provide the strongest evidence for providing a critically ill patient steroid replacement.
- The most common cause of relative adrenal insufficiency is exogenous steroid administration, though etomidate administration, traumatic brain

Contact information: Denver Health Medical Center, University of Colorado Health Sciences Center, 777 Bannock Street, MC 0206, Denver, CO 80204; Email: Daniel.Lollar@ucdenver.edu

injury, adrenal hemorrhage or infarction, and direct adrenal trauma should also be considered as potential etiologies. Dosing regimens equivalent to prednisone 7.5 mg daily (hydrocortisone 75 mg daily, dexamethasone 0.75 mg daily) for three weeks or longer significantly increases the likelihood that the HPA axis is suppressed and the patient is likely to develop relative adrenal insufficiency.

- Patients with a suspicion for adrenal insufficiency but whose clinical picture is unclear should be evaluated initially with a random serum cortisol level. Levels less than 15 mcg/dL require treatment with exogenous glucocorticoids (hydrocortisone) while levels >34 mcg/dL do not require therapy. Levels between 15–34 mcg/dL should be further evaluated with a Cosyntropin (synthetic ACTH or corticotropin) challenge with administration of 250 mcg of Cosyntropin. An increase <9 mcg/dL above baseline is an indication to start steroid supplementation.

- Patients in shock refractory to volume repletion and vasopressor therapy should be started empirically on replacement steroids. This is typically given as a bolus of hydrocortisone 100 mg IV followed by a continuous infusion of 12 mg/hr. If empiric therapy does not result in significant reduction in vasopressor intensity, consideration for cessation of empiric therapy should be given. However, the clinician should bear in mind that patients with untreated adrenal insufficiency have worse outcomes. Therefore, if there is uncertainty, treatment should be continued.

- While treatment of RAI should be initiated when needed, the clinician should recognize that steroid replacement has not been shown to definitively improve patient outcomes. RAI may be more a marker of disease severity than a distinct clinical entity.

Background

- The adrenal glands are paired organs that reside just above the kidneys in the retroperitoneal space. Each gland is composed of a three-layered cortex and an embryologically distinct medulla. The outer zona glomerulosa secretes aldosterone, while the zona fasciculata produces cortisol. The inner zona reticularis regulates sex hormone secretion primarily via production of dihydroepiandosterone. The adrenal medulla produces endogenous catecholamines in the form of epinephrine.

- Glucocorticoids play a significant role in maintaining glucose homeostasis and utilization. Stimulation of the anterior pituitary gland by the hypothalamus via corticotrophin-releasing hormone (CRH) causes secretion of adrenocorticotrophic hormone (ACTH). ACTH acts on the adrenal cortex causing release of cortisol. Cortisol is released in a diurnal pattern with maximum production around 8 am. Primary adrenal insufficiency refers to failure of the adrenal cortex to respond appropriately to ACTH stimulation whereas secondary adrenal insufficiency refers to lack of ACTH production from the pituitary.

- ACTH production is stimulated by hypotension, pain, anxiety and endotoxin. Additionally, cytokines released during stress such as TNF-α, IL-1β and IL-6 stimulate ACTH release. Cortisol produces negative feedback inhibition of ACTH production. Hence, endogenous steroid administration for longer than 3 weeks alters the HPA-axis decreasing ACTH synthesis which can last for up to a year after cessation.

- Free cortisol represents less than 10% of total plasma cortisol levels. Half of plasma cortisol is bound to cortisol-binding globulin (CBG) and an additional 40% is bound to plasma albumin during the non-stressed state. However, free cortisol is the physiologically active component and is rarely measured. Total cortisol levels do not accurately reflect the activity of free cortisol in critically ill patients who typically have elevated levels of free cortisol while having lowered levels of albumin and CBG.

- The half-life of cortisol is 60–120 minutes. The adrenal gland does not store glucocorticoids but can increase production substantially in response to ACTH. Cholesterol forms the precursor for glucocorticoids (and many steroid hormone molecules). High-density lipoprotein, the preferred cholesterol substrate, is converted to pregnenolone and then to the end-products of adrenal synthesis. Eighty percent of cortisol production is via this pathway.

- Cortisol is a steroid hormone which has both transmembrane and direct nuclear actions causing metabolic, cardiovascular, and immune effects. Metabolic effects include increasing glucose levels via hepatic gluconeogenesis, inhibition of insulin, peripheral lipolysis via increased lipocortin-1 and increased amino acid synthesis from protein breakdown. Cardiovascular effects of cortisol involve regulation of sodium and water and, importantly, the permissive interaction of cortisol with catecholamines on vasculature. Finally, cortisol affects immune function by regulation leukocyte production and migration, decreasing cytokine production and blocking eicosanoid action. The glucocorticoid receptor also plays a significant role iin modulating gene expression by inhibiting the action of nuclear factor κB (NF-κB).

Main Body

Glucocorticoids

- For the critical care clinician, adrenal insufficiency typically refers to insufficient production of glucocorticoids (cortisol) in response to a stress. Insufficient steroid production is a life-threatening complication and affects anywhere from 0–77% of the ICU population (depending on definition used); approaching 60% in patients with septic shock. In the literature, the concept of the adrenal gland not producing sufficient hormones in response to critical illness is variably referred to as relative adrenal insufficiency (RAI), critical illness-related corticosteroid insufficiency (CIRCI) or functional adrenal insufficiency.
- In critical illness, the pathophysiology of RAI is induced at multiple levels in the HPA-axis. One source has suggested 75% of RAI in patients with severe sepsis and septic shock is caused by cytokine mediated suppression of regulatory hormone release at the hypothalamic/pituitary level. However, additional mechanisms include insufficient uptake of cortisol production by the adrenal cortex, resistance of peripheral tissues to glucocorticoids, and intracellular resistance to glucocorticoid receptor actions.
- Signs and symptoms of adrenal insufficiency range from lethargy and low energy to hypotension and shock. Gastrointestinal symptoms include nausea and vomiting and dehydration. Fever may also be a part of the syndrome. Additionally, eosinophilia may suggest the diagnosis. Unfortunately, in patients who have RAI secondary to another process, symptoms may be indistinguishable from the primary problem (e.g. septic shock) and subtle signs and symptoms may not be elicited from an obtunded patient. Therefore, a high level of suspicion must be maintained.
- The effects of cortisol on vasculature are permissive with catecholamines. This means that without cortisol, catecholamines are ineffective in their vasoconstrictive actions. Therefore, the shock seen with RAI or with Addisonian crisis is a hyper-dynamic, distributive shock similar to that seen in sepsis. Administration of hydrocortisone will initially improve hemodynamic parameters within 10 minutes due primarily to its mineralocorticoid effects. Hemodynamic stability due to glucocorticoid action should be seen within 6 hours of initial dosing. Therefore, because all patients will respond to steroid replacement within 10 minutes, the determination to continue steroids should be assessed hours after initial dosing.
- The typical patient with RAI is an older, malnourished or alcoholic patient who presents with septic shock which is refractory to fluid resuscitation and

vasopressors. In this situation, the diagnosis of RAI is a clinical one and treatment should be started empirically. Laboratory diagnosis may be helpful in a patient who is in shock but either the etiology is unclear or the patient fails to improve despite appropriate therapy. A total cortisol level less than 15 mcg/dL strongly supports adrenal axis dysfunction as a causal mechanism while levels greater than 35 mcg/dL effectively rule out RAI. Levels that are in between these values should be further evaluated with a high-dose corticotropin (Cosyntropin) stimulation test. After a base line level is drawn, the patient is administered 250 mcg of cosyntropin via IV push. Cortisol levels are assessed 30 and 60 minutes after dosing administration. Patients who fail to respond with an increase more than 9 mcg/dL above the base line value are diagnosed with RAI and treatment should be started. The ACTH stimulation test should not be used in patients within three weeks of a pituitary insult such as surgery or infarction (apoplexy).

- Treatment of RAI is designed to replace the maximum physiologic response of the adrenal glands. Different regimens are used including a continuous infusion of hydrocortisone at 12 mg/hr, 100 mg q8 hrs or 50 mg q6 hrs. No dosing regimen has been shown to be superior to another. Therapy is continued throughout the acute phase of illness, typically for seven days and then discontinued. If the patient redevelops signs or symptoms of RAI, steroids are restarted and a formal wean is performed.

Mineralocorticoids

- The main mineralocorticoid is aldosterone which is secreted from the zona glomerulosa. Aldosterone action is controlled by the renin-angiotensin system. Production of aldosterone is via angiotensin II and while ACTH does induce production of aldosterone precursors, impaired ACTH production does not impair aldosterone production.
- Primary hypoaldosteronism is rarely seen in the ICU and is marked by hyperkalemia and hypotension. It should be remembered that hydrocortisone (cortisol) has significant mineralocorticoid effects at high levels.
- Patients with primary adrenal insufficiency or relative adrenal insufficiency not treated with hydrocortisone may require mineralocorticoid replacement with fludrocortisone 50 mcg/day, however this must be given orally.

Practical Algoritm(s)/Diagrams

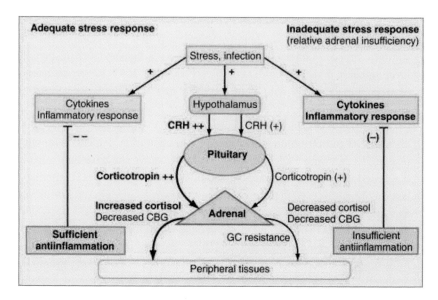

Fig. 1. Physiology and pathophysiology of cortisol release in response to stress. From Vincent *et al.*, *Textbook of Critical Care Medicine 6th ed.*, p. 1219.

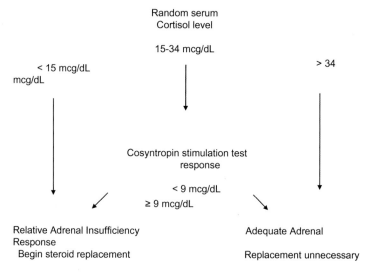

Fig. 2. Algorithm for laboratory analysis of adrenal insufficiency. Adapted from Cooper MS, *NEJM* 2003; **348**: 727–734.

Review of Current Literature with References

- In 2004, Hamrahian published a comparison of total cortisol, cortisol binding protein and free cortisol levels between normal controls and critically ill patients in the *New England Journal of Medicine*. In this prospective, observational study, the authors evaluated 33 normal controls matched to 66 critically ill patients (APACHE III score >15), 36 of whom had serum albumin levels less than 2.5 g/dL. The analysis revealed that patients with low albumin levels had lower total cortisol levels and a less robust response to an ACTH stimulation test. In fact, no patients with a serum albumin above 2.5 g/dL failed to mount a significant increase (>18.5 mcg/dL) to ACTH stimulation while 39% of the hypoalbuminemic patients did not mount an appropriate increase in response to ACTH. However, when free cortisol levels were examined, the baseline free cortisol level was almost identical. Additionally, the increase after ACTH stimulation was also similar. Levels of both total and free cortisol and response to ACTH stimulation were significantly greater in both critically ill groups versus the health volunteers. Of note, mineralocorticoid secretion was measured to be normal in all groups. The authors note that while critically ill patients mount an increase of free cortisol of 7–10× normal values, this is reflected in total cortisol levels of only 2–3× normal. They further concluded that total cortisol levels in patients with hypoalbuminemia can be misleading and encourage the use of free cortisol level measurements in critically ill patients.
- Hamrahian AH, Oseni TS, Arafah BM, Measurements of serum free cortisol in critically ill patients, *NEJM* 2004; **350**: 1629–1638.
- In a prospective, observation trial of 189 patients with septic shock admitted to two mixed ICU's in France, Annane evaluated each patient's cortisol level and their response to corticotropin stimulation. Patients were compared based on their initial total cortisol levels (>34 mcg/dL versus ≤34 mcg/dL) and their response to corticotropin stimulation test (increase ≥9 mcg/dL or <9 mcg/dL). The authors found the highest 28-day mortality (82%) in patients with an elevated cortisol level but who failed to increase their cortisol level in response to corticotropin stimulation. Intermediate outcomes were found in the group with either an elevated cortisol level and an appropriate response to corticotropin stimulation or a cortisol level less than 34 mcg/dL who did not respond to corticotropin stimulation. This cohort of patients had a 28-day mortality of 67%. The best mortality outcomes, at 26%, were with the cohort of patients who had a low cortisol level initially and who responded appropriately to corticotropin stimulation (i.e. an increase in cortisol level greater than

9 mcg/dL). The authors concluded that cortisol levels combined with a corticotropin stimulation test provides a good prognostic indicator for 28-day mortality outcomes.

- Annane D, Sébille V, Troché G *et al.*, A 3-Level prognostic classification in septic shock based on cortisol levels and cortisol response to corticotropin, *JAMA* 2000; **238**: 1035–1045.

- In a double-blind, placebo-controlled, randomized, parallel-group trial performed in 300 patients distributed across 19 mixed ICU's in France, Annane *et al.* examined whether replacement of hydrocortisone in patients with septic shock would improve mortality rates. Patients were included if they had sepsis with shock after being given fluid resuscitation and requiring vasopressor support. All patients had cortisol levels drawn before and during a corticotropin stimulation test. The treatment group received 50 mg of hydrocortisone every 6 hours for seven days after enrollment. Additionally, the treatment group received 50 mcg of fludrocortisone daily orally or via gastric tube. The results of the study found that patients who failed to respond to corticotropin stimulation with an increased cortisol level of more than 9 mcg/dL had the most improvement in mortality with treatment with an odds ratio of death of 0.54. In the group that did respond appropriately to corticotropin stimulation, there was no appreciable improvement in morality with treatment. In examination of the effect of treatment on duration of vasopressors, the authors found that all patients treated had a decreased duration of vasopressor use. This effect was pronounced in the non-responder group and was not seen in the responder group. The authors concluded that steroid replacement is beneficial in patients with septic shock, particularly those who do not respond to a corticotropin stimulation test.

- Annane D, Sébille V, Charpentier C *et al.*, Effect of treatment with low doses of hydrocortisone and fludrocortisone on mortality in patients with septic shock, *JAMA* 2002; **228**: 862–871.

- The CORTICUS study, published in 2008, examined the role of steroid replacement in a mixed ICU population of patients in septic shock. This trial randomized 499 patients into intention-to-treat groups of hydrocortisone 50 mg q6 hours versus placebo. There was no difference in the primary outcome of 30-day mortality between the two groups. Furthermore, all patients were given a corticotropin stimulation test. No difference in 30-day mortality was found between the group of patients that responded appropriately and the patients that did not respond to stimulation. In terms of secondary outcomes, the group treated with steroids did see an earlier resolution of shock by an average of three days. However, the incidence of superinfection or new episodes of septic shock were found to be higher with an odds ratio of 1.37 for the steroid group. Hyperglycemia was also more common. The authors conclude that there is no mortality benefit to treating patients in septic shock with steroid replacement regardless of their response to a corticotropin stimulation test.

- Sprung CL, Annane D, Keh D *et al.*, Hydrocortisone therapy for patients in septic shock, *NEJM* 2008; **358**: 111–124.

Chapter **11-(iii)**

Glycemic Control

Theresa L. Chin, MD, MPH*

*Surgical Resident, University of Colorado School of Medicine

Take Home Points

- Stress induced hyperglycemia is common in critically ill patients and is due to neurohormonal, nutritional, and iatrogenic factors. Insulin resistance with critical illness contributes to hyperglycemia.
- Hyperglycemia is associated with neuropathy, skeletal muscle wasting, increased growth hormone concentrations, increased susceptibility to infection, prolonged mechanical ventilation, and impaired neutrophil phagocytosis.
- To treat hyperglycemia in the ICU, intravenous insulin infusion should be the primary mode of glycemic control. A standard protocol should be used for monitoring and titration to avoid hypoglycemic episodes.
- Parenteral nutrition or enteral nutrition with a high carbohydrate load can affect glucose levels. Insulin should be titrated for initiation, alteration, or cessation of nutrition supplementation.
- Hypoglycemia, which occurs more frequently with intensive insulin therapy, has been associated with adverse outcomes and higher mortality. Hypoglycemic episodes should be avoided especially in patients with traumatic brain injury.

Contact information: Department of Surgery, 12631 East 17th Ave, C313; Email: Theresa.Chin@ucdenver.edu

- Once a patient is stable on insulin IV therapy and illness is improved, the patient can be assessed to determine if the patient requires long-term insulin coverage outside of the ICU. If the patient continues to require insulin therapy to control glucose levels, transition to basal/bolus insulin therapy.
- Intensive insulin therapy in critically ill patients has been shown to be associated with better morbidity and mortality, but on the contrary, other studies showed higher incidence and morbidity and mortality from hypoglycemia with intensive insulin therapy.

Background

- Hyperglycemia is common in the surgical ICU among postoperative, septic, and trauma patients and has been associated with worse outcomes, but may be related to the severity of illness.
- Neurohormonal factors contributing to hyperglycemia include increased cortisol after surgery or trauma, decreased peripheral glucose uptake from insulin antagonism from growth hormone and epinephrine, increased glucose production from glycogenolysis and enhanced gluconeogenesis.
- Other factors that increase glucose levels are administration of exogenous corticosteroids, certain vasopressors (epinephrine), and occult infection. Parenteral nutrition and IV solutions containing glucose contribute to hyperglycemia in the ICU.
- Protective effects of intensive glycemic control include endothelial protection and multiple organ failure, prevention of leukocyte dysfunction, decreased susceptibility to infection, improved myocardial function, and protection of liver mitochondrial ultrastructure and function.
- Hyperglycemia in patients with traumatic brain injury is associated with poor outcomes, and more recent studies have shown that intensive insulin therapy reduces brain glucose, increases intracranial hypertension and hypoglycemic episodes.

Main Body

Glucose monitoring

- Acutely, glucose control is similar in diabetics and is primarily based on point of care testing of blood glucose.
- Point of care glucose testing should be checked every hour until stable, at which point, monitoring can be changed to every two hours.

- Glucose levels should be checked every hour when there is a change in the insulin infusion rate, significant change in clinical status, especially requiring corticosteroid or vasopressor therapy or change in nutritional support.

Management of hyperglycemia

- All oral antihyperglycemic medications and subcutaneous insulin should be stopped for patients admitted to the ICU.
- Insulin therapy should be initiated for glucose >150 mg/dL and should be administered with a standard infusion protocol with goal range of 100–150 mg/dL. In most ICUs, glucose algorithms are managed by nurses. See *Practical Algorithm(s)/Diagrams* section for an example of an insulin infusion protocol.
- Insulin infusion adjustments must be made based on carbohydrate intake. If the dextrose infusion rate is changed via parenteral or enteral nutrition, or with medications in dextrose solutions, the insulin infusion will have to be adjusted to avoid hypoglycemia.

Nutrition

- Upon starting TPN, an intravenous regular insulin infusion or sliding scale with regular insulin can be started simultaneously to maintain glucose levels <= 140 mg/dL. One half to two thirds of the previous day's insulin requirement can be added to the TPN bag up to 40 units of regular insulin per liter of TPN. If the blood glucose remains high, dextrose concentrations levels can be reduced to 60–80% of the estimated needs until blood glucose levels are within range (Lange p. 128).
- TPN should be discontinued by decreasing the infusion rate incrementally to avoid rebound hypoglycemia.
- Nutrition, both parenteral and enteral, should be given continuously in the acute setting to avoid fluctuations in glucose levels and subsequent hypoglycemia. Cessation of nutrition intake should prompt modification of insulin dosing and timing. Hypoglycemic episodes are often due to interruption of enteral feeds.
- Renal and hepatic failure patients are most at-risk for hypoglycemia.
- Patients who are sedated or with altered mental status are unable to respond to hypoglycemia or show signs of hypoglycemia. Careful attention must be paid to these patients.

Hypoglycemia

- Glucose is the required substrate for the brain and hypoglycemia can lead to unresponsiveness, seizures, coma and death.
- Signs and symptoms of hypoglycemia include cold, clammy skin, palpitations, weakness, confusion and mood changes.
- Treat glucose <70 mg/dL with 12/5 grams of 50% dextrose IV (1/2 amp). Recheck glucose in 15 minutes and repeat as needed to reach blood glucose <100 mg/dL. Action should be taken to avoid further hypoglycemic episodes.
- Avoid glucose <100 mg/dL in traumatic brain injured patients.

Transition to SQ insulin

- Once the patient's condition is improved and can be discharged from the ICU, intravenous insulin can be transitioned to subcutaneous insulin. It would be ideal to wait until the patient is off vasopressors, peripheral edema has resolved and there are not planned interruptions.
- Consideration of prior history of diabetes and their home regimen, stress level, steroid use, and general clinical status is necessary when calculating the dosage. Long-acting insulin needs to be overlapped with discontinuation of the drip to prevent hyperglycemia.
- Transition from intravenous insulin therapy to subcutaneous insulin therapy once the patient has recovered from acute illness and is stable on insulin therapy. If the patient is not yet stable on insulin therapy, wait until glucose levels have stabilized. To transition, use basal/bolus concept. Sum the total number of units of insulin needed for a 24-hours period. Provide half of basal insulin using a long-acting insulin, such as NPH or glargine. Give a "bolus" of short-acting insulin at meals and at night.
- Several types of insulin can be used based on the onset and duration of action (see table).

Practical Algorithm(s)/Diagrams

Table 1. Denver Health insulin infusion protocol.

1. Start IV insulin infusion for critically ill when blood glucose >145 mg/dL.
2. Check glucose every two hours and every one hour as needed.
3. If tube feeds, TPN or D5W fluids are stopped, decrease insulin infusion rate by 50% and check glucose in one hour.
4. If blood glucose is elevated, continue current rate and check in one hour.
5. If blood glucose remains elevated or low, follow chart below and check glucose in one hour.
6. Do not bolus for serum creatinine >2.

Table 2. Initiation of blood glucose.

Blood glucose (mg/dL)	Bolus IV push (units)	Infusion rate (units/hour)
146–185	2	1
186–225	2	2
226–265	4	4
266–300	6	4
301–350	8	4
>350	10	4

Table 3. Continuation of insulin infusion.

Blood glucose (mg/dL)	Bous IV push (units)	Infusion rate (units/hour)
<60	0	Stop infusion; give one half amp of D50 IV push, recheck blood glucose in 30 minutes. If blood glucose >110, resume insulin infusion at 50% of previous rate
60–110	0	Stop infusion; recheck blood glucose in 30 minutes. If blood glucose >110, resume insulin infusion at 50% of previous rate
111–145	0	No change; if blood glucose continues to decrease within desired range over four hours, decrease rate by 20%.
146–175	2	Increase rate by 20%
176–215	4	Increase rate by 20%
216–245	6	Increase rate by 20%
246–295	8	Increase rate by 20%
296–345	10	Increase rate by 20%
>345	12	Increase rate by 20%

Table 4.   Types of insulin.

Insulin	Onset	Peak	Duration
Long acting insulins			
NPH	2–4 hours	6–10 hours	14–18 hours
Lente (X)	3–4 hours	6–12 hours	16–20 hours
Ultralente (X)	6–10 hours	10–16 hours	20–24 hours
Glargine	2 hours		24 hours
Short acting insulins			
Humalog/Lispro (rapid acting)	15 minutes	30–90 minutes	4–6 hours
Regular (short acting)	30–60 minutes	2–3 hours	8 hours

Review of Current Literature with References

- Often considered the landmark study of intensive glucose therapy, the group in Leuven, Belgium conducted a prospective randomized trial with 1,548 mechanically ventilated ICU medical-surgical patients. Patients randomized to intensive insulin therapy (glucose 80–110) had a lower mortality than patient treated with conventional glucose therapy (glucose <180). A second trial of 1,200 medical ICU patients conducted by the same group did not show a reduction in overall mortality and instead was associated with a higher rate of hypoglycemic episodes. The first study began the quest for the most beneficial glucose target in ICU patients (van den Berghe G, Wouters P, Weekers F *et al.* Intensive insulin therapy in critically ill patients. *N Engl J Med* 2001; **345**: 1359–1367).

- The normoglycemia in intensive care evaluation-survival using glucose algorithm regulation (NICE-SUGAR) trial is the largest trial of intensive insulin therapy in the ICU. Six thousand one hundered and four patients were randomized to intensive insulin therapy with glucose target of 81–108 mg/dL or conventional target of 180 mg/dL or lower. The intensive insulin therapy group had an increase in mortality at 90 days and increased incidence of hypoglycemia. This study suggests that moderate glycemic control may be as good or better (The NICE-SUGAR Study Investigators. Intensive versus conventional glucose control in critically ill patients. *N Engl J Med* 2009; **360**: 1283–1297).

- A meta-analysis of 26 clinical trials of intensive insulin therapy included over 13,000 patients. Intensive insulin therapy was not shown to affect overall mortality, and was also associated with severe hypoglycemia. Patients in a surgical ICU had a higher benefit from intensive insulin therapy than patients treated with conventional glucose levels (Griesdale DE, de Souza RJ, van Dam RM *et al*. Intensive insulin therapy and mortality among critically ill patients: a meta-analysis including NICE-SUGAR study data. *CMAJ* 2009; **180**: 821–827).

III: ICU Procedures

Chapter 12

Principles of Ultrasound

Paulo E. Jaworski, MD* Wilson R. Molina, MD[†]
and Fernando J. Kim, MD, FACS[‡]

*Urology Fellow, Denver Health Medical Center
[†]Assistant Professor of Surgery, University of Colorado School of Medicine
[‡]Professor of Surgery, University of Colorado School of Medicine

Take Home Points

- Ultrasonography uses mechanical energy in the form of high frequency longitudinal waves that interact with biological tissue and material.
- The piezoelectric effect, which occurs inside ultrasonic transducers, is the conversion of electric energy to mechanical energy in the form of sound waves, and vice-versa, by piezoelectric crystals.
- Reflected waves (echoes) from different body tissues are captured and processed according to their amplitude, assigning a graphic display to different types of echoes.
- Ultrasound (US) images are generated by the interpretation of emitted waves and reflected echoes using specific sound wave frequencies and intervals.

Contact information: Denver Health Medical Center, 777 Bannock St., MC 0206, Denver, C0 80204; Emails: fernando.Kim@dhha.org; Paulo.Jaworski@dhha.org; Wilson.Molina@dhha.org

- The higher the frequency, the shorter the penetration of sound waves and will result in higher quality images. Lower frequencies have deeper tissue penetration but poorer image resolution.
- Due to physical properties of the different materials and body tissues, wave interactions such as refraction, attenuation, or artifacts can alter the correct interpretation of US images.
- US images can be obtained using different modes according to the organ/tissue to be analyzed.
- A-mode gives information in a linear fashion with sound wave reflection of tissue and depth of each interface. This is mostly used in ophthalmology.
- In B-mode (Brightness Mode) or 2-Dimensional US, sound wave echoes are captured at a high refresh rate. An internal process builds a graphic representation of the structures with an illusionary effect of real-time scanning.
- M-mode interprets moving echoes to produce linear images. A line of scan is placed along the target area. The way structures move along the line of scan generates an image on the screen.
- The Doppler Effect allows for calculation of velocity of flow. Color Doppler applies a color map to the direction of the flow. Power Doppler is more sensitive to detect density of flow rather than direction or velocity.

Background

- Choosing the optimal ultrasound transducer is pivotal in improving efficacy of the sonographic study. The correct frequency and depth of sonogram will define the resolution of the anatomy and possible abnormalities.
- Sound waves are <u>mechanical waves</u> that can be transmitted through a medium (tissue, air or fluid). The audible sound frequencies are below 15 000 to 20 000 Hz, while diagnostic ultrasound is in the range of 2–20 MHz.[1,2]
- US waves propagate longitudinally, making particles move in one direction only. This produces areas of contraction and rarefaction within the medium particles, which can be graphically represented as a sine wave alternating up and down from a baseline.
- <u>Wavelength</u> corresponds to the distance between two peaks, and each interval between peaks is called cycle. The wavelength is inversely related to the frequency f by the sound velocity c: $c = 1f$. Meaning that the velocity equals the wavelength times the number of oscillations per second, and thus: $1 = c/f$.
- <u>Frequency</u> is the measurement of cycles per second. 1 cycle per second is referred as 1 Hz. The <u>amplitude</u> of a wave is the vertical range of the wave as it appears in the graphic.

- The velocity of a sound wave is constant to each medium or material and is calculated through the product of its frequency and wavelength. In soft tissues at 37 °C, sound travels at an average of 1540 m/s.[1]
- The sound velocity in a given material is constant (at a given temperature), but varies in different materials.

Medium or material	Velocity (m/s)
Air	330
Water	1497
Fat	1440
Average soft tissue	1540
Blood	1570
Muscle	1500–1630
Bone	2700–4100
Metal	3000–6000

- The US transducer contains either crystals or, more commonly, synthetic ceramic components that convert electrical energy to mechanical energy through the piezoelectric effect. These dipole crystals are organized in a way that, when voltage is applied, they contract and expand, producing a mechanical sound wave. Each group of wave cycles produced is called a pulse.[1,3]
- Pulses can normally contain from 2 to 4 wave cycles. After that, the transducer silences and works as a receptor of reflected waves. In fact, waiting for reflected echoes takes around 95% of the time during an entire ultrasound study. Through an inverted piezoelectric mechanism, reflected echoes are captured and transformed into electrical energy.[2,3]
- Information from the reflected echoes is processed and displayed up on the screen as a graphic representation of the mechanical interaction of the US waves with the body tissues.
- Some of the energy of the US is absorbed by the tissue, and converted to heat but the absorbed energy produced by the commercial sonogram equipment remains within limits that does not heat the tissue to dangerous temperatures.
- Attenuation of a tissue is a measure of how the energy of an US wave can be dissipated by that tissue, mainly due to absorption which is directly linked to the tissue's impedance. Attenuation also increases with both distance and frequency, and it limits penetration at any given frequency.[2,3,4]

- Attenuation can be dealt with by <u>gain</u>, Increasing overall gain, will increase the amplitude of the signal, and the structures at the bottom of the sector becomes more visible. However, increased gain increases signal and noise in the same manner.
- All commercial equipment today has a <u>time gain compensation</u> (TGC), increasing the gain of the reflected signals with increasing time from the transmitted pulse. This is equivalent to increasing the gain and depth. However, this is not a perfect solution, as the noise is constant with depth, while the reflected signals become weaker, and with TGC, the noise will be gained as well as the signal, and the signal-to-noise ratio will decrease, thus the resulting signal will become a grey blur at a certain depth.

Main Body

Artifacts

- <u>Acoustic shadowing</u> occurs when there is significant attenuation at a tissue interface, causing loss of information distally to that interface. For instance, in the examination of a kidney stone, waves striking that interface produce an anechoic or hypoechoic shadow.[2,3]
- Depending on the size and position, it may be difficult to obtain accurate measurements of the stone, structure, or even detail in the region of the shadow. Changing the angle of insonation usually overcomes that problem.
- <u>Increase through enhancement</u> occurs when sound waves pass through tissue with less attenuation than the surrounding tissue. For instance, a fluid-filled renal cyst has little attenuation and low reflection compared to the surrounding renal parenchyma.[4]
- When sound waves reach the posterior wall and underlying parenchyma, they are stronger/less attenuated compared to surrounding waves. That area reflects stronger echoes, making pixels brighter on the screen compared to the rest of the renal tissue, for example.
- Increase through enhancement can be overcome by changing the angle of insonation or adjusting the time-gain compensation settings.

A-Mode

- In <u>A-Mode</u> ultrasonography, only one pulse of ultrasound waves is emitted and the acoustical interfaces that reflect echoes are graphically represented as peaks along a line. The higher the peak, the greater the echo amplitude. The distance between peaks represents the distance between interfaces. This mode is currently used in ophthalmology for retina diseases.[2]

B-Mode

- In B-Mode (brightness), the transducer contains many crystals that are organized linearly. Simultaneous pulses are emitted side-by-side as a line of sight. After computer processing, a cross sectional graphic representation of the tissue's acoustic interaction is shown on screen.[1,2]
- The image is generated based on time of sound wave travel and echo intensity. Time is reproduced by position of the pixels on the monitor and intensity of echoes is represented by brightness of the pixels. The image refresh rate ranges from 15 to 40 frames per second.
- Abdominal and pelvic ultrasound use curvilinear transducers that cause a fanning out of the ultrasound beam, covering a field of view wider than the transducer footprint. Frequencies usually range from 1 to 8 MHz for evaluation of deeper structures.
- Straight linear array transducers produce waves in a straight line and work at higher frequencies (5–13 MHz), allowing better resolution and less penetration. Use includes skin, soft tissue, musculoskeletal and thrombosis evaluations, and vascular access.
- A key component of successful ultrasound imaging is to amplify attenuated echoes, adjusting the time-gain compensation. Higher frequencies are attenuated by tissue more than lower frequencies.[2,3]
- Adjusting the time-gain compensation allows a better visualization of structures far from the transducer, generating a more uniform image rather than an image that is too bright near the transducer that becomes progressively dark for further structures.

M-Mode

- A motion mode, M-Mode, is a continuous linear grey-scale display of amplitude from each depth along a scan line over time, with high temporal resolution due to a fast frame refresh rate.[5]
- Mostly used in echocardiography in order to measure cardiac parameters during the stages of the cardiac cycle.

Doppler

- The Doppler effect is a shift in the frequency of a transmitted sound wave based on the velocity of the reflecting object that it strikes. That shift depends on the angle of the transducer relative to the object in motion.[2]
- In most clinical circumstances, the angle between the transducer and the direction of motion should be less than or equal to 60° in order to get an accurate representation of flow characteristics. That can be achieved either manually or electronically steering the beam.[2,3]
- Spectral Doppler display is a graphic representation of flow in waveform. It is commonly used to provide information about peripheral vascular resistance of the tissues. The resistive index is the most used index of vascular resistance in clinical practice.
- Color Doppler allows for an evaluation of the velocity and direction of a moving object. It uses a color map superimposed to the real-time B-mode image: red is for motion towards the transducer and blue for motion away from it.
- In Color Doppler, the greater the velocity of the motion, the brighter is the color displayed. This mode is useful in characterizing blood flow in various organs and large vessels. It also detects fluid flow, i.e., ureteral jet flows of urine emerging from the ureteral orifices.[2,3]
- Power Doppler assigns the amplitude of frequency change to a color map. It does not allow evaluation of velocity or direction of the flow, but is more sensitive for detecting the density and presence of the blood to evaluate areas of ischemia.

Practical Algorithm(s)/Diagrams

Characteristic of an ultrasound wave

Number of cycles per second = frequency

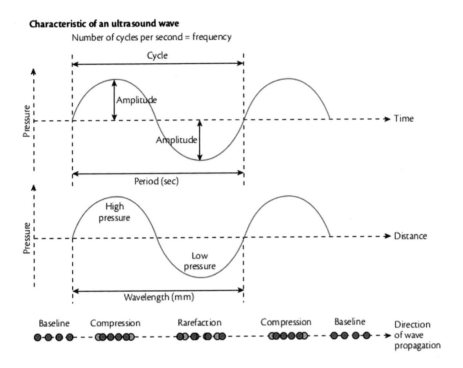

Fig. 1. Characteristics of an US wave.

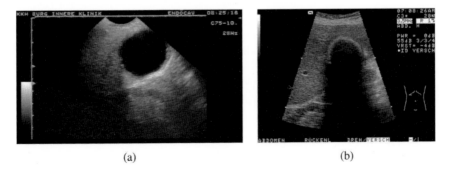

(a) (b)

Fig. 2. Artifacts in US — (a) Increased through transmission (pancreatic cyst); (b) Acoustic shadow (porcelain gallbladder).

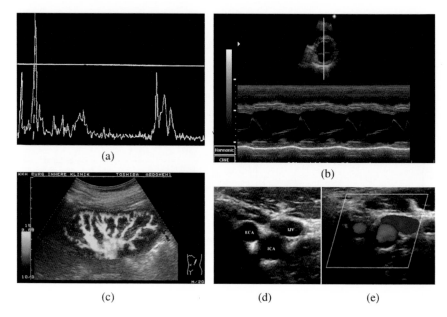

Fig. 3.　US Modes — (a) A-Mode (retina); (b) M-Mode (cross section of mitral valve); (c) Power Doppler (blood flow in the kidney); (d) B-Mode, (e) Color Doppler (internal and external carotid arteries and internal jugular vein).

Review of Current Literature with References

References

1. Wells, P.N. and H.D. Liang, Medical ultrasound: imaging of soft tissue strain and elasticity. *J R Soc Interface*, 2011, **8**(64): 1521–49.
2. Fulgham, P.F., Physical Principles of Ultrasound, in *Practical Urological Ultrasound*, P.F. Fulgham and B.R. Gilbert, Editors. 2013, Humana Press: New York.
3. Kim F.J., Rove K, and Sehrt D.E. Intraoperative urologic ultrasound, in *Practical Urological Ultrasound*, P.F. Fulgham and B.R. Gilbert, Editors. 2013, Humana Press: New York.
4. Terris, M.K., Principles of prostate ultrasound, in *Prostate biopsy*, J.S. Jones, Editor. 2008, Humana Press: Totowa, NJ.
5. Garbi, M., The general principles of echocardiography, in *The EAE Textbook of Echocardiography*, L. Galiuto, Editor. 2011, Oxford University Press: Oxford.

Chapter **13**

Echocardiography

*Greg Myers, MD**

**Assistant Professor of Surgery, University of Colorado School of Medicine*

Take Home Points

- Echocardiography should be performed by qualified physicians who are experienced in safe use of the equipment and interpreting the images.
- TTE (transthoracic echocardiography) and TEE (transesophageal echocardiography) should be considered when it may provide information for medical or surgical interventions.
- Echocardiography utilization starts in the emergency department (FAST — focused assessment with sonography for trauma) and continues in the OR and SICU.
- TTE is noninvasive and TEE is minimally invasive.
- Echocardiography is an invaluable tool that gives real-time, continuous information in the management of critically ill patients.
- The use of echocardiography helps not only to diagnose but also rule out clinically significant pathology. Because it is continuous, the response of the heart to interventions (e.g., volume loading, inotropes) may be assessed real-time.

Contact information: Denver Health Medical Center, 777 Bannock Street, Denver, CO 80204; Tel.: 303-602-1102, email: greg.myers@dhha.org

- Echocardiography helps provide information about regional and global cardiac function, valvular disease, pericardial pathology, pulmonary dysfunction and volume status.

Background

History

- TEE has been used in the operating room for three decades.
- Over the years many practice guidelines have been established by the American Society of Anesthesiologist (ASA) and Society of Cardiovascular Anesthesiologist (SCA) for perioperative TEE.
- The National Board of Echocardiography (NBE) has developed basic certification in TEE but is limited to anesthesiologists.

Indications

- TEE for noncardiac surgery (ASA):
  - o TEE may be used when the nature of the planned surgery or the patient's known or suspected cardiovascular pathology might result in severe hemodynamic, pulmonary, or neurologic compromise.
- Unexplained life-threatening circulatory instability.
- Unexplained persistent hypotension.
- Known or suspected CV pathology — hemodynamic, pulmonary, or neurological compromise.
- Persistent unexplained hypoxia.
- Evaluation of suspected aortic injury.

Safety

- TEE risk versus benefit should always be considered when placing a probe.
- Few contraindications exist for placement of the TEE probe and are associated mainly with esophageal or gastric pathology.
- Complications of TEE include dental, oropharyngeal, and esophageal trauma.
- Other complications such as cardiovascular stress, hypoxia and aspiration may be prevented by a secure airway and the use of appropriate sedation.
- Severe complications are rare with mortality of < 1 per 10,000 patients and morbidity of 2–5 per 1,000 patients (Scott T. Reeves *et al*. Basic perioperative

transesophageal echo. exam: A consensus statement of the ASE and the SCA. *J Am Soc Echocardiogr* 2013; **26**: 443–456).

Probe insertion

- The probe is inserted in the same manner as a gastroscope.
- If resistance is met, it may be necessary to perform a jaw thrust, change neck flexion or extension, or insert under direct view with a laryngoscope.

Probe manipulation

- Manipulation of the TEE probe can be performed by rotating, advancing, withdrawing, anteflexion or retroflexion (large circular knob), flexion to the right or left (small circular knob).

Multiplane imaging angle

- You can change the two-dimensional angle from 0° to 180° degrees.
- This will allow different cross sectional images at the same probe location.

Main Body

Transesophageal echocardiogram

Views

- American Society of Echocardiography and the Society of Cardiovascular Anesthesiologists recommend 11 views for the Basic Perioperative Transesophageal Examination (Fig. 1).
- Four main views with angle change or small adjustments will be sufficient in most clinical situations.
  - o **Mid-Esophageal Four Chamber (ME 4C–0°)**
    - ▪ Diagnostic information:
      - ⇨ Chamber volume
      - ⇨ Valvular function (Color Flow Doppler)
      - ⇨ Left Ventricular (LV) and Right Ventricular (RV) systolic function
      - ⇨ Regional Wall Function (infero-septal and anterolateral)
      - ⇨ Pericardial effusion

- Mid-Esophageal Long-Axis (ME LAX–120°)
    - By changing the angle (60–120°) you will acquire three views (ME Two Chamber, ME Mitral Commissure, ME LAX).
    - Diagnostic information
        - ⇨ Volume
        - ⇨ LV function
        - ⇨ Left Ventricular Outflow Track
        - ⇨ Aortic and Mitral Valve
- Transgastric Midpapillary Short-Axis (TG SAX – 0°)
    - **Advance the probe into stomach then slightly anteflex the probe.**
    - Diagnostic information.
        - ⇨ Volume
        - ⇨ LV function
        - ⇨ Regional Wall Abnormality
        - ⇨ Pericardial effusion
- Descending Aortic Short-Axis (– 0°)
    - **Obtain the Mid-esophageal four chamber view then rotate the probe toward patient's left posterior.**
    - Diagnostic information.
        - ⇨ Traumatic Aortic Rupture
        - ⇨ Dissection
        - ⇨ Pleural effusion

Transthoracic echocardiography

Views

- Windows
    - Parasternal
        - Short-Axis (papillary muscle) = TEE Transgastric midpapillary short-axis (TG SAX).
            - ⇨ Long-Axis = TEE Mid-esophageal long-axis (ME LAX)
    - Apical/Subcostal
        - ⇨ Four Chamber = TEE Mid-esophageal four chamber (ME 4C)

Pathology

- TEE/TTE can quickly detect and rule out clinically significant pathology.
- **Volume**
  - o Hypovolemia is a common cause of hemodynamic instability.
  - o TG Midpapillary SAX view is particularly useful in the diagnosis and treatment of hypovolemia and wall motion abnormalities.
  - o LV end-diastolic area is a good indirect measurement of LV preload.
- **Ventricular Function**
  - o **Left Ventricle**
    - Although quantitative measures of function are used, qualitative estimations of systolic function are extremely useful.
    - TG Midpapillary SAX view provides a global diagnostic evaluation of the LV and may identify which patients need inotropic intervention.
    - TEE provides early recognition of cardiac ischemia.
    - Concentric LV wall thickening (TG SAX) indicates good LV function.
  - o **Right Ventricle**
    - Evaluating the shortening of the corner of the tricuspid valve to the apex of the ventricle (ME 4C) helps assess the RV function.
    - RV dilation may indicate increased afterload (Pulmonary emboli), RV failure or volume overload.
- **Valvular Lesions**
  - o Color Flow Doppler should be utilized during evaluation of valves.
  - o Quantitative assessments of valves is not needed but visually being able to recognize significant valvular pathology will help in medically managing patients.
- **Pulmonary Embolism**
  - o TEE is not the gold standard for diagnosis of a pulmonary embolism but may help guide treatment in the acute situation.
  - o Saddle emboli may be visualized in the ME Ascending Aortic SAX but more likely to present with TEE finding of:
    - RV dilation and hypokinesis (four Chamber).
    - Possible LV hypovolemia, Tricuspid Regurgitation.
- **Aortic Trauma**
  - o TEE is considered a reliable accurate diagnostic tool for aortic trauma (traumatic aortic rupture, dissection, aneurysm) although visualization of

the distal ascending aorta and aortic arch can be technically difficult (bronchial air).

○ When evaluating for aortic trauma, verification of pathology in two views is suggested (ME Desc Aortic SAX and LAX).

- **Pericardial Effusion**

  ○ Presents as a hypoechoic outline of the heart (ME four chamber, TG SAX).

    ▪ Pericardial Tamponade — RA and RV collapsed with restrictive LV.

- **Pleural Effusion**

  ○ ME Descending Aortic SAX helps visualize and assess fluid accumulation in the lung fields.

Practical Algorithm(s)/ Diagrams

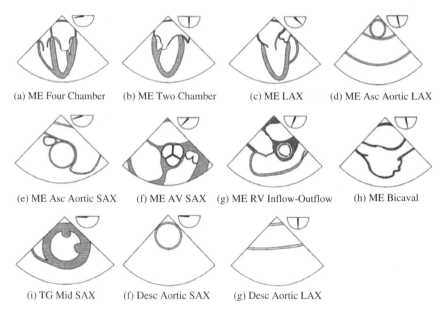

(a) ME Four Chamber   (b) ME Two Chamber   (c) ME LAX   (d) ME Asc Aortic LAX

(e) ME Asc Aortic SAX   (f) ME AV SAX   (g) ME RV Inflow-Outflow   (h) ME Bicaval

(i) TG Mid SAX   (f) Desc Aortic SAX   (g) Desc Aortic LAX

Fig. 1.   Commonly obtained echocardiographic views.

Review of Current Literature with References

- Catoire *et al.*: Prospective study of 70 trauma patients with multiple injuries.

Divided in two groups:

- o High suspicion group: patent or suspected thoracic or mediastinal injury
- o Low suspicion group: no sign of chest wall, pulmonary or cardiothoracic injury
    - TEE revealed new diagnoses in 70% of patients of Group 1 and 33% of Group II.
    - TEE both discovered and ruled out myocardial contusions and aortic injuries.
    - Severe hypovolemia, left ventricular dysfunction and pericardial effusions were commonly observed.

Authors concluded:

"TEE is of utmost importance in multiple injury patients, with or without any evidence of thoracic or mediastinal injury, providing safe and rapid examination of the mediastinal structures and evaluation of the hemodynamic status."

(Catoire, P, Orliaquet, G *et al.* Systematic transesophageal echocardiography for detection of mediastinal lesions in patients with multiple injuries. *J Trauma.* 1995; **38**: 96–102.)

- Richens *et al.*: Retrospective review of 132 cases of aortic rupture due to blunt chest trauma in MVCs in the UK.

Results:

- 2% survival rate for Blunt traumatic aortic rupture.
- TEE rapidly and accurately diagnosed these aortic injuries by direct visualization of dissection, intimal/medial flap, aortic wall hematoma or intraluminal thrombus or debris.

(Richens D *et al.* Rupture of the aorta following road traffic accidents in the United Kingdom 1992–1999. The results of the co-operative crash injury study. *Eur J Cardiothorac Surg* 2003; **23**: 143–148.)

- Memtsoudis and Rosenberger *et al.*: Retrospective review of 22 patients with intraoperative cardiac arrest during noncardiac surgical procedures who underwent TEE during the course of resuscitation.

Results:

- TEE established a suspected primary diagnosis in 19 of the 22 patients.
- Findings aided in further management in 18 patients, including specific surgical interventions in 12.
- Six had signs of MI on TEE, 3 underwent emergent CABP, 1 received IABP and medical management.
- Pulmonary emboli was diagnosed in 9 patients, 4 underwent emergent embolectomy.
- Two had pericardial tamponade treated with pericardiotomy.
- Two were diagnosed with hypovolemia leading to aggressive fluids.
- Overall, 14 of 22 patients survived the OR, 7 were discharged from the hospital.

(Memtsoudis, SD, Rosenberger, P *et al*. The usefulness of transesophageal echocardiography during cardiac arrest in noncardiac surgery. *Anesth Analg* 2006; **102**: 1653–1657.)

Chapter 14

Central Venous Cannulation

Molly E. W. Thiessen, MD* and Shea Cheney, MD†

**Assistant Professor of Emergency, University of Colorado School of Medicine,
†Emergency Department Resident, Denver Health Medical Center*

Take Home Points

- Central venous catheterization (CVC) is useful in the acute resuscitation and long-term management of patients.
- Select the appropriate site in each individual patient to avoid specific complications and common pitfalls, as well as minimize infection risk [Chapter 10-(viii)].
- Use real-time ultrasound guidance to decrease the risk of complication, line failure and procedure time.
- Use sterile technique and bundling measures to decrease the risk of catheter associated blood-stream infections.
- Place CVCs using the classically described Seldinger Technique.

Contact information: Denver Health Medical Center, Department of Emergency Medicine, 777 Bannock Street, Denver, CO 80204; Tel.: 303-602-7142, email: molly.thiessen@dhha.org; sheajcheney@gmail.com

Background

- Developed thirty years ago, CVC is a key tool in the management of patients with both life-threatening conditions and chronic illnesses.
- CVC is often used to aid in the resuscitation of several conditions such as hemorrhage, volume loss, hypothermia and sepsis. CVC also allows for the placement of transvenous pacemakers and pulmonary artery catheters to monitor hemodynamic and volume status [Chapter 5-(iii)].
- In several clinical scenarios, CVC is preferred to peripheral venous access such as in patients with major burns, intravenous drug users with difficult access, and patients requiring frequent, long-term blood draws.
- The incorporation of ultrasound has made attaining central access both safer and more successful.
- CVC is not without risk. Patients with distorted anatomy, bleeding disorders, anti-coagulation therapy and prior long-term venous cannulation may not be ideal candidates for CVC. Importantly, antibiotic-impregnated catheters should not be used in patients with allergies to the respective antibiotic.
- Preferred anatomical locations for CVC placement can vary based on the clinical scenario.

Main Body

Preparation

- **Gather Supplies:**
  - Most commercially available CVC kits will have all necessary supplies:
    - Chlorhexidene skin prep
    - Full-body fenestrated sterile drape
    - 1% lidocaine without epinephrine
    - 5 mL syringe for anesthetic
    - Needles for anesthetic
    - 5 mL syringe for venous puncture
    - 18 gauge needle for venous puncture
    - 11-blade scalpel
    - Dilator
    - Guidewire
    - Catheter
    - Catheter clamp
    - Suture

o Use a commercially available sterile ultrasound probe cover.

o Many kits do not contain hat, mask, sterile gloves and gown. These should be obtained and used for all CVCs.

o Use of a bundling system where these items are available in a central location or cart has been proven to decrease catheter-related infections.

- **Site Selection**

  o Internal Jugular (IJ) Vein

    ▪ The IJ vein has good external landmarks, decreased risk of pneumothorax [versus subclavian (SC) vein cannulation], and is an easily compressible site. With ultrasound guidance, it has improved success rates of placement than other locations.

    ▪ It may have a higher risk for infection and thrombosis than the SC vein.

    ▪ The IJ approach is contraindicated in patients with cervical trauma with swelling and anatomic distortion, and relatively contraindicated in patients with carotid artery disease.

  o Subclavian Vein

    ▪ The SC vein has good external landmarks in both the supra- and infra-clavicular approaches.

    ▪ It is considered a blind procedure, and compression of the vessels is not possible.

    ▪ The SC approach is contraindicated in patients with previous surgery or trauma involving the clavicle, first rib, or SC vessels, radiation in this area, chest wall deformities, marked obesity or thin stature. Acute penetrating thoracic injuries are not a contraindication unless injury to the SC vessels in suspected. When possible, SC access should be obtained on the side of the injury to avoid bilateral pneumothoraces.

  o Femoral Vein

    ▪ The femoral vein has good external landmarks, and given the easy access to the vessels for compression, is a good site for use in coagulopathic patients.

    ▪ Femoral central venous access has the highest risk for infection and thrombosis, and does not allow for reliable central venous pressure (CVP) monitoring.

    ▪ The femoral approach is contraindicated in patients with intraabdominal hemorrhage, injury to the IVC or to the pelvis or pelvic vessels, or deep venous thrombosis.

- **Use of Ultrasound vs. None**
  - o Use of ultrasound for placement of CVCs has been shown to
    - ▪ Increase the safety of the procedure.
    - ▪ Decrease complications associated with the procedure.
    - ▪ Decrease the time to completion of the procedure.
  - o A recent report from the Agency for Healthcare Research and Quality (AHRQ), which listed safety practices that were most highly rated in terms of strength of evidence, placed use of ultrasound for all CVCs eighth on their list.
  - o Ultrasound guidance should be used in the placement of all CVCs, unless the emergent nature of the procedure (i.e. cardiac arrest) precludes the use of ultrasound.

Technique

- Perform a "pre-scan" with ultrasound prior to sterile prep and drape to identify the target vessel and ensure its patency.
  - o Note that normal veins will collapse completely under pressure from the ultrasound probe, while arteries will remain patent and often pulsate under pressure from the probe.
- Perform a sterile prep of intended cannulation site, and place a full-body fenestrated drape.
- Don mask, hat, sterile gown and gloves.
- Prepare kit
  - o Flush each lumen of your catheter to ensure patency and functionality.
  - o Arrange items in kit in such a way that they are easily accessed during the procedure.
  - o Place sterile cover on ultrasound probe.
  - o Estimate depth of insertion of catheter using patient size/landmarks.
- Place patient in 10–20° of Trendelenberg.
- Use ultrasound to confirm your insertion site.
  - o Note the location of the vein relative to the artery, as well as its depth from the skin surface.
- Anesthetize the insertion site.

- Using ultrasound guidance, insert needle and syringe into skin, following their trajectory into the identified vessel. Apply steady negative pressure on the syringe as you advance the needle.
  - o Tissue motion will help you identify the path of the needle, and ring-down artifact will help you identify the needle itself (see Fig. 1). Identify your needle tip prior to advancement.
  - o If you cannot identify your needle tip, fan the probe to identify the needle, or pull the needle back to the skin and redirect it. Do not fan the needle through the soft tissues near large vessels.
  - o Short-Axis Cannulation:
    - ▪ View the vessel in the short-axis.
    - ▪ Measure the depth of the vessel on the screen.
    - ▪ If using the free-hand technique, insert your needle at the center of the probe (in line with the cord) the same distance from the middle of the probe surface as the depth of the vessel at a 45° angle. Based on the Pythagorean Theorem (a triangle of three equal angles has three equal sides), this will ensure that your needle will appear on screen as it pierces the superficial wall of the vessel (see Fig. 2).
    - ▪ If using a commercially available needle-guide, select the needle-guide that corresponds with the depth of the vessel on the screen, attach it to the probe and advance the needle in the trajectory of the needle guide. Note that this angle will be significantly steeper than with the free-hand technique to ensure that your needle will appear on screen as it pierces the superficial wall of the vessel.
  - o Long-Axis Cannulation:
    - ▪ View the vessel in the long-axis.
    - ▪ Insert your needle at the base of the end of the probe, directing it toward the desired vessel.
    - ▪ You should see the needle under the probe through its entire course, visualizing it as it moves through the soft tissues and enters the superficial vessel wall (see Fig. 3).
  - o Observe for aspiration of blood as the needle penetrates the vessel.
  - o Remove the syringe and cap the hub of the needle with your thumb.
  - o Confirm nonpulsatile flow.
  - o Introduce the curved end of the guide-wire into the hub of the needle and advance the wire.

- ■ If resistance is felt, do not force the wire further. Remove the wire and replace your syringe to confirm placement within the vein with aspiration or use of ultrasound.
  - ■ If you are unable to remove the wire because of resistance, remove the needle and the wire as a single unit.
- o Advance the guidewire until at least a quarter of the wire is in the vessel, but not more than 18 cm. If you observe premature ventricular contractions (PVCs) on the monitor, withdraw the wire until the PVCs resolve.
- o Once the wire is safely in the vessel, remove the needle from the skin, holding on to the wire at all times.
- o At this time, ultrasound confirmation of the wire within the compressible vein is recommended.
- o Make a small skin incision at the site where the wire enters the skin, taking care to not cut the wire with the scalpel.
- o Advance the dilator over the wire and through the skin incision with a spinning motion. Hold onto wire at all times.
- o Remove the dilator and thread the catheter over the wire, and advance until the wire protrudes from the distal port (remove this port's cover). Hold on to wire at all times. Advance the catheter to the depth previously determined.
- o For triple-lumen catheters, simply remove the wire, pulling it through the catheter. For sheath-introducers, remove the entire dilator and wire together.
  - ■ If the wire does not easily come out, remove the entire catheter-wire unit together.
- o Attach the catheter to the skin with sutures and commercially available anchoring device.
- o Draw and flush each port to ensure patency and functionality.
  - ■ Take care to not introduce air into the patient's vascular system by holding syringes upright.
- o Place a sterile, semi-permeable dressing over the cannulation site.
- o Dispose of all sharps in the appropriate containers.
- o For IJ or SC CVCs, order a chest X-ray to ensure appropriate placement and rule-out pneumothorax.
- • Site-specific ultrasound and landmark guidance
  - o Internal Jugular Vein

- Ultrasound Guidance:

    ⇨ Place the probe in a transverse position over the triangle formed by the clavicle and the sternal and clavicular heads of the sterno-cleidomastoid muscle. Compress to identify the IJ.

- Landmark Approach:

    ⇨ Puncture the skin lateral to the carotid pulse, at the apex of the triangle formed by the clavicle and the sternal and clavicular heads of the sternocleidomastoid muscle, with the needle directed caudally just lateral and parallel to the carotid artery.

o Subclavian Vein

- Ultrasound Guidance, Infraclavicular Approach:

    ⇨ Place the ultrasound probe in the midclavicular line such that the superior edge abuts the clavicle, getting a short-axis view of the clavicle and the vessels below it. Slide the probe medially and laterally until the vessels below the clavicle are identified. Rock the probe to collapse and identify the SC vein.

    ⇨ Once the vein is identified, rotate the probe to line up with the SC vein's long axis. This will usually then form a Y with the clavicle as the SC vein courses inferiorly and laterally. Then cannulate the SC vein in the long-axis from the lateral edge of the probe. This technique is typically more lateral than the traditional landmark approach, but provides excellent visualization of the axillary and SC vein (see Fig. 4).

- Ultrasound Guidance, Supraclavicular Approach:

    ⇨ Place the probe in the transverse (or short axis) over the IJ in the neck, then slide inferiorly until the junction with the SC vein is visualized.

- Infraclavicular Landmark Approach:

    ⇨ Puncture the skin at the lateral portion of the deltopectoral trian-gle, with the needle directed just superior and posterior to the suprasternal notch.

- Supraclavicular Landmark Approach:

    ⇨ Puncture the skin 1 cm posterior to the clavicle and 1 cm lateral to the clavicular head of the sternocleidomastoid muscle, with the needle directed just caudal to the contralateral nipple, bisecting the calvicosternomastoid angle.

o Femoral Vein

  ▪ US Guidance:

    ⇨ Place the probe in a transverse (or short-axis) orientation over the femoral artery just below the inguinal ligament. Slide superiorly and inferiorly to identify the ideal puncture site and relationship to the femoral artery.

  ▪ Landmark Guidance:

    ⇨ Palpate the femoral artery 2 fingerbreadths below the inguinal ligament, puncture the skin 1 cm medial to this point at a 45° angle, with the needle directed toward the umbilicus.

Common pitfalls

- Short-Axis US Cannulation (see Figs. 2, 5)
  - o When using US for venous access in the short-axis, the most common pitfall is misidentifying the location of your needle tip.
  - o The US cannot distinguish which slice of the needle it is visualizing. It is therefore imperative that you cannulate the superficial vessel wall with the needle tip directly under the US probe, watching it real-time on your screen.
  - o The most common difficulty in this orientation is where the needle has penetrated the vessel already and the US shows the mid-shaft of the needle in the vessel lumen on the screen. This is indistinguishable from the needle-tip. In this instance, your needle tip has penetrated the deep wall of the vessel.
  - o Use real-time US guidance as described above or a commercially available needle-guide to avoid this pitfall.
- Long-Axis US Cannulation (see Fig. 6)
  - o When using US for venous access in the long-axis, the most common pitfall is to misidentify the position of your needle relative to the vessel.
  - o The US will demonstrate anything under the probe in the same plane. If your needle is just to the side of the vessel it will project on screen as if your needle is in the same plane, when it is actually next to the vessel or near the vessel wall instead of in the lumen.
  - o Avoid this pitfall by placing the vessel directly under your probe and placing your needle into the skin directly under the middle of the US probe.

- Mis-identification of artery versus vein on US

  o The best way to distinguish between artery and vein on US is compressibility. Only cannulate vessels that easily, fully collapse.

  o Color-flow and pulse-wave Doppler may help distinguish between arteries and veins in some instances; however note that central vessels appropriate for central venous access lie on or near a large artery, and are near the right atrium, so they will have some pulsatile flow on US.

  o Do not place a central line in a vessel that does not easily, fully compress.

- Poor US machine placement

  o Always place the US machine so that it will be in your direct line of vision while placing the central venous catheter, such that you can look down at your procedure and easily glance up at the US screen. In some cases, this will be on the other side of the patient.

  o Have an assistant run the machine for you once sterile.

  o Do not place the ultrasound behind you or to your far right or left such that you have to turn away from your procedure to view the US.

- Lack of understanding/knowledge of classic anatomic landmarks and relationships/overreliance on US

  o Knowledge of classic anatomic landmarks and relationships is essential for placement of CVCs, to avoid complications and trouble-shoot when things do not go as planned.

- Lack of understanding of the physics behind needle guides

  o Commercially available needle guides are designed to help your needle tip penetrate the superficial wall of the vessel directly under the US probe.

  o These devices calculate the two other sides of a triangle based on the depth of the vessel.

  o Choose the device that will match the depth of the vessel under the probe, understanding that some fine adjustments will be necessary.

Practical Algorithm(s)/Diagrams

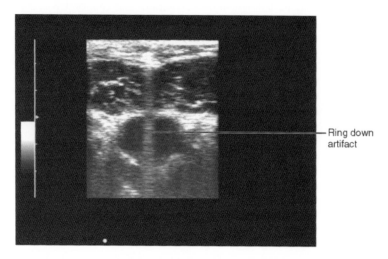

Fig. 1. An example of ring-down artifact during CVC placement.

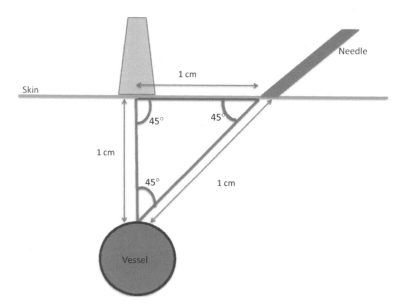

Fig. 2. For short-axis cannulation, measure the depth of your vessel, then insert the needle at a 45° angle at the same distance away from the probe, in this schematic 1 cm. This will ensure that your needle enters the vessel directly under the probe.

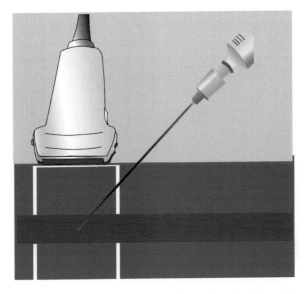

Fig. 3. For long-axis cannulation, insert the needle at the end of the probe, then watch it through its entire course as it traverses the soft tissues and enters the vessel.

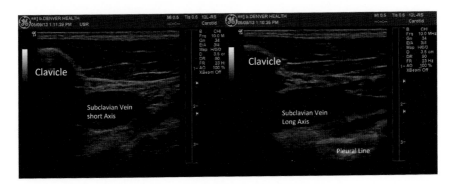

Fig. 4. The subclavian vein as visualized by US in its short- and long-axis. The vein should be localized in the short-axis, then cannulated in the long-axis.

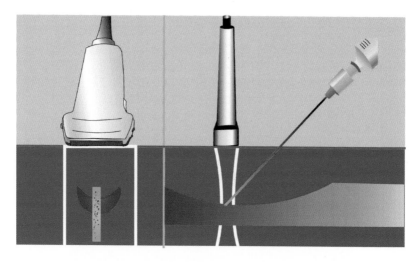

Fig. 5. Schematic demonstrating the appearance of the needle as it penetrates the superficial wall of the vessel directly under the US probe.

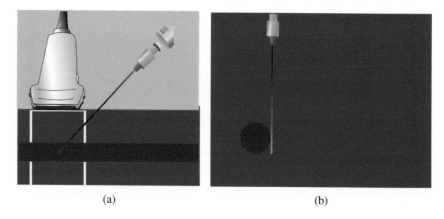

(a)   (b)

Fig. 6. In long-axis cannulation, if your needle is just to the side of the vessel it will project on screen as if your needle is in the same plane, when it is actually next to the vessel or near the vessel wall instead of in the lumen.

Review of Current Literature with References

Real-time two-dimensional US guidance for central venous cannulation — a meta-analysis

- Study Design
  - o All randomized studies that compared outcomes for patients undergoing CVC with either real-time US (RTUS) or landmark technique were pulled from PubMed, ISI Web of Knowledge, EMBASE and OVID EBM reviews through March 2012.
- Sample Size
  - o Twenty-six studies were included, with a total of 4,185 patients
- Results
  - o In adult patients, versus landmark technique, RTUS had pooled RR's:
    - Cannulation failure — 0.18 (95% CI: 0.10–0.32)
    - Arterial Puncture — 0.25 (95% CI: 0.15–0.42)
    - Hematoma — 0.30 (95% CI: 0.19–0.46)
    - Pneumothorax — 0.21 (95% CI: 0.06–0.73)
    - Hemothorax — 0.10 (95% CI: 0.02–0.54)
- Conclusions
  - o Real-time US guidance significantly decreases complications when used for placement of CVCs in adult patients.

Pulmonary artery catheters for adult patients in intensive care (Cochrane Review)

- Study Design
  - o All randomized controlled trials conducted in adults in ICUs, comparing management with and without a pulmonary artery catheter were included, based on usual Cochrane search methods.
- Sample Size
  - o Thirteen studies were included, with a total of 5,686 patients.
- Results
  - o Eight studies of high-risk surgery patients and five general intensive care studies were analyzed separately as subgroups for meta-analysis.

o Risk ratio (RR) for mortality in general ICU patients = 1.02 [95% confidence interval (CI) 0.96 to 1.09].

o RR for mortality in high-risk surgery patients = 0.98 (95% CI 0.74 to 1.29).

o Pulmonary artery catheters (PACs) did not affect general ICU LOS (four studies) or hospital LOS (nine studies).

o Four studies reported cost information, which was higher in the PAC groups. Of these four studies, two qualified for analysis. These did not show a statistically significant difference in hospital cost (mean difference USD 900, 95% CI -2620 to 4420, $p=0.62$).

- Conclusions

o Use of PACs does not improve mortality, hospital or ICU length of stay, or cost in ICU patients.

Catheter impregnation, coating or bonding for reducing central venous catheter-related infections in adults (Review)

- Study Design:

o Randomized controlled trials that compared any type of catheter with antimicrobial impregnation, bonding or coating to catheters with none of these modifications.

- Sample Size:

o Fifty-six studies were included, with a total of 16,512 catheters and 11 different types of antimicrobial impregnations.

- Results:

o Catheter impregnation reduced the rate of catheter-related blood stream infections:

▪ Absolute risk reduction = 2% (95% CI 3% to 1%)

▪ RR = 0.61 (95% CI 0.58 to 0.75)

o Catheter impregnation showed a significant reduction in the rate of catheter colonization in ICU patients:

▪ RR = 0.68 (95% CI 0.59 to 0.78).

o Catheter impregnation made no significant difference in:

▪ The rate of sepsis [RR 1.0 (95% CI 0.88 to 1.13)]

▪ Mortality [RR 0.88 (95% CI 0.75 to 1.05)]

- Conclusions:
  - o The use of impregnated catheters does reduce the risk of catheter-related blood stream infections and catheter colonization in hospitalized patients. However, the evidence shows that catheter impregnation has no significant effect on the reduction of clinically diagnosed sepsis or all-cause mortality in comparison to the use of non-impregnated catheters.

References

- Park, Robert S. *et al.* "Emergent procedures," Kendall and Cosby's the *Practical Guide to Emergency Ultrasound*, 1st Edition, Lippincott Williams & Wilkins, 2006.
- Lai NM, Chaiyakunapruk N, Lai NA *et al.* "Cather impregnation, coating or bonding for reducing central venous catheter-related infections in adults," (Review). *The Cochrane Collaboration* 2013; **6**, 1–175.
- Mallory DL, McGee WT, Shawaker TH *et al.* "Ultrasound guidance improves the success rate of internal jugular vein cannulation. A prospective, randomized trial," *Chest* 1990; **98**, 157–160.
- McNeil, Christopher R. *et al.* "Central venous catheterization and central venous pressure monitoring," Roberts & Hedges' *Clinical Procedures in Emergency Medicine*, 6th Edition, Chapter 22, Elsevier, Philadelphia, PA, 2014.
- Ma, John O., Mateer, James R. and Blaivas, Michael. "Vascular access," *Emergency Ultrasound*, 2nd Edition, McGraw Hill, 2008.
- Rajaram, Sujanthy *et al.* "Pulmonary artery catheters for adult patients in intensive care," (Review). *The Cochrane Collaboration* 2012: **2**, 1–59.
- Rothschild, Jeffrey M. "Ultrasound guidance of central vein catheterization," *Agency for Healthcare Research and Quality, Making Healthcare Safer: A Critical Analysis of Safety Practices*, Chapter 21, 2001, 245–253.

Chapter **15**

Arterial Cannulation

Bethany Benish, MD*

* Assistant Professor of Anesthesiology, University of Colorado School of Medicine

Take Home Points

- Peripheral arterial cannulation is a commonly performed procedure for monitoring critically ill patients.
- Arterial cannulation allows for continuous accurate blood pressure monitoring as well as vascular access for frequent blood sampling and repeat arterial blood gas analysis.
- An arterial catheter should be considered whenever continuous "beat-to-beat" assessment of blood pressure is necessary.
- The most frequent site of cannulation in both adult and pediatric patients is the radial artery but other sites including femoral, ulnar, axillary, brachial and dorsalis pedis can be considered.
- Arterial cannulation is considered a relatively safe bedside procedure. Potential complications of this procedure include air embolism, infection, hematoma formation, thrombosis, and hemorrhage.
- In addition to continuous blood pressure assessment, evaluation of the arterial waveform can provide information regarding myocardial contractility, hypovolemia, and hemodynamic changes related to cardiac arrhythmias.

Contact information: Denver Health Medical Center, 777 Bannock Street, Denver, CO 80204; Tel.: 303-602-1106, email: Bethany.benish@dhha.org

- The arterial waveform configuration changes as site of measurement moves more distal to the aorta. Peripherally measured systolic peak pressure is amplified and pulse pressure widens when compared to the central aortic pressure. This distal amplification must be considered when interpreting the displayed blood pressure.
- The incidence of arterial catheter related blood stream infections in the critically ill population is similar to that of short term central venous catheters. Aseptic technique should be taken during placement of arterial lines, especially when using a guidewire during placement. Further studies are necessary to determine whether chlorhexidine impregnated sponges at arterial catheter insertion site or antibiotic coated catheters would decrease blood stream infection rates.
- Ultrasound guided arterial cannulation improves first attempt success and may be especially useful in pediatric patients as well as critically ill patients with weak distal pulses.

Background

- **Principles of intra-arterial blood pressure monitoring**
  - o Direct arterial pressure monitoring consists of an arterial catheter, fluid-filled pressure tubing, a continuous-flush device and a pressure transducer.
  - o Intra-arterial blood pressure monitoring uses fluid filled tubing to transmit the force of the arterial pulse wave to a transducer. This transducer contains a diaphragm which is displaced in response to the applied pressure. This displacement is then converted into an electrical signal which, once amplified and processed, can be displayed as an arterial pressure tracing.
  - o Moving from the central aorta to peripheral arteries, the arterial pressure waveform becomes distorted. This progressive distortion is a result of both resonance (reflection of waves at arterial branch points) and changes in arterial wall compliance. As the pressure is transmitted distally, the systolic peak increases, pulse pressure widens, and the dicrotic notch is lost. This distal amplification is especially apparent when transducing the dorsalis pedis artery.
  - o The quality and accuracy of the transduced arterial waveform depends on the dynamic characteristics of the monitoring system (catheter, tubing, and transducer). System fidelity is affected by the stiffness of the catheter, tubing length (fluid mass), and number of connections and stopcocks in the system.

o Poor quality waveform (over/underdampened) can lead to a false reading and inappropriate interventions. An underdampened system (catheter whip) can lead to a falsely high systolic blood pressure while an over-dampened system underestimates the systolic and overestimates the diastolic blood pressure. Mean arterial pressure is least affected by the fidelity of the monitoring system.

o To avoid artifacts and inaccurate readings:

   ▪ Choose appropriate sized cannulas (20 g for radial/brachial/dorsalis pedis, 18 g for axillary/femoral).
   ▪ Use rigid tubing and minimize the length.
   ▪ Use only one stopcock per line and avoid air bubbles in tubing, stop-cock and dome.
   ▪ Use a continuous flushing system.
   ▪ Use a transducer with the highest frequency response.

o In order to ensure accurate arterial blood pressure reading, the transducer must be "zeroed" at the level of the right atrium or midaxil-lary line. Zeroing the system is performed by opening the transducer system to ambient atmospheric pressure. For sitting patients, the arterial transducer is placed at the level of the external auditory meatus (Circle of Willis).

o For every 15 cm in height that the transducer is moved up or down, there is a corresponding change of 10 mmHg in the blood pressure reading.

Main Body

Indications for invasive arterial blood pressure monitoring

• Anticipation of wide swings in blood pressure
• When tight blood pressure control is necessary
• Need for frequent blood draws or repeat analysis of arterial blood gases
• When noninvasive blood pressure monitoring is inaccurate (i.e., Morbid obesity, arrhythmias)
• Induced hypotension

Contraindications to invasive arterial blood pressure monitoring

• Inadequate circulation to the extremity
• Skin infection or burn at site of cannulation

Complications of invasive arterial blood pressure monitoring

- Distal ischemia
- Arterial thrombosis
- Hematoma formation
- Infection (catheter site or systemic)
- Air embolism
- Hemorrhage (due to disconnection)

Note: Severe atherosclerosis, diabetes, peripheral vasoconstriction (shock/ vasopressor use) all increase the morbidity of arterial cannulation.

- **Sites for arterial catheterization**
  - o Multiple arteries can be used for invasive arterial monitoring, including radial, ulnar, brachial, axillary, femoral, and dorsalis pedis. The radial artery is the preferred choice for invasive arterial monitoring due to its accessibility and collateral blood supply.
  - o Allen's test is used to evaluate the ulnar patency prior to radial artery cannulation. This test is performed by manually occluding both the radial and ulnar arteries at the wrist then releasing each artery to determine adequacy of collateral flow. If color returns to the hand within 5 secs, collateral flow is considered adequate. Although many clinicians use Allen's test prior to radial cannulation, the prognostic value of Allen's test has not been confirmed and there have been multiple reports of ischemic sequelae despite a normal Allen's test.
  - o Because of ischemic risk, ipsilateral ulnar cannulation should not be performed after multiple failed radial artery cannulation attempts.
  - o When evaluating alternative sites of arterial cannulation, there are specific clinical points to consider. The brachial artery does not have collateral circulation and risks median nerve injury. Axillary cannulation is considered safe for short-term use but, like the brachial artery, it does not have collateral circulation. The femoral artery is easily accessed particularly during low flow states, has low risk for ischemia but may have increased risk of infection. Dorsalis pedis artery does have collateral circulation (posterior tibial) but is relatively small making it difficult to cannulate and its distal location leads to artificially high systolic pressures.

- **Radial artery catheterization technique**
  - o Palpation of the peripheral pulse is necessary for percutaneous arterial cannulation. The use of doppler or ultrasound visualization may assist with identification of the artery when peripheral pulses are weak.

To cannulate the radial artery, the wrist is immobilized and dorsiflexed, the use of an arm board with rolled up towel or gauze can help with optimum positioning (Fig. 1).

o Prior to cannulation, the skin should be prepped using 4% chlorhexidine gluconate or povidone iodine and a sterile field should be created using towels or drapes (Fig. 2).

o The radial artery course is identified by palpation using the first and second fingers of non-dominant hand just lateral to the flexor carpi radialis tendon. It is best to cannulate the radial artery as distal as possible but at least 1 cm proximal to the styloid process to avoid penetrating the flexor retinaculum (Fig. 3). If the patient is awake, local anesthesia (1–2 mL of 1% lidocaine) can be used to infiltrate the skin over the anticipated site of cannulation.

o There are three techniques used for arterial cannulation: direct arterial puncture (catheter over needle), guidewire assisted (modified Seldinger technique), and transfixion-withdrawal. The guidewire assisted method is most commonly used in adults and large children. Commercially available kits with combined needle-guidewire-catheter system are commonly used (Fig. 4).

o Using sterile gloves, a 20 gauge arterial catheter is inserted at 30–45° angle to the skin toward the artery (Figs. 5 and 6). If using the commercially available arterial cannulation kits, a shallow skin nick using an 18 gauge needle can be used to prevent potential damage to the plastic arterial catheter on skin entry.

o The catheter apparatus is then advanced toward the artery until blood returns within the clear lumen of the catheter hub. The angle of insertion is then decreased slightly. Using the guidewire actuating lever, the guidewire is advanced into the vessel lumen. If resistance is met when advancing the guidewire, the needle is unlikely in the lumen of the artery and the entire apparatus should be withdrawn and cannulation should be reattempted.

o If using a 20 g angiocath, once a flash of blood is noted at the hub, the angle of insertion should be reduced slightly; the needle should then be advanced 1–2 mm to ensure that both the needle and the catheter tip are within the arterial lumen. The catheter is then advanced over the needle into the artery. If pulsatile blood returns but the catheter will not advance into the arterial lumen, a sterile guidewire can be advanced into the lumen of the artery, and the catheter advanced over the guidewire. Upon removal of the guidewire, pulsatile blood flow should be seen at the catheter hub.

o   An alternative technique involves transfixing the artery. Using this technique, the needle-catheter apparatus is advanced as above until an arterial flash is seen. The apparatus is then advanced completely through the front and back wall of the artery. The needle is removed from the catheter and the catheter is slowly withdrawn until pulsatile blood flow is obtained. The catheter is then advanced into the vessel lumen. As above, if the catheter will not advance easily into the arterial lumen, a sterile guidewire can be used.

o   Once arterial cannulation is confirmed, low-compliance pressure tubing should be tightly fastened to the catheter. The arterial catheter hub should then be secured with Steri-strips or sutures and covered with a clear sterile dressing.

Practical Algorithm(s)/Diagrams

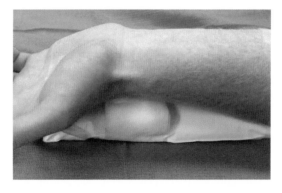

Fig. 1.   Dorsiflexion of wrist provides optimal position for radial artery cannulation.

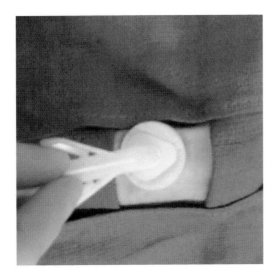

Fig. 2. Sterilize and drape area prior to procedure.

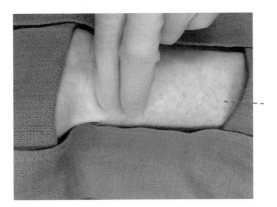

Fig. 3. Palpate radial artery using non-dominant hand.

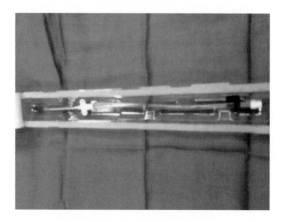

Fig. 4. Example of a commercially available combined needle-guidewire-catheter system.

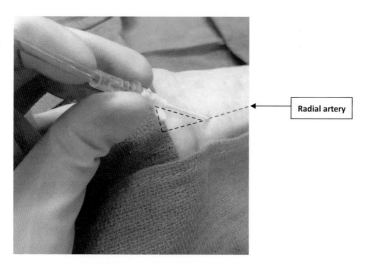

Fig. 5. Cannula is inserted at 30–45°. A shallow skin nick should be used to prevent potential damage to the plastic arterial catheter on skin entry if using the combined needle-guidewire-catheter.

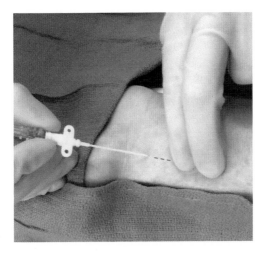

Fig. 6.

Review of Current Literature with References

- **Are arterial lines associated with blood stream infections?**
  - o In the past, arterial catheters were not considered a significant cause of bacteremia. Recent investigations however reveal that in critically ill patients who often require indwelling arterial catheters for >24 hrs, the risk of arterial catheter related blood stream infections approaches that of central venous line infections. To investigate this role, Esteve *et al.* performed a 2-year prospective non-randomized study of 1,456 ICU patients in which they evaluated the incidence of arterial catheter infections. They found an overall incidence of 3.53 per 1,000 arterial catheter days compared to 4.98 per 1,000 central venous catheter days. Days of insertion and ICU length of stay increased the risk of infection. They also compared radial and femoral arterial lines and found no significant difference in infection rates between the two sites. They did, however, find that femoral artery catheters were associated with more gram-negative arterial catheter related blood stream infections. This finding may affect the choice of therapeutic coverage in patients with an indwelling femoral line.
  - o Because of the significant role arterial lines may play in blood stream infection in the ICU setting, aseptic technique should always be used

during placement and some favor use of chlorhexidine impregnated sponges at the site of arterial cannulation.

Esteve, Francisco. Bacteremia related with arterial catheter in critically ill patients. *J Infection* 2011; **63**: 139–143.

Timsit JF, Schwebel C, Bouadma L, Geffroy A, Garrouste-Orgeas M, Pease S, Herault MC, Haouache H, Calvino-Gunther S, Gestin B, Armand-Lefevre L, Leflon V, Chaplain C, Benali A, Francais A, Adrie C, Zahar JR, Thuong M, Arrault X, Croize J, Lucet JC; Dressing Study Group. Chlorhexidine-impregnated sponges and less frequent dressing changes for prevention of catheter-related infections in critically ill adults: A randomized controlled trial. *JAMA* 2009; **301**: 1231–1241.

- **Ultrasound use has been shown to decrease complications in central venous line placement. What about arterial line placement?**
  - o Wan-Jie Gu and Jing-Chen Liu performed a meta-analysis of five randomized controlled trials, which included 370 patients, comparing ultrasound-guided arterial cannulation to traditional pulse palpation. When compared to palpation, ultrasound use was associated with an 84% improvement in first attempt success. Ultrasound guided radial catheterization significantly reduced the mean attempts as well as time to successful cannulation. It was also associated with a lower incidence of complication of hematoma. Overall, ultrasound was found to be superior to traditional pulse palpation in adults, children, and infants. Of note, the operators were experienced in ultrasound guided central line placement.

Wan-Jie Gu and Jing-Chen Liu. Ultrasound-guided radial artery catheterization: a meta-analysis of randomized controlled trials. *Intensive Care Medicine* 2011; **139**: 524–529.

  - o Others have found no significant difference in use of ultrasound vs. palpation of pulse, when evaluating the number of attempts at radial artery cannulation.

Edanaga M, Mimura M, Azumaguchi T, Kimura M, Yamakage M. Comparison of ultrasound-guided and blindly placed radial artery catheterization. *Masui.* 2012; **61**: 221–224.

  - o In pediatrics, the use of ultrasound for evaluation of radial artery diameter prior to arterial cannulation has been suggested to choose the appropriate catheter size. Varga *et al.* measured the distal radius internal diameter using ultrasound and found discrepancies between the diameter and the proposed catheter size in some individuals. Choosing the wrong size catheter could make cannulation more difficult and may increase potential injury to the artery.

Varga EQ, Candiotti KA, Saltzman B, Gayer S, Giquel J, Castillo-Pedraza C, Sanchez G, Halliday N. Evaluation of distal radial artery cross-sectional internal diameter in pediatric patients using ultrasound. *Paediatr Anaesth* 2013; **23**: 460–462.

Chapter 16

Tube Thoracostomy

Lisa S. Foley, MD*,† Michael J. Weyant, MD‡,§
Robert Meguid, MD**,†† and John D. Mitchell, MD‡‡,††

*Surgical Resident, University of Colorado School of Medicine
‡Associate Professor of Surgery, University of Colorado School of Medicine
**Assistant Professor of Surgery, University of Colorado School of Medicine
‡‡Professor of Surgery, University of Colorado School of Medicine

Take Home Points

- The goal of chest tube placement is to drain the pleural space.
- Air, blood, or fluid in the pleural space that impairs respiration requires evacuation.
- Larger tubes (32F) are useful for evacuating a hemothorax, whereas smaller tubes (24F) can be placed for pneumothoraces.

Contact information: University of Colorado Health Sciences Center, Division of Cardiothoracic Surgery, 12361 East 17th Avenue, C310, Aurora, CO 80045.
†Junior author, Tel.: 303-724-4682 (lab); 303-266-3667 (pager), 678-938-5967 (cell). Email: lisa.foley@ucdenver.edu
§Senior author, Tel.: 303-724-2800. Email: michael.weyant@ucdenver.edu
††Co-author, Tel.: 303-724-2799. Email: robert.meguid@ucdenver.edu, john.mitchell@ucdenver.edu

- Chest tubes should be placed under sterile conditions. In a conscious patient, local anesthetic is required for patient comfort, adequate dissection and controlled tube placement.
- Knowledge of anatomy and landmarks prevents complications. The ideal location for bedside chest tube placement is above the rib in the mid-axillary line of the 5th intercostal space. Counting rib spaces, marking the incision site, and/or draping in the nipple as a landmark can prevent malposition.
- Create an incision and subcutaneous tunnel that are wide enough to easily accommodate a finger and the chest tube. Palpation of the pleural surface ensures intrathoracic placement.
- Advancement of the tube should be in the posterior and superior direction, toward the apex.
- Securing the tube with heavy suture is an important step to prevent accidental removal.
- Complications of chest tube placement:
  - o Early:
    - Misplaced tube (kinked, too deep or too shallow, retroperitoneal, intraperitoneal, intercostal artery or nerve injury, pulmonary laceration).
    - Inability to evacuate pleural space (persistent pneumothorax, effusion, or hemothorax).
  - o Late:
    - Blocked tube
    - Empyema
- Common mistakes: inadequate local anesthetic, too small of an incision, inferior placement of incision, too narrow or excessively long subcutaneous tunnel, insufficient anchoring of the tube.

Background

- Respiratory mechanics rely on the bony and elastic components of the chest wall and lung. The smooth pleural surfaces of these two moving structures are directly opposed under normal conditions. This opposition is due to a negative intrapleural pressure (~2.5 mmHg at baseline, ~6 mmHg during inspiration) that keeps the lung fully expanded. Air, fluid, or blood in the pleural space diminishes the intrapleural force, allowing the lung to collapse away from the chest wall. The primary goal of chest tube placement is evacuation of the pleural space to restore respiratory mechanics.

- Tube thoracostomy indications can be broken down into four categories:

  o Pneumothorax: In general, moderate to large amounts of air in the chest cavity will impair respiration and require a chest tube. Exceptions to this rule can be made if the pneumothorax is very small and clinically insignificant or if it results from removal of a chest tube. On the other hand, a chest tube may be indicated to prevent a pneumothoraces in patients with multiple rib fractures on positive pressure ventilation.

  o Pleural Effusion: Edematous and parapneumonic effusions require drainage if there is significant lung compression or if there is concern for infection. Small, clinically asymptomatic effusions do not require intervention.

  o There is a lower threshold for evacuation of hemothoraces due to the greater risk of fibrinous consolidation, infection, and trapped lung.

  o The nature of pleural fluid can often be inferred by the inciting event. If it remains unclear, a chest CT can differentiate the fluid density and aid in decision-making.

  o Chest tubes should be left behind after any entry into the pleural space during an operation. Rarely, some surgeons suction out the pleural space and close it primarily at the end of a case; however, leaving a tube for drainage is the established practice.

  o Any pneumothoraces or effusions that do not require intervention should be followed with serial chest X-rays to monitor resolution.

- Special considerations:

  o Anticoagulated patients: Reversal of anticoagulation, if possible, is important prior to chest tube placement. The emergent nature of this procedure might prohibit reversal, in which case, extra precaution must be taken to avoid the neurovascular bundle.

  o Malignant pleural effusions: Effusions resulting from malignant processes have a tendency to reaccumulate after tube removal. In these cases, consideration should be given to placing a long-term tunneled pleural catheter or obliteration of the pleural space by pleurodesis.

Main Body

Preparation

- Review chest radiographs, reverse coagulopathy if present and patient is stable, obtain consent.

- Identify tube size (based on indications). Smaller tubes can be used for pneumothoraces, whereas larger tubes are required for viscous fluid.

Chest Tube Size	
Adult	24–36 Fr
Child	18–24 Fr
Newborn	12–14 Fr

- Collect necessary materials:
  - o For pre- and post-procedure: skin prep, mayo stand, drapes, pleural drainage system, dressing materials (xeroform, gauze, foam tape).
  - o Instruments for procedure: 10 or 11 blade scalpel, curved mayo scissors, hemostat, Kelly clamp, Adson or other skin forceps, needle driver.
- Position patient in the supine position with the ipsilateral arm maximally abducted.
- Mark the planned incision site, which should be located in the midaxillary line at the 5th intercostal space. Counting intercostal spaces is the most accurate way to find this location. It is often located slightly inferior to the nipple line, which can be used as a landmark.
- Prep and drape the chest wall.

Procedure

- Make a 2–3 cm incision overlying the 5th intercostal space in the midaxillary line. Carry this incision through the skin and subcutaneous fat.
- Sharply dissect with scissors to create a subcutaneous tunnel towards the rib and the intercostal space just superior to that rib. Explore the wound to assess depth and confirm appropriate direction of dissection. Continue dissection along the top of the rib, through the intercostal muscle layer.
- Switch to a blunt instrument, such as a Kelly or hemostat, to enter the pleural space. The dense parietal pleura requires considerable force to penetrate, so it is helpful to steady the non-operative hand against the patient, controlling entry. Once the pleural space has been entered, spread the clamp widely while withdrawing it to create an opening to accommodate the chest tube. Use the index finger to explore the wound and palpate the smooth pleural surface.
- Place a clamp on the distal end of the chest tube to occlude it during placement. Use a Kelly clamp on the perforated end of the tube to place it through the tunnel and direct it posteriorly and toward the apex. Advance the tube to

the apex and then withdraw it 2–3 cm. Ensure there are no chest tube holes outside of the chest wall. Note the centimeter mark on the tube that is at the skin.

- Secure the tube with heavy suture. Wrap xeroform around the base of the tube and cover that with sterile gauze. Apply tape over the entire incision and the tube at the chest wall to create an occlusive dressing and anchor the tube to the patient. Remove the distal clamp and connect the tube to the pleural drainage system. The tapered end of chest tubes is often not sized to fit the drainage system tubing and must be trimmed prior to joining the tubes.

- In general, newly placed chest tubes are put to −20 cmH$_2$O suction. This may vary depending on the indication. The chamber must always be kept below the level of the patient to prevent backflow into the patient. Bubbles in the pleural drainage chamber are often seen as the pleural space is evacuated. Persistent bubbling is indicative of an air leak.

- Obtain a chest X-ray to assess tube placement and improvement in condition. Most chest tubes have a radio-opaque line through along them that is interrupted by the most distal drainage hole. This hole must be within the chest to keep a closed system. If it is outside of the chest wall, the tube should be removed and a new one placed under sterile conditions.

Practical Algorithm(s)/Diagrams

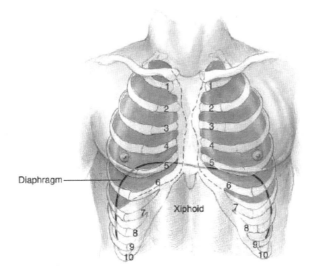

Fig. 1. Chest wall anatomy. This figure demonstrates relationships between anatomic landmarks and underlying structures.

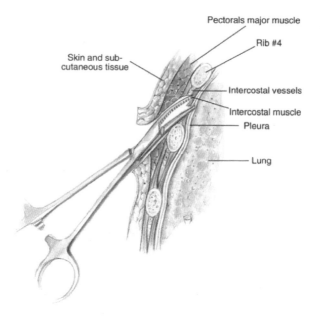

Fig. 2. Blunt dissection through chest wall. This cross-section demonstrates dissection planes encountered in creating the chest wall tunnel. It also highlights the importance of dissecting on the rib to avoid neurovascular injury.

Review of Current Literature with References

- Prophylactic antibiotics have not been shown to reduce pleural space infections following chest tube placement. A large prospective, randomized, double-blind, multi-center study of 224 patients undergoing chest tube placement for trauma indications evaluated rates of empyema in patients receiving cefazolin for the duration of the tube or for 24 hours surrounding placement. This study found a very low rate of empyema overall (2.6%) and failed to show a statistically significant reduction in empyema or pneumonia in patients receiving cefazolin prophylaxis, though no infectious complications occurred in the group receiving antibiotics for the duration of the tube. This study had insufficient patient accrual and was, therefore, susceptible to Type II error. A conclusion from this trial is that large numbers of patients would have to be treated to prevent one empyema due to the low rate of the complication.
- It is unclear if chest tube size (within the range appropriate for patient size) affects outcomes in patients with pneumothoraces or hemothoraces. One large

prospective observational study evaluated pain scales, tube related complications (pneumonia, empyema, retained hemothorax), and need for additional intervention in patients with small (28–32 Fr) versus large (36–40 Fr) chest tubes. Their study included 353 chest tubes placed in 293 patients and found no differences in numbers of small versus large tubes placed for each indication. Patients in both groups (small versus large) reported similar pain scores and had similar rates of retained hemothoraces (11.8% vs. 10.7%; adj. p 0.981). This study concluded that tube size for open thoracostomy did not affect outcomes. More studies are needed to address this question.

- o Data support the use of percutaneous pigtails catheters for pediatric patients and malignant pleural effusions. Urgency, severity of the pleural process, and availability of resources may prohibit percutaneous thoracostomy; however, greater consideration should be given to less invasive techniques in these populations.

- Chest tube complication rates are reported as occurring in 6% to 37% of procedures. A large, prospective and retrospective observational study of 242 tube thoracostomies performed by emergency medicine residents reported an overall complication rate of 37%. Of these complications, excessively deep tube advancement was the most common immediate complication, occurring in 10.7% of cases, and reaccumulation of pneumothorax was the most common delayed complication, occurring in 14.5% of cases. Tube manipulation or additional tube placement was only required in half of the reported complications (19%). Major complications requiring transfusion or surgical intervention were relatively rare (1.7%) and there were no deaths. This study identified the most common complications encountered and highlighted the relatively low rate of serious complications in a training environment.

References

- Sethuraman, K. N. *et al.* Complications of tube thoracostomy placement in the emergency department. *J Emerg Med* **40**, 14–20 (2011).
- Millikan, J. S., Moore, E. E., Steiner, E., Aragon, G. E. & Van Way, C. W. Complications of tube thoracostomy for acute trauma. *Am J Surg* **140**, 738–741 (1980).
- Maxwell, R. a. *et al.* Use of presumptive antibiotics following tube thoracostomy for traumatic hemopneumothorax in the prevention of empyema and pneumonia — a multi-center trial. *J Trauma Inj Infect Crit Care* **57**, 742–749 (2004).

- Fitzpatrick, C. & Brasel, K. J. Chest tube insertion. *Oper Tech Gen Surg* **5**, 129–133 (2003).
- Dull, K. E. & Fleisher, G. R. Pigtail catheters versus large-bore chest tubes for pneumothoraces in children treated in the emergency department. *Pediatr Emerg Care* **18**, 265–267 (2002).
- Inaba, K. *et al.* Does size matter? A prospective analysis of 28–32 versus 36–40 French chest tube size in trauma. *J Trauma Acute Care Surg* **72**, 422–427 (2012).
- Van Meter, M. E. M., McKee, K. Y. & Kohlwes, R. J. Efficacy and safety of tunneled pleural catheters in adults with malignant pleural effusions: a systematic review. *J Gen Intern Med* **26**, 70–76 (2011).

Chapter 17

Lumbar Puncture

Daniel Craig, MD* and Kathryn Beauchamp MD†

*Neurosurgical Resident, University of Colorado School of Medicine
† Chief of Neurosurgery, Denver Health Medical Center

Take Home Points

- Maintain sterile precautions at all times.
- Correct patient positioning is extremely important when measuring pressure.
- Patients with decompressive craniectomy may herniate when CSF is removed from lumbar region, therefore this is a relative contraindication
- When concerned about intracranial hypertension, image patient's brain prior to LP attempt.
- In the situation of traumatic tap, you may drain some of the bloody CSF prior to collection for the lab.
- Management of post-LP headache is with hydration, caffeine and in most extreme circumstances patients may need to undergo blood patching.

Contact information: Denver Medical Center, University of Colorado Health Sciences Center, 777 Bannock Street, MC 0206, Denver, CO 80204; Tel.: (Kathryn Beauchamp) 303-436-5842, email: daniel.craig@ucdenver.edu; Kathryn.beauchamp@dhha.org

Background

- History: performed since the late 19th century, widespread clinical use and continued mainstay of diagnosis in suspected meningitis, obsolete uses include pneumoencephalography (replaced by modern CT/MRI capabilities).
- Indications:[1,2,7,8] suspicion of meningitis, ICP measurement and symptomatic relief in non-obstructive hydrocephalus — specifically pseudotumor cerebri, diagnosis of sub-arachnoid hemorrhage, workup of inflammatory/neoplastic CNS disease, administration of intra-thecal medication or contrast (i.e. CT myelography).
- Contraindications:[1,2] most feared complication is downward herniation caused by pressure gradient across tentorium or foramen magnum. Thus radiographic contraindications on head CT include midline shift, basilar cistern effacement, obstructive hydrocephalus, posterior fossa mass. Clinical evidence of impending herniation — deteriorating consciousness, pupillary changes, irregular respiration. Relative contraindications related to pressure gradient include brain abscess/cerebral aneurysm with risk of rupture causing disseminated infection/bleed. Other relative contraindications include coagulopathy, thrombocytopenia, local skin breakdown or superficial infection at site. LP is relatively contraindicated in patients with decompressive craniectomy due to risk of paradoxical herniation away from craniectomy site.[3]
- Anatomy: selection of lumbar spinal level based on access to intrathecal cistern distal to conus medullaris (normally found at lower 3rd of L1 vertebral body, ranging from T12—top of L3). Target level is most commonly L3-4 or L4-5. L5-S1 may safely be used as well. L4 spinous process identified at level of iliac crest in axial plane. Ideal needle trajectory in midline sagittal plane passes through consistent tissue layers which can be felt during procedure by experienced physician and include — skin, subcutaneous tissue, supraspinous ligament, interspinous ligament, ligaentum flavum, dura/arachnoid (felt and crossed as one layer usually).
- Complications:[1,2] herniation is most feared but exceedingly rare, post-procedural headache is most common — caffeine can be effective treatment. Others include hematoma, infection, injury to nerve root or conus, CSF leak.
- Equipment: LP tray is commonly stocked in any intensive care unit and will include spinal needle (usually 22 gauge), lidocaine, CSF tubes, regular and fenestrated drape, iodine or other skin prep, three-way stop cock and manometer, extra tubing, syringe and needles (filtered for drawing from glass vial).
- Pre-LP CT Indications: age >60, immune compromised, known CNS lesion, seizure within one week, abnormal level of consciousness, focal neurologic deficit, papilledema or suspected elevated ICP.[4]

Main Body

Preparation

- Consent: once indication for LP is confirmed, patient or proxy should be consented, making sure to mention the probability (rather than possibility) of post-procedure headache as a complication in awake patients.
- Labs/Imaging: Current labs should be obtained and reviewed. This includes platelet count, ptt/inr (goals vary by institution, typically at Denver Health aim for platelets >80, INR <1.5), and blood glucose (to compare to CSF glucose). Relevant imaging should be reviewed, such as head CT (for risks as mentioned above), and L-spine imaging if available especially in post-surgical patients — to identify any anatomic abnormalities (i.e. previous laminectomy or fusion, missing or abnormal bony structures).
- Equipment: ensure LP tray available and obtain sterile gloves, hat/mask, additional lidocaine, larger spinal needle (i.e. 20 gauge, or longer needle for obese patients).
- Monitoring: RN available to assist in monitoring patient and administering medications, continuous pulse oximetry for any patient given sedation.
- Orders: place orders for CSF labs in advance so relevant labels printed and available, order additional lidocaine and desired sedation (commonly 25–100 mcg fentanyl and 0.5–2 mg ativan, or morphine and valium).

Procedure

- Checklist:
  - Confirm LP indication, review contraindications and relevant imaging/labs.
  - Obtain consent, order desired sedation/csf labs/additional pre-procedure labs if necessary.
  - Position patient (default Left Lateral Decubitus) and identify/mark L3-4 space.
  - Prep and drape area and infiltrate with 1% lidocaine.
  - Pass spinal needle, confirm CSF return, replace stylet and leave in place.
  - Remove stylet and measure opening pressure (adjust positioning).
  - Remove CSF for diagnostic tests and/or therapeutic pressure relief.
  - Measure closing pressure.
  - Remove needle (turn bevel parallel to caudal nerve roots first), hold pressure for 2–3 minutes, place dressing over site.

- <u>Positioning</u>: lateral decubitus position preferred (and required if measuring accurate ICP). Ensure perpendicular orientation of hips/shoulders and identify sagittal midline plane at multiple levels to avoid disorientation especially after draping. Have patient or assistant draw knees up toward chest to help spread spinous processes. You may also use seated position with patient leaning forward onto support such as Mayo stand.

- <u>Site Prep and Local Anesthetic</u>: identify L4 process from iliac crest level and choose either L3-4 or L4-5 space to target. Prep site with iodine or chlorhexidine and infiltrate 1% lidocaine working superficially to deep tissues, attempt to numb to depth of periosteum along spinous processes if possible and allow adequate time for medication affect. Place opaque drape tucked along flank under target site and fenestrated drape over site such that it allows for sterile palpation of iliac crest during procedure for re-orientation.

- <u>Spinal needle placement</u>: advance needle at desired level through tissue levels mentioned previously in mid-sagittal plane. Needle should be angled slightly cephalad, commonly oriented toward umbilicus, with bevel turned in parallel with spinal column to facilitate atraumatic passing through ligamentous fibers and caudal nerve roots. ALWAYS advance needle with stylet in place. If spinous process reached, walk needle in sagittal plane inferiorly to slip underneath it through posterior ligaments. Commonly mentioned "pop" at perforation of the dura is often not felt. Once CSF space is confirmed, immediately replace stylet to minimize drainage and rotate bevel 90° toward the head. Note: smaller gauge needles may decrease risk of post-procedure headache, but larger needles facilitate tissue layer identification and ICP measurement.

- <u>Sampling and Measurement</u>: always measure opening and closing pressure whenever possible. Prepare manometer and stop cock with additional tubing if desired. With stylet in place, secure needle and reposition patient with legs extended and bed horizontal. Give time for patient to relax if necessary and treat pain from needle placement. Measure OP and remember that results from manometer will be in cmH_2O, not mmHg. Once pressure obtained, sample CSF serially into provided tubes #1–4. Volume removed depends on indication — in cases of therapeutic tap for non-obstructive hydrocephalus plan to remove up to 35–40 cc. Measure closing pressure and note total volume removed. Remove needle and hold pressure with gauze for a few minutes before dressing site with bandage provided in LP tray.

Post-Procedure Management

Patients previously have been instructed to maintain bed rest in supine position post-LP to avoid/minimize post procedural headache and prevent CSF leak as dural defect heals. However, recent literature suggests that there is no evidence to continue this practice and that return to mobilization as tolerated is preferred especially in children/adolescents.[5,6] In our practice, awake patients are advised to lay flat for 1–2 hours only for symptom control (headache) if needed. Otherwise, awake patients may return to activity as tolerated. As noted above, caffeine can be an effective medication in addition to more typical prn's.

CSF results

- Cytology: traumatic tap introduces both RBC and WBC into CSF, approximately 1 WBC per 1,000 RBC can be considered traumatic rather than pathologic. Decreasing RBC in sequential CSF tubes indicates likely traumatic etiology rather than evidence of subarachnoid bleeding. Xanthochromia in spun samples is consistent with SAH. Elevated WBC suggests infection or less commonly inflammatory/neoplastic process. More specific cytology tests can be ordered depending on suspected pathology.
- Protein: normal levels vary by lab, typically 15–60 mg/dL. Increased levels can suggest infection, inflammatory process, or neoplasm. Electrophoresis and more specific profiles can be ordered depending on suspected pathology.
- Glucose: normal CSF glucose is approximately 60% serum glucose. Decreased CSF glucose is consistent with but not specific to bacterial infection. Elevated glucose is not correlated consistently with any specific diagnosis.
- Culture/Gram stain: any bacteria on gram stain is abnormal and should be treated as active infection pending final culture results.

Troubleshooting

- Dry Tap: if unable to obtain CSF return, always re-orient to your target and ensure proper patient positioning. Most commonly, needle trajectory is off laterally to midline sagittal plan. Adjust patient's hips and shoulders and focus on identifying individual tissue planes as needle advances, use larger gauge needle on re-attempt to better feel tissue layers. You may try different position (sitting vs lateral recumbent) or moving up one level to L3-4. Also consider low intrathecal CSF volume (i.e. in post-op patients or with recent EVD or lumbar drain placement), post-surgical or post-traumatic L-spine with abnormal dura. Dehydrated patient can contribute to low CSF volume and difficult tap — consider IV fluids to rehydrate prior to re-attempt.

- Bloody Return: exceedingly uncommon to encounter arterial blood, most likely needle tip has found epidural venous plexus. If this is suspected, slowly remove needle while frequently stopping to check for CSF return. You can also use manometer to check if pressure is consistent with venous tip location. Bloody CSF either from traumatic tap or in post-craniotomy patients can appear quite dark, and if blood has pooled in lumbar cistern due to bleeding elsewhere in CNS, it will not clear from tube to tube.

- Abnormal pressure: recheck patient position and be sure patient is not bearing down (vasovagal). Be sure that the manometer system is attached correctly and stopcock is open.

Practical Algorithm(s)/Diagrams

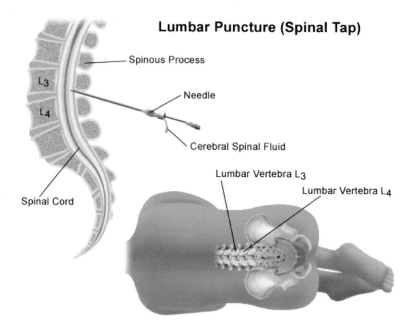

Fig. 1. Lumbar puncture [From HopkinsMedicine.org (http://www.hopkinsmedicine.org/healthlibrary/test_procedures/neurological/lumbar_puncture_lp_92,P07666/)].

Review of Current Literature with References

- Hasburn *et al.* review the utility of computed tomography of the head before lumbar puncture in adults with suspected meningitis (*New Engl J Med* 2001; **345**: 1727).

- Van Crevel *et al.* offer recommendations for indications to perform CT before lumbar puncture, grouped according to the safety and clinical utility of the procedure (*J Neurol* 2002; **249**: 129–137).

- D'Cruz and Vellore reported an awareness of the proper indications for lumbar punction both reduced the overall number of procedures performed and increased the number of positive procedures (*Acute Med* 2014; **13**: 113–117).

Bibiography

1. Cooper N. Lumbar puncture. *Acute Med.* 2011; **10**(4): 188–193
2. Wright BL, Lai JT, Sinclair AJ. Cerebrospinal fluid and lumbar puncture: a practical review. *J Neurol.* 2012; **259**: 1530–1545.
3. Oyelese AA, Steinberg GK *et al.* Paradoxical cerebral herniation secondary to lumbar puncture after decompressive craniectomy for a large space occupying hemispheric stroke: case report. *Neurosurgery.* 2005; **57**(3): E594.
4. Hasbun R, Abrahams J, Jekel J, Quagliarello VJ. Computed Tomography of the head before lumbar puncture in adults with suspected meningitis. *N Engl J Med.* 2001; **345**(24): 1727–1733.
5. Ebinger F, Kosel L, Pietz J, Rating D. Strict bed rest following LP in children in adolescents is of no benefit. *Neurology.* 2004; **62**(6): 1003–1005.
6. Teece S, Crawford I, Towards evidence based emergency medicine: best BETs from the Manchester Royal Infirmary: bed rest after lumbar puncture. *Emerg Med J.* 2002; **19**(5): 432–433.
7. Petzold A, Brettschneider J, Jin K *et al.* CSF protein biomarkers for proximal axonal damage improve prognostic accuracy in the acute phase of Guillian-Barre syndrome. *Muscle Nerve.* 2009; **40**(1): 42–49.
8. Chen JJ, Tubbs RS, Gordon AS, Dennithorne KH, Oakes WJ. Management of pediatric patients with pseudotumor cerebri. *Childs Nervous System.* 2012.
9. Spellberg B. Is computed tomography of the head useful for lumbar puncture? *Clin Infect Dis.* 2005; **40**(7): 1061.
10. Kastenbauer S, Winkler F. Cranial CT before lumbar puncture in suspected meningitis. *N Engl J Med.* 2001; **345**: 1727–1733.

Chapter 18

Inferior Vena Cava Filter

Charles J. Fox, MD,*

*Chief of Vascular Surgery, University of Colorado School of Medicine

Take Home Points

- Pulmonary embolism (PE) has been described as the third most common cause of death in patients who survive the initial 24-hour period after trauma.
- Certain subgroups of high-risk trauma patients are not candidates for deep vein thrombosis (DVT) prophylaxis or therapeutic anticoagulation.
- Retrievable inferior vena cava filters (R-IVCFs) presumably offer protection from PE during the post-traumatic period of greatest risk, while reducing the long-term complication (occlusion, migration, perforation) rate associated with permanent filter placement.
- Screening of high-risk patients, particularly those with spinal cord and/ or major pelvic/lower-extremity orthopedic injuries is thought to improve detection of DVT and reduce the risk of PE (0.14% vs. 0.22%).
- Patients who have a documented DVT (particularly those involving the popliteal or more proximal veins) and/or PE who cannot receive therapeutic anticoagulation are acceptable candidates for therapeutic filter placement.

Contact information: Denver Health Medical Center, University of Colorado Health Sciences Center, 777 Bannock Street, MC 0206, Denver, CO 80204; Tel.: 202-697-1456, email: Charles.fox@dhha.org

- Retrievable filters have gained popularity yet attempted retrieval is made in as few as one-quarter of patients, and technical issues (residual thrombus, angulation, in-growth) prevent retrieval in 10% to 25% of cases when attempts are made.
- One reason for filter displacement is inadvertent trapping of a wire during central line placement or exchange.
- Failures to retrieve filters have been attributed to tilt, strut malposition, detection of significant residual thrombus, or lack of follow-up.
- The rate of "loss to follow-up" was increased six-fold when the service of placing the filter was not responsible for the follow-up.

Background

- Trauma is known to be one of the strongest risk factors for pulmonary embolism (PE).
- A prospective study reported rates of deep venous thrombosis (DVT) as high as 58% among those who experience severe trauma without thromboprophylaxis.
- Current guidelines recommend low molecular weight heparin therapy for prevention of PE, but a small proportion of trauma patients who may be among the highest risk of venous thromboembolism (VTE) may have a definite contraindication to low-molecular weight heparin as a result of an ongoing risk of bleeding.
- The benefit of VTE prophylaxis in trauma patients may be overshadowed by the risk of excessive bleeding and opens the discussion for the placement of prophylactic inferior vena cava (IVC) filters.
- The increased use of IVC filters in trauma patients is well-documented and the Eastern Association for the Surgery of Trauma now promotes IVC filters in certain patients.

Main Body

- The use of IVC Filters in Trauma
  - Published clinical guidelines by the Eastern Association of Surgery of Trauma recommends insertion of prophylactic IVC filters in high-risk trauma patients who cannot receive anticoagulation therapy owing to bleeding risks and injury patterns associated with prolonged immobility. The introduction of temporary removable filters has been favorable as

long-term complication rates associated with lifelong indwelling devices have previously discouraged permanent filter placement for prophylactic indications. These concerns are particularly relevant to a young trauma population, and assume that temporary removable filters are actually removed in a timely manner. The decision to place a "prophylactic" vena cava filter (VCF) in a trauma patient requires a fundamental understanding of the risk/benefit ratio. In this review, the risk/benefit ratio is explored in the high-risk trauma patient.

- Scientific Evidence

  o Several reports now exist in the literature on the use of prophylactic vena cava filters in trauma patients. Six studies demonstrated a significant reduction in the incidence of PE in their trauma population compared with historical controls. Minimal insertion and short-term complications were reported, with 1-year patency rates ranging from 82% to 96%, and 2-year patency rates at 96% in prophylactic filters inserted in trauma patients. Moreover, a higher DVT rate was not seen in prophylactic filter patients compared with non-filter patients. A follow-up study with a minimum of 5 years in 199 patients showed that the filters were well-tolerated. Patients went on to live active lives, with a minimal migration of cava thrombosis. Prophylactic placement was associated with a low incidence of adverse outcomes and provided protection from fatal PE. The data presented herein would indicate that the risk/benefit ratio is favorable for the high-risk trauma patients. The problem is defining the high-risk patient. One trauma study identified four injury patterns that accounted for 92% of PEs: spinal cord injury with paraplegia or quadriplegia; severe closed head injury with a GCS score < = 8 for > than 48 hours; age > 55 years with isolated long bone fractures; and complex pelvic fractures associated with long bone fractures. Another retrospective review including 9,721 patients showed that the high-risk categories include head injury plus spinal cord injury, head injury plus long bone fracture, severe pelvic fracture plus long bone fracture, and multiple long bone fractures. These authors estimate that if they had used a prophylactic filter in these 2% of patients, a very dramatic reduction in PE would have been seen. They suggested that patients with an estimated risk of PE of 2% to 5%, despite prophylaxis, are reasonable candidates for prophylactic VCF placement, especially if conventional prophylactic measures cannot be used.

o Many years of experience with the Greenfield filter indicate that it has a patency rate of about 96%, a recurrent PE rate of 3% to 5%, and a caval penetration rate of about 2%. These complication rates were reasonable, but multiplied over the lifetime of a young patient, these rates could become important. One study indicated a significant amount of chronic venous insufficiency in long-term follow-up of prophylactic filter patients. However, with no non-filter group to compare with, whether the filter was the cause of this chronic venous insufficiency in this very high-risk group is not clear.

o The more recent literature on this subject discusses the bedside placement of filters. These studies showed that filters could be placed safely at the bedside, resulting in a decrease in operating room use and cost. The use of retrievable filters is particularly appealing to trauma surgeons whose patients are at high-risk for PE for a relatively short period. Few complications are reported with the retrievable filters yet poor follow-up and lack of actual retrieval have prevented their widespread application. To complicate matters, there is significant heterogeneity amongst studies with respect to complication rate and retrieval time.

o Overall, the current literature shows low complication rates with the use of prophylactic IVC filters in high-risk poly-trauma patients who may have contraindications to DVT prophylaxis. Filter-associated complications are uncommon and, when they do occur, they tend to be of limited clinical significance. Limited data supports a reduction in PE and PE-related mortality. Since the last systematic review, there has been increasing use of retrievable filters as well as the ability to safely retrieve them at longer intervals. Despite the addition of a few good matched-control studies, the literature is still plagued by a lack of high quality data, and therefore the true efficacy of prophylactic IVC filters for prevention of VTE in trauma patients remains unclear. Further studies are required to determine the true role of prophylactic IVC filters in trauma patients. For the moment, it appears that the use of IVC filters according to standardised protocols based on the existing EAST guidelines has resulted in a low rate of generally clinically insignificant complications (residual thrombus, tilt, migration), if not a definitive decrease in PE and PE-related death.

o No Class I studies exist to support insertion of IVC Filters in a trauma patient without an established DVT or PE. A fair amount of Class II and III data that may support IVC Filter use has been accumulated in "high-risk" trauma patients without a documented occurrence of a DVT or PE. High-risk injury patterns include severe closed head injury, spinal cord injury with paraplegia or quadriplegia, multiple long bone fractures or complex pelvic fractures with associated long bone fractures. At this time, we recommend consideration of IVC filter insertion in patients without a documented DVT or PE who meet high-risk criteria established by the Eastern Association for the Surgery of Trauma (EAST) and cannot be anticoagulated.

o Traditionally, IVC filters are placed using fluoroscopic guidance. Improvements in filter design and intravascular ultrasound technology has gained enthusiasm for intravascular ultrasound (IVUS) guided IVC filter insertion at the bedside. Although vena cavography is the standard imaging recommended by the Society of Cardiovascular and Interventional Radiology Standards of Practice Committee, the transport of critically ill trauma patients with high injury severity scores (ISS) on mechanical ventilation with invasive monitoring devices to and from the intensive care unit exposes the patient to excessive risk of iatrogenic complications. A number of reports have now shown that bedside insertion of IVC filters is safe, practical and cost-effective. IVUS localizes the renal veins with relative ease and is significantly more accurate than contrast venography for sizing the vena cava and determining the optimal site for filter placement while avoiding radiation iodinated contrast injections.

o The technique described by Jacobs and colleagues (*J Vasc Surg* 2007; **46**: 1284–6) is very reproducible. A 12.5-MHz IVUS probe (Volcano Therapeutics, Rancho Cordova, CA) is advanced transfemorally through the veins until cardiac motion is seen. The catheter is slowly retracted noting relevant venous anatomy (Fig. 1). The locations of the right atrium, the hepatic veins, and the right renal artery passing behind the cava are critically observed. The renal veins are typically 35–40 cm proximal and the iliac confluence is usually 15–20 cm from the femoral access. The IVUS is positioned just below the lowest renal vein and a sheath is advanced over the IVUS catheter until the sheath tip shadows the ultrasound image of the IVUS catheter. The sheath is then held in this position and the IVUS and wire are removed. The filter is advanced to the tip of the sheath and deployed once the sheath is withdrawn in pin-pull fashion. A radiograph confirms technical success. The required materials are summarized in Fig. 2.

- **Final Points**

  Pulmonary embolism remains such a high and constant threat in the trauma population, it is accepted that high-risk patients for DVT who cannot undergo prophylaxis are candidates for a vena cava filter placement. Likewise, those who have a documented DVT but cannot receive anticoagulation are candidates for a therapeutic vena cava filter. The perception that long-term complications are mitigated by temporary retrievable filters has resulted in widespread use. Data suggest that actual retrieval rates are significantly improved when the primary team ensures follow-up. Angulation, residual thrombus and in growth remain technical challenges that may prevent retrieval. Comparable long-term durability between permanent and temporary filters has not been proven. Although major complications (insertion DVT, recurrent PE, and caval thrombosis) remain low at 2–3%, filter migration and tilt may be underappreciated technical matters that render them ineffective for prophylaxis. Finally, there appears to be great practice variation with regard to screening for DVT, indications for vena cava filter placement, and the service responsible for the follow-up and removal. A prospective randomized clinical trial is needed to address many of these questions.

Practical Algorithm(s)/Diagrams

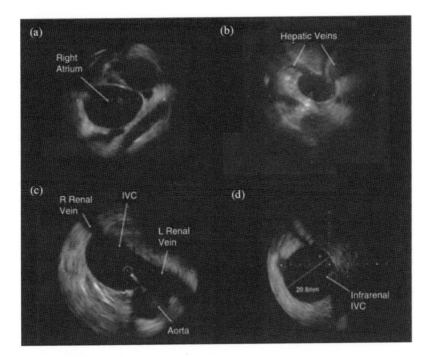

Fig. 1. Bedside IVUS guided inferior vena cava filter placement.
Imaging of IVC with IVUS to identify venous anatomic landmarks at the right atrium
(a) hepatic veins (b) renal veins (c) and infrarenal IVC above the iliac vein confluence
(d). (Reprinted with permission from: Passman MA, Dattilo JB, Guzman RJ, Naslund TC.
Bedside placement of inferior vena cava filters by using transabdominal duplex ultrasonography and intravascular ultrasound imaging. J Vasc Surg 2005; **42**: 1027–1032).

Materials for Bedside Placement
IVUS Machine, Volcano
8.2 Fr IVUS Catheter, Volcano
8 Fr 55 cm Brite Tip Sheath
Logiq E Portable Ultrasound, GE
US Probe Cover, Covidien
US Gel
Cook Celect IVC Filter, Femoral insertion
5 Fr. Pinnacle Precision Micropuncture Set, Terumo
Bentson Wire, 0.35", 260 cm
Heparinized Saline 5000 units/500 ml

Fig. 2. Inventory for bedside vena cava filter placement.

Review of Current Literature with References

- A retrospective review of retrievable vena cava filters in trauma patients evaluated practice patterns and outcomes as a AAST multicenter study. Of 446 filters, only 22% were actually retrieved and 31% were the result of no follow-up suggesting that the service placing the filter should be responsible for the follow-up and retrieval (*J Trauma* 2007; **62**: 17–25).
- A systematic review to compile the current literature on the usage of IVC filters for prophylaxis of venous thromboembolism in high-risk trauma patients. Twenty-four studies were included with the majority of the studies using the EAST guidelines to determine the need for IVC filter placement. IVC occlusion rate ranged 0–10%, among 16 of 1,430 patients across 12 studies (1.1%) concluding an overall low rate of filter-associated complications. Two studies reported tilt/migration rates of about 45% questioning the true effectiveness of prophylactic filters prompting the continued demand for high quality data (Injury, *Int J Care Injured* 2012; **43**: 542–547).
- A meta-analysis examining the comparative effectiveness of prophylactic IVC filters in trauma patients in eight controlled studies showing consistent reduction of pulmonary embolism and no significant difference in the incidence of DVT or mortality (*JAMA Surg* 2013).

- The Eastern Association for the Surgery of Trauma presented evidence-based clinical practice guidelines for the role of vena cava filter in the prophylaxis of PE. Authors concluded that no class I (prospective, randomized, controlled trial) studies exist to support the insertion of a vena cava filter in a trauma patient without an established DVT or PE. However, there was enough class II (prospectively collected or large retrospective with reliable data) and class III data to support its use in "high-risk" trauma patients. The working group recommended consideration of IVC filter insertion in those patients without a documented DVT or PE, who meet high-risk criteria and cannot be anticoagulated (*J Trauma* 2002; **53**: 142–164).

- A retrospective report the largest series of IVUS-guided IVC filter placement in a military multi-trauma population. The authors demonstrated that this technique is safe, expedient effective and should be used for critically ill patients who cannot be easily transported for minor procedures (*Vasc Endovascular Surg* 2009; **43**: 497–501).

- Haut E, Garcia L, Hasan S *et al.* The effectiveness of prophylactic inferior vena cava filters in trauma patients: A systematic review and meta-analysis. *JAMA Surg* 2014; **149**(2):194–202.

- Kindane B, Madani A, Vogt K *et al.* The use of prophylactic inferior vena cava filters in trauma patients: a systematic review. *Injury* 2012; **43**(5): 542–547.

- Riyad KJ, Jurkovich GJ, Velmahos GC *et al.* Practice patterns and outcomes of retrievable vena cava filters in trauma patients: an AAST multicenter study. *J Trauma* 2007; **62**(1): 17–24; discussion 24–25.

- Rogers FB, Cipolle MD, Velmahos G *et al.* Practice Management Guidelines for the Prevention of Venous Thromboembolism in Trauma Patients: The EAST practice management Guidelines Work Group. *J Trauma* 2002; **53**: 142–164.

- Aidinian G, Fox CJ, White PW *et al.* Intravascular ultrasound-guided inferior vena cava filter placement in the military multi-trauma patients: A single-center experience. *Vasc Endovascular Surg* 2009; **43**(5): 497–501.

- Jacobs DL, Raghunandan L, Motaganahalli MD *et al.* Bedside vena cava filter placement with intravascular ultrasound: A simple, accurate, single venous access method. *J Vasc Surg* 2007; **46**: 1284–1286.

Chapter 19

Percutaneous Tracheostomy

Clay Cothren Burlew, MD*

*SICU Director, Denver Health Medical Center,
Professor of Surgery, University of Colorado School of Medicine

Take Home Points

- Bedside percutaneous dilational tracheostomy (PDT) is a cost-effective and safe alternative to open tracheostomy.
- The ideal timing of tracheostomy remains a topic of debate.
- Patients with potential cervical spine injuries should not undergo tracheostomy until imaging is complete, injuries delineated, and treatment instituted.
- A step-wise technique by an experienced team of practitioners should be employed to minimize complications.
- To remember the critical steps at each part of the procedure, use the pneumonic "3 steps of 3."
- Bronchoscopy is essential throughout the procedure to confirm appropriate positioning prior to tracheal dilation as well as confirmatory placement of the tracheostomy tube.

Contact information: Department of Surgery, Denver Health Medical Center, 777 Bannock Street, MC 0206, Denver, CO 80204; Tel.: 303-602-1830, Fax: 303-436-6572, email: clay.cothren@dhha.org

Background

- Chevalier Jackson popularized tracheostomy in the early 20th century.
- Although originally described by Sheldon *et al.* in 1955, percutaneous tracheostomy was not routinely employed until the dilatational technique was reported by Ciaglia *et al.* in 1985.
- PDT has been shown to be a cost-effective and safe procedure when compared to open tracheostomy.
- Compared with surgical tracheostomy, PDT is relatively easy to perform, requires shorter procedure time, and obviates the transport of critically ill patients to the operating room.

Main Body

The Denver Health technique of PDT

- *Preparation*
  - Appropriate sedation (100–200 mcg fentanyl and 1–2 mg midazolam) and paralytics (typically 0.1 mg/kg vecuronium unless contraindicated) are administered.
  - In addition to Ciaglia Blue Rhino Percutaneous Tracheostomy kit (Cook Medical, Bloomington, IN), instruments should be readily available (Adson pickups, DeBakey's pickups, Seine retractors, needle driver, scissors, snaps).
  - The balloon of the tracheostomy tube should be tested to ensure there is no leak, and it should be appropriately loaded on the blue dilator.
  - 2–3 cc of water should be drawn up into the syringe that will be attached to the needle introducer.
  - An intrascapular rolled-up towel is used to "bump" the patient to facilitate hyperextension of the neck for adequate exposure.
  - Patients with cervical spine injuries are maintained in spine neutral position.
  - Although not considered a sterile procedure, the anterior neck is cleaned with hibiclens.
- *Initial Access to the Airway*
  - A 1–2 cm vertical incision is made just beneath the cricoid cartilage after infiltrating with 1% lidocaine with epinephrine.
  - Blunt dissection is performed with a snap until the tracheal rings are identified by palpation.

o Using a laryngoscope, the endotracheal tube is pulled back under direct vision until the balloon reaches the cords.

o The needle is then placed into the lumen of the airway between the first and second tracheal rings; aspiration of air through the saline in the attached syringe confirms intraluminal placement.

o The wire is advanced into the trachea; bronchoscopy is then performed to confirm two critical items: (1) the wire traverses into the lumen of the trachea and extends down to the carina; (2) the wire does not go through the Murphy eye of the endotracheal tube.

o Prior to tracheal dilation, repeat palpation of the anterior trachea is performed to ensure the wire goes into the anterior surface of the trachea in the midline and that it inserts approximately a fingertip beneath the cricoid cartilage (hence between the 1st and 2nd or 2nd and 3rd tracheal rings).

- *Dilation of the Trachea and Placement of the Tracheostomy*

  o Prior to Rhino dilation, three additional steps must be performed: (1) the tip of the Rhino dilator should be seated on the white inner cannula; (2) the sauter mark on the wire should be lined up with the distal portion of the white inner cannula; (3) the skin mark on the Rhino dilator should be observed as this is the limit of insertion into the trachea.

  o Following tracheal dilation, the tracheostomy tube is readied for insertion. Three final items are verified: (1) the tip of the dilator loaded with the tracheostomy tube should be seated on the white inner cannula; (2) the sauter mark on the wire should be lined up with the distal portion of the white inner cannula; (3) a 10 cc syringe is available to inflate the tracheostomy tube balloon after insertion.

  o Using an overhand pass, the tracheostomy tube is placed inside the airway.

  o Following tube placement, the dilator and wire are removed. Repeat bronchoscopy via the newly placed tracheostomy confirms proper placement within the trachea.

  o The tracheostomy is then sutured into placement at the four corners of the plastic flange and a tracheostomy tie is positioned.

  o Chest radiograph is not routinely performed post-procedure.

- *Avoiding Pitfalls*

  o Bronchoscopy is essential to the procedure to confirm that the wire is both in the trachea, and not through the Murphy eye of the endotracheal tube and back wall of the trachea into the esophagus. If the wire is through the Murphy eye and not detected by bronchoscopy prior to dilation and placement of the tracheostomy tube, decannulation of the endotracheal tube becomes impossible.

o Bronchoscopy is not used to determine how far back the endotracheal tube should be pulled, rather, direct vision with laryngoscopy is optimal; use of bronchoscopy alone can delude the operator into incorrect positioning of the endotracheal tube's cuff and potential loss of airway control.

o Leaving the bronchoscope within the tracheal lumen or inside the endotracheal tube increases the possibility of damaging the scope with the needle and impairs ventilation.

o The surgeon should not confuse a prominent thyroid isthmus for the cricoid cartilage.

o To remember the critical steps at each part of the procedure, use the pneumonic "3 steps of 3."

  ▪ First step of 3: (1) by bronchoscopy, the wire is identified in the lumen of the trachea and extends down to the carina; (2) by bronchoscopy, the wire does not go through the Murphy eye of the endotracheal tube; (3) digital palpation of the anterior trachea ensures the wire is no more than a fingertip beneath the cricoid cartilage and inserts into the trachea in the midline (Fig. 1).

  ▪ Second step of 3 — the 3 "S"s: (1) "seated" — the tip of the Rhino dilator should be seated on the white inner cannula; (2) "sauter" — the sauter mark on the wire should be lined up with the distal portion of the white inner cannula; and (3) "skin" — the skin mark on the Rhino dilator should be observed as this is the limit of insertion into the trachea (Fig. 2).

  ▪ Third step of 3 — the 3 "S"s: (1) "seated"; (2) "sauter"; and (3) "syringe". Steps 1 and 2 are identical while step 3 ensures the syringe is available to inflate the tracheostomy tube balloon.

o The endotracheal tube is not removed until the tracheostomy tube is confirmed to be satisfactory via bronchoscopy (Fig. 3).

o Any patient with an indeterminate spine status should not undergo tracheostomy until imaging is complete; any patient with an unstable cervical spine injury should have their tracheostomy delayed until the spine team determines stabilization and necessary treatment is instituted.

Practical Algorithm(s)/Diagrams

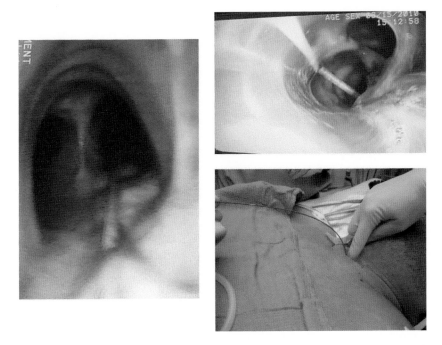

Fig. 1. The "first step of 3" — (1) by bronchoscopy the wire is identified within the lumen of the airway and (2) not through the Murphy eye. (3) Digital palpation confirms correct positioning of the wire.

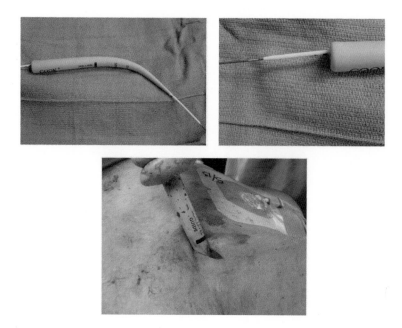

Fig. 2. The "second step of 3" — the 3 "S"s: (1) "seated" — the tip of the Rhino dilator should be seated on the white inner cannula, (2) "sauter" — the sauter mark on the wire should be lined up with the distal portion of the white inner cannula, and (3) "skin" — the skin mark on the Rhino dilator is the limit of insertion into the trachea.

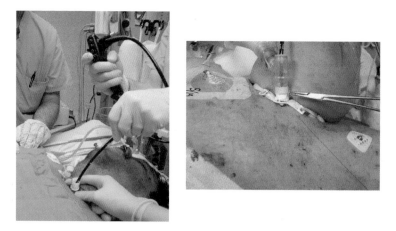

Fig. 3. Following placement of the tracheostomy tube, bronchoscopy confirms endotracheal location and the plastic flange is sutured to the skin after tracheostomy tie is secured.

Review of Current Literature with References

- Ciaglia *et al.* published the original description of the percutaneous dilatational tracheostomy (PDT) technique (*Chest* 1985; **87**(6): 715–719).
- Simon *et al.* published a systematic review of all publications reporting a PDT-related death; combining the data of 45 published studies with over 8,000 patients, they report a PDT-related death rate of 1 out of 600 patients. Hemorrhage, airway complications and tracheal perforation were the three most common causes of death in these patients (*Crit Care* 2013; **17**(5): R258).
- In a single institution study, Kornblith *et al.* reviewed 1,000 patients undergoing bedside PDT, including high-risk patients (cervical collar/halo, cervical spine injuries, systemic heparinization, PEEP >10 or $FiO_2 > 50\%$). Despite 48% of their patient population having at least one high-risk classification, only 1.4% of patients suffered a complication. They touted bedside PDT as the new gold standard for patients requiring tracheostomy for mechanical ventilation (*JACS* 2011; **212**: 163–170).
- Two of the largest published series (over 3,000 and 500 patients respectively) of the PDT technique demonstrate the technique is safe and easy to perform across a spectrum of critically ill patients [Dennis *et al.*, *JACS* 2013; **216**(4): 858–865 and Zagli *et al.*, *J Trauma* 2010; **68**(2): 367–372].

Chapter 20

Percutaneous Endoscopic Gastrostomy

James Haenel, RRT* Fredric M. Pieracci, MD, MPH†
and Ernest E. Moore, MD‡

*Surgical Critical Care Specialist, Denver Health Medical Center
†Acute Care Surgeon, Denver Health Medical Center
‡Professor of Surgery and Vice-Chair of Surgical Research, University of Colorado
School of Medicine

Take Home Points

- Enteral feeding via the stomach is usually well-tolerated in the critically ill or injured patient.
- Bedside percutaneous endoscopic gastrostomy (PEG) tube placement is a cost-effective, safe procedure for obtaining enteral access in the critically ill patient.
- Patient selection and timing for a PEG tube is individualized.
- Patient preparation consists of obtaining informed consent, physical exam review of exclusion criteria including coagulation status, assuring NPO status

Contact information: (Fredric M. Pieracci and James Haenel) Denver Health Medical Center, 777 Bannock Street, MC 0206, A388, Denver, CO 80206; (Ernest E. Moore) 655 Broadway, Ste. 365, Denever, CO 80203; Tel.: (Ernest E. Moore) 303-602-1820, email: Ernest.moore.@dhha.org; James.Haenel@dhha.org; Fredric.Pieracci@dhha.org

or gastric emptying prior to starting and antibiotic prophylaxis prior to procedure.

- Patients must be adequately monitored, sedated and paralyzed during the procedure. The combination of light transillumination with focal finger indentation of the anterior gastric wall (diaphonoscopy) minimizes inadvertent colon perforation.
- Strict attention must be paid to the positioning and tension applied to both the internal and external bumpers.
- Most common complications in the post-procedural period are preventable and minimized by appropriate monitoring of the external bumper position and cm marking of PEG tube.

Background

- Gauderer and Ponsky in 1980 reported performing a gastrosotomy without laparotomy, utilizing a percutaneous endoscopic technique.
- Although originally developed for children, PEG placement was quickly accepted by adult gastroenterologists as well as general surgeons familiar with endoscopy.
- Over the last quarter of a century since its introduction, insertion of a PEG has improved patient outcome by permitting a safe, cost-effective procedure for providing enteral access for nutritional support.
- Compared to a surgical laparotomy, bedside performance of a PEG has many advantageous, it is relatively simple, requires shorter procedure time, and obviates the transport of critically ill patients to the operating or GI suite and there is minimal discomfort post-procedure.

Main Body

- Indications
  - PEG tubes in the intensive care unit are commonly used to provide a route for enteral nutrition, hydration, gastric decompression and medication administration in patients with both short term and prolonged needs. Consideration should be given to those patients requiring enteral feeding for >3 weeks or those with complex pancreatoduodenal injuries or lesions anticipated to be associated with prolonged gastric ileus.
  - Surgical Intensive Care indications:
    - Head injury with GCS <8

- Severe facial fractures associated with jaw wiring
- Major burns
- Critical illness polyneuropathy
- Airway trauma associated (vocal cord paralysis or dysphagia >2 weeks)
- High cervical spinal cord injury
- Short bowel syndrome
- Head, neck and esophageal cancer
- Gastric outlet obstruction (for decompression)

- Medical Intensive Care indications:
  - Cerebral vascular disease
  - Severe dementia ±
  - Severe parkinson's disease
  - Severe cerebral palsy
  - Advanced multiple sclerosis
  - Anoxic injury post cardiac arrest
  - Amyotrophic lateral sclerosis
  - Polyneuropathy's

- Contraindications
  - Absolute
    - Major coagulation disorders (INR >2.0, PTT >50s, platelets <50,000/mm^3)
    - Severe ascites
    - Uncontrolled agitation/ICU delirium
    - Active peritonitis
    - Abdominal wall infection at insertion site
    - Hemodynamic instability
    - Elevated intracranial pressures (ICP)
    - Inability to pass scope through upper airway/esophagus
    - Limited life expectancy
    - Lack of informed consent

  - Relative
    - Portal hypertension with gastric varices
    - Hepatomegaly/Splenomegaly (review CT scan)
    - History of prior abdominal surgeries (concern for adhesions and bowel interposition)
    - Ventral hernia
    - Gastric bypass

- Laparotomies
- Colonic dilitation

- Preparation
  - Appropriate sedation and paralytics are administered in the intubated patient.
  - Ponsky Deluxe 20 F "Pull" peg kit at bedside (Bard Access Systems Salt Lake City, UT).
  - Place patient supine and elevated bed 30° to help with ICP control, for morbidly obese patients with significant panis and to "lower" the colon away from abdominal wall.
  - Ensure patient has been NPO for >4 hours or has gastric emptying via NG tube
  - Administer a first-generation cephalosporin such as cefazolin (2 g for patients <120 kg or 3 g if >120 kg) within 60 minutes of procedure. If penicillin-allergic, use 900 mg clindamycin within 60 minutes. For MRSA risk, use vancomycin 15 mg/kg infused over 60–90 minutes before procedure. If patient on antibiotics for other reasons, additional doses are unnecessary.

- Pull Technique (Gauderer-Ponsky)
  - The endoscopist performs upper endoscopy to ensure that there is no impediments to PEG placement (esophageal obstruction or ulcer at insertion site) then examination of gastric outlet and duodenum should be performed to rule out obstruction.
  - With the room lights dimmed, the assistant then identifies the appropriate insertion site on the abdominal wall (two fingerbreadths below the mid-portion of the inferior rib margin) by examining for transilliumination of light through abdominal wall.
  - Confirmation of proper positioning is performed by the assistant, who presses with one finger over the area of transillumination and a clear indentation of the gastric wall is visualized (diaphanoscopy).
  - Using sterile gloves, the assistant should prep the site with ChloraPrep solution and place a sterile drape over the abdomen, with the fenestration center over the chosen site.
  - The skin should be anesthetized with lidocaine.
  - Using the scalpel, an appropriate horizontal incision (0.5–1.0 cm wide) should be made at the site of infusion of the lidocaine.
  - The catheter-over-the needle from kit is inserted into the stomach. Needle insertion should not be done slowly as this will push the gastric wall away. It must be done with a firm quick push.

- o Just prior to needle insertion, the endoscopist inserts the snare down the channel of the endoscope into the stomach.
- o Once the needle/catheter are visualized in the stomach, the endoscopist will snare the catheter while the needle is removed.
- o The assistant then passes approximately 12 inches of the loop guidewire through the catheter and the endoscopist snares the wire.
- o The scope is then withdrawn from the patient ensuring that the wire is firmly snared. Upon scope removal from the mouth, the snare is released allowing the wire to be free.
- o The PEG tube is then secured to the looped end of the guidewire coming out of the patient's mouth. This is accomplished by passing the guidewire loop through the PEG loop and then passing the other end of the PEG tube through the guidewire loop and pulling the entire tube through it.
- o The assistant now pulls the guidewire exiting from the abdominal wall so that the PEG tube goes through the mouth, esophagus and stomach and out through the puncture site. Withdrawing the gastrostomy tube is terminated once the 5 cm mark is reached.
- o The endoscopist then reinserts the scope into the stomach and under direct visualization, the PEG is pulled back until the internal bolster is in contact with the gastric wall. This usually coincides with the PEG being at 3–4 cm from the patient's abdominal wall. Avoid applying too much tension i.e., blushing of the gastric mucosa.
- o The external bumper is passed over the PEG tube following cutting of the external wire. It is imperative to not place the bumper against the patient's skin. The external bumper should be 1–2 cm above the skin.
- o Cut the excess PEG tubing to leave approximately 8 inches of tube.
- o Insert the feeding tube adapoter provided in the kit.
- o Place a gauze roll directly next to the PEG tube so that the PEG is in a vertical position as it exits the abdominal wall. Tape the tube to the Roll and abdomen.

- PEG Complications
  - o Procedure-Related Complications
    - Aspiration — less likely in intubated patients but minimizing air insufflations of stomach and aspirating gastric contents before starting procedure is helpful.
    - Bleeding — occurs less than 1% of cases and less than 0.5% of all cases reported to require transfusion. Check coagulation profile before starting when indicated!

- Perforation of viscera — not to be confused with post-procedure pneumoperitoneum which may occur in as many as 56% of cases. Patients exhibiting post-procedure abdominal pain, leukocytosis, ileus and fever must be evaluated immediately. Either fluoroscopic imaging of the PEG tube using water soluble contrast or CT scan should be done.
- Prolonged ileus — tube feeds can usually be initiated within 4 hours post-PEG. In less than 2% of cases, a ileus precludes feeding.
- Cardiopulmonary changes — hypotension may result from over-sedation. Hypoxemia may also occur as a result of over-distention of abdominal contents, thus impeding the diaphragm.

o Post-Procedure Complications
  - Most post-procedure complications can be avoided!
  - PEG site infections (peristomal) are the most common complication and may occur in as many as 30% of cases. Pre-procedural antibiotics have been associated with reduced infections. Excessive pressure between the external and internal bolster is contributory. Loose contact of the outer bolster with the skin is necessary! Avoid excessive traction on the PEG tubing.
  - PEG site leakage-risk factors include infection, traction, increased gastric acid secretion and buried bumper syndrome.
  - Buried Bumper Syndrome — a rare but serious complication resulting in the partial or complete growth of gastric mucosa over the internal bolster or bumper and may occur in 2% of patients. The bumper may migrate back into the gastric wall or the tract. Early identification requires noting the position of the PEG tube at the skin level every day. This is preventable by avoiding excessive tension. During skin care, the PEG should be advanced 2–3 cm forward and then returned to original position. Correct position can be confirmed by endoscopy or radiographically.
  - Gastric ulcer/hemorrhage — rare.
  - Inadvertent removal — incidence is 2–4%. Tract maturation usually occurs within 10 days but may be delayed up to four weeks in the presence of malnutrition, ascites or steroids. Thus, in most patients a displaced tube can be replaced after two weeks at bedside. Prior to this if immediately recognized, it may be replaced endoscopically thus preventing the stomach and anterior abdominal wall from separating from each other, resulting in free perforation. Patients manifesting peritonitis require prompt surgical exploration.
  - Fistulous tract.

Practical Algorithm(s)/Diagrams

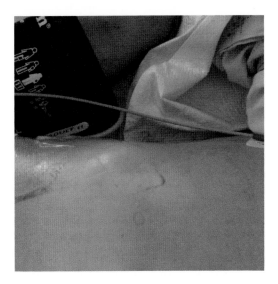

Fig. 1. Prior to opening the PEG kit, the ability to transilluminate is assessed. The location of the transillumination is then marked for the subsequent procedure.

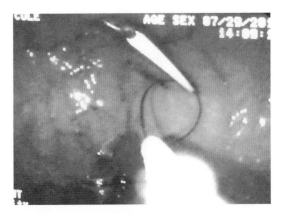

Fig. 2. The snare is placed over the predetermined location of gastric cannulation, such that the needle and catheter pass directly through the snare. The snare is then closed flush with the white catheter so that the wire may be safely passed.

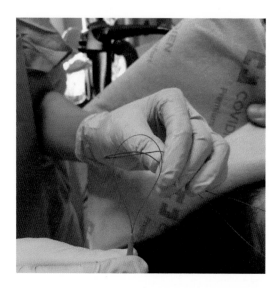

Fig. 3. Technique of passing the blue wire through the oval-shaped opening created by the wire at the end of the PEG tube. This sequence is remembered using the pneumonic, "the blue goes through."

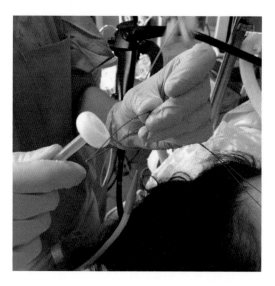

Fig. 4. The white PEG button then goes through the hole between the loop of the blue wire, thereby securing the silver wire of the PEG tube to the blue wire.

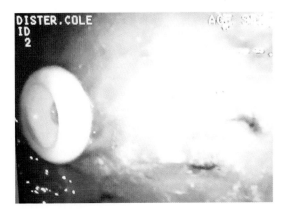

Fig. 5. The intra-gastric position of the white button is then confirmed endoscopically. Buckling of the surrounding gastric mucosa suggests that the tube is too tight and must be loosened. The white button should easily be able to perform a full rotation without movement of the underlying gastric mucosa.

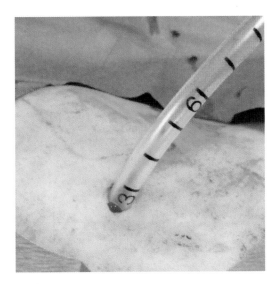

Fig. 6. The numeric position of the PEG tube at the skin is noted prior to applying the plastic buttress; this location is then noted each subsequent post-procedure day to confirm that tube migration (either into or out of the stomach) has not occurred.

Review of Current Literature with References

- Gauderer *et al.* published the original description of percutaneous endoscopic gastrostomy without the need for a laparotomy in 12 children and 19 adults (*J Pediatr Surg* 1980; **15**: 872–875).

- Tracheostomy and gastrostomy are frequent adjunct procedures required in the management of patients with severe brain injuries to facilitate neurorehabilitation. Moore *et al.* provided early evidence for the safety and efficacy in 27 brain injured patient's by performing a combined percutaneous tracheostomy followed by a percutaneous gastrostomy. Of note, there were no PEG related complications. [*J Trauma* 1992; **33**(3): 435–439].

- Percutaneous endoscopic gastrostomy is a surgical procedure and carries risk for soft tissue (peristomal) infection. Antibiotic prophylaxis remains controversial but the preponderance of evidence points to reduced infections following the administration of a single dose of a first generation cephalosporin or 15 ml/kg of vancomycin if MRSA is of concern (*Cochrane Database Syst Rev* 2013; **14**: 11).

- The European Society of Parenteral Enteral Nutrition (ESPEN) has developed a consensus statement for percutaneous endoscopic gastrostomy (PEG). This is a succinct review of indications, contraindications, technique and complications (*Clin Nutr* 2005; **24**: 848–861).

- Over the last 34 years, insertion of percutaneous endoscopic gastrostomy tubes has increased exponentially. Approximately 216,000 are performed annually. Lynch and Fang make an important contribution to this procedure by outlining strategies for prevention and management of complications associated with PEG tubes (*Practical Gastroenterology*, 2004).

- Replacement of an inadvertent dislodged gastrostomy tube is generally a safe and straight forward procedure if a mature tract is present (usually requires >4 weeks). The PEG tract differs from a surgical gastrostomy since there is no suture fixation of the gastric wall to the abdominal wall. Key principals for replacement involve. (1) Good control of the replacement tube with in the tract; (2) Using minimal insertion force; (3) Dependable process for ascertaining intragastric placement [*World J Gastrointest Endosc* 2013; **5**(1): 14–18].

Chapter 21

Difficult Urinary Catheterization

Paulo E. Jaworski, MD* Cole A. Wiedel, MD[†]
and Fernando J. Kim, MD, FACS[‡]

* Urology Fellow, Denver Health Medical Center
[†] Urology Resident, University of Colorado School of Medicine
[‡] Professor of Surgery, University of Colorado School of Medicine

Take Home Points

- First, one must assess the real need for urethral catheter placement.
- Urethral trauma is a contraindication for urethral catheterization by the novice. Urology consultation is mandatory.
- When facing a difficult catheterization, application of excessive pressure or force is not recommended. It may cause or increase magnitude of iatrogenic injury to the urethra.
- Difficult catheterization of female patients also represents a challenge and it is often due to patient's characteristics such as obesity, advanced age, or limitations in positioning. Urethral trauma in females is rare and when it occurs, it is associated with poor outcome.

Contact information: (Paulo E. Jaworski and Fernando J. Kim) Denver Health Medical Center, 777 Bannock St. MC 0206, Denver, CO 80204; (Cole A. Wiedel) 12631 East 17th Ave, MSC313, Aurora CO 80045. Email: Fernando.Kim@dhha.org; Paulo.Jaworski@dhha.org; Cole.Wiedel@ucdenver.edu

647

- Urethral strictures, sphincter spasm, prostate enlargement, phimosis, penile edema, and meatal stenosis are common causes of catheterization difficulty in men.
- Proper sterile technique with lubrication of the urethra with lidocaine gel is a key step to achieve successful catheterization and decrease chance of urinary tract infection.
- Contrary to common perception, larger diameter catheters (18–22 French) are preferable than smaller French catheters due to the firmness and better success rates.
- Flexible cystoscopy with catheter placement over a guidewire or suprapubic catheters are alternatives to a difficult urethral catheterization. These procedures must be performed by Urologists.

Background

- Several potential complications of difficult urinary catheterization (DUC) can cause acute and chronic complications, including rectal perforation, meatal and urethral erosions, infection, and chronic urethral strictures.
- The absolute need of indwelling urethral catheter placement must be assessed. Rates of unjustified catheterization can be as high as 50%.[1]
- Currently, blind urethral catheterization is contraindicated if a urethral injury is suspected since flexible endoscopy may be performed to diagnose and treat the injury.
- Complete urethral injuries are less frequent but when it occurs, patients may present with urinary retention, meatal blood, and high-riding prostate. Placement of supra pubic catheter may be needed and urethral realignment may be performed when patient is clinically stable.[2]
- Difficult catheterization in female patients is often due to patient characteristics such as morbid obesity, atrophic vaginitis, intravaginal retraction of the urethral meatus, and previous pelvic procedures.[3]
- The most common causes of DUC in men are urethral strictures and bladder neck contractures post-endoscopic procedures.
- Other causes of DUC in men include acute urinary retention caused by benign prostate hyperplasia (BPH) in older men >65 y.o., voluntary contraction of external sphincter, incorrect procedure technique, false passages, phimosis, meatal stenosis, etc.[3]
- When placing a Foley catheter, additional force to overcome any resistance may cause urethral trauma, bleeding, false passages, and future stricture formation.[3]

Main Body

Difficult female catheterization

- Obese females may require Lithotomy with Trendelenburg position for better exposure.
- A vaginal speculum can be used to press the posterior vaginal wall downwards and assistant retract the labia majora to expose the meatus. Similarly, in older postmenopausal women, the meatus may be retracted posteriorly towards the vagina. In these cases, insertion of the first and second fingers into the vaginal introitus may guide the insertion of the Foley catheter by locating the urethral meatus above the introitus and about 2–3 cm below the clitoris.
- Female meatus stricture can be secondary to previous instrumentation, injury and female circumcision. In these complex cases, urethral dilation with endoscopic approach is often necessary.

Difficult male catheterization

- In case of penile edema, hand compression of the distal half of the penis with gauze or application of loose fitting elastic dressings for 10–20 minutes can reduce the swelling and Foley catheter can be placed using standard sterile technique.
- Phimosis can make it difficult or impossible to visualize the meatus. Pulling the foreskin outward can open a passage that allows visualization. In severe cases of phimosis, blind or endocopic approach may be necessary to introduce the catheter aiming towards the 6 o'clock. Rarely, doral slit is indicated.[4]
- The Foley retention balloon can be inflated only after the Foley catheter is introduced into the bladder up to the Y-hub bifurcation of the catheter and drainage of urine is visualized.
- Bedside bladder ultrasound is recommended when in doubt of catheter's placement.[4]
- Lidocaine 2% gel is used as lubricant and local anesthetic. Better results are obtained using 20 mL of the gel at least 10 minutes prior to the procedure. If lidocaine gel is not available, plain lubricating gel can be used.[3,4]

Catheter selection

- The types of catheters used in common practice are: Latex or silicone catheters, two- or three-way Foley for continuous irrigation of the bladder, and

Coudé (curved tip) catheter. Catheter size is measured using the French scale, where 1 French equals 1/3 millimeter in diameter.

- Generally, the 16 or 18 French catheter are used for uncomplicated catheterization. Coudé catheters are used when patients are known to have a large prostate or history of difficult catheterization with clearance at 12 o'clock (high bladder neck). The tip should be directed anteriorly and upward in order to facilitate bypassing obstruction or false passages.[3–6]
- Council tip catheters are designed to be placed over a stiff guidewire pre-placed under cystoscopic guidance performed by the Urologist.

Flexible cystoscopy and dilatation

- Flexible cystoscopy can be performed in any setting under local anesthesia assisting the placement of Council tip catheters or supra-pubic catheters under direct visualization.
- Urethral dilation has traditionally been done blindly with metal Van Buren sounds. The use of such sounds is encouraged only for very distal strictures or meatal stenosis. Similarly, Filiforms and Followers can also be used but false passages may occur. Currently, the use of sequential urethral dilators over the guide wire under fluoroscopic guidance is often practiced.[3]

Suprapubic catheter

- A suprapubic catheter (SP) can be inserted percutaneously in cases of catheterization failure or when total urethral disruption is considered. SP tubes are placed using local anesthesia with or without the use of US 2 fingerbreadths above the pubic bone in the midline.[7]
- Contraindications for supra pubic tube placement include bladder cancer, unavoidable bowel injury due to previous surgery, uncorrected coagulopathies, and active anticoagulation and abdominal wall abscess or cellulitis.[4]

Practical Algorithm(s)/Diagrams

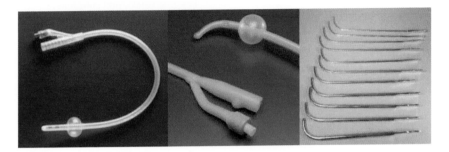

Fig. 1. Silicone Foley catheter; latex Coudé catheter; set of Van Buren sounds.

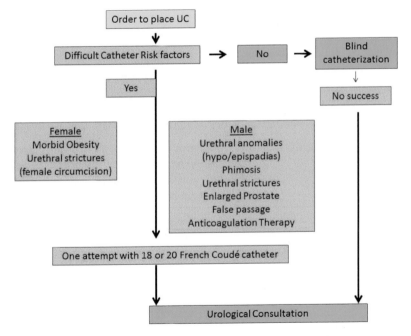

Fig. 2. Difficult urethral catheterization algorithm.[4]

Summary of possible issues with Urethral catheterization and solutions.

Issues	Possible causes and solutions
Difficulty to locate urethral meatus in females especially, when they are morbidly obese.	Use vaginal speculum or insert two fingers into the vaginal introitus to guide the insertion of the UC by locating the urethral meatus.
Pain or resistance early in placement, while in penile or bulbo-membranous urethra.	Urethral stricture or false passage may be the cause.
Resistance during passage through external sphincter or prostatic fossa.	Ask the patient to relax urinary sphincter muscles as if going to void, and reattempt passage.
	If substantial pain or resistance is encountered, the patient may have a bladder neck contracture or an enlarged prostate. The Coudé catheter can be attempted with generous lubrication. Reattempt catheterization with a 18 or 20 french Coudé catheter, with tip positioned upward.
Urine does not drain after full-length catheter insertion.	Gently palpate the bladder for fullness or flush catheter with saline. The lubricant gel may be blocking the catheter holes urine to open tip, which may be blocked with gel. Do not inflate the UC balloon until good drainage of urine is observed.
Difficulty to inflate the UC balloon.	Ascertain that the bladder is draining through the UC prior the balloon inflation. Immediately stop inflation if any difficulty, as tip of catheter may still be in urethra.

Always call the Urologist in case of problems. Ultrasound-guided Supra pubic catheters can be placed under local anesthesia.

Review of Current Literature with References

- In 2013, Kim *et al.* demonstrated that the success rate of early realignment was 100% in patients with total posterior urethral disruption. A total of 15 patients were treated within 5 days post-trauma.[2]
- Aaronson *et al.* conducted a meta-analysis: Does lidocaine gel before flexible cystoscopy provide pain relief? They concluded that urethral instillation

of lidocaine gel is more effective than plain lubricating gel in reducing the likelihood of moderate to severe pain during flexible cystoscopy.[5]

- In difficult cases of Foley placement, supra pubic catheters can be placed successfully using ultrasonography.[7]

References

1. Jain, P., *et al.*, Overuse of the indwelling urinary tract catheter in hospitalized medical patients. *Arch Intern Med*, 1995; **155**(13): 1425–1429.
2. Kim FJ, Pompeo A, Sehrt D, Molina WR, Mariano da Costa RM, Juliano C, Moore EE, Stahel PF. Early effectiveness of endoscopic posterior urethra primary alignment. *J Trauma Acute Care Surg.* 2013; **75**(2):189–194.
3. Ghaffary, C., *et al.*, A practical approach to difficult urinary catheterizations. *Curr Urol Rep*, 2013; **14**(6): 565–579.
4. Villanueva, C. and G.P. Hemstreet, Difficult catheterization: tricks of the trade. *AUA Update Series.* 2011: 41–48.
5. Patel, A.R., J.S. Jones, and D. Babineau, Lidocaine 2% gel versus plain lubricating gel for pain reduction during flexible cystoscopy: a meta-analysis of prospective, randomized, controlled trials. *J Urol*, 2008; **179**(3): 986–990.
6. Aaronson, D.S., *et al.*, Meta-analysis: does lidocaine gel before flexible cystoscopy provide pain relief? *BJU Int*, 2009; **104**(4): 506–509; discussion 509–510.
7. Kim FJ, Rove K, and Sehrt DE. *Intraoperative Urologic Ultrasound, in Practical Urological Ultrasound*, P.F. Fulgham and B.R. Gilbert, Editors. 2013, Humana Press: New York.

Chapter 22

Bedside Laparotomy

Clay Cothren Burlew, MD, FACAS*

*SICU Director, Denver Health Medical Center,
Professor of Surgery, University of Colorado School of Medicine

Take Home Points

- Bedside laparotomy (BL) is a reasonable option for the patient who requires immediate surgical intervention but is judged too unstable to tolerate transfer to the operating room (OR).
- Abdominal compartment syndrome (ACS) is likely the most common intraabdominal pathology resulting in an emergent BL.
- Other pathologic states that might require urgent BL include evaluation for ischemic bowel, septic source, or missed enteric injury. Rarely, re-opening of a prior laparotomy incision at the bedside is performed for hemorrhagic shock.
- Planned laparotomy at the bedside is performed at some institutions as a component of open abdomen management for (1) washout and replacement of temporary closure coverage; (2) partial fascial closure attempts; or (3) tightening of fascial retention devices.

Contact information: Department of Surgery, Denver Health Medical Center, 777 Bannock Street, MC 0206, Denver, CO 80204; Tel.: 303-602-1830, Fax: 303-436-6572. Email: clay.cothren@dhha.org

- Although minimal equipment may be necessary for the majority of cases, utilization of a full OR nursing team will ensure needed equipment should the unexpected arise.

Background

- Originally thought to be an act of heroism, BL in the intensive care unit (ICU) has become more commonplace in recent years.
- For patients who are too unstable for transport to the OR, operating room personnel and equipment can be transported to the ICU for a bedside procedure.
- Emergent BL typically requires minimal equipment: scalpel, suction, cautery, and abdominal temporary closure dressings. Rarely, bowel resections are required but can be performed with rapid excision using a GIA stapler, leaving the bowel in discontinuity.

Main Body

- Technique based upon etiology

  o Abdominal Compartment Syndrome: Decompressive laparotomy is easily accomplished at the bedside with minimal equipment. A midline incision into the peritoneal cavity permits evacuation of the viscera and intraabdominal fluid. Intraabdominal hypertension is immediately relieved, typically with improvement in the patient's hemodynamic status. Temporary visceral coverage is then performed.

  o Evaluation for ischemic bowel, septic source, or missed enteric injury: Laparotomy is performed through a midline incision using standard scalpel and electrocautery. Occasionally, BL for missed injury or ischemic bowel is performed in a patient who has already undergone abdominal exploration; in these cases, the midline incision is merely re-opened at the bedside. The viscera are explored for the suspected intraabdominal pathology. If a segment of ischemic or perforated bowel is identified, resection is rapidly accomplished using a series of GIA staplers, leaving the bowel in discontinuity. Alternatively, closure of any identified enterotomies may be performed using suture. Utilizing OR nursing personnel for these potentially more complex cases will ensure appropriate equipment is readily available. Drainage and temporary abdominal closure is then performed.

o Re-opening of a prior laparotomy incision for hemorrhagic shock: rarely, a patient may decompensate in the ICU due to intraabdominal hemorrhage necessitating BL. Scenarios in which this may occur include patients with bleeding from a known solid organ injury or patients with a postoperative bleed due to a suture coming off a tied vessel or other complications. Although transport to the OR for definitive intervention is probably more optimal, temporizing measures at the bedside should be in the surgeon's armamentarium. BL can afford direct control of the source of hemorrhage; for example, a Pringle maneuver performed digitally can markedly reduce bleeding in hepatic injuries while aortic cross-clamping at the diaphragmatic hiatus reduces hemorrhage while improving pressure above the diaphragm. Occasionally, directly tamponading a bleeding vessel is possible such as holding a bleeding splenic artery that a tie has come off following traumatic splenectomy.

o Planned laparotomy for open abdomen management: in some institutions, open abdomen patients have the majority of their operations performed at the bedside if the planned intervention is minimal (i.e. no enteric anastomoses, resections, stomas, vascular reconstructions, etc.). BL may entail simple removal of the temporary abdominal closure with abdominal washout and replacement of temporary closure coverage; this is often done in those patients who are too unstable for attempts at fascial closure or other planned interventions. In patients who are resuscitated, partial fascial closure attempts may be performed at BL; this may entail actual placement of permanent fascial sutures for closure (Fig. 2) or may consist of tightening of fascial retention devices.

- For patients undergoing initial laparotomy in the ICU, coverage of the abdominal contents may be necessary if the abdomen cannot be closed primarily. One option for temporary closure is 1010 steri-drape and Ioban closure [see Chapter 8-(vi)].

Practical Algorithm(s)/Diagrams

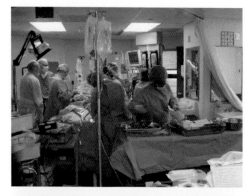

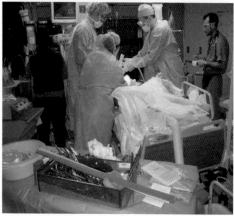

Fig. 1. Operating room equipment and personnel can facilitate bedside laparotomy in the ICU.

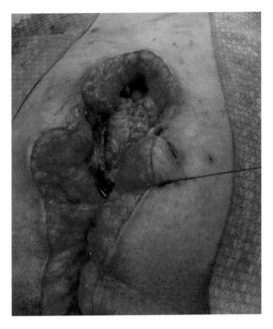

Fig. 2. Partial fascial closure of an open abdomen can be performed via BL in the ICU.

Review of Current Literature with References

- Diaz *et al.* has provided the only significant publications on the role of BL. Their initial publication in 2004 reported on 75 patients undergoing BL [*Surg Infect (Larchmt)*. 2004; **5**: 15–20]. The most common indications BL in this population were abdominal compartment syndrome (50%), suspected intra-abdominal infection (19%), and washout/pack removal (15%). These were acutely ill patients with a mean ISS of 51 and mortality rate of 49%; none of the deaths were attributed by the authors to BL. Subsequently, they published their results with a BL protocol (*Am Surg* 2005; **71**: 986–991)]; those patients with abdominal compartment syndrome, decompensation due to hemorrhage, washout/closure, and sepsis in a patient too unstable for transport to the OR were included. Over 75% of this protocolized group underwent BL for planned exploration and washout, resulting in a cost-effective management strategy.

IV: Special Populations

Chapter 23

Pediatric

Claudia Kunrath, MD* and Denis Bensard, MD[†]

*Assistant Professor of Pediatrics, University of Colorado School of Medicine
[†]Professor of Surgery, University of Colorado School of Medicine

Take Home Points

- Trauma is the leading cause of death for children 1–17 years.
- Trauma is the leading non-fatal injury treated in the emergency room: <1 year to 14 years.
- Multisystem trauma is the rule rather than exception.
- Kids are more susceptible to heat loss and hypothermia.
- Children are more susceptible to upper airway obstruction.
- Respiratory arrest usually precedes cardiac arrest.
- Hypotension is usually a late sign of hemorrhagic shock in children (loss of 30% or more of total blood volume).
- Traumatic brain injuries (TBI) are the most common cause of pediatric deaths.
- Trauma with degree of physical injury not explained by the history should be evaluated for non-accidental trauma (NAT).

Contact information: Denver Health Medical Center, University of Colorado Health Sciences Center, 777 Bannock Street, MC 0206, Denver, CO 80204; Tel.: 303-602-9169. Email: claudia.kunrath@dhha.org, denis.bensard@dhha.org

- Children do not enjoy more favorable outcome following cardiac arrest. In a study of pediatric hospital medical and surgical arrest, Matos *et al.* demonstrated that pediatric trauma patients survive less often and suffer worse neurologic outcome as compared to other etiologies of cardiac arrest.
- Children treated at designated pediatric trauma centers have better outcomes than predicted by trauma injury severity score (TRISS).

Background

- Children have unique anatomy and physiology that must be taken into consideration when treating their injuries.
- The force in any given trauma is more widely distributed throughout their bodies due to less fat and muscle mass, often resulting in more significant internal organ damage, often without signs of external injury.
- They have compliant chest wall, less rib fractures (<10 years old) with frequent pulmonary contusions. Presence of rib fractures is associated with significant risk of serious or life-threatening injury, not from the rib fracture, but rather the force imparted sufficient to fracture a rib.
- Children have a higher oxygen metabolism and are diaphragmatic breathers at baseline, therefore they have shorter safe apnea time and fatigue happens more quickly.
- Hemorrhagic shock is common in trauma; resuscitation should start with 20 ml/kg bolus of isotonic intravenous/intraosseous fluids. If no significant response has been achieved after two fluid boluses, reassessment and consideration of packed red cell transfusion should follow.
- The proportionately larger surface area of children's bodies to their weight exposes them to significant heat loss and secondary negative effects: decreased cardiac function, diminished platelet function and coagulopathy, altered renal and hepatic drug clearance, and a higher metabolic demand that potentiates metabolic acidemia.
- The head size is disproportionately larger, skull and scalp thinner, and affords less protection to the brain. Serious injuries can occur from fall, and although rare, upper cervical injuries must be considered. Intracranial bleeding can cause shock in infants.
- Children have low glycogen storage and high dependence on fat metabolism and thus are very sensitive to hypoglycemia that can potentiate persistent acidemia. Hypoglycemia can be more detrimental than hyperglycemia and can cause significant decrease in mental status.

- Hyponatremia should be avoided and the preferred fluids are $\frac{1}{2}$ NS, NS or ringers lactate to reduce the risk of hyponatremia induced seizure.

Main Body

- Airway/breathing/ventilation/sedation
  - o Indications for intubation: moderate to severe respiratory distress, declining mental status/severe head injury, shock, facial/airway trauma with increased risk of swelling, smoke inhalation/facial burns.
  - o During intubation, c-collar should be in place or another person hold in-line the C-spine, while the front of the cervical collar is released.
  - o Children become hypoxemic quickly and require careful preparation:
    - Have an oral airway and mask and ambu-bag appropriate for age — give minimal pressure to attain chest rise.
    - Have a rolled towel to put under shoulders.
    - Use a straight blade, OG to decompress stomach and colorimetric capnographyto confirm ET tube placement.
    - Before any attempt, pre-oxygenation is the key for success; oral intubation is the safest for children.
    - Age appropriate ET tube can be calculated using the formula: 4+ (age in years/4); when using cuffed ET tubes use 0.5 size smaller, keeping the cuff pressure at 25 mm H_2O.
    - Compare the ET tube with the fifth finger to see if adequate size and tape it at three times the tube size.
    - If no significant airway trauma or lung injury, an age appropriate LMA can be used if a difficult airway is encountered.
  - o The best drugs (hemodynamic profile) to use for intubation are:
    - Fentanyl IV 1 to 3 mcg/kg (needs to be given slowly to avoid chest rigidity).
    - Etomidate IV 0.1 to 0.3 mg/kg (can cause myoclonus, temporarily isoelectric EEG and decreases cortisol production for 2–24 hours).
    - If a paralytic needed, preference is given to rocuronium IV 1 mg/kg (succinylcholine: incidence of bradycardia and asystole is higher in children).
    - If a patient has increased intracranial pressure, give lidocaine 1 mg/kg IV prior to intubation.
  - o After intubation, propofol can be used temporarily for transport if patient is hemodynamically stable and in need of frequent neurologic exams.

Pediatric patients and teenagers are at a higher risk for propofol infusion syndrome (PRIS) so we try not to use it. We start with fentanyl 0.5 to 1 mcg/kg/hour and titrate up to 2 for goal sedation behavioral score (SBS) 0 to −1 before we start versed (higher incidence of delirium). We use remifentanil 0.05 to 1.3 mcg/kg/min if neurologic exams need to be done frequently.

o   Initial ventilator settings: 6–8 ml/kg of tidal volume, peep of 5, an initial rate of 20 works for most, but 30 for neonates and 15 to teenagers. If using pressure ventilation, 15 of peak pressure over 5 of peep is a good start aiming for an exhaled TV of 6–8 ml/kg. Sometimes as much as 10 ml/kg need to be given to improve hypercapnia.

o   Normal CO_2 is the goal for patients with traumatic brain injury (TBI) because hyperventilation can worsen neurologic outcomes. Protective ventilation strategies are similar to adults.

o   After intubation and OG placement, always do an X-ray to confirm placement of ET tube that should be at least 1 cm above the carina.

o   Chest CTs should be done selectively and only after a screening chest X-ray. Although CT will identify more injuries than chest X-ray, most are not life-threatening or alter management.

o   Pulmonary contusions are common without rib fractures, but ARDS is rare.

o   Hemothorax/pneumothorax with hemodynamic or respiratory compromise require a chest tube placement. Blood output more than 2 ml/kg/hour may require surgical intervention, but this is uncommon following blunt injury.

•   Circulation /venous access

o   Tachycardia is the first sign of volume loss in children and should be taken seriously. Pediatric patients have robust compensatory mechanisms that maintain the blood pressure in the normal range for a long period of time, despite intravascular volume deficits.

o   Signs of compensated shock include: tachycardia, cool and pale distal extremities, prolonged (>2 seconds) capillary refill (despite warm ambient temperature), weak peripheral pulses compared with central pulses, normal systolic blood pressure.

o   Decompensated shock is characterized by signs and symptoms consistent with inadequate delivery of oxygen to tissues (pallor, peripheral cyanosis, tachypnea, mottling of the skin, decreased urine output-less than 1 ml/kg/hour, metabolic acidosis, depressed mental status), weak or absent peripheral pulses, weak central pulses, and hypotension. The finding of decompensated shock suggests that greater than 30% of blood volume has been lost.

o The lower limit of normal systolic blood pressure in neonates is 60 mmHg. In children, it is 70 plus two times the age which provides a rapid estimate of normal systolic blood pressure.

o The goal of fluid resuscitation is to rapidly replace the circulating volume. An infant's blood volume can be estimated at 80 ml/kg and for a child 70 ml/kg. When shock is suspected, a bolus of 20 ml/kg of warm isotonic crystalloid (NS or lactate ringers) is needed and patient reacessed. If no improvement, a second and third bolus should be given with prompt involvement of a surgeon. If patient does not respond, then consider early use of 10 ml/kg of type specific or O-negative warmed packed red blood cells (PRBCs).

o Most common causes of pediatric trauma related shock are tension pneumothorax, abdominal trauma, or TBI (young children).

o If the weight of the child is unknown, a Broselow tape can be used to estimate weight.

o If patient develops cardiac arrest, pediatric advanced life support (PALS) guidelines should be used for patients less than 12 years and or less than 40 kg with use of weight dose for epinephrine and other vasoactive drugs if needed.

o If peripheral venous access cannot be obtained promptly (two attempts), intraosseous access with 18 gauge needle for infants and 15 gauge for children or other commercial devices should be attempted. Preferred site are: proximal medial tibial plateau, medial distal tibia and distal femur. If central access is attempted, use shorter catheter in order to give fluids more rapidly.

- Hematology

o Hemorrhage control: Local control, correct hypothermia, correct acidosis, normalize calcium.

o Obtain baseline PT/INR/PTT, fibrinogen, platelets, Ca^{2+}, rapid TEG; repeat every 30 minutes as needed. Follow Hct.

o Blood component therapy triggers: PT, PTT > 1.5 control or rapid TEG-ACT > 138 sec: 10 ml/kg plasma; platelet count < 50,000 or rapid TEG-MA < 53 mm: 1 unit of apheresed platelets/10 kg; fibrinogen < 100 mg/dl, rapid TEG-angle < 63 degrees: 10 ml/kg cryoprecipitate, hemoglobin (Hg) < 7: Packed red cells (PRBC) 10 ml/kg.

o The massive transfusion protocol should be initiated when ISS > 25, EBL > 4 mL/kg/hour and or, after crystalloid (50 mL/kg) SBP: > 10 years: SBP < 90 mmHg; one to 10 years: SBP < 70+ (2 × age years), one month to a year: SBP < 70, < 1 month: SBP < 60.

o Anticipated transfusion responses: 1 U(unit) PRBC or 5 mL/kg increases Hg by ~ 1g/dl; 1 U of Apheresis Platelets or 10 mL/kg increases Platelet Count by ~30,000–50,000; 10 U of Cryoprecipitate or 1 U/5 kg increases Fibrinogen by ~30–50 mg/dl; 2 U of plasma or 10 mL/kg provides ~ 20% of normal coagulation factors.

o Patients less than 13 years old (tanner 2 or below) do not require DVT prophylaxis unless previous history of it or have spinal cord injury (paralysis).

o Restrictive transfusion therapy is employed in stable patients with a transfusion trigger of < 7 gm/dl.

• Neurology

o Most pediatric traumatic brain injury are caused by fall, followed by car accidents and pedestrian injuries. In infants, in the absence of a verifiable history, NAT must be considered.

o MVC, > 3 feet fall and contact sports in children > 8 years old should have the neck immobilized with a C-collar. Patients with Trisomy 21, Klippel-Feil and Morquio Syndrome have an increased risk for C-spine injury.

o Prior to imaging, in select patients, the neck may be cleared clinically utilizing the Canadian C-Spine rules. Consider head CT/neck CT if significant trauma and: < 3 month old, full fontanel in children less than 1 year old, Glasgow score < 14 or any signs of altered mental status; any non-frontal hematoma in children less than 2 years old, signs of basilar skull fracture, falls more than 3 feet. MRI of the neck should be considered if persistent neurologic symptoms with normal cervical CT's and to rule out spinal cord injuries without radiographic abnormality (SCIWORA) that is more common in children less than 8 years old.

o Consider using Pediatric Glasgow score for patients less than 2/3 years old (Fig. 1).

o If patients requiring intracranial pressure (ICP) monitor, the goal ICP is less than 15 mmHg in children younger than 5 and less than 20 mmHg in patients above 5 years old.

o Supranormal BP in children (> 135 mmHg) in the first 72 h is associated with improved outcome; tolerate mild to moderate hypertension and treat pain/anxiety and possible high ICP prior to give antihypertensive medications.

o Avoid hypotension, hyperglycemia, hypoglycemia, hyperthermia and hyponatremia.

o In adequately sedated patients, elevated ICP should be treated with mannitol 0.25 to 1 gram/kg or 3% saline 1 to 10 ml/kg (maximum 100 ml). Consider early 3% saline infusion if persistent high ICP: 0.1 to 1 ml/kg/hour. Goal sodium is 145–160 meq/l and osmolality < 360 mOsm. When weaning hypertonic saline, the practitioner must ensure that serum sodium does not decrease more than 15 meq/day to avoid cerebral edema.

o EPTS (early post traumatic seizures) occur in 1.6–20% in children. The 2012 Pediatric Society for Critical Care Medicine Severe TBI guidelines states that the prophylactic treatment with Phenytoin may be considered to reduce the incidence of EPTS in pediatric patients with severe TBI. We suggest continuous EEG monitoring in the first 72 hours of PICU stay if patient intubated even if started any seizure prophylaxis.

• Fluids, endocrine and nutrition

o In children <13 years D5NS or D51/2NS should be utilized for maintenance fluids. Add KCL once adequate urine output is established and hyperkalemia has been excluded following crush injury or severe acidosis.

o If the patient has severe TBI, start D5NS at 80% maintenance if intubated (patient gets extra humidity from the ventilator) and write for a total IV fluid order.

o Check glucose q 2 hours with goal glucose 120 to 180 mg/dl. If glucose 200 mg/dl or above, repeat in 15 min, if still above 200 start insulin drip at 0.02 units/kg/hour. If glucose 300 or above, start insulin at 0.04 units/kg/hour. Check glucoses q1 hour and double the drip until drip is 0.1 units/kg/hour, after that increase the drip by 0.05 units/kg/hour.

o If a persistent acidosis is noted, first determine if the anion gap is normal (non-anion gap) or increased (>12). Non-anion gap metabolic acidosis is common due to excessive administration of normal saline solution. If an anion gap is present, attention should be directed to signs of ongoing bleeding, abdominal compartment syndrome, missed intra-abdominal injuries, or inadequate resuscitation.

o Once the patient is stable (not requiring urgent interventions) enteral feeds should be initiated. Bowel sounds do not predict readiness to feeding. Infants and patients that need heavy sedation may benefit from transpyloric feeding tubes.

o Regardless of gastric or transpyloric feedings, the monitoring of gastric residuals is unnecessary because they do not correlate with gastric volume or emptying, vomiting or aspiration risk. Abdominal circumference should be monitored once a shift to detect abdominal distention or feeding intolerance. If girth increase >10% rule out constipation or ileus with an abdominal X-ray, but continue feeds. If patient has emesis, NPO for 1 hour, restart feeds at the same rate. If reoccurs, NPO for 4 hours and decrease infusion rate.

o Start feeds at 0.5 to 1 ml/kg/hour max 20 ml/hour and advance every 4–8 hours the same volume. Infants should receive human milk or home formula. Kids above 1 and less than 25 kg should receive pediatric formula. Kids above 25 kg should receive adult formula to meet protein requirements. See Fig. 2 for caloric needs for pediatric patients.

Practical Algorithm(s)/Diagrams

PEDIATRIC GLASGOW COMA SCALE FOR NONVERBAL CHILDREN	
EYE OPENING	
Spontaneous	4
To speech	3
To pain	2
No response	1
VERBAL RESPONSE	
Coos, babbles	5
Irritable cry	4
Cries to pain	3
Moans to pain	2
No Response	1
MOTOR RESPONSE	
Follows commands	6
Localizes pain	5
Withdraws to pain	4
Decorticate flexion	3
Decerebrate extension	2
No response	1

Fig. 1. Pediatric glasgow coma scale for non-verbal children.

PEDIATRIC CALORIE GOALS		
Age	Acute Phase kcal/kg/day	Recovery Phase kcal/kg/day
0–1year	65–80	90–120
1–3years	65–70	80–100
4–6years	55–60	65–90
7–10years	50–55	55–70
11–14years	35–40	40–55
15–18years(BOYS)	35–40	40–47
15–18years(GIRLS)	30–33	35–40

Fig. 2. Pediatric calorie goals.

Review of Current Literature with References

- Bensard *et al.* reviewed all pediatric trauma evaluations over six years at an academic level trauma I center. Effective radiation dose was calculated. Fifty-seven of these (33%) had a chest CT. Fifty-five had a chest X-ray. All 7/57(12%) emergent or urgent chest interventions were based on information from chest X-ray and radiation dose was significantly greater from chest CT. This study suggests an opportunity to reduce radiation doses, using chest X-rays as a triage exam (*J Surg Res* 2013; **184**: 352–357).

- A prospective two-year study evaluated 194 injured children with a blunt mechanism and systolic hypotension and found 61% incidence of isolated head injury in children less than 5 years old, 31% in children 6 to 12 years old and 33% of children above 12 years old suggesting that systolic hypotension is a possible indicator of head injury in young trauma victims (*Am J Surg* 2002; **184**: 555–559).

- Gardner *et al.* did a retrospective review in a level one trauma center from January 2007 to December 2011. The goal was to find if isolated head injury was the most common cause of severe shock after trauma in children 0 to 15 years old. Thirty-one percent of 680 pediatric trauma patients presented with severe shock. Of these, 29% had isolated head injury. In kids less than 5 years old, 50% had isolated head injury and above 12 years none. This study suggests that isolated head injury is an important cause of severe shock in children less than 5 years old (*Pediatr Emerg Care* 2013; **29**: 879–883).

- A retrospective study reviewed records and imaging of all children with rib fractures over a six-year period. NAT was determined by the child advocacy and protection team. In children younger than 3 years of age, the positive predictive value (PPV) of a rib fracture as an indicator of NAT was 95%. The PPV increased to 100% once historical and clinical circumstances excluded all other causes for rib fractures. Rib fractures in young children without a reliable history should prompt practitioners to rule out NAT (*J Trauma* 2003; **54**: 1107–1110).

Chapter 24

Geriatric

Nicole T. Townsend, MD* and Thomas N. Robinson, MD†

*Surgical Resident, University of Colorado School of Medicine
†Professor of Surgery, University of Colorado School of Medicine

Take Home Points

- Hospital care for the geriatric patient involves closer monitoring of delirium, malnutrition, pain, sedation, polypharmacy, pulmonary complications, rehabilitation, and skin breakdown.
- Physiologic differences are in general marked by reduced physiologic reserve in all organ systems.
- Pre-existing frailty and geriatric syndromes, such as functional decline, delirium, falls and pressure ulcers, are associated with increased complications, morbidity, and mortality.
- Improved outcomes can result from system-wide interventions and programs addressing:
  - o Early mobility
  - o Malnutrition
  - o Delirium prevention

Contact information: 12631 East 17th Ave, MS C313, Aurora CO 80045. Email: Nicole.Townsend@ucdenver.edu; Thomas.Robinson@ucdenver.edu

o Sleep hygiene
o Reduction of polypharmacy
o Discharge planning

- Frailty is more predictive of complication length of stay, discharge disposition and mortality both postoperatively and in the ICU than other traditional
  measures.
- ICU care bundles, such as the ABDCE bundle (*Practical Algorithm(s)/
  Diagrams* and *Review of Current Literature with References* sections) can
  address multiple issues for the geriatric patient, improving quality of care for
  geriatric patients.

Background

- Americans older than 65 years are the fastest-growing segment of the
  population.
- Over one third of inpatient operations in the U.S. are in patients over the age
  of 65.
- Adults over the age of 65 have different healthcare priorities, including
  different physiology, different goals of healthcare outcomes, atypical disease
  presentations, different distribution of disease patterns, and higher social
  support needs.
- Functional disability is both more important to patients 65 years and older in
  addition to serving as a marker of chronic disease.
- Geriatric patients are at higher risk of infection and iatrogenic injury.
- Geriatric specialty care issues can and should be managed starting in the ICU.

The Geriatric Patient in the ICU

- Physiologic Differences: Aging can affect all organ systems. Below are critical differences in geriatric patients that reflect an increasing loss of
  physiologic reserve in geriatric ICU patients.

  o Neurological: Dementia effects over 5 million Americans over the age of
     65. The risk of the development of Alzheimer's is 1 in 6 for women and
     1 in 11 for men and is one of the strongest predictors for delirium (see
     below). Patients in this age group are also at high risk for cardiovascular
     disease and hypertension, with higher risk for stroke.
  o Pulmonary: Pulmonary function tests change with age, with decreased
     lung elasticity, decreased chest wall compliance, and skeletal changes

with loss of vertebral space. This places individuals at higher risk of pulmonary complication. The following clinical changes are characteristic of the effect of age on lung physiology:

- Decreased expiratory flow rates (FEV1)
- Larger residual volume (RV)
- Reduction in vital capacity (VC)

o Cardiac: Cardiac changes are characterized by decreased reserve, including a blunted response to adrenergic stimulation and inability to mount an appropriate cardiac response to hypovolemia or shock. Specific changes include:

- Decreased cardiac index
- Increased systemic vascular resistance
- Occult hypoperfusion, leading to prolonged acidosis, and higher mortality rates in trauma

o Renal: Glomerular filtration rate (GFR) declines with aging. This is accompanied by increased glomerulosclerosis and loss of nephrons, independent of co-morbid conditions. Thus, the estimated GFR (eGFR) should be used in lieu of creatinine to better dose drugs for geriatric patients.

- eGFR Calculation in ml/min/1.73 m^2: $186 \times$ (serum creatinine in mg/dl)$^{1.154} \times$ (age in years)$^{-0.203} \times$ (0.742 if female) $\times$ (1.21 if African American)

o Body Mass: Aging is associated with a significant decrease in total body water, as well as decreased muscle mass and increased fat mass. This can effect both drug metabolism, and ability to handle large fluid shifts.

- Frailty

o Frailty is a condition of decreased global physiologic reserve that is not related directly to chronologic age, but is an essential clinical assessment for community-dwelling seniors over the age of 65.

o There is no standard measurement of physiologic reserve; however the phenotype of frailty can be characterized by decline in five age-associated domains: shrinking (unintentional weight loss of >10 lbs in last 12 months), weakness (measured by grip strength), exhaustion (measured by questionnaire), low physical activity (measured by clinician inquiry), and walking speed (measured by 15 foot walking speed).

o Frailty predicts postoperative complications, length of stay, and discharge to nursing independently of other risk scoring mechanisms.

- o Frailty can predict ICU outcomes more effectively than other ICU illness scores, including SOFA and SAPS II.
- o The assessment of frailty should be used in discussions with patients and their families as an aspect of informed consent.
- Delirium
  - o Delirium is when a patient acutely experiences disturbed consciousness, cognitive changes, or perceptual disturbance. Delirium can be classified as hyperactive (5%), hypoactive (50%), or normal/mild (45%).
  - o Major risk factors for postoperative delirium include dementia, advanced age (>80), recent delirium, major cardiac or abdominal surgery, emergency surgery, major postaoperative complication (shock, prolonged intubation), and ICU stay of >1 day. Other risk factors to consider include polypharmacy (usually considered to be >5 medications, effecting 50% of patients over 65), comorbidities, poor pain control, poor sleep hygiene, history of alcohol use, general anesthesia, exposure to opiates or sedatives, any surgery, any ICU stay.
  - o Diagnosis of delirium is used with the confusion assessment method (CAM) for verbal patients or the CAM-ICU for nonverbal patients (see Figs. 1 and 2).
  - o Prevention of delirium is most effective using systematic preoperative risk evaluation, consultation or co-management with a geriatrics team, and nurse-run programs to evaluate for and prevent delirium (see *Review of Current Literature with References* section).
  - o Management of delirium focuses first on non-pharmacologic strategies (family presence, familiar pictures at bedside, use of eyeglasses/hearing aids, frequent reorientation, encourage day/night cycling, limit nighttime stimulation, early mobility during the day, distraction vests). Restraints should be avoided and reserved only if harm to the patient or caregivers is eminent. The symptom of agitation can be managed pharmacologically with haloperidol 0.5–1mg IV or PO can be given for acute agitated delirium if other interventions fail and if the patient's QTc is <500 ms. For frail older adults, the dosage of haloperidol should be as low as possible and discontinued as soon as possible.
- Medication Issues
  - o Outpatient polypharmacy in the elderly can increase therapeutic complications, increases costs, and is associated with higher rates of delirium in the hospitalized geriatric patient. Every effort should be made to eliminate unnecessary outpatient medications, and minimize introduction of new medications on discharge, starting in the ICU.

o The American Geriatrics Society (http://americangeriatrics.org) updates a list of medications to avoid or use with caution in the elderly called the Beers List. This list should be consulted before initiating new medications, however a partial list is included in Table 1 for common ICU medications.

• Hospital Systems to Address Issues: Geriatric patients are at higher risk to suffer from a variety of syndromes that can occur in the hospitalized and postoperative patient. For the older patient in the ICU, a multidisciplinary and systematic approach to the below issues will improve patient outcomes and adherence to evidence-based programs. Some of these interventions can be bundled together, such as the ABCDE bundle (see Fig. 3). Specific geriatric protocols and programs will be further explored in *Review of Current Literature with References* section.

o Malnutrition: Appropriate nutrition is essential to the critically ill older adult. Geriatric patients are at higher risk for malnourished states. As many as 25–30% of geriatric patients will have the syndrome of malnutrition (unintended weight loss, hypoalbumenemia), which is associated with worse outcomes and higher complication rates. Protein and energy supplements are associated with weight gain, shorter length of stay, and lowered mortality. In addition to appropriate nutrition (tube feeds, TPN, etc.) for the patient's clinical condition, all older adults should receive Vitamin D 800 IU/day and Calcium 1000 mg/day.

   ▪ WHO Energy Estimates for Adults Over 60 Years of Age:

   Women: $(10.5) \times (\text{weight in kg}) + 596$

   Men: $(13.5) \times (\text{weight in kg}) + 487$

o Pain control and sedation: Benzodiazepine use is a significant contributor to delirium in the ICU geriatric patient. Alternatives to sedation while the patient is mechanically ventilated include dexmedetomidine, which can decrease rates of delirium by 20%. Short-acting opiate should be used for pain control, with attention paid to any chronic kidney or liver disease in addition to the physiologic effect of aging on the kidney.

o Intra- and Post-Operative Coronary Events: Cardiac risk assessment should be performed for all geriatric patients as well as routine EKG.

o Skin Breakdown: Geriatric patients may have decreased mobility which impacts the development of skin ulcers, making these patients higher risk for the development of this hospital-associated complication. Routine nursing evaluation, frequent turning, and a protocol for assessment and treatment of skin breakdown decreases rates of iatrogenic skin breakdown.

- o Mobility: ICU patients experience cognitive and physical decline, with half of patients failing to return to baseline up to 1 year after hospitalization. Critically ill geriatric patients can participate in physical activity and mobility in spite of severe medical conditions and life-sustaining equipment, including ventilators. A protocol for early mobilization in this population will improve both functional and cognitive quality of life, which are priorities for the older population. It also improves discharge to home (compared to nursing home), decreases delirium, and decreases doses of pain and sedating medications. See *Review of Current Literature with References* section for further details.

- Social Issues

  - o Five percent of Americans older than 65 years live in nursing homes; however the population is increasing, indicating that although the rate has remained stable, the absolute number of Americans living in nursing homes is increasing.

  - o Discharge to home is a significant priority for geriatric individuals who were at home prior to hospitalization.

  - o Identification of patients at risk of being unable to discharge to home can be identified either preoperative or in the ICU using techniques described above (early mobilization, frailty, etc.). Discussions with patients at risk of being unable to discharge to home should occur as early as possible to prepare patient, family, and social work.

  - o Early discussions regarding goals of care may include significant change interventions and direction of care.

  - o More about capacity, DNR, and end of life discussions can be found in the Ethics and Behavioral Sciences chapters.

Practical Algorithm(s)/Diagrams

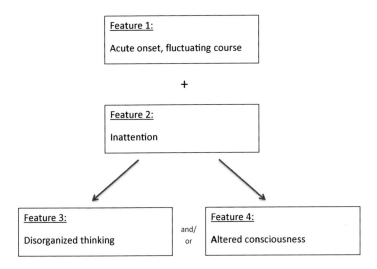

Fig. 1. Confusion assessment method (CAM).

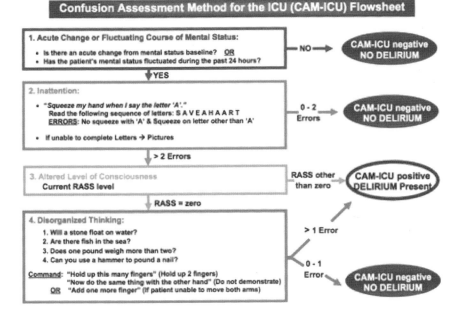

Fig. 2. CAM-ICU.

A	Spontaneous Awakening trials (SAT)	Daily sedation cessation, use of sedation scales for goal-directed therapy.
B	Spontaneous Breathing trials (SBT) in coordination with Awakening trials	Daily weaning trial, inter-professional coordination of SAT and SBT, protocol-driven wean from mechanical ventilation.
C	Choice of sedatives	Evidence-based choice of agent (avoid Beers List agents), intermittent v. continuous dosing, short-acting narcotic agents.
D	Delirium assessment and monitoring	Regular assessment for delirium, protocol to mitigate risk in all ICU patients.
E	Early mobility and Exercise	Daily exercise regimen for all ICU patients, ambulation for all appropriate patients (including ventilated patients).

Fig. 3. Awakening and Breathing trial coordination, Choice of sedatives and analgesics, Delirium monitoring, Early mobility and exercise (The ABCDE Bundle).

Table 1. Selection of medications from beers list to avoid in geriatric patients in ICU.

Drug Category	Specific Drugs to Avoid in ICU Care (and necessary comments)
Anticholinergics	Hydroxyzine
	Promethazine
Antispasmotics	Scopolamine
Alpha blockers (as first line antihypertensive)	Dexazosin
	Prazosin Terazosin
Alpha agonists	Clonidine
Antiarrhythmic drugs (as first line for new onset atrial fibrillation	Amiodarone (rate control has improved outcomes in geriatric population)
Antihypertensives	Nifedipine, immediate release
TCAs	Amitriptyline (strong anticholinergic effect)
	Doxepine
	Combination TCAs
Barbituates	Pentobarbital
	Phenobarbital
Benzodiazepines	Any type
Insulin, sliding scale	Insulin by protocol (higher risk of hypoglycemia)
Analgesics	Meperidine
	Non-COX-selective oral NSAIDs (can be given only if patient also on gastroprotective agent)
	Ketorolac

Review of Current Literature with References

- "Sedation, delirium and mechanical ventilation: the 'ABCDE' approach" Morandi A, Brummel NE, Ely EW. *Curr Opin Critical Care* 2011; **17**: 43–49.

  o Literature review of management of ventilated patients and strategies to improve outcomes.

  o The ICU 'ABCDE' bundle is an evidence-based interdisciplinary approach to ventilated patients.

  o Spontaneous awakening and breathing trials (the A and B) shorten duration of ventilation, ICU and hospital length of stay, and improve survival.

  o Choice of sedative (the C) to use an alpha-2 agonist reduces delirium and duration of ventilation.

  o Delirium monitoring (the D) improves diagnosis and intervention of delirium, although the optimal pharmacologic management is not yet determined.

  o Early mobility and exercise (the E) improves postoperative physical function and reduces delirium.

  o The 'ABCDE' bundle is an effective, evidence-based way to improve outcomes in the geriatric ICU population.

- "Dexmedetomidine vs lorazepam for sedation of critically ill patients: a randomized trial" Riker RR, Shehabi Y, Bokesch PM *et al.* JAMA 2009; **301**: 489–499.

  o Randomized controlled trial, double-blind, multicenter.

  o Sample size.

  o Patients sedated with dexemedetomidine had lower prevalence of delirium by >25% and two fewer days of mechanical ventilation.

  o Dexmedetomidine is appropriate for agitated and sedated ICU patients, especially those at high risk for delirium, like frail or geriatric populations.

- "ICU early mobilizations: from recommendation to implementation at three medical centers" Engel HJ, Needham DM, Morris PE, Gropper MA. *Critical Care Med* 2013; **41**: S69–S80.

  o Quality Improvement.

  o 860 patients from three academic center ICUs.

  o All ICUs found with limited additional personnel and limited additional resources, instituting early mobility was feasible and safe using the 'Plan-Do-Study-Act' implementation strategy.

o   All ICUs confirmed that early mobility was associated with decreased ICU and hospital LOS, decreased dosages of sedating medications and delirium rates, and net cost savings.

o   Early mobility is an achievable goal for all ICU patients and essential to improved outcomes.

- "Prevalence and impact of frailty on mortality in elderly ICU patients: a prospective, multicenter, observational study." Le Maguet P, Roquilly A, *et al*. *Intensive Care Med* 2014; **40**: 674–682.

o   Prospective, multicenter observational study.

o   196 patients in four ICUs.

o   Frailty was observed in 20–40% of patients admitted to the ICU. Frailty was associated with a hazard ratio (HR) of 3.3 for ICU mortality and HR of 2.4 for 6-month mortality.

o   Frailty is an accurate way to predict mortality in the critically ill patient.

- "Polypharmacy: the cure becomes the disease" Colley CA, Lucas LM. *J General Internal Med* 1993; **8**: 278–283.

o   Literature review.

o   Polypharmacy is when a medical regimen includes at least one unnecessary medication. Thirty-five percent of patients over the age of 85 leave encounters with three or more new prescriptions. Fifty percent of patients leaving the hospital have medication errors from changes to their drug regimen (including errors in drug selection and drug dosing), 12% of which could be potentially serious errors.

o   Polypharmacy leads to increased side effects (including serious adverse reactions), noncompliance with the medication regimen (estimates between 25–59% of elderly patients) and increased direct and indirect costs (10–17% of hospital geriatric admissions are related to adverse drug events).

o   Polypharmacy can be mitigated by eliminating pharmacologic duplication (using monotherapy, avoiding combinations with high risk of adverse interaction), decreasing the dosing frequency of medications, and a structured review of drug regimen at transitions of care (such as from the ICU) to make sure all agents are still needed and to simplify the regimen as much as possible.

Chapter 25

Bariatric

Fredric M. Pieracci, MD* and Jeffrey Johnson, MD†

*Acute Care Surgeon, Denver Health Medical Center

†Associate Professor of Surgery, University of Colorado School of Medicine

Take Home Points

- Most Americans are overweight, obese, or morbidly obese. The prevalence of obesity, morbid obesity, and bariatric surgery are all increasing exponentially; the number of these patients who will require critical care is thus expected to mirror these increases.
- Excess adipose tissue exerts deleterious effects on all organ systems through two basic mechanisms: increased mechanical load and secretion of active metabolites and hormones.
- Obesity is an independent risk factor for both morbidity and mortality during critical illness.

Contact information: (Fredric M. Pieracci) Denver Health Medical Center, 777 Bannock Street, MC 0206, A388, Denver, CO 80206. (Jeffery Johnson) MC 0206, 777 Bannock St., Denver CO 80204; Email: Jeffery.Johnson@dhha.org; Fredric.Pieracci@dhha.org

- Obesity does not equate with "over-nourishment." In fact, the opposite is true. Hyper-insulinemia and sedentary lifestyle result in protein catabolism and malnutrition.
- Early (2–4 hours postoperatively) and frequent ambulation is imperative for preventing complications in obese surgical patients.
- Large discrepancies between actual body weight (ABW) and ideal body weight (IBW) exist in morbidly obese patients. This discrepancy has implications for the ICU care of these patients, most importantly ventilator settings, caloric requirements, and drug dosing.

Background

- Obesity and morbid obesity are defined using the body mass index (BMI), which is equal to the weight in kilograms divided by the height in meter squared; normal BMI is 20–25 kg/m^2; overweight is defined as BMI 25–30 kg/m^2; obesity is defined as BMI 30–39 kg/m^2; morbid obesity is defined as either (1) BMI $\geq$40 kgm^2 or (2) BMI $\geq$35 kg/m^2 with one or more obesity-related comorbidities (discussed below).
- Excess adipose tissue exerts deleterious effects on all organ systems through two basic mechanisms: increased mechanical load and secretion of active metabolites and hormones.
- Recent cross sectional analyzes have reported that approximately 25% of critically ill patients are obese.
- Recent cohort series have reported that approximately 5% of laparoscopic and 15% of open bariatric surgery patients require $\geq$24 hours of ICU care. Risk factors for ICU admission after bariatric surgery include: male sex, age >50 years, BMI > 60 kg/m^2, diabetes mellitus, cardiovascular disease, obstructive sleep apnea syndrome, venous stasis, and intra-operative complications.
- Inflammation, hypercoagulability, and insulin resistance characterize obesity as a disease process that mimics critical illness.
- Adipose tissue is a potent source of both pro-inflammatory cytokines and pro-coagulants.
- Increased BMI requires increased cardiovascular, respiratory, and metabolic work, resulting in a markedly diminished physiologic reserve.
- Most studies have reported that the extremes of BMI (<15 kg/m^2 and >30 kg/m^2) are associated with mortality among critically ill patients. This potential increased risk appears to be mitigated in ICUs that care for a higher percentage of obese patients, suggesting that familiarity with the aforementioned pathophysiology may impact outcomes favorably.

Main Body

- Caring for the critically ill obese patient presents unique challenges regarding the management of each organ system, outlined below and summarized in Table 1.

Respiratory

- Obesity results in a restrictive lung pattern due to both increased pulmonary blood volume and increased chest wall mass from adipose tissue.
- Abnormal diaphragm position, upper airway resistance, and increased daily CO_2 production increase work of breathing.
- As a result, functional residual capacity is markedly decreased, resulting in rapid and potentially fatal desaturation following relatively brief periods of hypoxia (e.g., during induction of general anesthesia or bronchoscopy).
- Maneuvers to mitigate increased abdominal (and thus thoracic) pressure in the obese, ventilated patient include the addition of 10 mmHg of PEEP, and reverse Trendelenburg positioning at 45°.
- Obesity is correlated strongly with obstructive sleep apnea syndrome, and this diagnosis should be considered in all critically ill obese patients. Associated symptoms include snoring, systemic and pulmonary hypertension, gastro-esophageal reflux disease (GERD), and daytime somnolence. Apneic episodes occur with greatest frequency on post-operative day 5, which correlate with the resumption of rapid eye movement sleep. Current data suggest that mask delivery of continuous positive airway pressure (CPAP) does not increase the incidence of anastomotic leak.
- Percutaneous dilational tracheostomy (Chapter 19) may be performed safely in morbidly obese patients, provided that extra-long tracheostomy tubes are available.

Cardiovascular

- The majority of obese patients have one or more risk factors for coronary artery disease — hypertension and diabetes mellitus are most common. Due to a sedentary lifestyle, typical symptoms of angina or congestive heart failure may not be elicited easily; therefore, obese patients must be assumed to have coronary artery disease.
- Cardiovascular pathology from obesity is characterized by both diastolic dysfunction and pulmonary hypertension. These derangements are secondary to increased preload (due to increased circulating blood volume)

and afterload (due to increased concentrations of both catecholamines and mineralicorticoids).

- Noninvasive blood pressure monitoring is often inaccurate in obese patients due to cuff size mismatch, and an indwelling arterial catheter (Chapter 15) should be employed whenever hemodynamic stability is in question.
- β-blockade should be used cautiously in obese patients because of impaired ventricular contractility secondary to decreased β–adrenergic receptors.

Nutrition

- Obesity is characterized by the "metabolic X syndrome": insulin resistance, hyperinsulinemia, coronary artery disease, hypertension, and hyperlipidemia. Elevated insulin concentration suppresses lipid mobilization at the expense of protein catabolism to support gluconeogenesis.
- Obesity is characterized by protein-calorie malnutrition secondary to both low protein diet and the malabsorptive effects of inflammatory cytokines. Obese patients have increased resting energy expenditure secondary to increased BMI. Thus, contrary to popular belief, most obese patients are under-nourished.
- Nutritional requirements should approximate 30 kcal/kg/day and 2.0 g/kg/day of protein, and should be based on IBW [Chapter 8-(i)].
- Placements of a feeding gastrostomy should be considered during bariatric surgery when a period of critical illness is anticipated, or when the patient requires multiple enteral outpatient medications.

Thromboembolic disease

- Obesity is a thrombogenic state secondary to increased blood viscosity, decreased concentration of anti-thrombin-III, and increased concentrations of both fibrinogen and plasminogen inhibitor-1 produced by adipose tissue. Sedentary lifestyle, venous stasis, and pulmonary hypertension augment this risk.
- Several large series have identified obesity as a risk factor for venous thromboembolism (VTE) both after surgery and during critical illness.
- Obese patients should receive chemical prophylaxis against VTE as soon as possible, and preferably using goal-direction [Chapter 9-(ii)], as standard doses of pharmacoprophylaxis are usually inadequate. For example, one study found that morbidly obese, critically ill patients remained hypercoagulable as detected by thromboelastography, despite treatment with enoxaparin 40 mg SQ twice daily.

- VTE pharmacoprophylaxis should continue for at least 30 days post-operatively (or post-critical illness), as many fatal VTE-related events occur as outpatients during this time period.
- Prophylactic vena cava filter placement for bariatric patients at extremely high risk for VTE (BMI >50 kg/m^2) may be considered, though the efficacy of this strategy has not been proven.

Pharmacology

- Creatinine clearance of obese patients is highly variable: whereas obese patients with normal renal function have an increased glomerular filtration rate (and thus an increased clearance of drugs excreted by the kidney), underlying diabetes mellitus and hypertension may cause kidney dysfunction.
- Calculated and measured creatinine correlate poorly in obese patients: measured is preferred.
- Follow serum concentration of drugs whenever possible in obese patients.
- Lipophilic drugs accumulate in excess adipose tissue of obese patients, both increasing the volume of distribution and prolonging the elimination half-life. Thus, dosing of these drugs is best approximated using ABW.
- Conversely, dosing of hydrophilic drugs is best approximated using IBW because of poor penetration into adipose tissue.
- Dosing weights in obese patients for select drugs are summarized in Table 2.

Anastomotic leak after bariatric surgery

- Anastomotic leak after bariatric surgery is a devastating complication.
- Abdominal exam findings in morbidly obese patients are unreliable.
- The most sensitive findings are sustained tachycardia (HR >110 bpm) and respiratory failure.
- Because of the broad differential for the aforementioned signs in post-operative period, radiologic imaging of the stable bariatric patient in whom a leak is suspected is warranted. We favor computed tomography with oral contrast, as evaluation of the gastrojejunostomy, gastric remnant staple line, and jejunojejunostomy are all possible.
- If there is a strong clinical suspicion for anastomotic leak, or if the patient is unstable, imaging is contra-indicated and the next step is laparotomy.

Practical Algorithm(s)/Diagrams

Table 1. Major organ system derangements in obesity (reproduced with permission from Pieracci and Barie. *Crit Care Med* 2006; **34**: 1796).

Organ system	Pathology
Respiratory	↓ FRC, TLC, VC. IC. ERV
	↑ FEV$_1$/FVC
	Obstructive sleep apnea syndrome
Cardiovascular	↑ Blood volume
	↑ Vascular tone
	↓ Ventricular contractility
Renal	↑ Clearance of rertally excreted drugs
	Hypertensive and diabetic neptiropathy
Hematologic	↑ Fibrinogen
	↑ PAI-1
	AT-III
	Venous stasis
Gastrointestinal	Hiatal hernia
	↑ Gastric secretion volume
	↓ Gastric pH
Metabolic/Endocrine	↑ Resting energy expenditure
	Insulin resistance
	↑ Proteolysis
immunologic	↑ TNF-α
	↑ IL-6
	Impaired neutrophil function

Table 2. Dosing weights in obese patients for selected drugs used commonly in critical illness (reproduced with permission from Pieracci and Barie. *Crit Care Med* 2006; **34**: 1796).

Drug	Dosing weight
Propofol	ABW
Benzodiazepines	
Single-dosage	ABW
Continuous infusion	IBW
Fentanyl	$52/(1 + [196.4 \times e^{-0.025} ABW - 53.66]/100)$
Vancomycin	ABW
Aminoglycosides	IBW + (0.40 × [ABW – IBW])
Fluoroquinolones	IBW + (0.40 × [ABW – IBW])
Drotrecogin alfa (activated)	ABW

ABW, actual body weight; IBW, ideal body weight.

Review of Current Literature with References

- Naswraway *et al.* reported that morbid obesity was an independent predictor of mortality among a cohort of 1,373 critically ill surgical patients (*Crit Care Med* 2006; **34**: 964).
- In a series of 1,067 consecutive gastric bypass patients, Livingston *et al.* noted similar rates of anastomotic leak in patients receiving CPAP compared to those note receiving CPAP (*Ann Surg* 2002; **236**: 576).
- In a review of 210 consecutive laparoscopic gastric bypass patients, Hamilton *et al.* found severe tachycardia (heart rate >120 bpm) and respiratory failure (the development of an increasing oxygen requirement after discharge from the post-anesthesia care unit, SaO_2 <92% on room air, or respiratory rate >24 breaths/minute) to be the two most common presenting manifestations of anastomotic leak (*Surg Endosc* 2003; **17**: 679).

Chapter 26

Cardiothoracic

Ashok Babu* and Ryan Shelstad†

*Assistant Professor of Surgery, University of Colorado School of Medicine
†Cardiothoracic Surgery Fellow, University of Colorado School of Medicine

Take Home Points

- Hemodynamics define perfusion in the post-cardiac surgery patient.
- Cardiac surgery patients tend to have defined, often surgically treated, cardiac disease with predictable response to hemodynamic management.
- Resuscitation priorities include coagulopathy correction, preload restoration, and maintenance of hematocrit.
- Optimize preload and contractility/cardiac output with pressor support. Some cardiac patients will need pressor/contractility support regardless of preload.
- Fill the pump, push the pump, support the pump mechanically if needed.
- In the patient with failing ventricle, mechanic support can be a useful bridge to recovery or to advanced heart failure therapy.

Contact information: 12505 E. 16th Ave, Aurora, CO 80045; Email: Ashok.babu@ucdenver.edu, ryan.shelstad@ucdenver.edu

Background

- ICU Hemodynamics define perfusion.
- Swan-Ganz PA catheter:
    - CVP approximates RV preload, normal <15 mmHg.
    - PAD is closest to LEDP, so approximates LV preload; usually <15, but may need more if diastolic dysfunction present.
    - Mean PA-CVP >8 mmHg indicates adequate RV function.
    - Goal Cardiac Index: CI >2.2.
    - Mixed Venous saturation: normal 70%.
- Hemodynamic algorithm
- 1. Optimize preload: fill the pump
    - Fluid is almost always the answer.
    - Colloid over crystalloid.
    - If RV failing, then lasix
- 2. Optimize SVR: <700 or >1800 dynes-s/cm^{-5}
    - Vasopressin (0.04) especially if on ACE inhibitor preoperatively.
    - Rarely norepinephrine or phenylephrine.
- Contractility
    - Last line, Epinephrine 0.01–0.05 mg/kg/min if low SVR.
    - High or normal SVR→dobutamine (0–15 mcg/kg/min).
    - Still issues, then consider mechanical support (IABP).
    - Sinus rhythm is best (atrial kick provides 15–30% CO).
    - Pacing: Atrial is optimal; AV better than V alone.

Main Body

- Postop Valve CABG:
- Bleeding >200 ml/hr is concerning. Watch drain outputs. Maintain HCT >21.
    - Corrected coagulation mean normal fibrinogen, platelets >100, INR <1.6.
- Atrial fibrillation
    - Tachycardia is Atrial Fibrilliation until proven otherwise, usually occurs POD 3–5.
    - EKG for diagnosis. Adenosine 6 mg can differentiate SVT.
    - Goal is rate control <110, not sinus rhythm.

- o If BP unstable, then cardiovert per ACLS (rare).
- o If BP stable, IV metoprolol (5 mg IV × 3).
- o Amiodarone 150 mg load, plus 24 hour gtt or Diltiazem 2.5–15mg.

- Aortic Surgery (Root, ascending, arch, descending, thoracic).
- Bleeding: almost all will get transfusion. Correct coagulation **completely**.
- Neuro: at least hourly neurovascular checks.

- o Root to arch: CVA.
- o Arch to abdomen: paraplegia.

- Analgesia: most will need PCA due to extensive incision.
- Extubate ASAP; OOB and ambulate ASAP.
- Lumbar CSF drain: place preoperatively for high-risk paraplegia (Spinal perfusion = MAP-intrathecal pressure).

- o Level at Right Atrium.
- o If weak, drain to pressure 10 mmHg. Limit drainage to less than 20 ml/hr and 200 ml/day.
- o If not weak, clamp × 24 hours then remove (hold heparin × 12 hours for removal).

- Aortic Dissection
- All require ICU admission with a-line placement.
- Type B medical management.
- Type A (ascending) is a surgical emergency due to risk of tamponade/rupture, aortic valve insufficiency, and coronary dissection.
- Treatment goal is surgical restoration of flow to true lumen with separation of root from dissection.
- If unsure of diagnosis, transfer straight to OR and confirm with TEE.
- Type B (descending) are either complicated or uncomplicated.

- o Complicated: malperfusion requiring intervention to restore flow to end organ.
- o Uncomplicated: medical management.
- o Decrease HR <80 with esmolol, then control SBP <120 with nicardipine.

- Mechanical Circulatory Support
- Inta-aortic balloon pump (IABP):

- o Placed in descending aorta, fills in diastole and empties in systole.
- o Can be set to trigger by EKG or pressure (a-line).
- o Reduces afterload, augments pressure.

- Extra corporeal membrane oxygenation (ECMO).
- Veno-venous ECMO used to support pulmonary failure.
  - Best candidates have single organ pathology of reversible etiology.
  - Peripheral cannulation.
- Veno-arterial used to support cardiopulmonary failure.
  - Best candidates have single organ pathology and are potential transplant/ LVAD candidates.
  - Peripheral or central cannulation.

Practical Algorithm(s)/Diagrams

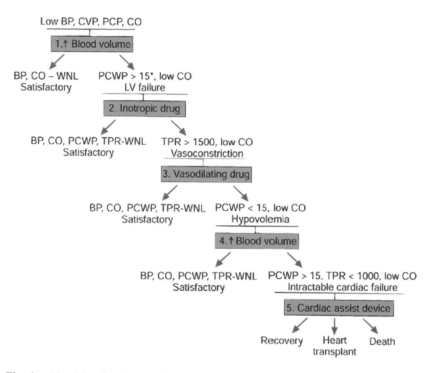

Fig. 1. Algorithm for therapy of low cardiac output. PAOP is an indirect measure of LVEDP; PAOP greater than 15 mmHg may be necessary in patients with a pressure gradient across the mitral valve and in those with elevated PAOP before surgery as a result of low ventricular compliance. BP, blood pressure; CVP, central venous pressure; PAOP, pulmonary capillary wedge pressure; CO, cardiac output; TPR, total peripheral resistance; WNL, within normal limits; ↑, increase. Measurement units are mmHg for pressure, dynes/cm^5/s for resistance, and L/min for CO.

Review of Current Literature with References

- Morales DA *et al*. A double-blind randomized trial: prophylactic vasopressin reduces postoperative hypotension following cardiopulmonary bypass. *Ann Thor Surg* **75** (3): 926–930, 2003.
- Randomized, blind study of 33 patients on ACE inhibitor therapy undergoing cardiopulmonary bypass. The study group required less norepinephrine and had physiologically normal levels of AVP. The study confirms the physiologic utility of vasopressin in the management of post-CPB vasodilation.

Chapter **27**

Obstetrics

Sara Mazzoni, MD, MPH*

*Assistant Professor of Obstetrics and Gynecology, University of Colorado School of Medicine

Take Home Points

- Pregnancy is a time of profound physiologic change.
- Vital signs and laboratory values are altered by pregnancy.
- Maternal well-being is the first priority in the pregnant critically-ill patient. Diagnostic or therapeutic interventions (such as imaging and medications) should not be delayed or avoided due to concerns about the fetus.
- Obstetric hemorrhage remains the most common reason for admission to the surgical intensive care unit in developed countries and one of the most common causes of maternal death. Massive transfusion protocol is not altered by pregnancy.
- Care of the pregnant trauma patient must include a multi-disciplinary team with maternal stabilization as the primary goal.

Contact information: Denver Health Medical Center, University of Colorado Health Sciences Center, 777 Bannock Street, MC 0660, Denver, CO 80204; Tel.: 303-602-9733, email: Sara.mazzoni@dhha.org

Background

- Pregnancy-induced changes in physiology and anatomy must be considered during the evaluation and management of a critically-ill gravida. Important changes by system include:
  - Cardiovascular
    - ↑ cardiac output
    - ↑ blood volume (by 50%)
    - ↑ heart rate (by 5–15 beats per minute)
    - ↓ systemic vascular resistance
    - ↓ blood pressure by 10–15 mmHg
    - ↓ venous return from the lower extremities
    - ↑↑ uterine blood flow (up to 600 mL/min)
  - Respiratory
    - ↑ minute ventilation
    - ↓ functional residual capacity
    - Arterial blood gas changes (respiratory alkalosis):
      - ⇨ ↑ PaO_2
      - ⇨ ↑ PCO_2
      - ⇨ ↓ base deficit
    - Elevation of the diaphragm (important for chest tube placement)
  - Gastrointestinal
    - ↓ gastric motility and emptying
    - Bowel crowded in to upper abdomen
  - Coagulation
    - ↑ clotting factors I, VII, VIII, IX, X and fibrinogen
    - ↑ risk for thromboembolic disease
  - Renal
    - ↑ renal plasma flow and glomerular filtration rate
    - ↑ ureteral dilation
  - Laboratory
    - ↓ serum creatinine, blood urea nitrogen (BUN), hemoglobin and hematocrit
    - ↑ white blood cell count, alkaline phosphatase level, fibrinogen, D-dimer and erythrocyte sedimentation rate

- A fetus is considered viable, or able to survive after delivery, at 24 weeks gestation.

Main Body

- Hemorrhage
  - o Obstetrical hemorrhage is the second most common cause of all ICU admissions during pregnancy, and the most common reason in the SICU. Although the patient is postpartum upon admission to the ICU, her physiology is still that of pregnancy.
  - o A pregnant woman can lose up to 30% of her blood volume before demonstrating changes in her vital signs.
  - o Hemodynamic changes during the immediate postpartum period include increased cardiac preload due to autotransfusion of blood from the uterus back to the intravascular space with a resulting increase in cardiac output and stroke volume, both of which normalize gradually. Diuresis normally occurs between day 2 and 5 postpartum to allow for loss of excess extracellular fluid.
  - o Blood product transfusion protocol as covered in Chapter 9-(i) is not altered by pregnancy.
  - o Medications routinely used during an obstetric hemorrhage include Pitocin (synthetic oxytocin), misoprostol/Cytotec and Hemabate (prostaglandins), and methylergonovine/Methergine (an ergot derivative).
  - o Surgical procedures commonly performed by the obstetric team during a hemorrhage include
    - B-Lynch suture — a uterine compression suture.
    - O'Leary stitch — uterine artery ligation.
    - Bakri balloon — a silicone balloon attached to a catheter filled to a maximum of 500 cc with sterile saline to provide tamponade. Uterine bleeding will continue to drain from the catheter.
    - Selective uterine artery embolization — performed by interventional radiology.
    - Hysterectomy (removing the uterine body, leaving the ovaries and cervix).
- Trauma during pregnancy
  - o Traumatic injuries are the most common cause of non-obstetrical maternal death. The most frequent traumas in pregnancies are motor vehicle

crashes, falls and assaults. The most common obstetrical complications of trauma are placental abruption, preterm labor and fetal loss.

o Maternal and fetal risks following the injury depend on the timing of pregnancy.

- In the first trimester, the risk of direct trauma to the uterus is very low since the uterus is still protected in the bony pelvis, yet the developing fetus will be affected by maternal hypovolemia since the blood flow to the uterus is not autoregulated.
- In the second trimester, abdominal organs are misplaced. Uteroplacental circulation can now be compromised in the supine position due to aortocaval compression and pregnant women should be placed in the lateral decubitus position.
- In the third trimester, the risk of direct injury to the uterus and fetus are greatest, yet vital maternal organs are protected by the uterus.

o Considerations of specific types of injury:

- **Blunt** trauma to the maternal abdomen can cause placental abruption due to shearing forces on the uterus and attached placenta. This obstetrical complication can result in life-threatening hemorrhage for both the mother and fetus.
- **Fractures** are most common in the lower extremities, yet pelvic fractures are most likely to result in an adverse outcome for both the mother and fetus due to the hypertrophy of the pelvic retroperitoneal vasculature. A pelvic fracture is not necessarily a contraindication to a vaginal delivery.
- **Penetrating trauma** is less likely to result in death in pregnancy due to the protection of vital organs by the gravid uterus. Wounds to the upper abdomen can result in complex bowel injury.
- **Burns** carry the same prognosis during pregnancy, yet require more aggressive fluid resuscitation due to physiologic changes of pregnancy (increased blood volume, decreased colloid osmotic pressure and increased body surface area).

o Assessment and management of the pregnant trauma patient begins in the emergency department and should include coordination of emergency medicine physicians, trauma surgeons and obstetricians. The equipment to perform a Cesarean delivery should be readily accessible, and personnel to perform neonatal resuscitation on stand-by.

- **Maternal well-being and stabilization are the first priority.** Initial assessment of the woman is not altered by pregnancy other than left lateral displacement of the gravid uterus. After the primary survey and stabilization of the mother, assessment of the pregnancy includes ultrasound to determine fetal viability and gestational age (this can be done following a maternal FAST scan).

- Secondary obstetric assessment includes fetal and uterine contraction monitoring to evaluate for fetal well-being and signs of placental abruption or preterm labor (such as vaginal bleeding or loss of fluid). This should occur in the emergency department if the patient remains there undergoing additional evaluation, and otherwise should occur on labor and delivery for at least 4 hours following the trauma.
- In addition to routine laboratory testing, a blood type should be ordered to assure that Rh negative women receive Rhogam.

- Surgery during pregnancy
  - In the latter half of pregnancy, the gravid uterus compresses the IVC requiring that the patient be placed in a left **lateral tilt** during surgery.
  - Exposure to anesthetic agents is safe during pregnancy. Pregnant patients are at increased risk of aspiration and are more difficult to intubate.
  - The early second trimester is the ideal time to perform non-emergent operations that cannot be delayed until postpartum.
  - Continuous intraoperative fetal monitoring is not essential. The decision to monitor the fetus should be made in consultation with the obstetric team and depends on factors such as gestational age, type of surgery and maternal condition.
  - Laparoscopy is safe during any trimester of pregnancy. Insufflation pressures should be kept below 15 mmHg.

- Intensive Care Unit
  - Cardiopulmonary arrest in pregnancy is very rare, and as such, there is limited data. CPR during pregnancy is made more difficult by anatomic and physiologic changes. Modifications include:
    - Left uterine displacement either manually, tilting the table upon which the patient is positioned or placing a wedge under the right hip.
    - Aggressive airway management because of increased oxygen utilization, risk of aspiration and difficult intubations due to edema.
    - Increase in chest wall compression force due to anatomic changes.
    - Use higher doses of medications if the patient does not respond to standard doses to account for the expanded plasma volume of pregnancy.

- Begin Cesarean delivery in 4 minutes if spontaneous circulation is not restored; mostly to aid in maternal resuscitation with the possible benefit of infant survival.
- **Maternal resuscitation takes precedence over the fetus.**

- Radiology
  - Concerns regarding exposing the developing fetus to ionizing radiation should never delay medically indicated imaging of pregnant women. All risks and benefits must be considered, including the risks to both mother and fetus of incorrect or delayed diagnosis.
  - Ultrasound and magnetic resonance imaging (MRI) are the imaging modalities of choice during pregnancy when possible as neither are associated with known adverse fetal effects. Gadolinium, the contrast medium used for MR, is not recommended in pregnancy.
  - A plain X-ray generally exposes the fetus to very small amounts of radiation. With the exception of barium enema or small bowel series, most fluoroscopic examinations result in fetal exposure of millirads. Radiation exposure from computed tomography (CT) varies depending on the number and spacing of adjacent image sections but is also minimal when not involving the abdomen or pelvis.
  - Women may breastfeed after receiving iodinated contrast media.

Review of Current Literature with References

- Chames MC, Pearlman MD. Trauma during pregnancy: Outcomes and clinical management. *Clin Obstet Gynecol* 2008; **51**: 398–408.
- Chen MM, Coakley FV, Kaimal A, Laros RK. Guidelines for computed tomography and magnetic resonance imaging use during pregnancy and lactation. *Obstet Gynecol* 2008; **112**: 333–340.
- Foley MR, Strong TH, Garite TJ. *Obstetric Intensive Care Manual, Fourth edition*. New York: McGraw-Hill Education, 2014.
- Management of Intrapartum Fetal Heart Rate Tracings. *ACOG Practice Bulletin Number 116*, November 2010.
- Pearlman MD, Tintinali JE, Lorenz RP. A prospective controlled study of outcome after trauma during pregnancy. *Am J Obstet Gynecol* 1990; **162**; 1502–1507.
- Vanden Hoek TL, Morrison IJ, Shuster M *et al*. Part 12: Cardiac arrest in special situations: 2010 American Heart Association guidelines for cardiopulmonary resuscitation and emergency cardiovascular care. *Circulation* 2010; **122**: S829–S861.

V: Special Issues

Chapter 28

Burn

Gordon Lindberg*

*Associate Professor of Surgery, University of Colorado School of Medicine

Take Home Points

- Skin is the largest solid organ in the body and is very sensitive to thermal injuries.
- Burn units treat thermal, chemical and electrical injuries.
- Burn care is referral-based and burn care begins in the field, continues during transport to the hospital, in the emergency department and in the Burn Unit.
- A good history of the injury and physical exam can often predict the need for emergency surgery and the need for grafting before the patient arrives at the burn unit.
- The burn patient is, first and foremost, a trauma patient and trauma injuries need to be ruled out before concentrating on the burn.
- Burn patients require aggressive, but appropriate fluid resuscitation.
- Escharotomies need to be performed on all full thickness circumferential burns and many non-circumferential near-full thickness burns.
- Inhalation injuries occur in triad of smoke inhalation, enclosed space and elevated carboxy-hemoglobin.

Contact information: Medical Director Burn Unit, University of Colorado. 1635 Aurora Court, Aurora, CO 80045; Email: Gordon.Lindberg@ucdenver.edu

- Chemical burns require immediate irrigation for best outcomes.
- Electrical injuries often have associated trauma and affect almost every organ system in the body.

Background

- There are 450,000 burn injuries requiring medical attention each year in the United States.
- Burn injuries are a significant part of any mass casualty disaster or terrorist attack.
- These patients need to be referred to a burn unit within 24 hours of the injury for best outcomes.
- Burn referral criteria are:

  o >10% Total Body Surface Area partial thickness burns.
  o Any third-degree burn.
  o Any burn to the hands, feet, face, perineum, genitalia or across major joints.
  o Burns associated with pre-existing major medical conditions.
  o Burns associated with trauma.

Main Body

- **The patient is a trauma patient first — Primary Survey**
- Approach the burn patient as you would any trauma patient. Make sure it is safe and employ Universal Precautions.
- The burn patient will be alert and oriented, answering questions, and be tachycardic and hypertensive. If the patient is hypotensive, there are intoxicants present or there is a trauma injury.
- If there is suspicion for trauma, ignore the burn and concentrate on trauma workup:

  o Place the patient in a c-spine collar and use log roll precautions.
  o Obtain an abdominal FAST exam.
  o Obtain plain films per trauma protocol.

- Place two large bore IV's. You can go through burn if you need to, do a saphenous venous cut down, place central lines and even use interosseous infusions if is a need.
- Place Foley.

- You can start the Parkland Resuscitation while the patient is in the CT scanner to rule out trauma.
- **Rule out and treat Inhalation Injuries**
- Inhalation injuries occur in the triad of breathing smoke in an enclosed space, real carbonaceous sputum and an elevated carboxy-hemoglobin.
- Asking the patient to speak and if his voice is abnormal, suspect an inhalation injury.
- If the carboxy-hemoglobin is high, or if the patient is acidotic, treat for cyanide toxicity using a cyanokit, which is hydroxocobalamin (a Vitamin B-12 precursor).
- Intubate if needed using as large an ETT tube as possible.
- Place NGT if intubating.
- **Parkland Resuscitation**
- For burns less than 30% total body surface area (TBSA), start Normal Saline or Lactated Ringers at maintenance fluid amounts, based on the patients weight.
- For burns greater than 30% TBSA Parkland Resuscitation is divided into two phases: pre-hospital and upon arrival to the hospital. The pre-hospital fluids are based on age:
  - o <5 years get 125 cc's/hour, Children must have dextrose added to their fluids.
  - o 6–13 years get 250 cc's/hour,
  - o >14 years get 500 cc's/hour.
- In-hospital fluids, over the first 24 hours, are based on age of patient, weight and the size of the burn:
  - o Anyone >14 y/o or >40 kgms: 2 cc's LR times weight in kgms times % TBSA
  - o Anyone <14 y/o or <40 kgms: 3 cc's LR times weight in kgms times % TBSA
  - o Electrical injuries 4 cc's LR times weight in kgms times % TBSA

Half of this fluid is given in the first eight hours <u>after the time of the burn</u> (not after they arrive in the hospital) and the second half is given over the next 16 hours, <u>after the time of the burn</u>.

The burn size is determined by a Lund Browder Diagram or by the rule of nines (see figures). For irregular shapes, the person's hand is 1% of their TBSA.

Note, the fluid administration is the same for 2nd (partial thickness) and 3rd (full thickness burns). This is not a mistake.

- **Secondary Survey**
- Complete Head to Toe exam, time to rule out extremity injuries.
- Remove finger rings, necklaces and any constricting jewelry.
- Send off labs: CBC, ABG with carboxy-hemaglobin, serum chemistries, toxicology screen, blood alcohol level, coagulation labs (TEG, PT, PTT, INR), type and cross for blood and FFP, Urinalysis, CXR.
- Additional X-rays as needed for trauma workup.
- Start pain control using fentanyl/dilaudid and versed/ativan.
- For large burns, dress with warm sheets and do not use saline soaked gauze (it will cause hypothermia). Place warm blankets over the patient. Use fluid warmers and heat the room.
- Now is also the time to get a thorough history, list of medications, past medical history and elucidate more clearly the circumstances surrounding the burn.

    o Fire Burn: Were there other people injured? Was patient ambulating? Was patient trapped near fire? Was there trauma?
    o Scald Burn: What liquid? What temperature? How much liquid? Was the patient wearing clothes? Were they cooled off in the field?
    o Chemical Injury: How long was the patient exposed to the chemical? What was the chemical and concentration? Was there decontamination?
    o Electrical Injury: Direct or indirect current? What voltage current? Was the patient thrown? Was there loss of consciousness? CPR in the field?
    o Is the history consistent with the burn? This is an important consideration with children.

- Now is also the time to differentiate partial thickness from full thickness burns. Partial thickness burns are weepy, tender and blanch. Full thickness burns are non-tender and do not blanch, even when they are red. Note: Full thickness burns induces pain and need to be treated with narcotics.
- Also make note if there are circumferential burns to extremities or torso.
- Past Medical History, use AMPLET

    o Allergies
    o Medications
    o Past Medical History, Pregnancy
    o Last Meal
    o Events
    o Tetanus and immunizations

- **Transferring to a Burn Unit**

- Burn patients develop a severe ileus if feeding is not started within six hours of injury, it is acceptable to gastric feed using NGT.
- Call nearest Burn Unit for transfer arrangements and ask to speak to the attending.
- When giving report on the patient, please give the details of the accident, the events in the field and ED, the trauma workup, the resuscitation to date and the patient's past medical history. Also mention if you think the patient may need escharotomies.

Practical Algorithm(s)/Diagrams

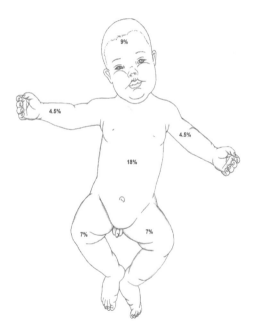

Fig. 1. Estimated percentage total body surface area for infant (front).

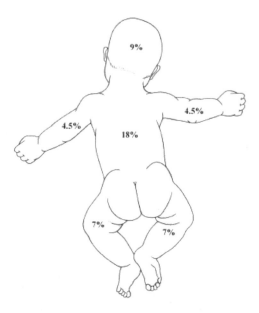

Fig. 2. Estimated percentage total body surface area for infant (back).

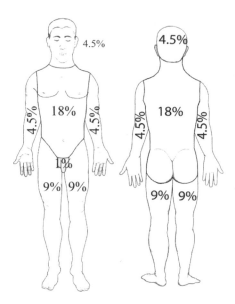

Fig. 3. Estimated percentage total body surface area for adult.

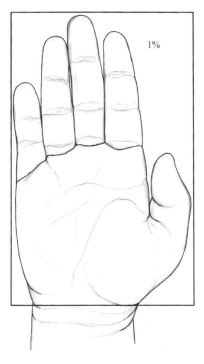

Fig. 4. Estimated percentage total body surface area for hand.

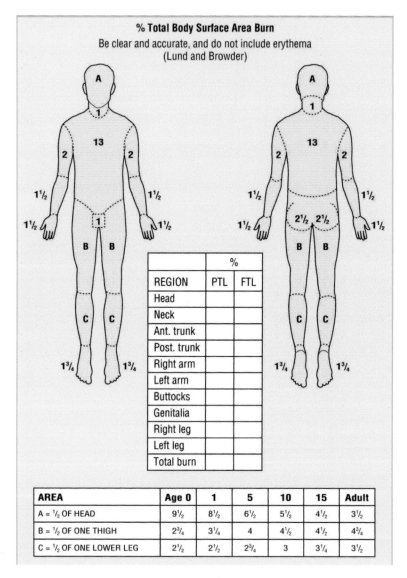

Fig. 5. Lund and Browder worksheet for calculating total body surface area burned. (PTL, partial thickness; FTL, full thickness).

Chapter 29

Hypothermia

Michael J. Schurr, MD*

*Professor of Surgery, University of Colorado School of Medicine

Take Home Points

- Hypothermia is defined as core body temperature less than 35°C. The symptoms and treatments of accidental hypothermia depend on the severity of the temperature drop.
- The use of passive versus active rewarming will depend on the core body temperature and the clinical scenario; however, cardiopulmonary bypass is the most effective technique for rewarming in the presence of full arrest.
- The amputation rate associated with frostbite may be reduced by infusion of TPA within the first 24 hours.
- Intraoperative and postoperative hypothermia is common in surgical patients and is associated with wound infections and adverse cardiac events.
- Hypothermia after trauma results in a cascade of shock and coagulopathy and the inability to rewarm the patient is a major risk factor for death.

Contact information: University of Colorado, Denver, 12631 E 17th Avenue, Aurora, CO 80045; Email: Michael.j.schurr@ucdenver.edu

Background

- The effect of body temperature on outcomes has largely been underestimated. The cascade of shock, coagulopathy, and hypothermia is a recognized complication of uncontrolled hemorrhage and best practices have included patient rewarming, control of coagulopathy with infusions of fresh frozen plasma and platelets, and damage control surgery to prevent the cascade from spiraling out of control. However, operating rooms have typically been adjusted to minimize the discomfort of the surgical team and the emergency room evaluation of patients has been performed with little thought to temperature control. Recent data has become convincing that hypothermia impacts patient outcomes on multiple levels from coagulopathy, to postoperative wound infection, pain control, and adverse cardiac events. The surgical care improvement project (SCIP) has recognized the importance of temperature control and the effectiveness of temperature control measures are being tracked on a local and national level. As these data are collected and analyzed, further definitive patient management recommendations should be forthcoming.
- Hypothermia intentionally induced for cerebral, cardiac and spinal cord protection is being used with increasing frequency. Three randomized trials of 383 patients evaluated therapeutic hypothermia in patients after cardiac arrest. With cooling, patients were 55% more likely to leave the hospital without major brain damage. The exact indications, contraindications, and cooling protocols are under development and beyond this discussion.

Main Body

Hypothermia

- The human body is skilled at maintaining homeostasis across a wide range of conditions. Temperature control is as tightly regulated as pH or intra/extra cellular electrolyte concentrations. Normal body temperature varies less than 1°C throughout a diurnal cycle. There is tremendous ability to cool oneself through evaporative loss; however, body warming depends primarily on behavioral change. These include moving to warmer environments and donning of insulating layers. Heat loss is complex, and the degree of heat transfer by conduction, radiation, or convection will depend on temperature, humidity, wind speed, presence of a wet environment, direct contact with cold surfaces, etc. The physiologic changes designed to warm the body may have significant associated morbidities, especially in the diseased or injured. The initial response is one that mimics sympathetic stimulation with tachycardia, tachypnea, vasoconstriction with shunting to vital organs, and dramatic increase in oxygen consumption secondary to shivering. These efforts, especially shivering, are effective at generating heat and warming the body; however, one can see how these responses would be harmful in a variety of medical conditions. For example, the increases in heart rate and cardiac output can lead to decompensation of the injured myocardium. Likewise, the patient with large total body surface area burns will convert second-degree burn to third-degree burn if allowed to become hypothermic with resulting in shunting of blood away from the skin.

- The human response varies with the degree of hypothermia (mild, 32°C to 35°C; moderate 28°C to 32°C; severe <28°C). If the cooling insult is not reversed or the physiologic changes fail to maintain temperature, the level of consciousness becomes depressed, the cardiac output begins to drop, bradycardia develops, the QT interval becomes prolonged, and rhythm disturbances or asystole results. The ability to shiver is lost and the cooling process accelerates. The loss of compensatory mechanisms occurs with moderate hypothermia (somewhere around 30°C) which then rapidly progresses to severe hypothermia if rewarming is not started.

- Accidental hypothermia is often associated with drug or alcohol intoxication, but medical illnesses such as hypothyroidism, hypoglycemia, myocardial infarction, stroke and others should be considered at the time of initial evaluation. The elderly are particularly susceptible and should be evaluated for sepsis as the underlying etiology. The mortality in this group is particularly high. The symptoms and treatment (passive versus active rewarming) depend on the severity of the drop in core body temperature and the clinical scenario. Passive rewarming techniques are effective for mild hypothermia. There are a variety of techniques such as forced air systems, warm blankets, infrared lights, warm intravenous fluids, warm ventilator circuits, etc. These efforts are designed to rewarm the patient over a period of several hours. Active rewarming consists of a variety of more invasive techniques such as warm nasogastric or bladder lavage. Similarly, the peritoneal and thoracic cavities can be lavaged through small incisions. Often these patients will be dehydrated due to prolonged exposure, associated illnesses and cold dieresis, so skilled resuscitation during the rewarming process is essential to avoid circulatory collapse. Cardiopulmonary complete or partial bypass is the most effective technique and good outcomes can occur despite the presence of full arrest, prolonged CPR, and fixed dilated pupils. The major advantage of bypass is that tissue perfusion and oxygenation are maintained during the warming process. Cardiopulmonary bypass resuscitation is recommended for hypothermic patients in arrest and for all patients with core temperatures lower than 25°C. Patients with a rhythm and temperature between 25°C and 28°C can be treated with cardiopulmonary bypass or active warming techniques.

Frostbite

- Frostbite occurs from cold exposure to exposed body parts. It is also often associated with drug or alcohol ingestion or other causes of altered mental status such as trauma or severe hypothyroidism. The severity of injury to the exposed area depends on multiple factors such as the absolute and wind chill temperatures and wet versus dry conditions. The body's response to cold is vasoconstriction which, if unchecked, will lead to cellular dehydration, ice crystal formation, and necrosis of skin, subcutaneous tissue, muscle and/or bone. Previous cold injury is associated with an increased risk of amputation if there is reexposure of the body part. Tobacco use is another amputation risk factor. Unfortunately, the social conditions associated with frostbite injury are not easily changed and reexposure is always a concern.
- Early treatment consists of rapid rewarming by immersion in a warm bath utilizing narcotic analgesics to control the severe pain associated with the rewarming process. Multiple freeze and thaw cycles should be avoided and are associated with an increased rate of amputation. Partial rewarming in the field should not delay transfer to an environment where definitive rewarming can occur. Blisters that form may contain vasoactive substances and should be debrided and dressed with a moist/nonadherent dressing. Several adjuncts have been advocated in an effort to reduce the amputation rate (aspirin, high dose vitamin C, topical aloe vera). These seem reasonable in patients with mild injury where the concern for amputation is not high.
- The amputation rate associated with severe frostbite may be reduced by infusion of recombinant tissue plaminogen (TPA) activator within the first 24 hours after rewarming. TPA is designed to prevent thrombosis of the injured vessels that can occur during the reperfusion phase of frostbite injury. TPA should be considered in those with absent or weak pulses on Doppler examination. Alternatively, a bone scan that shows lack of perfusion to the affected area is an indication, but often skilled clinical assessment that the patient is at high risk for amputation is used as an indication for therapy. Contraindications are evident and include recent surgery, trauma, hemorrhage, pregnancy, prolonged INR, etc. Frostbite specific contraindications include multiple freeze and thaw cycles, more than 48 hours of cold exposure,

and delay of TPA infusion more than 24 hours after rewarming. The risk benefit discussion should also consider the functional aspects of the amputations. For example, finger amputations have a much greater long term loss of function than toe amputations. After TPA, systemic heparin is typically administered for five additional days and the patient is discharged on daily aspirin.

- Frostbite injury slowly demarcates and delay in surgical intervention often preserves length. This is vitally important with hand and multiple finger involvement in order to maximize hand function. There is no real advantage to early operative intervention and definitive amputation, if required, can be safely delayed for a couple of months in most circumstances. Hand therapy to preserve range of motion is essential and often the pain is difficult to control which limits these efforts.

Intraoperative hypothermia

- Intraoperative hypothermia is a risk factor for a variety of avoidable complications. Anesthetics blunt the shivering response, patients are exposed for long periods of time and the operating rooms are cool to maintain the comfort of the surgical and operating room staff. Patients often lose body heat during surgical procedures and this effect is more pronounced with an open body cavity such as with laparotomy or thoracotomy. These procedures last for more than one or two hours and have progressive heat loss if not carefully monitored and treated. Patient warming in the perioperative period has been shown to reduce surgical site infections after colorectal as well as after clean surgical procedures. The mechanism of action is not completely clear; however, vasoconstriction may reduce blood flow to the incision, and human enzymes and adaptive physiologies are impaired in the setting of reduced body temperature. Perioperative maintenance of normothermia also reduces the incidence of postoperative cardiac events likely due to avoidance of the tachycardia and increased oxygen consumption induced by hypothermia.
- The SCIP has recognized these data and has a focus on the avoidance of intraopeative hypothermia. A review of 19 randomized, controlled warming trials showed that perioperative warming of surgical patients is effective for reducing postoperative wound pain, wound infection and shivering. Generalized warming options exist, including increasing the temperature of the room, the intravenous fluids, and the inspired gases. Forced air warming is readily available and easy to use during the operation and afterwards, during the recovery period. Early efforts at preventing heat loss are often easier

than attempts to rewarm the patient. In particular, it is important to keep the patient covered and warm during anesthesia induction and patient preparation prior to sterile draping.

Hypothermia and acute illness

- Hypothermia is part of the cascade of shock and coagulopathy that develops after major trauma, gastrointestinal hemorrhage and other clinical scenarios such as long operative cases with ongoing hemorrhage. Hypothermia interferes with platelet and clotting cascade function and hemorrhage results in a dilutional coagulopathy resulting in further blood loss, worsening hypothermia and worsening coagulopathy. Although the incidence of hypothermia in trauma increases with increasing injury severity score, hypothermia is often preventable by careful attention to patient temperature during the evaluation and resuscitation phases of patient care. The concept of damage control surgery stems from these findings. Early temporary control of hemorrhage with packing and rapid abdominal closure may allow for resuscitation in the intensive care unit, rewarming and control of coagulopathy prior to returning to the operating room for definitive control of hemorrhage. Ideally the operative conditions and the chances for success would be higher in the warm, reuscitated and non-coagulopathic patient. In a study of hip arthroplasty patients, a decrease in core temperature of 1.6°C increased blood loss by 500 mL and increased the need for blood transfusion. There is some data, however, to suggest that the hemorrhage associated with hypothermia may be exacerbated by acidosis and minimized in the patient with normal serum pH. As with a number of critical patient situations, best outcomes are associated with a global approach to the patient and management of the fine details.
- There is a higher mortality in trauma patients with hypothermia; however, hypothermia is more common in more severely injured patients so the clinical significance of the hypothermia is difficult to determine. Is hypothermia simply a marker of severity of injury as are so many trauma-related outcomes? A randomized, prospective clinical trial attempted to determine whether hypothermia during resuscitation is protective or harmful to critically injured trauma patients. Active arteriovenous rewarming techniques rewarmed patients faster than control. Actively rewarmed patients also required less fluid during resuscitation. This study did show that the inability to rewarm was associated with death in all patients who failed to reach 36°C.
- The concept of intentional hypothermia for brain protection after trauma has been studied and a recent review reported on 23 trials with a total of 1,614

patients. These trials showed no decrease in the likelihood of death in patients treated with intentional hypothermia and questionable reduction in other unfavorable outcomes such as severe disability or vegetative state. There has been some concern as to the increase in incidence of pneumonia in hypothermic patients. Intentional hypothermia after cardiac arrest seems reasonable in a careful protocolized fashion; however, intentional hypothermia after trauma cannot be recommended without further data defining the risks and benefits.

Review of Current Literature with References

- No controlled studies comparing cardiopulmonary bypass for warming of severely hypothermic patients have been done; however, data on 68 patients treated with cardiopulmonary bypass were analyzed from the literature. Most patients were hypothermic from alcohol, drug abuse, or mental illness. The mean core temperature was 21°C and 90% were in full arrest. Overall survival was 60% with 80% returning to their previous level of function.

  Vretenar DF, Urschel JD, Parrott JC, Unruh HW. Cardiopulmonary bypass resuscitation for accidental hypothermia. *Ann Thorac Surg* 1994; **58**: 895–898.

- TPA and IV heparin were used in 19 patients with severe frostbite. All patients had severe frostbite not improved by rapid rewarming, absent Doppler pulses in distal limb or digits, no perfusion by bone scan, and no contraindication to TPA. The outcomes were compared to historic bone scan data that suggested that 174 digits were at risk for amputation without TPA infusion. In this study, only 33 digits were amputated suggesting a fairly dramatic reduction in amputation rate. Arterial TPA was associated with bleeding site complications, so the final stages of the study was completed with systemic intravenous TPA administration.

  Twomey JA, Peltier GL, Zera RT. An open-label study to evaluate the safety and efficacy of tissue plasminogen activator in treatment of severe frostbite. *J Trauma* 2005; **59**: 1350–1354; discussion 1354–1355.

- Two hundred patients undergoing colorectal surgery were randomly assigned to routine intraoperative thermal care or additional warming in a double-blind fashion. The mean core temperature was 34.7°C in the routine group and 36.6°C in the warming group ($p < 0.001$). Surgical-wound infections were found in 18 of 96 patients (19%) in control, but in only 6 of 104 (6%) patients assigned to warming ($p = 0.009$). The duration of hospitalization was prolonged by 2.6 days control group ($p = 0.01$)

Andrea Kurz, MD, Daniel I., Sessler, MD, and Rainer Lenhardt, MD. for the Study of Wound Infection and Temperature Group. Perioperative normothermia to reduce the incidence of surgical-wound infection and shorten hospitalization. *N Engl J Med* 1996; **334**: 1209–1216.

- In another randomized controlled trial comparing routine care to additional warming, 300 patients with either coronary artery disease or at high risk for coronary artery disease were evaluated. All underwent abdominal, thoracic, or vascular surgical procedures. The core temperature after surgery was lower in the control group (35.4°C) than in the warming group (36.7°C) ($p < 0.001$). Perioperative cardiac events occurred less frequently in the warming group than in the control group (1.4% versus 6.3%; $p = 0.02$). By multivariate analysis hypothermia was an independent predictor of adverse cardiac events with 55% reduction in risk with perioperative warming.

Frank SM, Fleisher LA, Breslow MJ, Higgins MS, Olson KF, Kelly S, Beattie C. Perioperative maintenance of normothermia reduces the incidence of morbid cardiac events. A randomized clinical trial. *JAMA* 1997; **277**: 1127–1134.

- In a randomized study of arteriovenous rewarming of trauma patients, arteriovenous techniques rewarmed significantly faster the control patients and had less early mortality. The patients who underwent arteriovenous rewarming also required less fluid during resuscitation. Only 2 of 29 patients who underwent arteriovenous rewarming failed to warm to 36°C and both died, whereas 12 of 28 control patients failed to reach 36°C, and all 12 died. This study consists of a unique subset of trauma patients that were resuscitated with a Swan Ganz catheter, so the results may be confined to this unique group and not be translatable across a variety of patients.

Gentilello LM, Jurkovich GJ, Stark MS, Hassantash SA, and O'Keefe GE. Is hypothermia in the victim of major trauma protective or harmful? A randomized, prospective study. *Ann Surg* 1997; **226**: 439–449.

Chapter 30

Orthopaedics

James R. Bailey, MD* and Cyril Mauffrey, MD†

*Orthopaedic Surgery Fellow, University of Colorado School of Medicine
†Associate Professor of Surgery, University of Colorado School of Medicine

Take Home Points

- Orthopaedic emergencies are rare, but if you work in Trauma and Critical Care, you are likely to see a few of them.
- Fracture stabilization should take priority as soon as possible after immediate life-saving efforts, for unattended pelvic and long bone fractures can lead to hemorrhage, fat emboli, uncontrolled pain, permanent deformity, loss of limb, and possible loss of life.
- Patients presenting with an open fracture require antibiotics as soon as possible. This should be the priority. Any loose gravel or gross contamination should be removed from the wound with copious irrigation at bedside, the wound should be covered with a sterile dressing (and not removed again until seen by an orthopaedic surgeon), the limb should be splinted and the patient given tetanus prophylaxis.
- Injuries to the extremities with tight compartments and pain out of proportion should be treated as compartment syndrome until ruled out by an

Contact information: Denver Health Medical Center, 777 Bannock St. MC 0188, Denver, CO 80204; Email: James.Bailey@dhha.org; Cyril.Mauffrey@dhha.org

orthopaedic surgeon, needle pressure-measuring device, or surgically released. Compartment syndrome is a surgical emergency.

- Rapidly progressing soft tissue infections should be watched with great vigilance. The margins of the infection should be marked on the skin and treated as necrotizing fasciitis until proven otherwise.
- Patients with long bone fractures should be carefully examined for other associated smaller bone fractures as these are often missed due to the distracting injury, concomitant head injury and/or in intubated patients.
- A single radiograph is never adequate. Every bone of concern should have orthogonal radiographs or other form of advanced imaging. Never clear a bone based on one radiographic view. If the middle of a bone is broken, obtain radiographs of the joint above and below. If a bone is broken into a joint, obtain radiographs of the bone above and below.
- Joint infections rapidly degrade cartilage and should be evaluated and diagnosed without delay.

Background

- Orthopaedic surgery, a field of medicine once managed by General Surgeons has broken off into a distinct field of practice leading to many different specialties — from trauma to microsurgery. And with this emergence of specialty, training has seen a rapid increase in the science of our field.
- While many of our previously viewed orthopaedic emergencies are becoming more appreciated as urgencies, there are still critical point-of-care steps that can be taken which have a positive effect on the patient's long-term outcome and function.
- The orthopaedic surgeon should be viewed as part of the trauma and critical care team whose main goal is to restore life, limb, and function as soon as safely possible.
- The treatment modality of fractures depends on the displacement at the fracture site, the degree of comminution, associated soft tissue injury, anatomical location, patient's age and associated injuries. In this chapter, we will review just a few of the more concerning injuries in our field and highlight some of their treatment principles.

Main Body

- Pelvis fractures
  - o Usually secondary to high-energy mechanisms. Usually NOT in isolation. Look for internal injuries, head injuries, and concomitant fractures.

o Can lead to life-threatening bleeding from presacral and peri vescical venous plexuses. Once identified, the pelvis should be "closed down" with the use of sheets tied or snapped together at the level of the femoral greater trochanters.

o The stability of the pelvis should only be assessed once by the trauma team (if the orthopaedic surgeon is not present to perform this action) and once by the orthopaedic team. Repetitive stressing of the pelvis leads to disruption of blood clots within the pelvic floor.

o The most common source of bleeding associated with pelvic fractures is from a venous source.

o Early application of pelvic external fixation is recommended for mechanically unstable pelvic fractures with hemodynamic instability. This device rarely compromises access to the abdomen for simultaneous or delayed general surgical procedures.

- Hip fractures/dislocations

  o Hip fractures include femoral neck fractures, intertrochanteric hip fractures, and subtrochanteric hip fractures.

  o Approximately 80–90% of hip dislocations are posterior.

  o Posterior hip dislocations present with a hip in the position of flexion, internal rotation, and adduction. Anterior hip dislocations rest in slight flexion, external rotation, and abduction. It is important to note the direction of dislocation for the appropriate reduction maneuver.

  o Hip fractures and dislocations in young patients is a surgical emergency. The longer the femoral head remains dislocated and/or the femoral neck fracture not reduced, the risk of osteonecrosis of the femoral head significantly increases. In all patients, every effort should be made to reduce a dislocated hip as soon as possible.

  o After a hip dislocation has been reduced, a CT scan should be obtained to ensure there are no loose bodies in the joint. Depending on the size and location, the loose body may need to be surgically removed.

- Femoral fractures

  o These are usually seen in young males following high energy trauma or in older females following a low energy fall (bimodal distribution).

  o The femur is subject to extremely high mechanical and muscular deforming forces. Length and anatomical alignment should be restored provisionally using traction if the patient is not going to the operating room imminently. In cases where distal blood supply is compromised, the fracture should be reduced and stabilized urgently.

o   Long bone fractures are often associated with a blood loss of 1 liter.
o   Femoral shaft fractures are often found in association with spine, pelvis, and ipsilateral lower extremity fractures. All trauma patients with a femur fracture should get a fine cut CT scan to exclude an ipsilateral femoral neck fracture, which can be present in 10% of cases and missed in 50%. This finding does change the treatment modality and the technical difficulty of the surgery.
o   The majority of these fractures can be definitely treated with intramedullary nailing once the patient is stable.

- Knee dislocations
  o   Even if the knee self-reduced, providers must have an extremely high suspicion for vascular injuries associated with knee dislocations.
  o   An ankle brachial index (ABI) should be performed as soon as possible and followed over time, even if palpable pulses are identified. If the ABI is <0.9, a CT angiography should be performed and vascular surgeon consulted if a vascular injury is identified.
  o   Stability of the knee is often hard to assess at time of presentation due to pain and effusion. It should be examined as soon as possible. If grossly unstable, the knee should be stabilized provisionally with a splint, brace or ideally with a spanning external fixation and an MRI should be obtained.

- Tibia fractures
  o   Fractures of the tibia and fibula are the most common long bone fractures.
  o   Alignment must be re-established with adequate length and rotation restoration. This maneuvre will unkink vessels, improve blood flow to distal structures, improve pain, and help prevent further neurovascular injury.
  o   Closed and open tibia fractures are at high-risk of developing compartment syndrome. Crush injuries and revascularized extremities should also be a warning sign for potential raised intra-compartmental pressures.
  o   Although cast treatment followed by functional bracing can be used successfully in many of these fractures, the majority of tibial fractures are treated with operative fixation using either an intramedullary nail or plates and screws. This is even more common in the poly-trauma setting. If the patient is not stable enough for definitive fixation, external fixation methods can be used to provisionally or definitively treat many of these injuries.

- Spine fractures [see also Chapter 4-(iii)]
  o   All trauma patients have a spine injury until proven otherwise; however, a hard C-collar and backboard are not benign treatment modalities.

The patients' spine should be cleared as soon as possible. Delayed clearance has been associated with multiple complications including decubitus ulcers and respiratory compromise.

o Spine clearance, especially in the obtunded patient, is often a point of controversy. Multiple algorithms have been designed to help with this decision-making process to include the national emergency X-radiography utilization study (NEXUS) protocol, the Canadian C-spine Rule, and the eastern association for the surgery of trauma (EAST) guidelines.

o If a fracture is noted on imaging in one area of the spine, there is a high rate of noncontiguous spine fractures at other levels. Imaging should be carefully scrutinized.

o Pediatric and adult spines are very different entities. Special precautions must be taken during immobilization due to a large head/body ratio in children. The child's body should be raised on an additional board or a pediatric-specific back board with a head cut out should be used. If these measures are not in place, the child's neck will be hyperflexed.

- Shoulder dislocations

o Shoulder trauma radiographs must include an axillary view to rule out shoulder dislocation. This cannot be adequately assessed with an AP and scapular-Y views. If the patient is unable to cooperate with an axillary view, a Velpeau axillary view or a CT scan must be obtained.

o The combination of shoulder's anatomy and the classical mechanisms of shoulder dislocation make the anterior dislocation far more common than its posterior counterpart. This latter is usually secondary to seizures, lightning strikes or electrocution. The direction of dislocation is crucial as it guides the reduction maneuver. An uncommon form of shoulder dislocation occurs when the humeral head dislocates inferior to the glenoid. The arm is usually locked in full abduction and forward elevation (also known as luxatio erectae).

o The glenohumeral joint must be reduced as soon as possible. The reduction can be accomplished on a sedated patient or with the use of intra-articular lidocaine injection.

o Once reduced, post-reduction radiographs must be obtained and the shoulder splinted in a position of stability. For anterior shoulder dislocations, this is usually accomplished by a simple sling with the arm adducted and internally rotated. For posterior shoulder dislocations, the shoulder is placed in slight abduction and in neutral to external rotation. Special "gun-slinger" slings or slings with side bumps can also be used.

- Humerus fractures
  - o Proximal, diaphyseal, and distal humerus fractures are separate entities and treatment is often tailored to the specifics of those locations.
  - o Until seen by the orthopaedic surgeon, most proximal humerus fractures are treated initially with a sling while diaphyseal and distal humerus fractures usually require stiffer immobilization (splint or surgical fixation).
  - o The majority of humeral shaft fractures can be treated nonoperatively even when associated with a radial nerve palsy.
- Open fractures
  - o Open fractures are defined as a wound with direct communication with the underlying fractured bone. This is not to be confused with a fracture that has an associated soft tissue injury but no communication. However, often it can be difficult to truly assess if there is a communication. If so, one should err on the side of caution.
  - o Time to antibiotics has shown in multiple studies to be the most important predictor to long-term outcome in these fractures. Allergies should be reviewed and if able, all open fractures should receive a 1st generation cephalosporin IV. Higher grade injuries should have the addition of an aminoglycoside IV. Intravenous penicillin or Clindamycin should be added to any wound with farm contamination or bowel contamination to cover clostridium.
  - o All open fractures should have their tetanus status updated.
  - o Bleeding should be controlled with compression or a tourniquet. These wounds should then be assessed for size, depth, and extent of underlying damage. They should have any gross contamination removed or irrigated out of the wound with sterile saline and then covered with a sterile dressing. This dressing should not be removed until seen by an orthopaedic surgeon.
  - o Low velocity gunshot wounds associated with fractures can be treated as closed fractures unless they carry with it a piece of soiled clothing or pass through bowel content.
- Compartment syndrome
  - o Compartment syndrome is a surgical emergency.
  - o Even open fractures can develop compartment syndrome.
  - o The most common locations for compartment syndrome are the lower leg, thigh, buttock, forearm, hand, and foot. Each have very specific compartments that need to be surgically released.

o Although technical tools are available for the monitoring of compartment pressures, the syndrome remains a clinical diagnosis based on history and clinical findings. Clinical signs include pain out of proportion with the injury, pain with passive motion of the joint above or below (usually flexion/extension of the great toe for calf compartment syndrome), paresthesia, paralysis, pallor, and/or a pulseless extremity — although these four latter signs are associated with delayed presentation and poor prognosis. Pain with passive stretch is the most sensitive finding.

o The diagnosis of compartment syndrome is often difficult to establish in the obtunded or over-sedated patient. If the injury or exam is concerning compartment syndrome, compartment pressures should be evaluated with a monitoring device. Most agree that compartments should be released if the absolute value is greater than 30 mmHg or is within 30 mmHg of the patient's diastolic blood pressure (the so-called delta P).

o If there is concern for compartment syndrome, do not elevate the leg above the level of the heart. This exacerbates the situation.

o Most missed compartment syndromes (>12–24 hrs from symptoms) should not undergo fasciotomies. The risk of infection, amputation, and death is much higher than supportive management.

• Necrotizing soft tissue infections [see also Chapter 10-(ix)]

o Necrotizing fasciitis is a fast-spreading, life-threatening infection of the body's deep tissues and fascia.

o The boundaries of any suspected infection should be marked on the patient with the time and date. This allows for rapid assessment of propensity to expand or decrease.

o Necrotizing fasciitis is usually polymicrobial and patients should be started on broad spectrum antibiotics immediately.

o Definitive diagnosis is made by fascial biopsy but wide operative debridement should not be postponed if the diagnosis of necrotizing fasciitis is suspected.

o The LRINEC score can be used as a tool to help the provider diagnose necrotizing fasciitis. The score is calculated using CRP, WBC, hemoglobin, sodium, creatinine, and glucose.

Practical Algorithm(s)/Diagrams

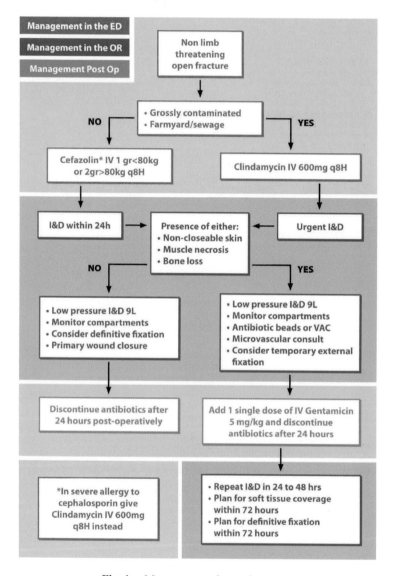

Fig. 1. Management of open fractures.

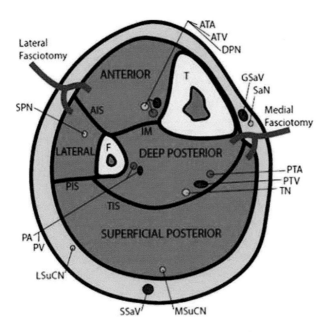

Fig. 2. Axial depiction of 4-compartment lower extremity compartment release. ATA, anterior tibial artery; ATV, anterior tibial vein; DPN, deep peroneal nerve; GSaV, greater saphenous vein; SaN, Saphenous nerve; PTA, posterior tibial artery; PTV, posterior tibial vein; TN, tibial nerve; MSuCN, medial sural cutaneous nerve; SSaV, small saphenous vein; LSuCN, lateral sural cutaneous nerve; PA, peroneal artery; PV, peroneal vein; SPN, superficial peroneal nerve.

Review of Current Literature with References

- Egol KA, Koval KJ, Zuckerman JD, eds. *Handbook of Fractures*. 4th ed. Philadelphia: Lippincott Williams and Williams; 2010.

  o Excellent pocket-sized orthopaedic reference resource for fracture management.

- Mauffrey C, Bailey JR, Bowles RJ, Price C, Hasson D, Hak DJ, Stahel PF. Acute management of open fractures: proposal of a new multidisciplinary algorithm. *Orthopaedics* 2012; **35**: 877–881.

  o Review article and proposed algorithm for the acute treatment of open fractures.

- Mauser N, Gissel H, Henderson C, Hao JD, Hak D, Mauffrey C. Acute lower leg compartment syndrome. *Orthopedics* 2013; **36**: 619–624.

  o Review article for the diagnosis and treatment of acute lower leg compartment syndrome.

- Routt MLC, Falicov A, Woodhouse E, Schildhauer TA. Circumferential pelvic antishock sheeting: a temporary resuscitation aid. *J Orthopaedic Trauma* 2006; **20**: S3–S6.

  o Technical trick paper on proper way to apply a pelvic sheet in the trauma bay.

- www.orthobullets.com

  o Excellent web-based resource for general orthopaedic knowledge.

- www.wheeless.com

  o Excellent web-based resource for general orthopaedic knowledge.

Chapter **31**

Pharmacology

Candine R. Preslaski, PharmD*

*Clinical Pharmacy Specialist, Denver Health Medical Center

Take Home Points

- Critically ill patients have altered pharmacokinetics (larger volumes of distribution, decreased protein binding, delayed metabolism and excretion) which can lead to drug accumulation and oversedation.
- The overall goal of pain, agitation, and delirium (PAD) management is to maintain an optimal level of comfort and safety for critically ill patients.
- PAD should be assessed using validated scales and scores:

    o Pain: A numerical scale (0–10) or visual analog scale.
    o Agitation: Richmond agitation and sedation scale (RASS).
    o Delirium: Confusion assessment method for the ICU (CAM-ICU).

- Strategies for treating PAD should follow a pain first approach to minimize the use of hypnotic sedative agents.

Contact information: Denver Health Medical Center, 777 Bannock St., MC, Denver, CO 80204; Tel.: 303-602-9200, email: candice.preslaski@dhha.org

- Opioids are the most commonly used analgesic; however, adjunctive therapies such as acetaminophen, non-steroidal anti-inflammatory drugs, and agents for neuropathic pain may help minimize opioid use.
- When sedative agents are necessary, target light sedation (RASS −1 to +1) unless contraindicated, utilize intermittent dosing and daily awakenings to minimize drug accumulation.
- Benzodiazepines should be used judiciously to minimize risk of delirium.
- Non-benzodiazepine sedative agents (propofol, dexmedetomidine) are alternative agents that can be used in specific patient populations.
- Non-pharmacologic strategies to minimize the risk of development of delirium should be employed in all patients:
    o Maintenance of a night/day, sleep/wake cycle.
    o Daily awakening and spontaneous breathing trials.
    o Provision of glasses and hearing aids.
    o Early mobilization.
- Patients with a positive CAM-ICU should have their benzodiazepines minimized or discontinued and may receive pharmacologic treatment with antipsychotic agents: haloperidol (acutely, for patients exhibiting unsafe behaviors) or quetiapine.

Background

- All critically ill trauma patients will experience pain, anxiety, and agitation due to their injuries, procedures, routine nursing care, and prolonged immobility.
- The universal goal for critical care practitioners is to maintain an optimal level of comfort and safety for critically ill patients.
- Sedative and analgesic agents are among the most frequently used medications in the intensive care unit (ICU).
- Although general guidelines can be written, not all patients will fit the guidelines; therefore, these guidelines are to be considered recommendations for the management of pain, agitation, and delirium in the adult ICU patient.
- Critically ill patients have altered pharmacokinetics (larger volumes of distribution, decreased protein binding, delayed metabolism and excretion) which can lead to drug accumulation, oversedation, and increased risk of adverse effects.

Main Body

Pharmacokinetic alterations in critically ill surgical patients

- Absorption
  - o Most medications are primarily absorbed in the small intestines; however, a few medications are absorbed in the stomach and more distally.
  - o Absorption of oral medications is affected by GI tract function (ileus, bowel obstructions), alterations in GI pH (continuous feeding, stress ulcer prophylaxis), anatomical changes, unavailable GI route (NPO).
  - o Transdermal, subcutaneous, and intramuscular medications have variable and sometimes unpredictable absorption in the critically ill surgical patients due to edema, and/or skin breakdown.
- Volume of distribution
  - o Amount of bodily fluid that a medication is distributed to produce a serum concentration: Dose/Vd = serum concentration.
  - o Surgical critically ill patients have larger volumes of distribution due to large volume intake (resuscitation) and/or leaky capillaries.
  - o Hydrophilic medications have smaller volumes of distribution, are maintained more intra-vascularly, and therefore are more affected by changes in volume of distribution (e.g. antibiotics).
  - o Hydrophobic medications are more widely distributed throughout the body, have larger Vd and less affected by alterations (e.g. sedative agents).
- Protein binding
  - o Many medications are bound to serum proteins.
  - o For medications with a narrow therapeutic index, protein binding changes can greatly impact the amount of free (or unbound) drug available leading to either decreased efficacy or increased toxicity (e.g. digoxin, phenytoin, warfarin).
  - o Critically ill patients tend to have decreased protein binding secondary to availability of serum proteins, reduced dietary protein intake, and/or reduced hepatic synthesis thus lending itself towards increased risk of adverse effects.
  - o When serum levels are available, careful consideration should be made to whether the lab is reporting TOTAL or FREE levels.
  - o Examples:
    - Phenytoin

⇨ Corrected phenytoin levels are calculated by: PHT/[(0.2*albumin) + 0.1].

⇨ Goal free phenytoin levels 1–2 mcg/mL, if patient is clinically stable, can use free fraction to calculate future levels from total.

- Calcium

  ⇨ Calcium levels can be corrected for albumin using the following equation: calcium + 0.8*(4-albumin).

  ⇨ Ionized calcium is a more accurate indicator of critically ill patients available calcium, especially in patients receiving blood products where calcium becomes bound to citrate.

- First pass metabolism

  o Fraction of drug lost during the process of absorption through metabolism by the liver or similar enzymes that can be found in the gut wall.

  o Drugs that experience extensive first pass metabolism have decreased oral bioavailability and therefore larger oral doses are required to obtain similar systemic concentrations to IV dosing.

  o Critically ill patients may have alterations in first pass metabolism secondary to liver dysfunction or genetic variability.

- Hepatic metabolism

  o Phase 1 metabolism is through enzymatic processes (oxidation, reduction, or hydrolytic reactions) primarily due to the cytochrome P450 system and usually results in drug inactivation.

    - Liver dysfunction secondary to hypoxia, sepsis, shock, cardiac dysfunction; alterations in blood flow, altered protein binding (free drug is available for metabolism).

  o Phase 2 metabolism are conjugation reactions (sulfonation, glucuronidation) that facilitate the elimination by improving water solubility.

    - Phase 2 metabolism is less affected by liver dysfunction.

- Excretion

  o The primary route of elimination for most medications is renal excretion.

  o Most medications are weak acids or bases; therefore excretion is affected by alterations in acid-base status.

  o In critically ill patients experiencing renal dysfunction secondary to shock, medication related kidney injury (i.e. from antibiotics, IV contrast), cardiac dysfunction, or incomplete resuscitation excretion may be decreased leading to accumulation of parent drug and both active and inactive metabolites.

o Accumulation of active metabolites can lead to prolonged action of medications and even toxic effects.

o Medications that rely on renal excretion either of the parent drug or an active metabolite should be adjusted for renal dysfunction to avoid untoward effects.

- Examples of medications that should be adjusted in renal dysfunction include antibiotics, sedative agents (particularly midazolam and morphine), insulins.

• Drug-drug interactions

o Critically ill patients are often on more medications than less ill patients and therefore are more prone to drug-drug interactions.

o Interactions result from inhibition or induction of metabolizing enzymes or displacement of bound medications from serum proteins.

o Drug-drug interactions can cause increased unbound drug concentrations and decreased metabolism leading to an increased risk for adverse effects and prolonged action.

Protocols, tools, and assessments for pain, agitation, and delirium

• Pain, agitation and delirium should be routinely monitored in all ICU patients.

• Self-report is the most reliable form of pain assessment.

• For non-verbal patients, the face legs activity cry consolability (FLACC) scale, numerical scale (0–10), or visual analog scale should be utilized to assess pain.

• Goal of sedation in the ICU is to provide comfort and anxiolysis, and facilitate mechanical ventilation or procedures.

• Richmond agitation and sedation scale (RASS) should be followed for everyone on sedation and sedative medications should be adjusted to target minimal sedation (RASS −1 to +1).

• Vital signs should not be used as a sole assessment of pain and agitation, but can be used as a cue to begin further assessment in these patients.

• The confusion assessment method for the ICU (CAM-ICU) or the intensive care delirium screening checklist (ICDSC) should be used to assess for delirium.

• Protocolized sedation has been shown to improve compliance with guidelines, decrease mechanical ventilation time, and decrease drug cost.

Analgesics

- Opioids are the most commonly used analgesic therapy.

  - Mechanism of action: act on μ and κ receptors both centrally and peripherally to decrease perception of pain.
  - Morphine has an active metabolite that can accumulate during renal dysfunction resulting in prolonged somnolence/sedation. Additionally, morphine can lead to hypotension from histamine release which is often problematic in the hemodynamically labile critically ill patient.
  - Hydromorphone is often chosen for intermittent dosing or patient controlled analgesia.
  - Fentanyl is the most common opioid used in the ICU due to its availability as a continuous infusion. Hypotension is possible with bolus dosing; however the cardiac effects are less than those of morphine. Additionally, there have been reports of chest wall rigidity with high doses.

- Opioid side effects should be anticipated and treated.

  - Constipation: requires a preventative approach, all patient in the ICU who are receiving opioids should receive a bowel regimen which consists of laxatives and/or stool softeners.
  - Respiratory depression: stop the infusion and give Naloxone as 100 mcg IV push. May repeat every 3 minutes to reverse profound respiratory depression.
  - Nausea/vomiting: metoclopramide 10 mg intravenous (IV) every 4 hours as needed (PRN), ondansetron 4 mg IV every 6 hours PRN or droperidol 0.25–1.25 mg IV every 4 hours PRN.
  - Pruritus: diphenhydramine 25–50 mg oral (PO) or IV every 6 hours PRN or nalbuphine 2.5–5 mg IV every 6 hours PRN.
  - If side effects cannot be controlled with adjuvant drugs, consider switching to a different opioid or an alternative method of analgesia.

- Tapering the dose quickly without replacement opioid therapy may result in symptoms of withdrawal with long-term use (>7 days).

  - Signs and symptoms include: dilation of the pupils, sweating, lacrimation, rhinorrhea, tachycardia, vomiting, diarrhea, hypertension, fever, tachypnea, restlessness, irritability, increased sensitivity to pain, cramps, muscle aches and anxiety.
  - Taper analgesic doses by 10–25% per day (over 4–10 days) or substitute a long-acting agent at 50% of the equipotent dose and then taper.

- Scheduled oxycodone: administer every 4–6 hours.
- Transdermal fentanyl: stop opioid infusion 6–12 hours after applying the patch.
- Methadone: initial dosing should be every 8–12 hours, as drug begins to accumulate, daily dose can be utilized.

- Adjunctive therapies such as acetaminophen, non-steroidal anti-inflammatory drugs (NSAID), and agents for neuropathic pain can be used and may help minimize opioid use.

  o Doses of acetaminophen should not exceed 2,000 mg per day in patients with liver dysfunction or 4,000 mg per day in all other patients due to the risk of hepatotoxicity. Additionally, patients receiving scheduled acetaminophen should be monitored for signs of infection other than fever due to acetaminophens antipyretic effects.

  o In patients receiving NSAID therapy (ibuprofen, ketorolac), renal function should be monitored. NSAIDs should be avoided in patients with active bleeding or increased risk of gastritis due to gastrointestinal bleeding risk.

  o If neuropathic pain is suspected, agents such as gabapentin or tricyclic antidepressants are potential adjunctive therapies.

Sedatives

- The preferred method of sedation is through intermittent dosing. If dosing required to keep patients within their sedation goal is more frequent than every 2 hours, continuous infusions should be utilized.
- To prevent over-sedation on a continuous infusion, daily "wake up" should be attempted in most intensive care unit patients.

  o Patients should have their continuous infusion discontinued every morning (alternatively the infusion can be decreased by 50% every morning), so mental status assessments may be made during patient care rounds.

    - Patients who should <u>not</u> have their infusions decreased include:
      ⇨ Paralyzed patients
      ⇨ Prone position patients
      ⇨ Patients with PEEP requirements >8 cmH$_2$O
      ⇨ Patients on pressure control with inverse ratio ventilation (IRV)

  o If patients need to be re-sedated after the "wake up" due to agitation or noncompliance with the ventilator, the sedative infusions should be restarted at half the previous rate and titrated to the patient's goal Ramsey score.

- When sedative agents are necessary, benzodiazepines should be used judiciously to minimize their risk of the delirium.
- Benzodiazepines
  - o Mechanism of action: acts on GABA receptors to produce anxiolytic effects and anterograde amnesia.
  - o Lorazepam is the most common benzodiazepine in the ICU.
  - o Midazolam is shorter acting than lorezepam when given as an intermittent bolus; however, active metabolites begin to accumulate with continuous infusions or in patients with liver or renal dysfunction leading to prolonged sedation. Additionally, midazolam has a higher incidence of hypotension than lorazepam.
  - o Diazepam is the longest acting intravenous benzodiazepines and has active metabolites, which accumulate in the elderly or patients with liver and/or renal dysfunction.
  - o Benzodiazepines have been associated with an increased risk of the development of ICU delirium and should be minimized in all patients especially those with other risk factors for the development of delirium:
    - ▪ History of dementia
    - ▪ History of hypertension and/or alcoholism
    - ▪ High severity of illness at admission
- Non-benzodiazepine sedative agents (propofol, dexmedetomidine) are alternative agents that can be used in specific patient populations.
- Propofol
  - o Mechanism of action: short-acting, lipophilic, primarily thought to act on $GABA_A$ receptors or through blockade of glutamatergic activity on NMDA receptors.
  - o Often used in patients with intracranial hypertension due to its ability to decrease intracranial pressures and its quick on/off action to allow for neurologic assessment.
  - o Hypotension is a common adverse effect of propofol.
  - o Monitor for elevated triglycerides every 48–72 hours while on propofol infusions due to 10% lipids vehicle; enteral and parenteral nutrition rates may need to be adjusted while on propofol.
  - o Doses >83 mcg/kg/min and with use >4 days have been associated with cardiac failure (resistant bradycardia/hypotension) called propofol related infusion syndrome (PRIS).
    - ▪ Monitor for unexplained metabolic acidosis (positive anion gap), hypotension or increased vasopressor need, arrhythmias (bradycardia, PR or QT interval prolongation) and/or rhabdomyolysis.

- Elevations in lactate, CK, and/or triglycerides may be a sign of developing cardiac failure.
- Glucagon may be useful for refractory hypotension due to propofol's beta-blocker and calcium channel blocker effects.

- Dexmedetomidine
  - Mechanism of action: selective alpha2-adrenoceptor agonist targeting receptors in the brainstem resulting in inhibition of norepinephrine release.
  - Does not cause respiratory depression, patients need not be intubated or may be extubated while on infusion.
  - Patients are easily arousable and go back to being sedated after stimulus removed.
  - Potentiates effects of opioids, benzodiazepines and propofol, anticipate a decreased need and decrease doses by ~50% or discontinue.
  - Hypotension and bradycardia are the most common adverse effects of dexmedetomidine and may limit its use in a hemodynamically labile critically ill patient.
  - If difficulty weaning or signs/symptoms of withdrawal occur, may consider the addition of clonidine.
- Withdrawal may occur with long-term use (>7 days) of infusion of all sedative agents.
  - Signs and symptoms of withdrawal include: dysphoria, tremor, headache, nausea, sweating, fatigue, anxiety, agitation, increased sensitivity to light and sound, paresthesias, muscle cramps, myoclonus, sleep disturbances, delirium and seizures.
  - Taper sedative doses by 10–25% per day (over 4–10 days) or substitute a long-acting agent and taper.
  - If symptoms of agitation appear while tapering sedatives, increase medication to the previous dose that controlled symptoms.
- With high-dose sedative use (i.e. midazolam >8–10 mg/hr or propofol >50–60 mcg/kg/min), consider adding an agent from another class to wean down the high-dose agent.

Delirium

- Principles of prevention and therapy are:
  - Avoid factors known to cause or aggravate delirium
  - Identify and treat underlying acute illness

o   Provide support and restorative care to prevent further decline

o   Control dangerous and disruptive behaviors

• Patients with a positive CAM-ICU should have their benzodiazepines minimized or discontinued. If sedation is necessary, dexmedetomidine or propofol may be administered.

• There have been no studies to show that the administration of haloperidol reduces the duration of delirium in ICU patients. Therefore, haloperidol is recommended for the acute management of delirium in patients exhibiting behaviors that are dangerous to themselves or medical staff.

o   Mechanism of action: blocks dopaminergic D_1 and D_2 receptors in the brain.

o   Acute: start at 2 mg IV and double the dose every 30 minutes until the patient is calm (maximum: 40 mg/dose, 200 mg/day).

o   Higher doses may cause paradoxical delirium.

o   Once controlled, start quetiapine with as needed haloperidol OR consider maintenance haloperidol dose: give ½ of dose that controlled patient every 4 or 6 hours and taper over several days.

o   Haloperidol side effects

   ▪   QT prolongation, including torsades de pointes, is dose dependent, monitor for EKG changes daily and optimize serum potassium (>4 mEq/mL) and magnesium (>2 mEq/mL).

   ▪   Monitor for extrapyramidal side effects including pseudoparkinsonism, akathisia, and dystonia. Discontinue if symptoms develop.

   ▪   Constipation due to anticholinergic effects.

• Atypical antipsychotics (particularly quetiapine) may reduce the duration of delirium and improve sleep/wake cycles.

o   Mechanism of action: primarily blocks dopaminergic D_2 and serotonergic 5-HT2 receptors in the brain, may also exhibit action on other serotonergic and dopaminergic receptors.

o   50 mg every 12 hours, titrated daily by increments of 50 mg based on as needed haloperidol use (Recommended maximum dose: 200 mg q12 h).

o   Adverse effects are similar to those of haloperidol, but typically with lesser incidence.

Practical Algorithm(s)/Diagrams

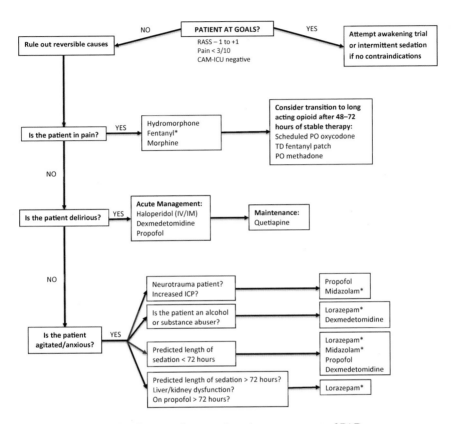

Fig. 1. Suggested approach to the management of PAD.

*Intermittent dosing preferred, may use continuous infusion if more frequent than q2h.

Table 1. Properties of common analgesics used in ICU patients.

Agent	Equianalgesic dose	Half-life	Adverse effects	Intermittent dose (usual)	Infusion dose range (usual)
Morphine	10 mg	3–7 hrs	Histamine release, active metabolites	1–4 mg Q1-2hr	1–10 mg/hr
Hydromorphone	1.5 mg	2–3 hrs	************	100–400 mcg Q1-2hr	0.2–2 mg/hr
Fentanyl	200 mcg	1.5–6 hr	Chest wall rigidity with high doses	25–50 mcg Q30 min–1hr	25–200 mcg/hr

Table 2. Properties of common sedatives used in icu patients.

Agent	Equipotent dose	IV Onset	Half-life (parent)	Unique properties	Intermittent dose (usual)	Infusion dose range (usual)
Midazolam	2–3 mg	2–5 min	3–11 hr	Active metabolite	1–4 mg Q30 min–2 hr	1–10 mg/hr
Lorazepam	1 mg	5–20 min	8–15 hr	Acidosis/renal failure from propylene glycol diluent	1–2 mg Q2–6 hr	1–8 mg/hr
Diazepam	5 mg	2–5 min	20–120 hr	Phlebitis, active metabolite	5–10 mg Q1–6 hr	Not done
Propofol	Not applicable	1–2 min	26–32 hr	Increased triglycerides Propofol-related infusion syndrome	Not done	5–50 mcg/kg/min
Dexmedetomidine	Not applicable	30 min	2–5 hr	Hypotension, bradycardia	Not recommended	0.2–1.4 mcg/ kg/hr

Review of Current Literature with References

- A landmark randomized, controlled trial involving 128 mechanically venti-lated adult patient in the medical ICU receiving continuous sedative infusions were randomized to daily interruption of sedative infusions versus a control group in which the infusions were interrupted at the discretion of the ICU clinicians. The patients in the daily awakening group had decreased mida-zolam requirements, decreased duration of ventilation, and decreased ICU stay (*NEJM* 2000; **342**: 1471–1477).

- A randomized, controlled trial of 336 mechanically ventilated patients who were randomized to either spontaneous awakening trials plus a spontaneous breathing trial versus spontaneous awakening trials alone. All patients received sedation per usual care. Patients who received both spontaneous awakening and spontaneous breathing trials had more ventilator-free days and shorter ICU and hospital lengths of stay. There were more self-extubations in the intervention group; however the rate of re-intubation was similar (*Lancet* 2008; **371**: 126–134).

- A randomized trial of 140 mechanically ventilated patient who were expected to need ventilation for >24 hours were randomized to either a no sedation or sedation (using propofol or midazolam) protocol. Both groups received morphine as their primary pain control agent. Patients in the no sedation group had significantly more days without mechanical ventilation, shorter ICU stays, and a higher incidence of agitated delirium. There was no differ-ence between the groups with regard to accidental extubations, need for CT or MRI brain scans, or development of ventilator associated pneumonia (*Lancet* 2010; **6**: 475–480).

- A two-phase multicenter, randomized, double blind trial that compared mida-zolam to dexmedetomidine and propofol to dexmedetomidine for maintenance of sedation of 897 mechanically ventilated patients. No differences were seen between the midazolam/dexmedetomidine or propofol/dexmedetomidine groups with regard to time at target sedation. Patients in the dexmedetomi-dine groups had shorter duration of mechanical ventilation compared to the midazolam group but not the propofol group. ICU length of stay and mortal-ity were similar between all groups. The only other notable difference was a higher incidence of hypotension and bradycardia in the dexmedetomidine group when compared to midazolam (*JAMA* 2012; **307**: 1151–1160).

- A prospective cohort study of 275 mechanically ventilated medical or coro-nary ICU patients comparing 6-month mortality and length of stay between patients that developed delirium and those that did not. Eighty-two percent of patients developed delirium at some point during their ICU stay defined as a positive CAM-ICU. The development of delirium was found to be associated with significantly higher 6-month mortality and longer ICU length of stay. This was the first study to directly link the development of ICU delirium to major clinical outcomes such as mortality (*JAMA* 2004; **291**: 1753–1762).

- A prospective study of 100 surgical or trauma ICU patients requiring >24 hours of mechanical ventilation found the prevalence of delirium to be 73% in the surgical ICU and 67% in the trauma ICU. The strongest predictor of the development of delirium was midazolam exposure, which is consistent with other similar studies performed in the medical ICU population (*J Trauma* 2008; **65**: 34–41).

- A randomized, placebo controlled trial of 36 ICU patients with delirium (defined as ICDSC score >= 4). Patients were randomized to receive either quetiapine 50 mg every 12 hours (titrated daily) or placebo. Both groups could also receive as needed haloperidol. Quetiapine added to as needed haloperidol resulted in faster delirium resolution, less agitation, and a greater rate of transfer to home or rehab. This was a small study with results that suggest there may be a role for the atypical antipsychotic agent, quetiapine, for the treatment of ICU delirium; however, there is a need for a larger study to confirm these results (*Crit Care Med* 2010; **38**: 419–427).

Chapter 32

Free Flap Monitoring

Raffi Gurunluoglu, MD, PhD*

*Professor of Surgery, University of Colorado School of Medicine

Take Home Points

- A free tissue transfer entails the harvest of skin, fascia, muscle, and bone or various combinations of these components along with a designated pedicle (blood vessels) and restoration of perfusion through microvascular anastomoses using recipient site blood vessels.
- A free tissue transfer is required when local and/or regional reconstructive options are not applicable or when a free flap is considered to provide the best reconstructive solution.
- Free flaps are frequently used for head and neck reconstruction, breast reconstruction, upper/lower extremity and trunk reconstruction.
- Outcomes depend on vigilant preoperative assessment, patient selection and careful preoperative planning, flap selection, delicate surgical technique obeying the principles of microvascular surgery, selection of proper recipient site blood vessels, and postoperative care.

Contact information: 777 Bannock St., MC 0206, Denver, CO 80204; Email: Raffi.Gurunluoglu@dhha.org

- Immediate postoperative care requires availability of qualified personnel and intensive care unit to monitor free flaps and patients undergoing free flap surgery.
- Patients receiving free flap surgery should be closely monitored for vital signs, pain control, urine output, drain output at reconstruction site, proper positioning of the reconstruction as well as flap donor site. Suboptimal hemodynamic parameters and improper positioning may influence flap perfusion.
- Capillary refill (flaps that have a skin paddle), color, pin-prick, temperature, turgor, and skin graft adherence (muscle flaps resurfaced with skin graft) are used for clinical assessment of perfusion into a free flap.
- Adjunctive methods for flap monitoring include handheld Doppler device, implantable Doppler, Duplex ultrasound, Laser Doppler, tissue oxygenation probe, near infrared angiography, and microdialysis.
- Implantable Doppler may be instrumental for free flap cases where regular clinical assessment cannot be pursued such as in the case of buried free flap.
- Clinical assessment remains the mainstay in monitoring free flaps that are not buried.
- All personnel (physicians, mid-level providers, and nursing staff) responsible for flap monitoring should be knowledgeable in differentiating between a healthy free flap and a flap with compromised perfusion.
- Timely intervention and re-exploration may salvage a failing free flap with compromised perfusion.
- Leech therapy may be indicated in certain situations to decongest a congested free flap.

Background

- The concept of the *reconstructive ladder* was introduced in 1982. The goal of the ladder was to guide the surgeon to consider options for wound closure in a systematic way. The steps of the ladder were arranged to allow procedures from simple to complex in an ascending order: direct closure, skin graft, local flap, distant flap, tissue expansion, and free flap. The ladder concept offered treatment strategies by identifying the simplest procedure suitable for a problem and by eliminating unnecessarily complicated approach.
- If a local flap is available and satisfies all criteria to provide the best functional and aesthetic outcomes, this will always be preferable to avoid the vagaries and risks of a microsurgical tissue transfer. This option can be especially

valuable if the patient has multiple co-morbidities precluding any lengthy surgical procedures, the allocation of resources, including time, is limited or the requisite technical expertise is absent.

- With the progressive use of microsurgical flaps, higher rungs of the ladder have become possible strategies when lower rungs fail to provide optimal solutions. The principles and practice of plastic surgery may be better reflected in the phrase *reconstructive elevator*. The reconstructive elevator implies that in the era of form and function, simplest is not necessarily always the best. As an example, if a patient desires autologous breast reconstruction following mastectomy, sequential thought would indicate that a technically feasible pedicle flap is always better than a free flap. But clearly there are cases where a free deep inferior epigastric artery perforator (DIEAP) flap is a better option than a pedicled transverse rectus abdominis myocutaneous (TRAM) flap. The reconstructive elevator accommodates a wider spectrum of options striving for optimal form and function.

- The rate of successful free tissue transfer currently averages greater than 95%. Nevertheless every case can potentially fail. Free flap failure is a traumatic experience for patient, surgeon, nursing staff, and all involved in the care of a particular patient who has undergone free flap surgery. Not only has the reconstruction failed but now a donor site morbidity is present. In addition, the best reconstructive option usually has already been utilized for the primary procedure. Additional operations are likely required and unfortunately, these secondary methods are less likely to achieve all of the goals originally intended. Furthermore, the cost associated with operative take-backs for flap take-down and additional procedures, becomes an important issue.

- It is prudent to take appropriate measures in every case to minimize the risk of free flap failure. Imperative steps such as careful preoperative planning, successful surgical execution, and intimate postoperative care and flap monitoring should be employed.

Preoperative Phase

- Preoperative planning includes assessment of patient for fitness for anesthesia, selection of donor flap and its characteristics (size, color, texture, thickness, innervated, buried, vascular pedicle length), selection of recipient vessels taking into account zone of injury, radiation, infection, possible need for vein grafts, and timing of surgery (inadequately debrided wound bed or excessive waiting prior to wound coverage).

Intraoperative Phase

- Surgical execution is the next prerequisite for a successful free flap transfer. Technical expertise of the surgeon was identified as the most critical factor related to improved flap success rates.
- Ideally, two venous anastomoses should be considered for tissue transfer, whenever possible to reduce flap loss. However, two recipient veins that are close together and two flap veins may not be available.
- Traumatic dissection of vessels, poor blood flow from the recipient artery, vessel size mismatch, short pedicle, pedicle tension, kinking and torsion, poor operative setting, uncomfortable positioning, poor anastomotic technique (traumatic vessel preparation, catching back wall, improper visualization of vessel lumens), delaying the restoration of perfusion which eventually may lead to ischemia reperfusion injury and the no reflow phenomenon have been shown to increase flap failure.
- The tolerated ischemia time varies according to the composition of the tissues. In general, skin flaps tolerate longer periods of ischemia (up to 4 hours) than musculocutaneous flaps. Musculocutaneous flaps do not tolerate prolonged ischemia times because of the metabolic requirements of muscle tissue. The maximum time tolerated is about two hours of ischemia. Likewise, in jejunal intestinal flaps, the tolerance for anoxemia reduces to two hours.
- Peripheral vasoconstriction as a consequence of hypotension, hypothermia, or anemia is highly undesirable intraoperatively. The patient must be well-hydrated and relaxed. In addition, prolonged surgery increases the risk of deep vein thrombosis and pulmonary embolus. Therefore, administration of prophylactic heparin subcutaneously prior to induction of anesthesia may be considered in patients undergoing free flap surgery. The use of low-dose heparin does not seem to increase significantly the risk of hematoma or intraoperative bleeding. In addition, a cause-and-effect relationship between the use of anticoagulants and flap loss or prevention of anastomotic thrombosis is not established.
- Use of prophylactic anticoagulants in uncomplicated cases widely varies among microsurgeons. Nevertheless, the author's preference includes intraoperative IV heparin bolus of 5000 U five minutes prior to flap harvest. Use of 4% Xylocaine for topical vasodilation, and heparin solution (100 U/ml) for irrigation of vessel lumen during microvascular anastomoses is a common practice. Other medications that may be used include Decadron, 4–8 mg to reduce edema and swelling especially for reconstructions of the head.

- Following completion of the microvascular anastomoses, the flap must be properly set which requires adherence to some basic principles. The vascular pedicle should be inspected to avoid kinks, twists, compression, and tension. The flap should be inspected for bleeding, capillary refill, color, and temperature. Handheld Doppler unit can be used to assess the blood flow through the pedicle. Intraoperatively, near infrared angiography can be used as an adjunctive method to confirm patency of arterial and venous anastomoses and perfusion of tissue.

Postoperative Phase

- Hemodynamic status of the patient undergoing free tissue transfer may impact the perfusion of the flap. Vital signs and urine output should be closely monitored. Hypertension, hypotension, hypothermia, or anemia should be avoided. In adults, urine output should be directed at greater than 30 cc/hr. The patient should be kept warm and pain free postoperatively to avoid vasoconstriction. Vasopressors should not be used unless no other option is available to maintain blood pressure.
- Using postoperative medications to inhibit clot formation at the anastomosis is controversial. Studies evaluating the efficacy of heparin, dextran, and aspirin have demonstrated that none are absolutely necessary for an uncomplicated case. Use of such medications seems to be at the discretion of the microsurgeon. The author prefers to run heparin subcutaneously at DVT prevention dosage and aspirin 325 mg/day for three weeks postoperatively.
- Microvascular free tissue transfer is a reliable method for reconstruction of complex surgical defects. However, there is still a small risk of flap compromise necessitating urgent re-exploration. Studies suggest that the great majority of circulatory compromises occur within the first 72 hours.
- Therefore, monitoring the free flap during the early postoperative period is critical to ensure flap survival. Availability of experienced nursing staff and intensive care unit may be limited and frequency of flap monitoring may vary from institution to institution and surgeon to surgeon. The cost-effectiveness of postoperative monitoring of free flaps is greatest during the first two days, after which it decreases significantly. It is recommended that free flaps are monitored intensively during the first 24 hours on a half-hourly basis, for the next 24 hours (day 2) on an hourly basis, for the next 24 hours (day 3) every two hours and finally at day 4, 4 hourly. Cases of late arterial and venous thrombosis beyond five days have been reported, but these are rare. Therefore, flap monitoring can be discontinued at about 5–6 days postoperatively.

- The time of presentation of flap compromise is a significant predictor of flap salvage outcome. Intensive flap monitoring at a special microsurgical intensive care unit by well-trained nurses and surgeons allows for early detection of vascular compromise, which leads to better outcomes. When recognized early and managed promptly (<6h), compromised free flaps have a 75% salvage rate when taken back to the operating room.

- It is important to avoid circumferential bandaging of limbs or tracheostomy tapes around the neck for head and neck flaps and to have full exposure of the whole flap so as to detect any changes in a timely manner.

- Techniques and parameters used for monitoring the free flap depend on the tissue characteristics. Flaps including skin paddles (musculocutaneous, fasciocutaneous, adipocutaneous, and osteocutaneous flaps) in their composition can be inspected to assess surface characteristics. These include evaluation of *capillary refill, color, surface temperature, presence of bleeding when pinpricked* (Table 1).

- Normal flap color is similar to that of the donor site. The pale flap postoperatively must be interpreted as arterial thrombosis until proven otherwise. The skin of some free flaps is normally pale and this may elicit confusion during assessment. Evaluation of capillary refill provides a valuable adjunct especially in such cases. Normal capillary refill is 1–2 seconds. Visualizing the capillary refill is easier in shaded light. A useful technique to detect subtle capillary return in pale flaps is to press on the flap with the handle part of a scissors. The blenched halos created using the scissors held flat against the skin surface will allow visualization of return of capillary fill (Table 1).

- Arterial blood supply can also be assessed by pricking the flap with a needle or rubbing a raw wound edge with gauze. These maneuvers should provoke bright red bleeding (Table 1).

- Surface temperature of the flap can be measured with a surface monitor or back of the hand. This is aided by a self-adhesive temperature tab that is applied to the flap with a control on the adjacent normal skin. A difference of 2°C between the two indicates vascular compromise. However, there are many technical factors that can adversely affect surface temperature. Marked improvements in the specificity and sensitivity of temperature monitoring can occur when this modality is combined with clinical observation (Table 1).

- High drain output and excessively saturated bandage with dark colored blood at a reconstruction site may suggest circulatory problems (Table 1).

- Problems with arterial inflow are suggested when the flap is cool to touch, pale relative to donor site, and when there is sluggish or absent capillary refill and no bleeding on pin-prick (Table 1).
- Problems with venous outflow are suggested when the flap is congested, swollen, and when the capillary return is brisk and rapid. Color and appearance of congested flaps can vary depending on the severity of the congestion and ranges from a mild bluish hue to dark blue or purple color (Fig. 1). A congested flap will immediately start oozing dark colored blood on pin-prick (Table 1).
- Muscle flaps covered with a skin graft are evaluated using color, turgor, and skin graft adherence. Surface temperature and capillary refill are not used in these situations. Signs of arterial occlusion include a pale flap without turgor, poor graft adherence, no bleeding on pinprick and failure to contract upon stimulation. Venous outflow obstruction is suggested when the flap is congested and swollen, when there is excessive bleeding from the flap edge and dark blood on pinprick (Table 1).
- External Doppler — The handheld Doppler (5–8 MHz) is the most widely used device for assessment of flap perfusion. This very sensitive device produces a different acoustic signal for arterial and venous flow in a flap pedicle. Normal arterial flow is characterized by triphasic flow pattern i.e. prominent systolic forward flow, early diastolic flow reversal, and a second phase of forward flow throughout the rest of diastole. The use of stereo earphones to listen to the audio signal is helpful to assess triphasic flow because forward flow is heard in one ear and reverse flow in the other. The type of arterial signal can be distinguished by an experienced person where a triphasic signal that becomes a biphasic or monophasic one may indicate a change in the status of the flap. An audible sharp arterial flow with increased velocity results by inflow against resistance secondary to blood stasis in the flap or stenosis at the artery. Nevertheless, handheld Doppler monitoring is less effective for determining the status of the venous anastomosis. Venous obstruction may be present while the arterial pulse is still present. A significant amount of delay may be found between a venous obstruction and loss of the arterial signal in large flaps (Table 2).
- Surface Doppler assessment for flaps may yield a false positive result by picking up signals from surrounding or deep vessels instead of the flap's vascular pedicle. This may mislead the observer to believe that the flap's pedicle is patent. It is recommended that accurate marking of the location of the pedicle be performed intraoperatively. A marking suture is often placed for later use in locating the Doppler signal by the nurses.

- Implantable Doppler — A deep or buried flap is the most difficult one to monitor. A small skin portion of the flap can be exposed and used as a monitor of buried flap if there is a skin component e.g. adipocutaneous or fasciocutaneous flap.
- Buried flaps (e.g. free fibular bone flap devoid of skin paddle) are reliably monitored by implantable Doppler probe placed adjacent to the artery and vein at the time of operation. A 20 MHz Doppler crystal implanted on a silicone cuff is placed around the artery and/or vein distal to anastomotic site for direct vessel monitoring of microvascular anastomosis. The probe is safely disengaged with only 1/10lb pressure at about 5–6 days postoperatively. The implantable Doppler can measure blood flow across a microvascular anastomosis and is an effective tool to monitor flap perfusion and improve salvage rates. (Table 2).
- The internal Doppler probe has low subjectivity and allows inexperienced nursing staff to quickly detect a perfusion problem in the flap, but the probe is costly and can malfunction or become displaced during the early postoperative course.
- Laser Doppler — Light from a helium neon laser that penetrates 1.5 mm below the surface of the flap is reflected by the red blood cells circulating in the capillaries. Laser Doppler values differ depending on tissue type, and perfusion readings may fluctuate for every patient. Therefore, the observer must monitor the trend rather than the absolute values. This fact is of particular importance during venous occlusions when a drop in value is not as sudden and steep as compared to arterial obstruction. The system may be helpful in darkly pigmented skin where clinical evaluation is not straight forward. Numerous clinical series demonstrated the use of the laser Doppler as a valuable postoperative monitor after free-flap transfers. However, a laser Doppler device is expensive (Table 2).
- Tissue oxygenation — the partial oxygen pressure of the flap can be continuously monitored using a microprobe. This technique only monitors the circulatory changes or failures of the tissue near the probe, and may miss other areas of ischemia. As seen with the internal Doppler, the partial oxygen pressure drops rapidly after an arterial inflow problem and gradually in cases of venous thrombosis. Several perfusion probes are available on the market. Expensiveness is a distinct disadvantage of these probes. Therefore, these probes are not recommended routinely where clinical surveillance is easily performed. The only discrete indication for their use is in skin grafted muscle/ fascia flaps or buried flaps (Table 2).
- Duplex ultrasound — Duplex US offers a safe, quick, and non-invasive method for the assessment of pedicles in buried free flaps. If available, an experienced

radiologist should apply this modality in order to visualize the vessels' course, diameter, and flow. The information retrieved is highly accurate. However, this technique provides a static evaluation and is not a form of continuous monitoring (Table 2).

- Microdialysis — This is a relatively new approach for monitoring free flap perfusion. A double-lumen microdialysis catheter with a dialysis membrane at the end is introduced into the tissue to monitor glucose, glycerol, and lactate concentrations. During anoxia, the glucose concentration drops, while lactate and glycerol levels rise. The technique also has the distinct disadvantage of measuring tissue perfusion only at the site of catheter implantation (Table 2).
- Near infrared angiography — This technique is based on the detection of a systemically administered dye (indocyanine green) by exposing the tissue to near-infrared light and detecting emitted signals through an optic filter. This modality is not applicable in the case of a buried flap (Table 2).

Leech Therapy — Key Practice Guidelines

- Surgical exploration is the first-line approach in flaps demonstrating signs of venous compromise (Fig. 1). Leeches are not beneficial in a blue flap. Nevertheless, the use of medicinal leeches, Hirudo medicinalis, has demonstrated value in the treatment of venous congestion in an otherwise well-perfused flap. Application of leech therapy protocol may salvage free tissue transfers with venous obstruction that are otherwise unsalvageable by surgical exploration.
- After many years of use, Hirudo medicinalis received official FDA approval as a medical device in 2004. The mechanism of action is based on the active agent, hirudin, which is a selective thrombin inhibitor.
- A type and screen (crossmatch) should be sent before the onset of leeching and kept up to date. Blood transfusion may be required due to the continuous blood loss during and for several hours following leech therapy. It is advised to check the full blood counts of patients before and after leech therapy.
- Leeches should not be administered to patients unwilling to have a blood transfusion if there is any other alternative available — and if it is necessary, there should be a well-documented discussion of the risks.
- Prophylactic antibiotics should be administered to all patients being treated with leeches. The antibiotic treatment should be initiated along with leech application and may be discontinued 24 hours after the last application. The antibiotic susceptibility testing on water collected from the leeches may guide antibiotic regimen of choice for leech therapy.

- Although optimal practice has not been established, sulfamethoxazole-trimethoprim (SXT) and fluoroquinoles seem to be consistently active against Aeromonas infection (Aeromonas hydrophila, Aeromonas veronii). Ciprofloxacin is also commonly used against this pathogen although resistance has been reported.
- Leeches can only be applied to free flaps that have a skin paddle in their composition.
- A blunt forceps can be used to grasp the leech from its container.
- Anchorage of leeches to the skin surface of the flap may be facilitated by pinpricking the skin prior to application. Inability of getting a leech to start sucking may indicate compromised arterial inflow.
- It is critical to keep the leech in the designated flap region. The application site should be kept clean of ointment or gel (Doppler) as these will repel the leeches. However, leeches can be surrounded by moist gauze to contain them. In addition, some type of tape can be used to block off the surrounding skin from the leech. Traveling of leeches applied over a flap close to any orifice should be prevented.
- The number of leeches used is highly variable, ranging from one leech per day to as many as two every hour.
- The time interval between applications is similarly varied, ranging from hourly to once a day for several days.
- Leeches will detach themselves when full. This usually takes about half an hour. They need to be monitored closely as they get detached. Then the leech is sacrificed by submerging it in an alcohol filled container.
- The suction sites will ooze after the leech is detached, which is normal. The flap should be cleaned with wet gauze frequently.
- Flap perfusion (color of the skin paddle, capillary refill, color of the blood oozing from suction sites) should be assessed every 30 min or hourly after the detachment of the leech. Re-application should be considered if necessary based on the assessment of parameters.

Closing Remarks

- During the first 48 hours, it is preferable to monitor free flaps in the surgical intensive care unit. On day 3, when the monitoring interval is every 2 hours, the patient can be transferred to the progressive unit.
- Combination of clinical assessment tools remains the mainstay of free flap monitoring. However, most surgeons rely on adjunctive methods to optimize flap salvage because continuous observation by the surgeon is currently not

possible. Inhouse conferences and bedsite discussions in order to train nursing staff are critically important.

- Documentation of findings according to a prearranged list of criteria and detailed algorithm (which may be slightly different in every institution) is critical to note any alterations. Misinterpretation of clinical signs and symptoms may commonly occur as a result of a shift change in nursing staff. Therefore, calls from nursing staff to the surgeon-in-charge should be encouraged if any doubt about perfusion of the flap exists.

- Essential to successful flap salvage are the recognition of the existence of a problem and an early call made to the surgeon (Fig. 2). Exclusion of problems related to external effects (compressive dressing, posture etc.) and to the hemodynamic status of the patient (hypotension, hypothermia, anemia with hemoglobin <9 g/dl) is extremely important and these factors should be dealt with prior to surgical exploration.

- If surgical exploration is deemed necessary, an expedient transport of the patient, communication with the operating room staff and preparation of the patient (i.e. obtaining the consent for the operation, including the possibilities of the need for vein grafts, alternative options skin grafts or local tissue harvest) should be initiated.

Practical Algorithm(s)/Diagrams

Table 1. Monitoring free tissue transfer.

Clinical assessment	Arterial compromise	Venous compromise	Normal perfusion	Frequency	Darkly pigmented skin	Buried flap	Skin-grafted muscle flap	FC, MC, OC flaps
Capillary refill	>2 seconds, none	brisk	1–2 seconds	Intermittent*	Difficult to interpret or N/A	N/A	N/A	Applicable
Turgor	Flaccid, flat, decreased	Tense, bulging, increased	Normal tissue turgor	Intermittent*	Applicable	N/A	Applicable	Applicable
Color	Pale, mottled, bluish	Bluish, purplish	Similar to donor site	Intermittent*	Difficult to interpret or N/A	N/A	Not reliable	Applicable
Temperature	Cool (>2°C difference compared to surrounding control)	Cool (>2°C difference compared to surrounding control)	Similar to surrounding tissue	Intermittent*	Applicable	N/A	Applicable, Not reliable	Applicable

Needle stick test	Minimal amount of blood, none or serous drainage	Abrupt bleeding of dark blood	Bright red bleeding	Intermittent*	Applicable	N/A	Applicable But not very reliable	Applicable
Skin graft adherence	No adherence	Adherent until arterial compromise	Adherent	Intermittent*	N/A	N/A	Reliable	N/A
Dressing	Too clean, no drainage	Saturated	Mildly stained	Intermittent*	Applicable	N/A	Applicable	Applicable
Drain output	Too little, none	High output with dark blood	Mild-moderate serosanginous	Intermittent*	Applicable	Applicable	Applicable	Applicable

*Intermittent per monitoring protocol. FC: fasciocutaneous, MC: Musculocutaneous, OC: Osteocutaneous.

Table 2. Monitoring free tissue transfer.

Assessment using device	Arterial compromise	Venous compromise	Normal perfusion	Frequency	Darkly pigmented skin	Buried flap	Skin-grafted muscle flap	FC, MC, OC flaps	Other features
Hand-held external Doppler	Biphasic or monophasic arterial signal	Absence of continuous venous signal,	Triphasic arterial signal, continuous venous signal	Intermittent*	Applicable	Rarely applicable	Applicable	Applicable	Inexpensive/ widely used
Implantable Doppler	Biphasic or monophasic arterial signal	Absence of continuous venous signal,	Presence of normal arterial and venous signals	Continuous	Preferable	Preferable	Applicable	Applicable	Expensive, objective,
Duplex Ultrasound	Decreased flow	Decreased flow	Normal flow	As needed	Reliable if applicable	Reliable if applicable	Reliable if applicable	Reliable if applicable	Requires experienced radiologist, evaluation at one particular point in time

Laser Doppler	Abrupt and steep drop trend in values (50% or more decrease in perfusion values)	Gradual drop trend in values	No drop in perfusion values	Continuous	Preferable	N/A	Applicable	Applicable	Expensive, objective
PO$_2$ Probe	Rapid drop in tissue PO$_2$	Gradual drop in tissue PO$_2$	Gradual and slow decrease in values on a daily basis**	Continuous	Applicable	Preferable	Preferable	Applicable	Monitors tissue near the probe
Near Infrared Angiography	Gray-black	Gray-black	Bright white	N/A	Applicable	N/A	Applicable	Applicable	Intraoperative, evaluation at one particular point in time
Microdialysis	Decrease in glucose and increase in lactate and glycerol concentrations	Decrease in glucose and increase in lactate and glycerol concentrations	No significant change in glucose, lactate and glycerol concentrations	Continuous	Applicable	Applicable	Applicable	Applicable	Expensive, variability in concentrations, monitors tissue near the probe

*Intermittent per monitoring protocol. **Normal pattern due to fibrin apposition to the probe. FC: fasciocutaneous, MC: Musculocutaneous, OC: Osteocutaneous.

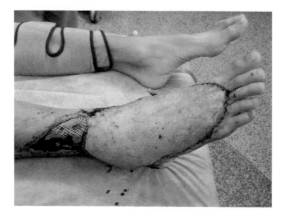

Fig. 1. A congested anterolateral thigh flap secondary to venous compromise. The anterolateral thigh free flap was utilized for the reconstruction of an extensive dorsal foot and ankle wound with exposed tendons and vasculature that resulted from serial debridements for necrotizing fasciitis.

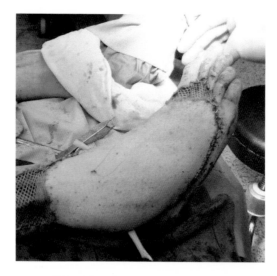

Fig. 2. Salvage was possible with early recognition of the problem and expedient transport of the patient to the operating room. Exploration, venous thrombectomy, and saphenous vein grafting were performed to restore perfusion.

Review of Current Literature with References

- Gurunluoglu R, Glasgow M, Williams SA, Gurunluoglu A, Antrobus J, Eusterman V. Functional reconstruction of total lower lip defects using innervated gracilis flap in the setting of high-energy ballistic injury to the lower face: Preliminary report. *J Plast Reconstr Aesthet Surg* 2012; **65**: 1335–1342.

- Sacak B, Gurunluoglu R. Innervated gracilis muscle flap for microsurgical functional lip reconstruction: Review of the Literature. *Ann Plast Surg* [Epub ahead of print] 2013; PMID: 23804028.

- Gurunluoglu R, Spanio S, Rainer C, Ninkovic M. Skin expansion before breast reconstruction with the superior gluteal artery perforator flap improves aesthetic outcome. *Ann Plast Surg* 2003; **50**: 475–479.

- Ninkovic M, Moser-Rumer A, Ninkovic M, Spanio S, Rainer C, Gurunluoglu R. Anterior neck reconstruction with pre-expanded free groin and scapular flaps. *Plast Reconstr Surg* 2004; **113**: 61–68.

- Gurunluoglu R, Shafighi M, Schwabegger A, Ninkovic M. Secondary breast augmentation with deepithelized free flaps from lower abdomen for treatment of intractable capsular contracture and maintenance of breast volume. *J Reconstr Microsurg* 2005; **21**: 35–41.

- Gurunluoglu R. The ascending branch of the lateral circumflex femoral vessels: review of the anatomy and its utilization as recipient vessel for free-flap reconstruction of the hip region. *J Reconstr Microsurg* 2010; **26**: 359–366.

- Gilman K, Ipaktchi K, Moore EE, Barnett C, Gurunluoglu R. Reconstruction of an emergency thoracotomy wound with free rectus abdominis flap: Anatomic and radiologic basis for the surgical technique. *World J Emerg Surg* 2010; **7**(5): 12.

- Gurunluoglu R. Experiences with waterjet hydrosurgery system in wound debridement. *World J Emerg Surg* 2007; **2**(2): 10.

Chapter 33

Ethics of Surgical Critical Care

Thomas M. Dunn, PhD* and Abraham M. Nussbaum, MD†

*Associate Professor of Psychological Science, University of Northern Colorado
†Assistant Professor of Psychiatry, University of Colorado School of Medicine

Take Home Points

- This chapter provides guidance to a surgeon facing clinical ethical questions that often present during a case.

  o This is not an exhaustive guide that covers systemic ethical issues, such as physician behavior, billing and insurance questions, gifts, or organizational systems.

- Clinical ethical questions usually arise when the right course of action for a patient is unknown or unclear.

  o These questions are often experienced as disagreements about what is best for a patient:

    ▪ A patient wishes to pursue treatment that a surgeon believes is not indicated.

Contact information: Denver Health Medical Center, 777 Bannock St. Denver, CO 80204; Email: Thomas.Dunn@dhha.org; Abraham.Nussbaum@dhha.org

- A surgeon believes that a patient would benefit from a procedure, yet the patient declines, preferring an outcome that may lead to disability or death.
- A patient is incapable of making or communicating a medical decision, and there are no advance directives or proxy decision-makers available to substitute for the patient's judgment.
- Proxy decision-makers disagree about what treatment a patient would want and cannot adequately guide the surgeon.
- Advance directives conflict with what proxy decision-makers believe is in the patient's best interest.
- There is conflict between members of the treatment team about the care being given.

o Additional ethical questions may arise when there are two (or more) equally defensible treatment approaches that could be considered and there is conflict about which approach is best.

o Often, questions that present as ethical questions are actually symptoms of communication breakdown.

- The treatment team has not properly communicated futility to the patient or her family.
- Family members disagree about care for a loved one because they are talking with different providers, at different times, and not talking between themselves.
- Risks are inadvertently presented as being far more likely to occur than what typically happens in the common case.

- When should you call an ethics consult?

o Whenever there is a question regarding whether the care of a patient is being performed ethically **and** if providers are unable to reach a satisfactory solution that is agreeable to the surgeon, the patient, family members, and other members of the treatment team.

o Ethics committees are composed of a variety of providers, from different disciplines, who are both physician and non-physicians.

- Ethics consults may be called by anyone, including any member of the surgical treatment team, the patient, the patient's friends or family, or anyone interested in ethical treatment.
- A hospital ethics committee (or a sub-committee) provides an independent evaluation of the ethical question in order to promote the good of the patient. Clinical ethical consultants do not make decisions

on behalf of the treatment team, but attempt to clarify issues and improve communication to help a patient, her representatives, and her surgical treatment team arrive at an agreeable outcome.

- To help guide the surgeon to take the necessary steps to assure ethical care of their patients prior to calling a consult, we review:
  o The major bioethical theories.
  o How culture and religion can affect patient decisions.
  o Advance directives.
  o Common ethical questions.
  o When to seek expert consultation regarding ethical issues.

Background

- Ethics guide decision-making as we strive to do what is "right."
  o Generally, people have a sense of what is right and wrong.
  o It is believed that physicians behave ethically when practicing medicine.
  o Many organizations have ethics codes that apply to their members.
- Biomedical ethics is the application of ideas from a broader body of work encompassing moral philosophy with major theoretical views, including:
  o Utilitarianism — the ethical choice is one that results in the greatest good for most people. Whether a decision is the right decision is determined by its outcome, not by the actions taken to arrive there. Also called the consequentialist theory of ethics. John Stuart Mill is considered the paradigmatic utilitarian philosopher.
  o Deontology — the ethical choice is one that follows predetermined moral rules. The features of the action itself, and not the consequences of the decision, determine its morality. Also called rules-based ethics. Immanuel Kant is considered the paradigmatic deontological philosopher.
  o Virtue Ethics — the ethical choice is the choice that a good person would make. The ethical choice is not determined by its outcome or by its adherence to moral rules, but its correspondence to the actions undertaken by a good or virtuous person. In virtue ethics, a surgeon strives to achieve the character traits that will prepare him/her to make ethical decisions. Also called character ethics. Aristotle is considered the paradigmatic virtue philosopher.
  o Principle Theory — established by Beauchamp and Childress for bioethical decision-making, their tenets are abstracted from the major

bioethical traditions. They are widely taught in contemporary medicine. The tenets are:

- Autonomy: Respecting the right of an individual to make an informed decision.
- Beneficence: Decisions are guided by doing what is in the best interest of the patient.
- Non-maleficence: Basis for the well-known principle — first, do no harm.
- Justice: The emphasis that decisions are guided by fairness and what is equitable.

- Ethical questions often arise during end-of-life treatment. In such instances, the surgeon may find that the guiding principles of autonomy, beneficence, non-malfeasance, and justice are in conflict.

  o For example, a patient may make a treatment decision that the surgeon believes may lead to a bad outcome, including death. In this instance, the autonomy of a patient conflicts with the pursuit of beneficence and non-maleficence.

  o In other instances, the patient may be unable to communicate a choice about end of life care and there is conflict regarding what treatment should be provided. In this instance, proxy decision-makers may substitute their judgment for what care the patient would choose.

    - Family members may pursue treatment options that the surgeon believes are futile.
    - The surgeon may believe that there are treatment options that will benefit the patient, yet proxy decision-makers decline such treatment on behalf of the patient.
    - Family members disagree among themselves about what treatment the patient would want, leaving the surgeon without a clear sense of how to act with beneficence and respect for patient autonomy.

- Such conflicts can often be alleviated, or at least simplified, if patients take steps in advance to make decisions about what care is desired in the event they are rendered unable to make or communicate a decision.

  o Collectively known as "advance directives," such advance decision-making can take many forms and helps provide guidance to providers about what treatment the patient wants and does not want:

    - The physician and the patient agree that resuscitation should not be attempted and a "Do Not Resuscitate" (DNR) order is written.

- The patient creates a living will, specifying the care desired that covers a wide range of medical conditions, including mechanical ventilation, a persistent vegetative state, antibiotics, etc.
  - The patient and his or her physician sign a "no CPR" document.
  - Wishes about end of life care are specified in a document such as "Allow Natural Death," or "Five Wishes."
  o Patients may also formally designate a proxy decision-maker to make medical decisions on their behalf in the event they are incapable of voicing their wishes.
    - The medical durable power of attorney is one type of proxy decision-maker.

- Some surgeons may be uncomfortable when patients make decisions about their healthcare based on religious beliefs or cultural standards.
  o While lists or descriptions of ethical principles associated with major religious tradition and cultural standards can be found, the best counsel is to assume nothing about a patient's belief or culture. Patients may have unexpected religious and cultural practices than present at first glance.
  o Instead, consider asking questions like: "Are there particular religious traditions or cultural practices that we should consider in your care? Does your religious tradition or cultural practices require or forbid certain treatments?"
  o It is often helpful to seek the guidance of someone who is a more experienced navigator of cultural and religious difference. In some hospitals, this can be a chaplain or member of the surgical treatment team. However, you should consider asking a patient or her representatives if there is a leader in her cultural or religious community who can provide guidance to the treatment team.

Main Body

- The decision that a surgical procedure is indicated for a particular patient will inevitably result in informing the patient of the risks and benefits of the surgery.
  o Such a conversation is typically done using layperson's terms and results in the documentation that the patient is making an informed decision regarding surgery.
    - The conversation demonstrates the autonomy of a patient.

o Rarely do any issues arise from a patient agreeing to a procedure that the surgeon believes is necessary to perform.

  ▪ Although some cases may present an ethical challenge, particularly if the patient agrees to a procedure when he or she cannot understand the risks associated with it.

o It is often when the patient is at odds with the surgeon about the procedure that ethical questions arise.

  ▪ Some issues may be straightforward to solve. For example, a surgeon is not obligated to perform a surgical procedure simply because the patient requests a procedure.

  ▪ In this instance, the surgeon's commitments to beneficence and non-maleficence take priority over the autonomy of a patient.

o It is particularly problematic when a patient declines life- or limb-saving surgery with obvious benefits and acceptable risks.

o However, part of the informed consent process is to allow a patient to make an informed decision about whether they accept the surgeon's recommendation.

  ▪ When a patient declines a recommended treatment, this is not, in itself, evidence that a patient's ability to make informed decisions is impaired.

  ▪ Avoid passing judgment on a patient's decision. "Everyone has the right to make a bad decision," is judgmental. Instead, say something like, "Everyone should make informed decisions about their health and well-being."

o Assessing a patient's capacity for making decisions is often complex and sometimes requires expert consultation. However, capacity assessments are also implicit in any informed consent process. When a physician seeks the consent of a patient to perform a procedure, the physician implicitly believes the patient is capable of making medical decisions. A review of assessing decision-making capacity follows.

  ▪ While some will discuss whether the patient is "competent" to make decisions, this term is technically incorrect. Competency is a legal term determined by a judge which reflects a global inability to make decisions. Clinicians assess "capacity" to make specific decisions at a particular time.

o Young children, adults with a clear intellectual disability, or adults with a court appointed guardian do not make their own decisions and a proxy decision-maker instead gives informed consent.

  ▪ Older children may be mature and sophisticated enough to make their own medical decisions. Often, state law and hospital policy will dictate how the surgeon proceeds in these cases.

o Legal adults who can <u>communicate a choice</u> about the treatment they desire is the first step in assessing decision-making capacity.

  ▪ Providing care to patients who speak a language other than the surgeons can be complicated, as differences in language can inhibit a conversation regarding informed consent.

    ⇨ Surgeons are encouraged to use an approved interpreter whenever possible and avoid using family members or those who are not credentialed by the hospital to provide such services.

o Patients should be able to <u>understand relevant information</u> in order to demonstrate to the surgeon that they are informed.

  ▪ Caution should be used if the patient presents with impaired capacity to manipulate information.

    ⇨ Particularly patients with altered mental status.
    ⇨ Some psychiatric disorders can impair decision-making ability, such as psychosis and severe depression, but having a psychiatric disorder does not itself constitute impaired capacity.

  ▪ Patients should be able to demonstrate in their own words their understanding of their medical condition and why surgical intervention is indicated.
  ▪ A clear understanding of the risks of surgery should be demonstrated, as well as the benefits of surgical intervention.
  ▪ Finally, the patient should be able to clearly articulate what might happen if they choose not to proceed with surgery.

    ⇨ "I could die," while true, may not totally capture possible negative outcomes. Patients should articulate their understanding of long-term suffering, lengthy hospitalization, and severe disability, (if such are possible) in addition to death.

- o Patients also need to <u>demonstrate their ability to assign personal value</u> to their situation by showing an appreciation for their condition and the treatment that is recommended.
  - ▪ In essence, they have to believe that everything that has been discussed applies to them personally.
  - ▪ Some patients may be able to clearly articulate risks and benefits of the procedure, but are unable to appreciate how it applies to them.
    - ⇨ There are instances when patients do not believe risks apply to them, particularly when refusing a procedure against medical advice.
  - ▪ A patient who has been told that death is a very probable outcome of refusing a situation and can demonstrate personal value might start making arrangements for hospice, for example. Another patient, unable to assign personal value, may believe he will be returning to work soon.
- o Finally, it is important that the patient's decisions is <u>rational and stable over time</u>.
  - ▪ A surgeon should ask her patient how she reached her decision.
    - ⇨ Well-reasoned, well-thought out choices that indicate deliberation are indicative of rational decisions.
    - ⇨ Decisions that are irrational may be based on faulty reasoning, intense fear, delusions, or may seem odd and atypical.
  - ▪ Stable decisions are ones that are enduring and pervade across multiple decisions.
    - ⇨ A decision that is suddenly in conflict with years of previous choice suggests instability.
    - ⇨ A patient who cannot seem to make up their mind about their choice also suggests decisions that are unstable over time.
- o Patients whose decisions will lead to severe outcomes (death, permanent disability) should demonstrate high functioning decision-making capacity that may not be required for less consequential decisions (such as a venipuncture for blood draw).
- o Patients can simultaneously be capable of making some medical decisions and not others.
  - ▪ Similarly, they can be capable at some times and not others. Assessments of capacity apply to a specific patient, decision, and time.

- o Complicated cases may require expert consultation, and psychiatry/ psychology consultations may help clarify a patient's capacity.
    - Mental health professionals can also determine if depression or other mental illness is impairing a patient's decision-making.
- If a patient is found to lack decision-making capacity for a procedure, there are a variety of additional considerations:
    - o In emergent situations, particularly those involving trauma, there is much greater emphasis on performing the standard of care and acting in what is believed to be in the patient's best interest.
        - In these instances, the surgeons are guided by the principal of benefi- cence and perform life- or limb-saving surgery with the belief this is what patients would want if they were capable of making an informed decision.
    - o In non-emergent situations, the surgeon should first look to advance direc- tives for guidance.
        - Living wills, for example, take precedence over decisions that might be made by proxy decisions-makers.
    - o If there are no advance directives, or if the particular advance directive does not apply to the current clinical situation, then a proxy decision- maker is identified.
        - A durable medical power of attorney is designed to make medical decisions on behalf of the patient when it is deemed the patient is incapable.
        - If no formal proxy decision-maker is identified, then often a family member is designated as such.
            - ⇨ Who may be designated a proxy decision-maker may be governed by state law and hospital policy.
            - ⇨ While often spouses and adult children, decision-makers can be romantic partners, siblings, or other individual who presents themselves to be an interested party.
            - ⇨ The surgeon should carefully consider whether the proxy decision- maker is acting in the patient's best interest.
        - If an appropriate proxy cannot be identified, or if the interested par- ties cannot reach a consensus, a court appointed guardian may be necessary.

o Common ethical questions occur when it is unclear whether a particular advance directive should be in force for a specific patient presentation, when proxy decision-makers attempt to override advance directives, and when proxy decision-makers are making decisions that are at odds with the recommended treatment.

- It may be necessary to suspend advance directives, such as a DNR, for patients who are undergoing surgery.

  o Some patients have made advance directives with the intention that they do not wish heroic measures to be undertaken at the end of their lives.

  o However, such heroic measures, such as defibrillation, may be necessary to correct a common complication while undergoing surgery and general anesthesia.

    ▪ Such measures, meant to correct a transient occurrence with a high likelihood of a patient returning to baseline, are obviously in the best interest of the patient.

    ▪ Suspending the DNR removes ambiguity while in the OR.

  o If the DNR is to be suspended, the following is recommended:

    ▪ A clear proxy decision-maker should be identified in the even that the patient emerges from the procedure as incapable of making medical decisions.

    ▪ There should be a clear time that the DNR is again in force.

    ▪ If some common complications can be foreseen and the patient wishes can be determined to cope with specific circumstances, then this should be well-communicated to other members of the operative team, including nursing.

- Common ethical questions

  o A 68-year-old male with a history of colorectal malignancy and recent CVA presents with abdominal pain, nausea, vomiting and hemtochezia. His workup is positive for a recurrence of colon adenocarcinoma (stage IIC) with complete small bowel obstruction. The patient is admitted to the surgical service and a right hemicolectomy is recommended.

    ▪ During the consenting process, a surgeon determines the patient lacks medical decision-making capacity due to severe cognitive decline following his CVA. The patient states he does not desire surgery.

    ▪ After previous abdominal surgery, the patient made a living will saying that the only care he wished for was antibiotics, pain control, and did not want cardiovascular resuscitation attempted.

- The patient's adult son, an attorney, presses the surgical team to complete the procedure, saying that the procedure will alleviate pain and extend his father's life. He states that his father's living will does not prohibit surgery and that the patient has grandchildren who love him dearly.

  ⇨ The son offers to be the proxy decision-maker and says that he knows what is best for his father and offers to consent on behalf of the patient.

- The surgery team is conflicted, as the procedure will likely lead to a good outcome, but if the condition is left untreated, it will lead to the patient's demise.
- Conflict between the patient's advance directive and family's wishes are common ethical dilemmas.
- Surgeons are caught between respecting patient autonomy and practicing with beneficence.

  ⇨ The patient has stated his wishes in a living will about what he would like done in the event he is unable to make his own medical decision.

  ⇨ However, the patient would likely benefit from the procedure and a family member is asking that surgery be performed.

  ⇨ Living wills often do not address every possible medical situation that a patient may face and must sometimes be interpreted.

- There are two defensible approaches to managing this patient.

  ⇨ An ethics consult is called and ethics consultants meet with the family and members of the surgical treatment team. It is pointed out that the patient has been through abdominal surgery before and afterwards made it clear that he wanted comfort care measures only.

  ⇨ The son is encouraged to consider what his father meant by requesting comfort care measures only in a living will. He stops pursuing surgical options. The patient is transferred to medicine and is made comfortable before he eventually succumbs on hospital day 4.

o A 55-year-old homeless man with a long history of alcohol use disorder, hypertension, schizophrenia, and 4 weeks status post deep frostbite to his left foot presents to the emergency department with pain in his lower left extremity and difficulty in walking. Physical exam reveals the frostbitten foot now has demarcation of healthy tissue from eschar with purulent discharge. Osteomyelitis is diagnosed in all of the metatarsals and tarsus; the patient is admitted to the surgical service for amputation of his foot at the distal tibia and fibula.

- The patient rejects surgical options, believing that the surgeons are going to sell his foot on the internet.
  - ⇨ Psychiatry is consulted and they note the patient has fixed delusions refractory to antipsychotic medication.
  - ⇨ The patient is deemed incapable of making medical decisions as he does not appreciate his condition. The patient believes if he is given enough IV fluid, his desiccated foot will regenerate.
  - ⇨ He will accept oral antibiotics and pain medication.
  - ⇨ There are no family members available to act as proxy decision-makers.

- While it is believed that the foot will auto-amputate, there is concern that the patient will become septic, with risk of multi-organ failure and death.

- Again, the surgery team is caught between two seemingly defensible choices:
  - ⇨ Honor the patient's autonomy and not perform surgery over his objections.
  - ⇨ Act with beneficence and intervene on behalf of the patient who is unable to make his own decision.

- An ethics consultation is sought, and they observe that the patient lacks decision-making capacity and needs a proxy decision-maker to consider his best interests.
  - ⇨ These interests may include performing a non-emergent lifesaving procedure.
  - ⇨ A court appointed guardian is appointed who consents to amputation.

o A 24-year-old female suffers a stab wound to the anterior chest during a robbery at the convenience store where she works. She is found in extremis in the field and transported emergently to a trauma center. While en route, she suffers full cardiopulmonary arrest. CPR is started, she is intubated and aggressive fluid resuscitation is attempted. Upon arrival at the ED, trauma surgeons perform left anterior thoracostomy and repair a laceration to the right ventricle. After reperfusion and ventricular fibrillation, there is successful defibrillation into a sinus rhythm.

- Despite rapid surgical intervention, the patient shows no pupillary light reflex. On postoperative day three, her motor response is consistent with decorticate posturing. CT shows diffuse cerebral edema and neurology diagnoses hypoxic encephalopathy.
- On postoperative day four, she enters status epilepticus. An EEG reveals electrocerebral silence and neurology declares the patient to be brain dead.
- The patient has no advance directives.
- Her brother is her only living family member and is made her proxy decision-maker. The primary team frankly describes the futility of her situation and advises him that she will require extensive measures to keep her alive.
- The brother states that the patient has repeatedly told him that she would not wish to be kept alive in such a situation. He requests that treatment be withdrawn after the patient's boyfriend has a chance to say goodbye.
- The following day, the brother returns and directs the primary team to "do whatever it takes" to keep the patient alive. When a social worker asks what has changed, the brother says that he lives with the patient, but is not on her lease. Upon her death, he will be evicted from her apartment. "I am not going to lose my place over this," he states.
- An ethics consult is called.
    - ⇨ In this instance, the question is how to honor the patient's autonomy despite the direction being given by the proxy decision-maker.
    - ⇨ Providers may be directed to perform care that is in conflict with the patient's beliefs.
    - ⇨ In this instance, the patient's wishes were clearly communicated to the treatment team. Despite acting as her proxy, the team has the obligation to honor what they believe to be patient's wishes.
    - ⇨ Treatment is withdrawn.
- Before calling an ethics consult.
    - o Many conflicts that arise may be due to lack of communication between the interested parties.
        - Between the primary team and consultants.
        - Between family members/proxy decision-makers.
        - Between the primary team and family members/proxy decision-makers.

- o Despite busy schedules and demands on the surgeon's time, a multidisciplinary meeting with all interested parties may ultimately save time in the end by clarifying treatment goals and options.
- o The patient (if able to participate) should meet with the primary team, representatives from consulting services, family members and proxy decision-makers.
  - It may be helpful, with multiple family members/proxies, to have the interested parties appoint a spokesperson.
- o Often, the futility of the patient's condition has not been properly communicated.
- o It may help if proxy decision-makers are reminded that it is not their wishes that are to be honored, but to help the team understand what the patient would want.

Practical Algorithm(s)/Diagrams

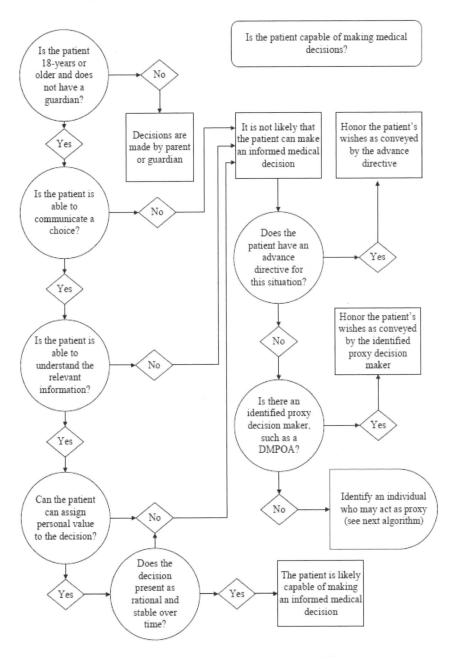

Fig. 1. Algorithm for decision-making capability.

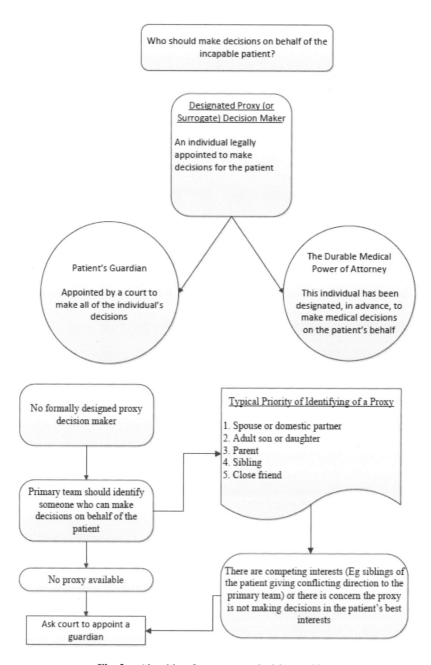

Fig. 2. Algorithm for surrogate decision-making.

Review of Current Literature with References

- Advance directives and outcomes of surrogate decision-making before death (*N Engl J Med* 2010; **362**: 112–1218).

  o A study exploring the prevalence of lost decision-making capacity in adults over age 60, the preferences documented in advance directives, and the outcome of proxy decision-making. A sample of 3,746 individuals was identified who had died between 2000 and 2006.

  o In this sample, 1,536 (41%) were required to make a medical decision in the days preceding death. Data were available for 1,409 of these patients to determine whether a proxy decision-maker was required.

    - Of these, 999 of the 1,409 (70.3%) had a decision made by a proxy.
    - A living will and or appointed durable medical power of attorney was not available in 38% of patients.
    - Of those who had prepared a living will, only 1.9% requested that all care possible be given.
    - People with medical durable power of attorney appointed were less likely to die in the hospital.

  o Interestingly, a large proportion of patients at the end of their lives were asked to make a medical decision. Of those required to make a decision, a plurality were incapable of doing so.

    - Being critically ill is a risk factor for being incapable.
    - Finally, the presence of living will is strongly associated with a patient who has determined that they do not want all care possible.

      ⇨ Where the patient's choice is unclear, the living will may signal to providers that the patient most likely did not want aggressive care.

- On consent forms (*J Med Ethics* 2011; **37**: 187–189 and *Ann R Coll Surg Engl* 2007; **89**: 66–69).

  o A British study examined 100 consecutive consent forms to repair a hip fracture.

    - Thirty-one forms were completed by people who were unable to unable to consent.
    - All 100 were correctly filled in, but 2 were illegible.
    - The total number of complications listed in the risk section by the surgeon ranged from 4 to 11.
    - Thirty different complications were recorded, some only appearing once.

- o A similar study reviewed 173 case notes for femur fracture requiring surgical intervention. One hundred and two met inclusion criteria.
  - ▪ The number of risks also showed variability ranging from 0 to 9.
  - ▪ No risks were recorded in two.
  - ▪ Sixty-two forms contained the phrase "risks from GA" and another 85 forms indicating risk as "DVT/PE."
    - ⇨ A majority of consent forms listed risks that were not spelled out in layperson's terms.
- o Standardizing consent documents for common procedures by using pre-printed forms listing the most common risks will lead to improvement in patients making informed choices.
- The American College of Surgeons has several resources available for further learning.
  - o The Code of Professional Conduct can be found online at http://www.facs.org/memberservices/codeofconduct.html.
  - o The ACS also publishes a journal, *Issues in Surgical Ethics*, which explores surgical ethics questions.

Index